STEP-UP
TO
PEDIATRICS

STEP-UP
TO
PEDIATRICS

Samir S. Shah, MD, MSCE
Director, Division of Hospital Medicine
Attending Physician, Divisions of Hospital Medicine and Infectious Diseases
Cincinnati Children's Research Foundation Endowed Chair in Hospital Medicine
Cincinnati Children's Hospital Medical Center
Professor, Department of Pediatrics
University of Cincinnati College of Medicine
Cincinnati, Ohio

Jeanine C. Ronan, MD
Assistant Professor of Clinical Pediatrics
Co-Director, Pediatrics Clerkship
Perelman School of Medicine at the University of Pennsylvania
Attending Physician
Division of General Pediatrics
Children's Hospital of Philadelphia
Philadelphia, Pennsylvania

Brian Alverson, MD
Director, Division of Pediatric Hospital Medicine
Hasbro Children's Hospital
Associate Professor, Department of Pediatrics
The Warren Alpert School of Medicine at Brown University
Providence, Rhode Island

Wolters Kluwer Health | Lippincott Williams & Wilkins
Philadelphia • Baltimore • New York • London
Buenos Aires • Hong Kong • Sydney • Tokyo

Publisher: Michael Tully
Acquisitions Editor: Tari Broderick
Product Development Editor: Jennifer Verbiar
Marketing Manager: Joy Fisher-Williams
Designer: Holly Reid McLaughlin
Production Manager: Priscilla Crater
Compositor: Absolute Service, Inc.

1st Edition

351 West Camden Street
Baltimore, MD 21201

Two Commerce Square
2001 Market Street
Philadelphia, PA 19103

Printed in China

9 8 7 6 5 4 3 2 1

Library of Congress Cataloging-in-Publication Data

Shah, Samir S., author.
Step-up to pediatrics / Samir S. Shah, Jeanine C. Ronan, Brian Alverson. -- First edition.
p. ; cm. -- (Step-up series)
Includes index.
Summary: "A guide for third year medical students preparing for the end-of-rotation NBME shelf exam, the pediatrics clerkship, and the USMLE Step 2 CK"--Provided by publisher.
ISBN 978-1-4511-4580-9 (paperback)
I. Ronan, Jeanine C., author. II. Alverson, Brian., author. III. Title. IV. Series: Step up series.
[DNLM: 1. Pediatrics--Outlines. 2. Pediatrics--Problems and Exercises. WS 18.2]
RJ48.2
618.9200076--dc23

2013032140

DISCLAIMER

Care has been taken to confirm the accuracy of the information present and to describe generally accepted practices. However, the authors, editors, and publisher are not responsible for errors or omissions or for any consequences from application of the information in this book and make no warranty, expressed or implied, with respect to the currency, completeness, or accuracy of the contents of the publication. Application of this information in a particular situation remains the professional responsibility of the practitioner; the clinical treatments described and recommended may not be considered absolute and universal recommendations.

The authors, editors, and publisher have exerted every effort to ensure that drug selection and dosage set forth in this text are in accordance with the current recommendations and practice at the time of publication. However, in view of ongoing research, changes in government regulations, and the constant flow of information relating to drug therapy and drug reactions, the reader is urged to check the package insert for each drug for any change in indications and dosage and for added warnings and precautions. This is particularly important when the recommended agent is a new or infrequently employed drug.

Some drugs and medical devices presented in this publication have Food and Drug Administration (FDA) clearance for limited use in restricted research settings. It is the responsibility of the health care provider to ascertain the FDA status of each drug or device planned for use in their clinical practice.

To purchase additional copies of this book, call our customer service department at **(800) 638-3030** or fax orders to **(301) 223-2320**. International customers should call **(301) 223-2300**.

Visit Lippincott Williams & Wilkins on the Internet: http://www.lww.com. Lippincott Williams & Wilkins customer service representatives are available from 8:30 am to 6:00 pm, EST.

CCS1013

Section Editors

GIL BINENBAUM, MD, MSCE
Diseases of the Eye
Assistant Professor
Department of Ophthalmology
Perelman School of Medicine at the
University of Pennsylvania
Attending Surgeon
Department of Ophthalmology
Children's Hospital of Philadelphia
Philadelphia, Pennsylvania

APRIL O. BUCHANAN, MD
Diseases of the Gastrointestinal System
Associate Professor of Clinical Pediatrics
Academic Director, Years 3 and 4
University of South Carolina School of Medicine
Greenville
Pediatric Hospitalist
Department of Pediatrics
Greenville Health System
Greenville, South Carolina

DOUGLAS W. CARLSON, MD
Infectious Diseases
Professor of Pediatrics
Department of Pediatrics
Washington University
Director, Division of Hospital Medicine
Department of Pediatrics
St. Louis Children's Hospital
St. Louis, Missouri

DANIEL T. COGHLIN, MD
Fluids and Electrolytes
Clinical Assistant Professor of Pediatrics
The Warren Alpert School of Medicine
at Brown University
Pediatric Hospitalist
Department of Pediatrics
Hasbro Children's Hospital
Providence, Rhode Island

AMY ELIZABETH FLEMING, MD
Dermatologic Conditions
Associate Professor
Division of Hospital Medicine
Director of Medical Student Education
Department of Pediatrics
Vanderbilt University School of Medicine
Monroe Carell Jr. Children's Hospital
Nashville, Tennessee

MATTHEW GARBER, MD
Diseases of the Pulmonary System
Associate Professor
Department of Pediatrics
University of South Carolina School of Medicine
Director of Pediatric Hospitalists
Department of Pediatrics
Palmetto Health Children's Hospital
Columbia, South Carolina

DOUGLAS HARRISON, MD
Hematologic Diseases
Oncologic Diseases
Assistant Professor of Pediatrics
The Warren Alpert School of Medicine
at Brown University
Pediatric Hematologist Oncologist
Department of Pediatrics
Hasbro Children's Hospital
Providence, Rhode Island

MEENA IYER, MD
Neurologic Disorders
Assistant Professor of Pediatrics
Department of Pediatrics
University of Texas Southwestern–Austin
Medical Director, Hospital Medicine
Dell Children's Medical Center of Central Texas
Austin, Texas

ELIZABETH A. JAMME, MD
Developmental and Behavioral Disorders
Clinical Assistant Professor
Department of Pediatrics
Perelman School of Medicine at the
University of Pennsylvania
Pediatric Hospitalist
Department of General Pediatrics
Children's Hospital of Philadelphia
Philadelphia, Pennsylvania

LEONARD J. LEVINE, MD
Diseases Unique to Adolescent Medicine
Associate Professor of Pediatrics
Assistant Chair for Medical Student Education in Pediatrics
Director, Pediatrics Clerkship and Pediatrics Pathway
Director, Program for Integrated Learning Small Group Process
Drexel University College of Medicine
Philadelphia, Pennsylvania

VINEETA MITTAL, MD, FAAP
Diseases Unique to the Newborn
Associate Professor of Pediatrics
Department of Pediatrics
Academic Colleges Mentor
University of Texas Southwestern Medical Center
Pediatric Hospitalist
Department of Pediatrics
Children's Medical Center
Dallas, Texas

FRANCES M. NADEL, MD, MSCE
Emergency Medicine, Critical Care, Toxicology, and Child Abuse
Professor of Clinical Pediatrics
Department of Pediatrics
Perelman School of Medicine at the
University of Pennsylvania
Attending Physician
Division of Emergency Medicine
Children's Hospital of Philadelphia
Philadelphia, Pennsylvania

JENNIFER K. O'TOOLE, MD, MEd
Diseases of the Renal and Genitourinary System
Associate Director, Internal Medicine and Pediatrics Residency Training Program
Medical Director of Education, Division of Hospital Medicine
Cincinnati Children's Hospital Medical Center and
The University of Cincinnati Medical Center
Assistant Professor of Internal Medicine and Pediatrics
University of Cincinnati College of Medicine
Cincinnati, Ohio

RICARDO A. QUINONEZ, MD, FAAP, FHM
Allergic and Immunologic Disorders
Associate Professor of Pediatrics
Chief
Division of Pediatric Hospital Medicine
Children's Hospital of San Antonio
Baylor College of Medicine
San Antonio, Texas

JOSE BERNARDO QUINTOS, MD
Endocrine and Metabolic Diseases
Assistant Professor of Clinical Pediatrics
Department of Pediatrics
Division of Pediatric Endocrinology
The Warren Alpert School of Medicine
at Brown University
Pediatric Endocrinologist
Division of Pediatric Endocrinology
Rhode Island Hospital
Providence, Rhode Island

STACEY R. ROSE, MD
Disorders of the Ear, Nose, and Throat
Clinical Assistant Professor of Pediatrics
Department of Pediatrics
Perelman School of Medicine at the
University of Pennsylvania
Attending Physician
Division of General Pediatrics
Children's Hospital of Philadelphia
Philadelphia, Pennsylvania

MARK W. SHEN, MD
Neurologic Disorders
Associate Professor of Pediatrics
Department of Pediatrics
University of Texas Southwestern–Austin
Pediatric Hospitalist
Dell Children's Medical Center of Central Texas
Austin, Texas

NATASHA SHUR, MD
Dysmorphology and Genetic Disorders
Assistant Professor
Department of Pediatrics
The Warren Alpert School of Medicine
at Brown University
Attending, Clinical Geneticist
Department of Pediatrics
Rhode Island Hospital
Providence, Rhode Island

JENNIFER BETH SOEP, MD
Rheumatologic Disorders and Orthopedic Conditions
Associate Professor
Department of Pediatric Rheumatology
University of Colorado
Children's Hospital of Colorado
Aurora, Colorado

SUSAN WU, MD
Diseases of the Cardiovascular System
Assistant Professor of Clinical Pediatrics
Department of Pediatrics
University of Southern California
Keck School of Medicine
Department of Pediatrics
Division of Hospital Medicine
Children's Hospital Los Angeles
Los Angeles, California

Contributing Authors

DIANNE ABUELO, MD
Associate Professor
Department of Pediatrics
The Warren Alpert School of Medicine
at Brown University
Director, Genetic Counseling Center
Department of Pediatrics
Rhode Island Hospital
Providence, Rhode Island

ENITAN ADEGITE, MD, MPH
Assistant Professor
Department of Pediatrics
Drexel University College of Medicine
Attending Physician
Department of Adolescent Medicine
St. Christopher's Hospital for Children
Philadelphia, Pennsylvania

SOUMYA ADHIKARI, MD
Assistant Professor of Pediatrics
Division of Endocrinology
Department of Pediatrics
Pediatric Clerkship Director
Department of Pediatrics
University of Texas Southwestern Medical Center
Attending Physician
Department of Pediatrics
Children's Medical Center
Dallas, Texas

LILLIAM V. AMBROGGIO, PhD
Assistant Professor of Pediatrics
Division of Hospital Medicine
Cincinnati Children's Hospital Medical Center
Department of Pediatrics
University of Cincinnati College of Medicine
Cincinnati, Ohio

ZOLTAN ANTAL, MD
Assistant Professor
Department of Pediatric Endocrinology
Weill Cornell Medical College
Attending Physician
Department of Pediatric Endocrinology
NewYork Presbyterian Hospital
New York, New York

MAROUN AZAR, MD
Assistant Professor
Department of Medicine
The Warren Alpert School of Medicine
at Brown University
Nephrologist
Department of Medicine
Rhode Island Hospital
Providence, Rhode Island

FRANCES BALAMUTH, MD, PhD
Assistant Professor
Department of Pediatrics
Perelman School of Medicine at the
University of Pennsylvania
Attending Physician
Division of Emergency Medicine
Children's Hospital of Philadelphia
Philadelphia, Pennsylvania

M. RYAN BALLARD, PA-C
Faculty
Department of Pediatric Orthopedics
University of Colorado
Physician Assistant
Department of Pediatric Orthopedics
Children's Hospital of Colorado
Aurora, Colorado

KATHLEEN W. BARTLETT, MD
Associate Professor
Department of Pediatrics
Duke University School of Medicine
Pediatric Hospitalist
Department of Pediatrics
Duke University Medical Center
Durham, North Carolina

KEVIN BARTON, MD
Instructor of Pediatrics
Division of Hospitalist Medicine
Washington University School of Medicine
St. Louis, Missouri

KATHLEEN J. BERG, MD
Assistant Professor
Department of Pediatrics
University of Mississippi Medical Center
Blair E. Batson Hospital for Children
Jackson, Mississippi

ELIZABETH M. BIRD, MD
Assistant Professor
Department of Pediatrics
The Warren Alpert School of Medicine
at Brown University
Pediatric Hospitalist
Department of Pediatrics
Hasbro Children's Hospital
Providence, Rhode Island

MERCEDES BLACKSTONE, MD
Assistant Professor of Clinical Pediatrics
Department of Pediatrics
Perelman School of Medicine at the
University of Pennsylvania
Attending Physician
Division of Emergency Medicine
Children's Hospital of Philadelphia
Philadelphia, Pennsylvania

AIDA BOUNAMA, MD
Resident in Ophthalmology
Scheie Eye Institute
Perelman School of Medicine at the
University of Pennsylvania
Philadelphia, Pennsylvania

CHRISTINA CASTRICHINI BOURLAND, MD
Assistant Professor of Pediatrics
Department of Pediatrics
University of Texas Southwestern Medical Center
Pediatric Hospitalist
Department of Pediatrics
Children's Medical Center
Dallas, Texas

MICHAEL D. BRYANT, MD, MBA
Assistant Professor of Clinical Pediatrics
Department of Pediatrics
University of Southern California
Keck School of Medicine
Division Head
Department of Pediatrics
Division of Hospital Medicine
Children's Hospital Los Angeles
Los Angeles, California

APRIL O. BUCHANAN, MD
Associate Professor of Clinical Pediatrics
Academic Director, Years 3 and 4
University of South Carolina School of Medicine
Greenville
Pediatric Hospitalist
Department of Pediatrics
Greenville Health System
Greenville, South Carolina

HEATHER LEE BURROWS, MD, PhD
Clinical Assistant Professor
Department of Pediatrics and Communicable
Diseases
University of Michigan
Ann Arbor, Michigan

MELISSA L. CAINE, AuD
Audiologist
Children's Hospital of Philadelphia
Philadelphia, Pennsylvania

LYNN R. CAMPBELL, MD
Assistant Professor
Department of Pediatrics
University of Texas Southwestern–Austin
Pediatric Hospitalist
Department of Pediatrics
Dell Children's Medical Center of Central Texas
Austin, Texas

J.B. CANTEY, MD
Fellow
Department of Pediatrics
Division of Infectious Diseases and Neonatology
University of Texas Southwestern Medical Center
Department of Pediatrics
Children's Medical Center
Dallas, Texas

WILLIAM CAREY, MD
Clinical Professor of Pediatrics
Department of Pediatrics
Perelman School of Medicine at the
University of Pennsylvania
Senior Physician
Department of General Pediatrics
Children's Hospital of Philadelphia
Philadelphia, Pennsylvania

SCOTT CARNEY, MD
Assistant Professor of Clinical Pediatrics
Department of Pediatrics
University of South Carolina
Palmetto Health Richland
Columbia, South Carolina

DAVID CHAO, MD
Assistant Professor
Department of Pediatrics
Children's Hospital of Nevada
Assistant Professor
Department of Emergency Medicine
University of Nevada School of Medicine
Emergency Medicine Physicians
Las Vegas, Nevada

SUNITA CHERUVU, MD
Fellow
Division of Endocrinology
Department of Pediatrics
The Warren Alpert School of Medicine
at Brown University
Rhode Island Hospital
Providence, Rhode Island

STEPHANIE L. CLARK, MD, MPH
Chief Resident
Department of Pediatrics
Cincinnati Children's Hospital Medical Center
University of Cincinnati College of Medicine
Cincinnati, Ohio

DAVE FITZGERALD CLARKE, MD, MBBS
Associate Professor
Department of Pediatric Neurology
University of Texas Southwestern-Austin
Director
Comprehensive Epilepsy Program
Dell Children's Medical Center of Central Texas
Austin, Texas

WILLIAM B. CUTRER, MD, MED
Assistant Professor
Department of Pediatrics
Division of Pediatric Critical Care
Vanderbilt University School of Medicine
Nashville, Tennessee

MEGHAN DAVIGNON, MD
Fellow
Department of Behavioral Pediatrics
Children's Hospital of Philadelphia
Philadelphia, Pennsylvania

SHELLEY DELL'ORFANO, RN, MSN, CPNP, ND
Faculty
Department of Orthopedics
University of Colorado at Denver
Nurse Practitioner
Department of Orthopedics
Children's Hospital of Colorado
Aurora, Colorado

BRADLEY D. DENARDO, MD
Fellow, Pediatric Hematology/Oncology
Department of Pediatric Hematology/Oncology
Hasbro Children's Hospital
The Warren Alpert School of Medicine
at Brown University
Providence, Rhode Island

PREEYA JEYAPAUL DESH, MD
Fellow
Department of Pediatric Hematology/Oncology
Rhode Island Hospital
Providence, Rhode Island

JON A. DETTERICH, MD
Associate Professor
Department of Pediatrics
University of Southern California
Keck School of Medicine
Assistant Professor
Department of Pediatrics
Division of Cardiology
Children's Hospital Los Angeles
Los Angeles, California

ERIN PETE DEVON, MD
Clinical Assistant Professor of Pediatrics
Department of General Pediatrics
Children's Hospital of Philadelphia
Philadelphia, Pennsylvania

MICHAEL J. DOUGHERTY, DO
Assistant Professor of Clinical Pediatrics
Department of Pediatrics
University of South Carolina School of Medicine
Greenville
Faculty
Department of Pediatric Gastroenterology
Greenville Health System
Greenville, South Carolina

MICHELLE DUNN, MD
Clinical Assistant Professor of Pediatrics
Department of General Pediatrics
Children's Hospital of Philadelphia
Philadelphia, Pennsylvania

LINDSAY E. ELTON, MD
Child Neurologist
Dell Children's Medical Center of Central Texas
Austin, Texas

M. KHURRAM FAIZAN, MD, FAAP
Clinical Assistant Professor
Department of Pediatrics
The Warren Alpert School of Medicine
at Brown University
Division Director, Pediatric Nephrology
Department of Pediatrics
Hasbro Children's Hospital
Providence, Rhode Island

EZAM GHODSI, MD
Child Neurologist
Dell Children's Medical Center of Central Texas
Austin, Texas

MONIKA GOYAL, MD, MSCE
Assistant Professor
Departments of Pediatrics and Emergency Medicine
Children's National Medical Center
George Washington University
Washington, District of Columbia

KRISTIN GREENE, MS
Senior Speech-Language Pathologist and Outpatient Coordinator
Department of Speech-Language Pathology
Children's Hospital of Philadelphia
Philadelphia, Pennsylvania

JEFFREY GRILL, MD
Associate Professor
Department of Pediatrics
University of Louisville School of Medicine
Pediatric Hospitalist Director
"Just for Kids" Hospitalist Service
Kosair Children's Hospital
Louisville, Kentucky

MATTHEW PAUL GRISHAM, MD
Assistant Professor of Clinical Pediatrics
Department of Pediatrics
University of South Carolina School of Medicine
Greenville
Faculty
Department of Pediatrics
Greenville Health System
Greenville, South Carolina

RUCHI GUPTA, MD
Assistant Professor of Pediatrics
Department of Pediatrics
Baylor College of Medicine
Pediatric Hospital Attending
Department of Pediatric Hospital Medicine
Texas Children's Hospital
Houston, Texas

DOUGLAS HARRISON, MD
Assistant Professor of Pediatrics
The Warren Alpert School of Medicine
at Brown University
Pediatric Hematologist Oncologist
Department of Pediatrics
Hasbro Children's Hospital
Providence, Rhode Island

ERIKA V. HAYES, MD
Assistant Professor of Pediatrics
Department of Pediatrics
Washington University School of Medicine in St. Louis
St. Louis, Missouri

TRAVIS HEARE, MD
Associate Professor
Department of Orthopedic Surgery
University of Colorado
Director, Orthopedic Oncology Program
Department of Orthopedic Surgery
Children's Hospital of Colorado
Aurora, Colorado

FRED M. HENRETIG, MD
Professor
Department of Pediatrics and Emergency Medicine
Perelman School of Medicine at the
University of Pennsylvania
Attending Physician
Division of Emergency Medicine
Children's Hospital of Philadelphia
Philadelphia, Pennsylvania

LAURIE HOFFMAN, MD
Pediatric Resident PGY3
Department of Pediatrics
The Warren Alpert School of Medicine
at Brown University
Pediatric Resident (House Officer)
Department of Pediatrics
Hasbro Children's Hospital
Providence, Rhode Island

MAMBARAMBATH A. JALEEL, MD
Associate Professor
Division of Neonatology
Department of Pediatrics
University of Texas Southwestern Medical Center
Medical Director
Neonatal Intensive Care Unit
Parkland Health and Hospital Services
Attending Neonatologist
Department of Pediatrics
Children's Medical Center
Dallas, Texas

ANNE K. JENSEN, MD
Resident in Ophthalmology
Scheie Eye Institute
Perelman School of Medicine at the University of Pennsylvania
Philadelphia, Pennsylvania

THANAKORN JIRASEVIJINDA, MD
Associate Professor
Department of Pediatrics
Director, Pediatric Undergraduate Medical Education
Weill Cornell Medical College
NewYork Presbyterian Hospital/Weill Cornell Medical Center
New York, New York

JEFFREY KANE, MD
Clinical Associate Professor
Department of Pediatrics
University of Texas Southwestern–Austin
Section Chief
Department of Pediatric Neurology
Dell Children's Medical Center of Central Texas
Austin, Texas

KAREN KEOUGH, MD
Child Neurologist and Epileptologist
Department of Child Neurology
Pediatric Surgical Subspecialties
Staff
Department of Child Neurology
Dell Children's Medical Center of Central Texas
Austin, Texas

EMILY N. KEVAN, MD
Assistant Professor of Clinical Pediatrics
Department of Pediatrics
University of South Carolina School of Medicine Greenville
Faculty, Staff Physician
Department of Pediatric Gastroenterology
Greenville Health System
Greenville, South Carolina

MONICA KHITRI, MD
Attending Ophthalmologist
Jules Stein Eye Institute
University of California Los Angeles
Los Angeles, California

JANE ELIZABETH KIFF, MD
Assistant Professor of Clinical Pediatrics
Division of Pediatric Critical Care Medicine
The Warren Alpert School of Medicine at Brown University
Rhode Island Hospital
Providence, Rhode Island

MELISSA D. KLEIN, MD, MEd
Associate Program Director, Pediatric Residency Training Program
Director Education Section, Division of General and Community Pediatrics
Cincinnati Children's Hospital Medical Center
Associate Professor of Pediatrics
University of Cincinnati College of Medicine
Cincinnati, Ohio

ANSON KOSHY, MD
Assistant Professor of Pediatrics
The University of Texas Health Science Center at Houston
Department of Developmental and Behavioral Pediatrics
Children's Learning Institute
Houston, Texas

MICHAEL KOSTER, MD
Assistant Clinical Professor of Pediatrics
The Warren Alpert School of Medicine at Brown University
Division of Pediatric Hospital Medicine
Hasbro Children's Hospital
Providence, Rhode Island

HILLARY KRUGER, MD
Clinical Associate Professor of Pediatrics
Department of Pediatrics
Perelman School of Medicine at the University of Pennsylvania
Attending Physician
Department of Child Development
Children's Hospital of Philadelphia
Philadelphia, Pennsylvania

GRACE KUNG, MD
Associate Professor
Department of Pediatrics
University of Southern California
Keck School of Medicine
Department of Pediatrics
Division of Cardiology
Children's Hospital Los Angeles
Los Angeles, California

JULIE YOU KWON, MD
Resident in Ophthalomology
North Shore Long Island Jewish Health Care System
Great Neck, New York

BENJAMIN LASKIN, MD, MS
Attending Physician, Division of Pediatric Nephrology
Children's Hospital of Philadelphia
Assistant Professor of Clinical Pediatrics
Perelman School of Medicine at the University of Pennsylvania
Philadelphia, Pennsylvania

BENJAMIN C. LEE, MD
Associate Professor
Associate Director, Pediatric Clerkship
Department of Pediatrics
University of Texas Southwestern Medical Center
Pediatric Hospitalist
Department of Pediatrics
Children's Medical Center
Dallas, Texas

LEONARD J. LEVINE, MD
Associate Professor of Pediatrics
Assistant Chair for Medical Student Education in Pediatrics
Director, Pediatrics Clerkship and Pediatrics Pathway
Director, Program for Integrated Learning Small Group Process
Drexel University College of Medicine
Philadelphia, Pennsylvania

HUAY-YING LO, MD
Assistant Professor
Department of Pediatrics
Baylor College of Medicine
Texas Children's Hospital
Houston, Texas

SHARYN MALCOLM, MD, MPH
Fellow in Adolescent and Young Adult Medicine
Children's National Medical Center
Washington, District of Columbia

RACHEL M. MARANO, BA
Medical Student, Class of 2014
The Warren Alpert School of Medicine at Brown University
Providence, Rhode Island

CIANA T. HAYES MAXWELL, MD
Pediatrician
Advocare Delran Pediatrics
Delran, New Jersey
Attending Physician
Department of Pediatrics, Section of Emergency Medicine
St. Christopher's Hospital for Children
Philadelphia, Pennsylvania

LAURIE MERCURIO, BS
Medical Student
The Warren Alpert School of Medicine at Brown University
Researcher
Department of Pediatrics
Rhode Island Hospital
Providence, Rhode Island

ANGELA MIHALIC, MD
Associate Professor of Pediatrics
Department of Pediatrics
Academic Colleges Mentor
Associate Dean for Student Affairs
University of Texas Southwestern Medical Center
Attending Physician
Children's Medical Center
Dallas, Texas

AARON S. MILLER, MD, MSPH
Assistant Professor
Department of Pediatrics
Washington University
St. Louis Children's Hospital
St. Louis, Missouri

RYAN MOONEY, PA-C
Clinical Instructor
Department of Orthopedics
University of Colorado School of Medicine
Physician Assistant
Department of Orthopedics
Children's Hospital of Colorado
Aurora, Colorado

SAGE MYERS, MD, MSCE
Assistant Professor
Department of Pediatrics
Perelman School of Medicine at the University of Pennsylvania
Attending Physician
Division of Emergency Medicine
Children's Hospital of Philadelphia
Philadelphia, Pennsylvania

SAROJ NIMKARN, MD
Pediatric Endocrinologist
Bumrungrad International Hospital
Bangkok, Thailand

KATHLEEN M. OSTROM, MD
Assistant Professor of Clinical Pediatrics
Department of Pediatrics
University of Southern California
Keck School of Medicine
Department of Pediatrics
Division of Hospital Medicine
Children's Hospital Los Angeles
Los Angeles, California

STACI OTTO, MS, CCC-SLP
Speech-Language Pathologist
Inpatient Coordinator
Department of Speech-Language Pathology
Children's Hospital of Philadelphia
Philadelphia, Pennsylvania

REINA PATEL, DO
Assistant Professor of Pediatrics
Department of Pediatrics
University of Texas Southwestern Medical Center
Pediatric Hospitalist
Department of Pediatrics
Children's Medical Center
Dallas, Texas

CHANIKA PHORNPHUTKUL, MD
Associate Professor
Department of Pediatrics
The Warren Alpert School of Medicine
at Brown University
Division Director
Division of Human Genetics
Department of Pediatrics
Rhode Island Hospital
Providence, Rhode Island

ELISE C. PIEBENGA, MD
Pediatric Hospitalist
Bryn Mawr Hospital
Nemours/Alfred I. duPont Hospital for Children
Wilmington, Delaware
Pediatrician
Wayne Pediatrics
Wayne, Pennsylvania

STACY B. PIERSON, MD
Assistant Professor
Department of Pediatrics
Baylor College of Medicine
Attending Physician
Department of Pediatric Hospital Medicine
Texas Children's Hospital
Houston, Texas

KARI R. POSNER, MD
Assistant Professor of Pediatrics and Emergency Medicine
Department of Emergency Medicine
New York University School of Medicine
Attending Physician, Pediatric Emergency Medicine
Department of Emergency Medicine
NYU Langone Medical Center
New York, New York

JAY D. PRUETZ, MD
Assistant Professor
Department of Pediatrics
University of Southern California
Keck School of Medicine
Department of Pediatrics
Division of Cardiology
Children's Hospital Los Angeles
Los Angeles, California

CASSANDRA M. PRUITT, MD
Assistant Professor
Department of Pediatrics
Washington University School of Medicine
Pediatric Hospitalist
Department of Pediatrics
St. Louis Children's Hospital
St. Louis, Missouri

KRIS P. REHM, MD
Assistant Professor
Department of Pediatrics
Vanderbilt University School of Medicine
Director, Division of Hospital Medicine
Department of Pediatrics
Monroe Carell Jr. Children's Hospital
Nashville, Tennessee

MADELINE H. RENNY, MD
Attending Physician, Urgent Care
Division of Emergency Medicine
Children's Hospital of Philadelphia
Philadelphia, Pennsylvania

KYUNG E. RHEE, MD, MSC
Assistant Professor of Pediatrics
Department of Pediatrics
University of California, San Diego
La Jolla, California
Assistant Professor and Hospitalist
Department of Pediatrics
Rady Children's Specialists of San Diego
San Diego, California

SCOTT RICKERT, MD
Acting Director of Pediatric Otolaryngology
Department of Otolaryngology
New York University
Attending Physician
Department of Otolaryngology
New York University Langome
New York, New York

CATHERINE RILEY, MD
Attending Physician
Department of Child Development
Children's Hospital of Philadelphia
Philadelphia, Pennsylvania

STACEY R. ROSE, MD
Clinical Assistant Professor of Pediatrics
Department of Pediatrics
Perelman School of Medicine at the
University of Pennsylvania
Attending Physician
Division of General Pediatrics
Children's Hospital of Philadelphia
Philadelphia, Pennsylvania

CHRISTOPHER JOHN RUSSELL, MD
Assistant Professor of Clinical Pediatrics
Department of Pediatrics
University of Southern California
Keck School of Medicine
Department of Pediatrics
Division of Hospital Medicine
Children's Hospital Los Angeles
Los Angeles, California

KOURTNEY KUSS SANTUCCI, MD
Assistant Professor of Pediatrics
Department of Pediatrics
University of Tennessee College of Medicine
Pediatric Hospitalist
Department of Pediatrics
Children's Hospital at Erlanger
Chattanooga, Tennessee

NADINE SAUER, MD
Fellow
Division of Pediatric Hematology/Oncology
The Warren Alpert School of Medicine
at Brown University
Hasbro Children's Hospital
Providence, Rhode Island

JOCELYN HUANG SCHILLER, MD
Clinical Associate Professor
Department of Pediatrics
University of Michigan Medical School
Pediatric Hospitalist
Department of Pediatrics
C.S. Mott Children's Hospital
Ann Arbor, Michigan

DANA ARONSON SCHINASI, MD
Clinical Instructor
Northwestern University Feinberg School of
Medicine
Attending Physician
Division of Emergency Medicine
Ann & Robert H. Lurie Children's Hospital of
Chicago
Chicago, Illinois

CINDY L. SCHWARTZ, MD, MPH
Alan G. Hassenfeld Professor of Pediatrics
Department of Pediatrics
The Warren Alpert School of Medicine
at Brown University
Director, Pediatric Hematology/Oncology
Department of Pediatrics
Hasbro Children's Hospital
Providence, Rhode Island

HALDEN F. SCOTT, MD
Assistant Professor
Department of Pediatrics
University of Colorado School of Medicine
Attending Physician
Department of Pediatrics, Section of Emergency
Medicine
Children's Hospital of Colorado
Aurora, Colorado

LUIS SEGUIAS, MD
Assistant Professor of Pediatrics
Department of Pediatrics
University of Texas Southwestern Medical Center
Pediatric Hospitalist
Department of Pediatrics
Children's Medical Center
Dallas, Texas

DOROTHY M. SENDELBACH, MD
Associate Professor
Associate Residency Director
Department of Pediatrics
Academic Colleges Mentor
University of Texas Southwestern Medical Center
Attending Physician
Children's Medical Center
Dallas, Texas

PURVI PATEL SHAH, MD
Instructor, Pediatrics
Department of Pediatrics
Washington University School of Medicine
St. Louis Children's Hospital
St. Louis, Missouri

LETICIA SHANLEY, MD
Assistant Professor of Pediatrics
Department of Pediatrics
University of Texas Southwestern Medical Center
Pediatric Hospitalist
Department of Pediatrics
Children's Medical Center
Dallas, Texas

DOUGLAS SHEMIN, MD
Associate Professor of Medicine
The Warren Alpert School of Medicine
at Brown University
Medical Director of Dialysis Services
Rhode Island Hospital
Providence, Rhode Island

JACQUELINE SIVAHOP, MS, PA-C
Clinical Coordinator
Assistant Professor
Department of Pediatrics
University of Colorado
Physician Assistant
Department of Rheumatology
Children's Hospital of Colorado
Aurora, Colorado

CHARLRE' E. SLAUGHTER-ATIEMO, MD
Attending Physician
Department of Pediatrics
St. Christopher's Hospital for Children
Philadelphia, Pennsylvania

ELVERA SOFOS, MD
Resident
Department of Pediatrics
Children's Hospital and Research
Center Oakland
Oakland, California

LAUREN G. SOLAN, MD
Fellow, Division of Hospital Medicine
Cincinnati Children's Hospital Medical Center
University of Cincinnati College of Medicine
Cincinnati, Ohio

KARTHIK SRINIVASAN, MD
Assistant Professor
Department of Pediatrics
University of Texas Southwestern Medical Center
Pediatric Hospitalist
Children's Medical Center
Dallas, Texas

ANGELA M. STATILE, MD, MEd
Pediatric Hospitalist, Division of Hospital Medicine
Cincinnati Children's Hospital Medical Center
Assistant Professor of Clinical Pediatrics
University of Cincinnati College of Medicine
Cincinnati, Ohio

SHARON W. SU, MD, FAAP
Clinical Assistant Professor of Pediatrics
Department of Pediatrics
Division of Pediatric Nephrology
The Warren Alpert School of Medicine
at Brown University
Hasbro Children's Hospital
Providence, Rhode Island

MICHELLE ELIZABETH SUTTER, RN, C-PNP
Instructor of Pediatrics
Department of Pediatrics
University of Colorado
Pediatric Nurse Practitioner
Department of Allergy/Immunology/Rheumatology
Children's Hospital of Colorado
Aurora, Colorado

JOANNA E. THOMSON, MD
Fellow
Division of Hospital Medicine
Cincinnati Children's Hospital Medical Center
University of Cincinnati College of Medicine
Cincinnati, Ohio

LYNN THORESON, DO
Assistant Professor
Department of Pediatrics
University of Texas Southwestern–Austin
Pediatric Hospitalist
Dell Children's Medical Center of Central Texas
Austin, Texas

NDIDI I. UNAKA, MD
Associate Program Director, Pediatric Residency
Training Program
Pediatric Hospitalist, Division of Hospital Medicine
Cincinnati Children's Hospital Medical Center
Assistant Professor of Clinical Pediatrics
University of Cincinnati College of Medicine
Cincinnati, Ohio

NEIL G. UPSAL, MD
Assistant Professor
Department of Pediatrics
University of Washington
Attending Physician
Division of Emergency Medicine
Seattle Children's Hospital
Seattle, Washington

JOYEE G. VACHANI, MD, MEd
Assistant Professor
Department of Pediatrics
Baylor College of Medicine
Director of Quality Improvement and Patient Safety
Section of Pediatric Hospital Medicine
Associate Director of Pediatric Hospital Medicine
Fellowship Department of Pediatric Hospital
Medicine
Texas Children's Hospital
Houston, Texas

MARIA VOGIATZI, MD
Associate Professor
Department of Pediatric Endocrinology
Weill Cornell Medical College
NewYork Presbyterian Hospital
New York, New York

COLLEEN M. WALLACE, MD
Assistant Professor
Department of Pediatrics
Washington University School of Medicine
St. Louis Children's Hospital
St. Louis, Missouri

SOWDHAMINI WALLACE, DO
Assistant Professor
Department of Pediatrics
Baylor College of Medicine
Faculty
Department of Pediatric Hospital Medicine
Texas Children's Hospital
Houston, Texas

SUSAN CHU WALLEY, MD
Associate Professor
Department of Pediatrics
University of Alabama at Birmingham
Children's Hospital of Alabama
Birmingham, Alabama

JENNIFER GREENE WELCH, MD
Assistant Professor
Department of Pediatrics
The Warren Alpert School of Medicine
at Brown University
Attending Physician
Department of Pediatric Hematology/Oncology
Hasbro Children's Hospital
Providence, Rhode Island

CRAIG BRYAN WODA, MD, PhD
Clinical Fellow
Department of Medicine
Harvard Medical School
Pediatric Nephrology Fellow
Department of Nephrology
Children's Hospital Boston
Boston, Massachusetts

MARGARET WOLFF, MD
Assistant Professor of Pediatrics and Emergency
Medicine
Associate Program Director, Pediatric Emergency
Medicine Fellowship
University of Michigan School of Medicine
Attending Physician
C.S. Mott Children's Hospital
Ann Arbor, Michigan

MARK R. ZONFRILLO, MD, MSCE
Assistant Professor
Department of Pediatrics
Perelman School of Medicine at the
University of Pennsylvania
Attending Physician
Associate Director of Research
Division of Emergency Medicine
Children's Hospital of Philadelphia
Philadelphia, Pennsylvania

Reviewers

ALEX BROTHERS
Medical Student
Jefferson Medical College
Thomas Jefferson University
Philadelphia, Pennsylvania

TYFFANY CHEN
Medical Student
Vanderbilt School of Medicine
Nashville, Tennessee

CHANCEY CHRISTENSON
Medical Student
Tulane University School of Medicine
New Orleans, Louisiana

JOY ALISON COOPER
Medical Student
Fogarty International Clinical Research Scholar
Howard University School of Medicine
Washington, District of Columbia

KATIE DONAHUE
Medical Student
Michigan State University College of Osteopathic Medicine
East Lansing, Michigan

MEENA HASAN
Medical Student
Michigan State University College of Human Medicine
East Lansing, Michigan

CHRISTOPHER HOM
Medical Student
Meharry Medical College
Nashville, Tennessee

LIYING LOW
Medical Student
University of Glasgow
Glasgow, United Kingdom

BRANDON MAULDIN
Medical Student
Florida State University College of Medicine
Tallahassee, Florida

USKER NAQVI
Medical Student
Robert Wood Johnson Medical School
New Brunswick, New Jersey

ALLISON PRICE
Medical Student
University of Miami Leonard M. Miller School of Medicine
Miami, Florida

REEM SABOUNI
Medical Student
The University of Texas Medical School at Houston
Houston, Texas

Preface

This book is intended to be a study guide for medical students as they prepare for their clinical experiences in pediatrics. Pediatrics is an evolving and exciting field in medicine where students have the opportunity to integrate basic sciences and clinical knowledge to develop an approach to common childhood complaints and illnesses.

Leaders in pediatrics and pediatric medical education wrote this book as a collaborative effort. Each section contains high-yield information that is representative of the content necessary for success in all pediatric clinical settings.

Each section is divided into three major components. First, approaches to the common complaints and problems within that organ system are discussed. Then, relevant information about each individual topic is further explored in detail. Finally, a bank of multiple-choice style questions with comprehensive explanations is provided.

We hope this book will serve you well as you develop your clinical skills in pediatrics. We would like to extend our heartfelt gratitude to all of our section editors and chapter authors. Without their participation and contribution, this would not have been possible.

Samir S. Shah
Jeanine C. Ronan
Brian Alverson

Dedication

We would like to dedicate this book to Dr. Stephen Ludwig,
our beloved mentor and colleague. He has been our role model as a
clinician and educator.

We would like to thank our families for their continued support:
Kara, Siddharth, Avani & Anika
Rebecca, Lorelei & Morgan
Tim, Madelyn, Natalie & TJ

Contents

Chapter 8. Fluids and Electrolytes

Chapter 9. Hematologic Diseases

Chapter 10. Infectious Diseases

Chapter 11. Allergic and Immunologic Disorders

Chapter 12. Dermatologic Conditions

Chapter 13. Diseases Unique to Adolescent Medicine

Chapter 14. Diseases Unique to the Newborn

Chapter 15. Developmental and Behavioral Disorders

Chapter 16. Dysmorphology and Genetic Disorders

Chapter 17. Diseases of the Eye

Chapter 18. Emergency Medicine, Critical Care, Toxicology, and Child Abuse

Chapter 19. Disorders of the Ear, Nose, and Throat

Chapter 20. Oncologic Diseases

1 Diseases of the Cardiovascular System

SYMPTOM SPECIFIC

I. Approach to the Cyanotic Infant

A. Background and differential diagnosis
   1. Bluish discoloration of the skin, which can be caused by (Box 1-1)
      a. Presence of at least 3–5 mg/dL deoxygenated hemoglobin due to
         i. Shunting of blood from right to left side of heart
         ii. Hypoventilation
         iii. Ventilation/perfusion ($\dot{V}/\dot{Q}$) mismatch in lungs
         iv. Problems with diffusion of oxygen (O_2) through alveolar–capillary membrane
         v. Poor oxygen affinity to hemoglobin
      b. Poor peripheral circulation resulting in increased O_2 extraction from blood
         i. Venous stasis from poor cardiac output (e.g., congestive heart failure [CHF])
         ii. Peripheral vasoconstriction (e.g., sepsis)

B. Historical findings
   1. Age of onset (Table 1-1)
   2. Birth history: fetal distress, prolonged rupture of membranes (sepsis), meconium-stained amniotic fluid (associated with pulmonary hypertension and fetal distress), maternal sedation or drugs of abuse
   3. Associated symptoms: cough, difficulty breathing, fever, hypotonia, tachypnea
   4. Prenatal risk factors
      a. Congenital heart disease (CHD): maternal age, diabetes, teratogen exposure (alcohol, medication)
      b. Central nervous system (CNS) disease: abnormal fetal movements, advanced maternal age
      c. Pulmonary disease: prematurity, oligohydramnios, polyhydramnios
      d. Sepsis: prematurity, group B *Streptococcus* status, fetal distress
   5. Family history: CHD, blood disorders, asthma, birth defects, genetic syndromes

C. Physical examination findings
   1. Cyanosis detection dependent on multiple factors
      a. May be more difficult to appreciate in darkly pigmented patients
      b. Degree of cyanosis may not correlate with degree of hypoxemia: factors that shift hemoglobin dissociation curve to the right (e.g., fever, sepsis, acidosis) cause greater cyanosis at a higher partial pressure of oxygen in arterial blood (PaO_2)
   2. Inspection of skin and extremities: distribution of cyanosis
      a. Differential cyanosis between upper extremities (UE) and lower extremities (LE)
         i. UE hypoxemia and LE normal: transposition of great arteries (TGA)
         ii. UE normal and LE hypoxemia: patent ductus arteriosus (PDA) with right (R)→left (L) shunt (usually in setting of persistent pulmonary hypertension of the newborn [PPHN]), aortic coarctation, or interrupted aortic arch [IAA])

QUICK HIT

Carbon monoxide toxicity does not produce cyanosis; it causes hemoglobin to bind O_2 more tightly at the remaining 3 O_2 binding sites, preventing delivery to the tissues. The patient may be a bright red color.

QUICK HIT

Acrocyanosis (hand, foot, and perioral cyanosis) is usually normal in the newborn period. It results from poor perfusion and increased venous pressure and can be accentuated by polycythemia.

MNEMONIC

The "5 T's and HOPE" of Cyanotic Heart Disease

Truncus arteriosus
Transposition of the great arteries (TGA)
Tricuspid atresia
Tetralogy of Fallot (TOF)
Total anomalous pulmonary venous return (TAPVR)
Hypoplastic left heart syndrome (HLHS)
Other forms of single ventricle
Pulmonary atresia
Ebstein anomaly of the tricuspid valve (TV)

QUICK HIT

Differential cyanosis: upper and lower extremities appear different; is seen in right to left shunting through a PDA.

QUICK HIT

Cyanosis depends on hemoglobin level, so it is more readily apparent in patients with polycythemia and difficult to recognize in patients with severe anemia.

QUICK HIT

Cyanosis is best seen in mucous membranes (nose, mouth, tongue) and periorally.

BOX 1-1

Differential Diagnosis of Cyanosis in the Newborn

Cardiovascular	Cyanotic congenital heart disease with right to left shunting Severe congestive heart failure • Myocardial disease • Significant left to right shunt resulting in severe pulmonary edema Low cardiac output
Central nervous system	Central hypoventilation or apnea • Perinatal asphyxia • Intracranial hemorrhage • Seizures • Exposure to maternal sedatives • Structural brain abnormalities • Metabolic disorders • Congenital central hypoventilation syndrome
Pulmonary	Pulmonary vascular disease • Persistent pulmonary hypertension of the newborn • Pulmonary atrioventricular malformations (sometimes present in infants with hepatic disease) Anatomic upper airway abnormalities (Pierre-Robin, choanal atresia, laryngomalacia, vascular malformations) Parenchymal lung disease • Pneumonia • Respiratory distress syndrome • Meconium aspiration • Pulmonary interstitial emphysema • Congenital cystic adenomatoid malformation Diffusion capacity abnormalities • Bronchopulmonary dysplasia • Pulmonary edema Pleural effusions Diaphragmatic hernia
Hematologic	Methemoglobinemia Hemoglobinopathies
Other	Acrocyanosis Sepsis Metabolic disorders

TABLE 1-1 Age of Symptom Onset for Cyanotic Congenital Heart Lesions

Neonatal period	• Transposition of the great arteries • Hypoplastic left heart syndrome • Obstructed total anomalous pulmonary venous return • Severe Ebstein anomaly • Critical pulmonary stenosis or aortic stenosis
Infancy	• Tetralogy of Fallot with moderate pulmonary stenosis • Truncus arteriosus • Transposition of the great arteries with ventricular septal defect
Beyond infancy	• Mild tetralogy of Fallot, total or partial • Unobstructed totally anomalous pulmonary venous return • Single ventricle with pulmonic stenosis

QUICK HIT

Apnea, hypotonia, and lethargy with shallow irregular breathing imply CNS pathology, sepsis, or severe acidosis.

3. Lung exam: breathing pattern (tachypnea, shallow, irregular), respiratory distress (grunting, retractions), auscultation for diminished breath sounds, rales, wheeze, or rhonchi
   a. Tachypnea without respiratory distress is a common presentation of cyanotic cardiac disease ("**happy tachypnea**")
   b. Tachypnea with respiratory distress is usually indicative of lung disease, but occasionally seen with cardiac disease (total anomalous pulmonary venous return [TAPVR])
4. Cardiac exam
   a. Inspection and palpation of precordium (sternal heaves, thrills)
   b. Auscultation: S1, S2, murmurs (systolic, diastolic, and continuous)
      i. Systolic ejection murmurs: aortic stenosis (AS), pulmonary stenosis (PS), and tetralogy of Fallot (TOF)
      ii. Holosystolic murmurs: tricuspid atresia (from ventricular septal defect [VSD]), Ebstein anomaly (from tricuspid regurgitation)
      iii. Continuous murmurs (from PDA): ductal dependent lesions, such as TGA, hypoplastic left heart syndrome (HLHS), and coarctation of the aorta

D. Laboratory testing and radiologic imaging
1. Obtain arterial blood gas (ABG)
   a. If no hypoxemia, then suspect acrocyanosis, hematologic causes
   b. If hypoxemia confirmed, suspect pulmonary versus cardiac cause
   c. Hypercarbia may be seen with pulmonary causes
   d. Acidosis may be seen in sepsis, shock, critical coarctation, TGA
2. **Hyperoxia test** can be performed by administering 100% FiO_2 for 10 minutes and rechecking ABG
   a. PaO_2 >200 mm Hg = cardiac lesion very unlikely and highly suggests pulmonary or neurologic disease
   b. PaO_2 50–150 mm Hg = suggests mixing cardiac lesion without restrictive pulmonary blood flow (truncus arteriosus, tricuspid atresia)
   c. PaO_2 <50 mm Hg = indicates cardiac lesion with parallel circulation (TGA) or mixing cardiac lesion with ductal dependent pulmonary blood flow
3. Complete blood count (CBC): assess for anemia, polycythemia
4. Chest x-ray (CXR): assess for visceral situs inversus, aortic arch shape/configuration, cardiac size/shape, lung fields, and pulmonary vasculature (Figure 1-1)
   a. Pulmonary: pneumonia, pneumothorax, effusion, atelectasis, congenital diaphragmatic hernia
   b. Cardiac: see Figure 1-1
5. Electrocardiogram (ECG, or EKG): usually nonspecific
   a. Increased right forces with right axis deviation, right atrial enlargement (RAE), and/or right ventricular hypertrophy (RVH): TOF, truncus arteriosus, HLHS, Ebstein anomaly, severe PS, TAPVR, and pulmonary hypertension
   b. Increased left forces with left axis deviation, left atrial enlargement (LAE), and/or left ventricular hypertrophy (LVH): tricuspid atresia, critical AS, and coarctation of aorta
6. Echocardiogram (Echo)
   a. Most often confirms diagnosis of CHD
   b. Can be helpful in evaluating PPHN

II. Approach to Chest Pain

A. Background and differential diagnosis (Box 1-2)
1. Common reason for emergency room (ER) visits: ~650,000 per year among ages 10–21 years
2. Main concern on part of family is cardiac origin; however, that is rare
   a. Most common listed diagnosis is "idiopathic"
3. Originates from musculoskeletal, pleural, cardiac, and referred sources
   a. Broad differential diagnosis covers large range of benign and malignant conditions

QUICK HIT

Heart murmurs can be absent in many serious forms of cyanotic CHD such as in HLHS.

QUICK HIT

Most cyanosis is not detectable on exam until O_2 saturation is <85%.

QUICK HIT

Differential cyanosis can be detected by routinely screening infants for CHD with pulse oximetry on the right hand and the foot between ages 24 and 48 hours. Lower saturation in the leg than in the right hand suggests right to left shunting.

QUICK HIT

Diminished femoral pulses and upper extremity blood pressure >10 mm Hg more than lower extremity blood pressures suggest coarctation of the aorta.

QUICK HIT

Prostaglandin infusions are lifesaving for ductal dependent lesions in the neonate, until surgical interventions are performed.

QUICK HIT

Most common identified source of chest pain is musculoskeletal.

FIGURE 1-1 **Radiographic approach to cyanotic congenital heart lesions.**

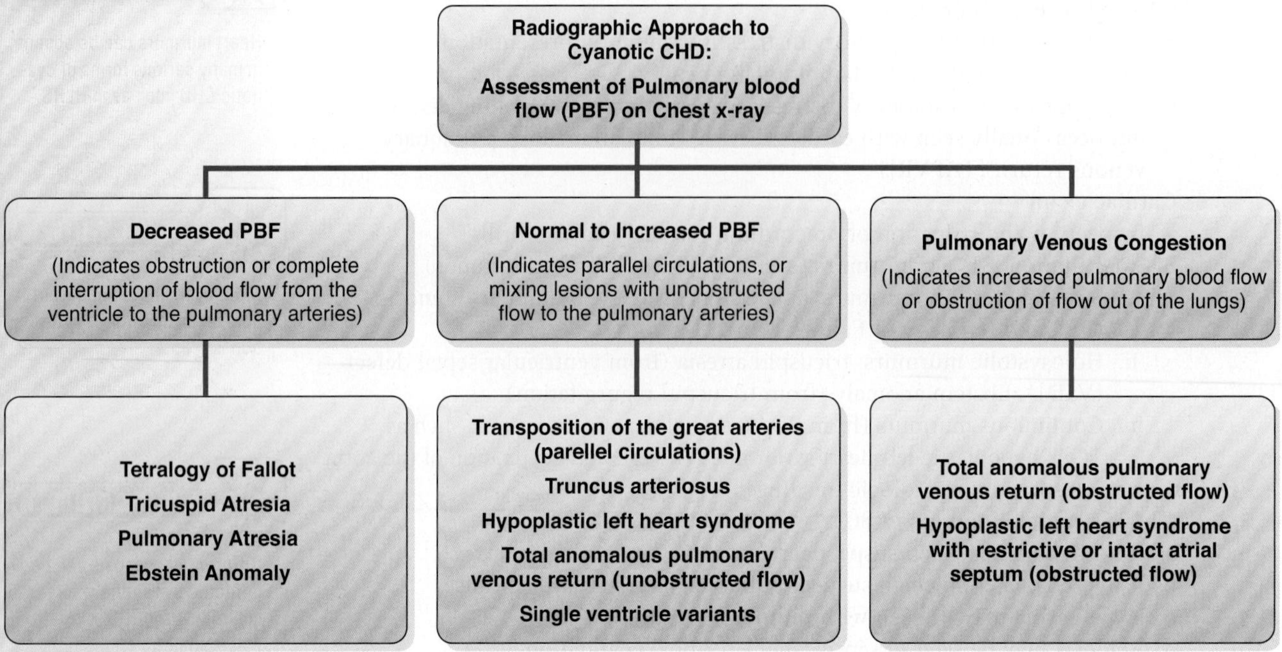

QUICK HIT

Although cardiac origin is the most frequent concern and musculoskeletal origin is the most common source, there are more ominous disease conditions that can present with chest pain.

QUICK HIT

Cardiac causes of chest pain are more likely to occur with exertion, and arrhythmias *rarely* present with chest pain.

B. Historical findings
   1. When did the pain first occur, and how frequently is it occurring?
   2. Are there other symptoms associated with the chest pain, such as fever, lethargy, poor appetite, difficulty breathing, or recent illness?
      a. Benign musculoskeletal pain does not have associated fever, weight loss, or other constitutional symptoms
      b. Difficulty breathing/wheezing or coughing is common finding with asthma or other respiratory complaints
      c. Fever and/or rash may occur with inflammatory conditions, myocarditis, pericarditis, pleuritis, or oncologic conditions

BOX 1-2

Chest Pain: Differential Diagnosis

Musculoskeletal
- Costochondritis
- Slipping rib syndromes
- Precordial catch

Infectious
- Pneumonia
- Bronchitis
- Pleural effusion
- Herpes zoster
- Coxsackie virus ("devil's grip")

Respiratory
- Asthma
- Pneumothorax/pneumomediastinum
- Pleuritis

Gastrointestinal
- Esophagitis
- Gastroesophageal reflux
- Biliary disease
- Pancreatitis

Psychiatric
- Conversion disorder
- Hyperventilation

Idiopathic

Breast
- Thelarche
- Breast tenderness (menses/pregnancy)
- Mastitis
- Gynecomastia

Cardiac
- Pericarditis
- Myocarditis
- Left ventricular outflow obstruction
- Aortic root dissection
- Coronary anomaly
- Coronary vasospasm
- Tachyarrhythmia

Toxins
- Cocaine

d. Syncope and/or palpitations concerning for underlying arrhythmia
e. Association with eating concerning for gastroesophageal reflux, esophagitis, or gastritis
3. How long do the episodes last?
4. Is it associated with activity?
5. Where is it located, and does it move?
6. Does it change with position?
7. Was there any preceding event (e.g., trauma, stressor, ingestion)?
8. Is there an underlying medical problem?

C. Physical exam findings
1. Chest exam focuses on maneuvers to reproduce musculoskeletal chest pain
a. Palpate for tenderness at costochondral junction, muscles, breasts
b. Respiratory exam may reveal asymmetric decreased breath sounds, wheezing, rhonchi, or rales in the setting of underlying pulmonary disease
2. Cardiac exam
a. Tachycardia
b. Murmurs due to valvular disease or outflow obstruction
c. Rubs suggest pericardial effusion
3. Abdominal exam
a. Pain on palpation implies gastrointestinal (GI) cause
b. Some patients with pneumonia will have pain on palpation of upper abdomen

D. Lab testing and radiologic imaging
1. Limited evaluation is needed if physical exam is normal, family history negative, and history is not suggestive of underlying disease
2. CXR, ECG, Echo: if needed to evaluate for underlying pulmonary or cardiac disease

QUICK HIT
Costochondritis presents with sharp midsternal chest pain without radiation that is worse with inspiration and reproducible on exam.

QUICK HIT
Chest pain with pericarditis improves when leaning forward.

QUICK HIT
Rubs may not be audible with large pericardial effusions because inflamed surfaces are no longer in contact.

QUICK HIT
Normal heart rate varies by age. Infants have a higher heart rate than older children.

III. Approach to Tachycardia

A. Background and differential diagnosis
1. Abnormally high heart rate for age
2. Should be measured for full 60 seconds
3. Life-threatening cardiac causes of tachycardia
a. Supraventricular tachycardia (SVT, or narrow complex tachycardia; see Tachyarrhythmia, page 22)
i. Presentation in infants may be asymptomatic or nonspecific, including feeding problems and increased fussiness
ii. Older children complain of palpitations, chest pain, and shortness of breath
b. Atrial flutter: rapid heart rate with sawtooth pattern seen on ECG
c. Ventricular tachycardia (VT; see Tachyarrhythmia, page 22)
i. Can be asymptomatic in otherwise healthy children
4. Life-threatening noncardiac causes of tachycardia: shock
a. Septic shock (tachycardia due to vasodilation, hypotension, and increased metabolic demand)
b. Hypovolemic shock (diarrhea, vomiting, blood loss)
c. Anaphylactic shock: **IgE mediated** (**type 1 hypersensitivity**)
5. Non–life-threatening causes of tachycardia
a. Stimulants cause direct, adrenergic stimulation of sinoatrial (SA) node, leading to sinus tachycardia and risk for life-threatening arrhythmias that cause tachycardia
b. Nonstimulant medications
i. Tricyclic antidepressants, antihistamines, antipsychotics, and other medications have **anticholinergic effects**
ii. Hypoglycemics (sulfonylureas) increase metabolic demand
c. Other causes
i. Anemia (due to decreased O_2-carrying capacity)
ii. Hyperthyroidism
iii. Pheochromocytoma (adrenergic effects)
iv. Hypoglycemia

QUICK HIT
Pathophysiology of tachycardia may involve increased firing of the sinoatrial (SA) node (the pacemaker), an ectopic focus, or aberrant conduction tissue due to increased stimulation.

QUICK HIT
A key aspect of evaluating tachycardia is to decide whether the tachycardia arises from above the ventricles (supraventricular or "narrow complex") versus those arising within the ventricles (ventricular or "wide complex").

QUICK HIT
Common stimulants include cocaine, amphetamines (e.g., attention deficit hyperactive disorder [ADHD] medications, diet pills, crystal methamphetamine), caffeine, and albuterol.

QUICK HIT

SVT usually presents with a nonvariable heart rate and absence of P waves.

QUICK HIT

Consider SVT in infants with heart rate >200 bpm or in children with heart rate >180 bpm.

QUICK HIT

Vagal maneuvers and adenosine may be attempted for patients with stable SVT; any patient with unstable SVT requires prompt cardioversion.

QUICK HIT

Sustained tachycardia with a wide QRS complex is VT until proven otherwise and requires immediate intervention to prevent transition into ventricular fibrillation (VF).

QUICK HIT

Most tachycardia in children is noncardiac in origin.

QUICK HIT

Before conducting a thorough history and physical, always assess the ABCs (airway, breathing, and circulation) to determine if immediate interventions are necessary.

QUICK HIT

Treat any fevers with antipyretics to assess if tachycardia has cause other than fever.

v. Infection (usually with fever, often viral)
vi. Anxiety

B. Historical findings
1. Have there been any other systemic symptoms (pain)?
 a. Respiratory issues may point to pneumonia
 b. Fever points to infectious etiology
2. Are there any signs of dehydration?
 a. Vomiting or diarrhea
 b. Decreased oral intake or low urine output
3. Is there sweating with feedings, color changes or cyanosis, or complaints of chest pain or palpitations? (Suggests underlying cardiac disease)
4. Are there possible medication exposures or medications around the home?
5. Are there comorbid psychiatric issues that may lead to anxiety?
6. Any history of cardiac issues or surgeries? (Increased risk of arrhythmias if CHD present, even if corrected)
7. Family history of cardiac issues or sudden death in the family? (Suggests structural heart abnormalities or hereditary arrhythmias)

C. Physical examination findings
1. Vital signs
 a. Heart rate and rhythm: evaluate if rate is regular versus irregular
 b. Blood pressure: low pressure suggests hypovolemia, possible shock
 c. Temperature: fever can cause or worsen underlying tachycardia
 d. **Pulse oximetry**: hypoxia causes tachycardia to increase end-tissue O_2 delivery
2. Head, eyes, ears, nose, throat, and neck
 a. **Exophthalmos** is seen in Graves thyroiditis (hyperthyroidism)
 b. Enlarged or tender thyroid suggests thyroid inflammation
 c. Dry mucous membranes suggest hypovolemia and dehydration
 d. Conjunctival or tongue frenulum pallor suggests anemia
 e. Nasal flaring, grunting, or retractions point to underlying lung disease
3. Chest and lung
 a. **Tachypnea** is common in lower respiratory tract infections
 b. Increased work of breathing (e.g., retractions)
 c. Auscultate for wheezing, rales, or focal crackles
4. Cardiovascular
 a. Palpate point of maximal impulse (PMI), assess for hyperdynamic precordium
 b. Auscultate for murmurs, extra heart sounds
5. Extremities
 a. Warm versus cool extremities
 b. Peripheral pulses: bounding versus diminished
 c. Capillary refill: brisk versus delayed

D. Laboratory testing, radiologic imaging, and ancillary studies
1. Laboratory evaluation
 a. CBC to evaluate hemoglobin (anemia)
 b. Chemistry to evaluate for electrolyte abnormalities, particularly
  i. Bicarbonate for signs of acidosis
  ii. Potassium
  iii. Calcium and magnesium if tachycardia is cardiac in origin
  iv. Glucose for evaluation of hypoglycemia
 c. Consider toxicology screening
 d. Cultures as indicated (blood, urine, cerebrospinal fluid [CSF])
 e. For shock, consider disseminated intravascular coagulation (DIC) studies: prothrombin time (PT), partial thromboplastin time (PTT), international normalized ratio (INR), fibrinogen, D-dimers
 f. Consider thyroid-stimulating hormone, free thyroxine (T_4)
2. Imaging and ancillary studies
 a. CXR: evaluate heart size, lung parenchyma
 b. ECG: assess for dysrhythmias, discussed earlier
 c. Echo: to directly visualize heart anatomy, evaluate ventricle function

IV. Approach to Syncope

A. Background and differential diagnosis (Table 1-2)
  1. Neurologic
    a. Vasovagal syncope
      i. >50% of syncope seen in pediatric ERs, particularly in teenagers
    b. Breath-holding spells
      i. Typically ages 6 months to 5 years (peak at age 2 years)
      ii. May result in unconsciousness and cyanosis but requires behavioral intervention only
    c. Seizure disorder and CNS mass (see Chapter 5)
  2. Cardiovascular
    a. Cardiac arrhythmias (see bradyarrhythmia, tachyarrhythmia, long QT)
      i. SVT (e.g., Wolff-Parkinson-White [WPW])
      ii. VT
      iii. Long QT syndrome
    b. Poor contractility
      i. Myocarditis: due to decreased cardiac output
      ii. Dilated cardiomyopathy leads to syncope through arrhythmias or poor cardiac output
    c. Outflow obstructive lesions
      i. Right ventricular outflow tract obstructions
        (a) Pulmonary hypertension
        (b) PS
        (c) Pulmonary embolism
      ii. Left ventricular outflow tract obstructions
        (a) Hypertrophic cardiomyopathy (HCM): history of syncope increases risk of death in HCM 5-fold
        (b) AS
        (c) Rare: atrial myxoma
  3. Other causes
    a. Orthostatic hypotension
      i. Postural drop in blood pressure when moving from laying or sitting to standing, resulting in decreased cerebral perfusion
      ii. Patients may only complain of antecedent light-headedness
      iii. May be due to hypovolemia, decreased vascular tone, and associated decreased venous return
    b. Hypoglycemia

QUICK HIT

If a patient continues to have symptoms, consider cardiology referral for Holter or event monitor placement.

QUICK HIT

Syncope is the transient loss of consciousness and postural tone due to inadequate cerebral perfusion (cerebral blood flow <50% leads to syncope).

QUICK HIT

Orthostatic hypertension recovers spontaneously without intervention.

TABLE 1-2 **Differential Diagnosis of Syncope**

Cardiovascular	*Neurologic*
Primary electrical disorder	Vasovagal syncope
Supraventricular tachycardia	Orthostatic hypotension
Ventricular tachycardia	Postural orthostatic tachycardia syndrome
Long QT syndrome	Seizures
Brugada syndrome	Migraine
Poor contractility	Breath-holding spells
Congestive heart failure	Central nervous system lesion
Myocarditis	*Other*
Dilated cardiomyopathy	Anemia
Outflow tract obstruction	Hypoglycemia
Pulmonary hypertension	Medication ingestions
Pulmonary stenosis	Drugs of abuse
Hypertrophic obstructive cardiomyopathy	Pregnancy
Aortic stenosis	Panic attacks
	Conversion disorder

QUICK HIT

Approximately 15% of children will experience syncopal episode.

QUICK HIT

Vasovagal syncope is a diagnosis of exclusion.

QUICK HIT

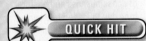

Cardiac causes lead to syncope through sudden decreases in cardiac output and resultant decreased cerebral perfusion.

QUICK HIT

Ask specifically for family history of motor vehicle accidents, drowning, or unexplained childhood death that may represent sudden cardiac death.

QUICK HIT

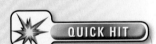

Make sure to take orthostatic vital signs: heart rate and blood pressure in supine, sitting, and standing positions at 2, 5, and 10 minutes.

QUICK HIT

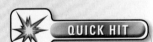

A sustained drop in blood pressure between supine and standing positions of more than 20 mm Hg systolic or 10 mm Hg diastolic defines orthostatic hypotension.

QUICK HIT

HOCM murmur increases in intensity as preload decreases, such as from squatting to standing or with Valsalva maneuver, because there is less blood flow to overcome the obstruction.

TABLE 1-3 Historical Factors Indicative of a Life-Threatening Cause of Syncope

Absence of prodrome
Syncope during exercise
Cardiac symptoms (e.g., chest pain, palpitations)
Family history of heart disease (e.g., arrhythmias, cardiomyopathy) or sudden death
History of congenital heart disease or cardiac surgery

c. Pregnancy
d. Ingestion

B. Historical findings (Table 1-3)
1. What is the description of the event?
a. Shorter (<1 minute) duration of unconsciousness suggests noncardiac causes
b. Inciting or predisposing emotional events suggest neuropsychiatric cause
c. Presence of prodrome suggests neurologic cause
d. Syncope related to exercise suggests cardiac outflow tract obstruction
2. Were there symptoms of dehydration, vomiting, and diarrhea suggesting hypovolemia?
3. Was there associated chest pain, palpitations, or rapid heart rate suggesting cardiac causes associated with ischemia or arrhythmias?
4. Is there a history of cardiac issues or surgeries?
5. Is there a history of sudden death in the family?

C. Physical examination findings
1. Vital signs
2. Mucous membranes: hydration status, pallor suggesting anemia
3. Cardiac
a. Systolic ejection murmurs: AS, hypertrophic obstructive cardiomyopathy (HOCM)
b. S3 and S4 suggest heart failure
4. Neurologic: focal deficits, signs of increased intracranial pressure (ICP)/papilledema

D. Laboratory testing, radiologic imaging, and ancillary tests
1. Laboratory tests
a. Glucose and electrolytes may be useful immediately after the event
b. Hematocrit if history or physical examination suggests anemia
c. Urine pregnancy test
d. Consider urine toxicology
2. ECG: evaluate for rate, rhythm, and conduction abnormalities
a. In particular: WPW pre-excitation, long QT, heart block
b. Holter monitor or event monitor for infrequent events
c. Echo: if needed, to evaluate for obstruction, structural abnormalities

DISEASE SPECIFIC

V. Truncus Arteriosus

A. Definitions
1. Single arterial trunk with single semilunar valve supplying the systemic, pulmonary, and coronary circulations (instead of distinct pulmonary artery and aorta)
2. Truncus overrides VSD and receives blood from both right and left ventricles (Figure 1-2)

B. Cause/pathophysiology
1. Genetic associations: DiGeorge syndrome
2. Immediately after birth, pulmonary blood flow is normal; as pulmonary vascular resistance decreases over first few weeks of life, more blood flows to lungs causing pulmonary overcirculation and CHF

FIGURE 1-2 **Truncus arteriosus.**

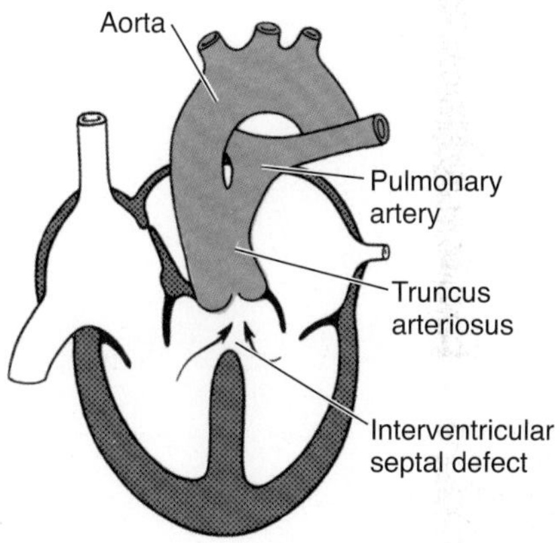

(From Sadler T. *Langman's Medical Embryology*, Ninth Edition Image Bank. Baltimore: Lippincott Williams & Wilkins; 2003.)

C. Clinical presentation
  1. Signs of CHF within the first month of life (tachycardia, dyspnea, poor feeding, hepatomegaly)

D. Testing
  1. CXR: cardiomegaly, possible right aortic arch, **increased pulmonary vascularity**
  2. Echo: demonstrates large truncal artery overriding VSD

E. Therapy
  1. Surgical repair
  2. Supportive therapy for management of CHF (see Congestive Heart Failure, page 16)

VI. Transposition of the Great Arteries *(Figure 1-3)*

A. Definitions
  1. Aorta arises from right ventricle (RV), and pulmonary artery arises from left ventricle (LV)
  2. Systemic and pulmonary circulations are parallel circuits
  3. Often associated with VSD, coronary abnormalities, aortic arch abnormalities

B. Cause/pathophysiology
  1. Parallel circuits: deoxygenated blood from body returns to right heart and gets pumped through aorta back into systemic circulation
  2. Oxygenated blood from lungs returns to left atrium (LA) and gets pumped through pulmonary artery back to lungs

C. Testing
  1. Hyperoxia test: PaO_2 <150 mm Hg after administration of 100% O_2
  2. Echo: usually will confirm transposed vessels
  3. Cardiac catheterization: evaluate coronary anatomy

D. Therapy
  1. Immediate goal: allow oxygenated blood to reach systemic circulation
    a. **Start prostaglandin (PGE_1)** to keep PDA open
    b. May also need emergent balloon atrial septostomy
  2. Surgical repair usually done in the first 2 weeks of life
    a. Divide aorta and pulmonary artery and re-anastomose to correct position
    b. Coronary arteries removed and reimplanted in the "neoaortic" root

VII. Total Anomalous Pulmonary Venous Return

A. Definitions
  1. Rare form of CHD, ~1%–2% of total
  2. Pulmonary veins do not drain to LA, but rather via an anomalous pathway to systemic venous system and eventually back to right heart
    a. **Supracardiac** (50%) drains **above diaphragm**
    b. **Infracardiac** (20%) drains **below the diaphragm**

> **QUICK HIT**
> Truncus arteriosus is associated with cyanosis in the newborn period.

> **QUICK HIT**
> Second most common cyanotic CHD in newborns (~5%).

> **QUICK HIT**
> TGA is not compatible with life unless desaturated and oxygenated blood can mix through openings at one or more levels (i.e., VSD, patent foramen ovale [PFO], and/or PDA).

FIGURE 1-3 Transposition of the great arteries.

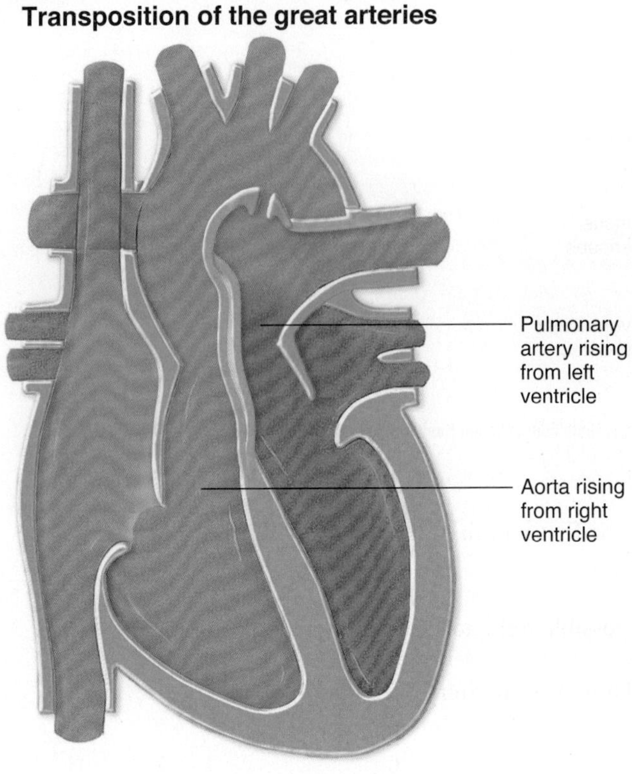

(Asset provided by Anatomical Chart Co.)

> **QUICK HIT**
> CXR shows cardiac shadow, which may have the classic "egg-on-a-string" appearance with a narrow upper mediastinum and increased pulmonary vascularity.

> **QUICK HIT**
> Obstructed TAPVR: pulmonary venous return unable to leave lungs, resulting in severe pulmonary hypertension.

> **QUICK HIT**
> Obstructed TAPVR is one of the only forms of CHD that remains a true surgical emergency that presents at birth since the routine use of PGE_1.

> **QUICK HIT**
> Using PGE_1 in obstructed TAPVR can cause decompensation by flooding the lungs with more pulmonary blood flow that cannot get out, causing increased pulmonary congestion and making it more difficult to ventilate/oxygenate the patient.

c. **Cardiac** (20%) drains directly to the right atrium (RA) or coronary sinus
d. **Mixed type** (10%) involves combination of any of above types

3. Pulmonary veins may be unobstructed or obstructed

B. Pathophysiology: pulmonary veins return oxygenated blood to RA where it mixes with deoxygenated blood

C. Clinical presentation
1. **Obstructed TAPVR: presents immediately after birth with profound cyanosis and respiratory distress; poor prognosis**
2. Unobstructed TAPVR: increased work of breathing, tachypnea, growth failure

D. Testing
1. CXR: cardiomegaly, prominence of right heart border, increased pulmonary vascular markings ("snowman" shape to heart)
2. ECG: right axis deviation, RAE, RVH; sometimes right bundle branch block
3. Echo: evaluate pulmonary veins, atrial shunting, pulmonary hypertension

E. Therapy
1. Unobstructed TAPVR: surgical repair
2. Obstructed TAPVR: immediate intervention with ventilator support, supplemental oxygen, PGE_1 infusion, correction of acidosis, volume resuscitation and inotropes; **emergent surgical repair usually within first 24 hours of life**

VIII. Tricuspid Atresia *(Figure 1-4)*

A. Definitions
1. No connection from RA to RV
2. RV often hypoplastic
3. VSD usually present but of variable size

B. Cause/pathophysiology: due to failure of tricuspid valve (TV) formation or fusion of leaflets

FIGURE 1-4 **Anatomy of tricuspid atresia.**

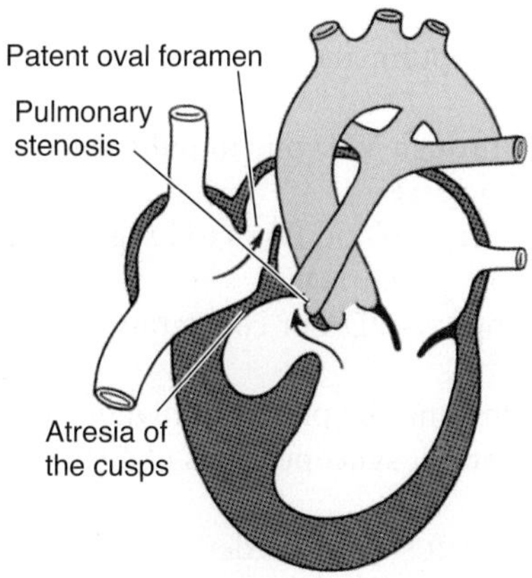

Blood flow from the right atrium to the right ventricle is obstructed, so it must flow through the patent foramen ovale to the left atrium, and reach the pulmonary circulation through either the ventricular septal defect (VSD) or the patent ductus arteriosus (PDA). (From Sadler T. *Langman's Medical Embryology*, Ninth Edition Image Bank. Baltimore: Lippincott Williams & Wilkins; 2003.)

C. Clinical presentation
   1. Cyanosis at birth (degree depends on VSD size, severity of pulmonic stenosis)
   2. CHF (fatigue, dyspnea, tachypnea, poor feeding)

D. Testing
   1. CXR: either poor circulation (restricted pulmonary blood flow) or congestion (excessive pulmonary blood flow) with cardiomegaly/right heart prominence

E. Therapy
   1. **Start PGE_1 immediately to maintain pulmonary blood flow**
   2. Typical 3-stage repair for single-ventricle physiology over the first several years of life

IX. Tetralogy of Fallot

A. Definitions
   1. Includes 4 primary anomalies ("tetralogy") (Figure 1-5)
      a. Obstruction to RV outflow (pulmonary stenosis)
      b. VSD

FIGURE 1-5 **Tetralogy of Fallot is characterized by the combination of 4 defects: (1) pulmonary stenosis, (2) ventricular septal defect, (3) overriding aorta, and (4) right ventricular hypertrophy.**

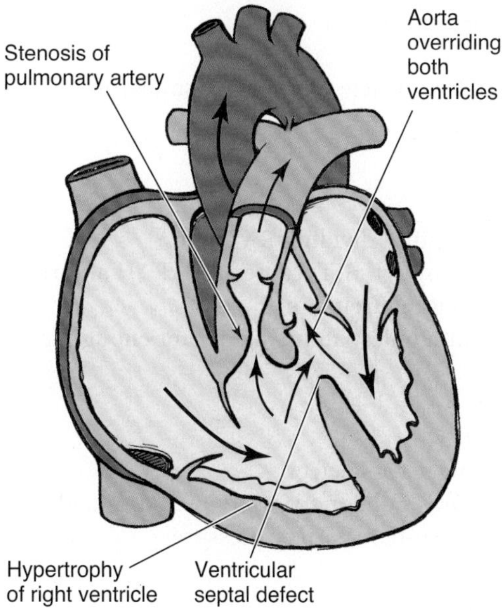

QUICK HIT

Tricuspid atresia blocks flow from right atrium to right ventricle. An atrial septal defect or patent foramen ovale must be present for survival.

QUICK HIT

ECG shows LVH with left axis deviation, which distinguishes tricuspid atresia from most other forms of cyanotic heart disease.

QUICK HIT

TOF is the most common *cyanotic* congenital heart defect in newborns.

QUICK HIT

TOF may be associated with DiGeorge, Down, or fetal hydantoin syndrome.

QUICK HIT

"Tet spells," or hypercyanotic spells, occur when there is suddenly increased resistance to pulmonary blood flow, causing more deoxygenated blood to flow through the VSD and aorta to the systemic circulation (e.g., during crying).

QUICK HIT

Treatment of "tet spells" is aimed at decreasing pulmonary outflow tract obstruction (calming measures, such as morphine and β-blockers) and increasing systemic venous return as well as systemic resistance (knee–chest position, squatting, phenylephrine) to encourage blood flow to the lungs.

QUICK HIT

Only 1% of CHD but has highest mortality from CHD in 1st month of life

QUICK HIT

Neonates with HLHS must have an atrial communication and PDA to survive. If the atrial septum is intact, the baby is usually critically ill at birth and requires emergency surgery to decompress the LA and allow egress of pulmonary venous return.

QUICK HIT

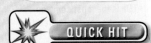

Neonates with HLHS will present with shock shortly after birth.

QUICK HIT

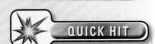

Ironically, excessive O_2 administration at birth for cyanosis may lead to systemic hypotension, because it dilates the pulmonary vessels, and blood then preferentially goes to lungs instead of the systemic circulation.

QUICK HIT

A wide, fixed split S2 due to right-sided volume overload is pathognomonic for ASD, especially if associated with midsystolic murmur at the right upper sternal border or RV heave.

c. Dextroposition of aorta overriding VSD
d. RVH

B. Cause/pathophysiology
1. Results from abnormal rotation of conotruncal septum and malalignment with intraventricular septum
2. Blood flows from RA → RV → preferentially through VSD due to pulmonic stenosis → deoxygenated blood mixes in LV → aorta
3. If pulmonic obstruction is mild/moderate, sufficient blood flows to lungs to get oxygenated → balanced shunt (acyanotic or "pink" TOF)
4. If obstruction is severe, blood must flow to lungs via PDA or collaterals

C. Clinical presentation
1. If right outflow obstruction is mild: cyanosis may not be present initially
2. If obstruction is severe: cyanosis in neonatal period, syncope, signs of CHF (difficulty feeding, failure to thrive)
3. Loud/harsh systolic murmur (possible thrill) at left sternal border
4. "Tet spell": dyspnea, tachypnea, worsening cyanosis, fussiness, syncope

D. Testing
1. CXR: **"Boot-shaped" heart** due to right ventricle enlargement (RVE), clear lung fields (secondary to decreased pulmonary blood flow)
2. ECG: right axis deviation and RVH
3. Echo: assess degree of pulmonary obstruction

E. Therapy
1. PGE_1 to keep PDA open and maintain pulmonary blood flow
2. Patients with severe outflow tract obstruction or pulmonary atresia need surgical repair

X. Hypoplastic Left Heart Syndrome

A. Definitions (Figure 1-6)
1. Underdeveloped, small LV
2. LV inflow obstruction (mitral stenosis or atresia)
3. LV outflow obstruction (AS or atresia)
4. Hypoplastic ascending aorta and aortic arch

B. Clinical presentation
1. In newborns: cyanosis, respiratory distress, shock once PDA closes
2. *Murmur may be absent*
3. Single loud S2, hyperactive precordium with palpable sternal heave

C. Testing
1. CXR: mild cardiomegaly (right heart border), pulmonary congestion
2. Echocardiogram

D. Therapy
1. Mechanical ventilation, inotropes, correct acidosis
2. *Immediately begin PGE_1 infusion*
3. Surgery is a 3-stage palliation for single-ventricle physiology (similar to tricuspid atresia)
4. Heart transplant is an option

XI. Atrial Septal Defect (ASD)

A. Definition: abnormal communication in septum dividing RA and LA

B. Cause/pathophysiology: L → R shunting through ASD causes RAE/RAH and right heart overload, which may lead to tricuspid regurgitation

C. Clinical presentation: may be asymptomatic unless shunt significant enough to cause CHF

D. Testing
1. ECG: RV conduction delay, RAE, RVH
2. Echo: right heart enlargement, shunting across defect
3. Cardiac catheterization: directly measures pulmonary artery pressures and compares pulmonary artery pressure to systemic artery pressure

E. Therapy
1. Most ASDs <8 mm spontaneously close
2. Definitive repair indicated for symptomatic patients

FIGURE 1-6 **Circulation in hypoplastic left heart syndrome.**

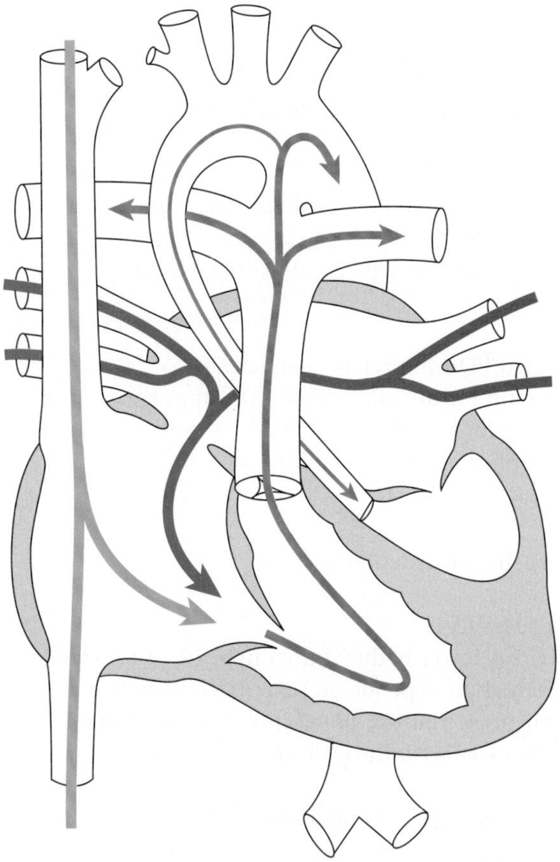

Oxygenated blood (red) returns from the lungs to the left atrium, but left ventricle and aorta are obstructed and hypoplastic so blood must flow through atrial defect to the right atrium where it mixes with deoxygenated blood (blue), then through the pulmonary artery (purple) either back to the lungs or through the patent ductus arteriosus to supply the systemic circulation.

XII. Ventricular Septal Defect

A. Definition
1. Abnormal communication in septum dividing RV and LV
2. ~75% of VSDs are membranous
3. Other types include muscular, atrioventricular (AV) canal type, or outlet septum

B. Cause/pathophysiology
1. Abnormal formation of ventricular septum in embryologic development
2. Higher LV pressures cause blood flow from LV → RV
3. Increased pulmonary flow causes pulmonary congestion and CHF

C. Clinical presentation
1. Heart murmur develops after birth when pulmonary artery resistance drops
2. CHF (see page 16)
3. If not corrected, can lead to Eisenmenger syndrome

D. Testing
1. CXR: cardiomegaly, increased pulmonary vascularity/pulmonary edema
2. Echo: directly visualize VSD and assess LV size and pressure gradient

E. Therapy
1. *~75% of small VSDs close without intervention,* especially muscular defects
2. Symptomatic patients managed with anticongestive medication to increase cardiac output and reduce pulmonary edema (see Congestive Heart Failure, page 16)
3. Surgical repair indicated if still symptomatic despite medical management and should be done in first year of life to prevent pulmonary vascular disease

QUICK HIT

As RA/RV pressures increase, pulmonary hypertension may develop, and shunting transitions from L → R to R → L (**Eisenmenger syndrome**).

QUICK HIT

Eisenmenger syndrome: dyspnea, fatigue, palpitations, cyanosis, hypoxemia, clubbing, ↑ jugular venous pressure

QUICK HIT

Patients with paradoxical embolic events (e.g., stroke from deep vein thrombosis [DVT]) should be evaluated for presence of ASD and Eisenmenger syndrome.

QUICK HIT

Patients with right heart enlargement are at risk for developing tachyarrhythmias, such as atrial fibrillation or atrial flutter.

QUICK HIT

VSDs are the most common isolated CHD (~20%) and are associated with several genetic conditions (e.g., trisomy 21).

QUICK HIT

In general, a smaller VSD will have a higher pitch (frequency) on auscultation, usually localized to the lower left sternal border. A murmur from a very large VSD may be low pitched and difficult to hear.

QUICK HIT

A PDA may be life preserving and kept open with prostaglandins at birth if in the presence of other CHD (e.g., TGA).

QUICK HIT

Prognosis is poor if pulmonary vascular disease/Eisenmenger physiology is present.

QUICK HIT

Most common coarctation site = juxtaductal

QUICK HIT

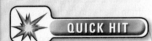

Among aortic coarctation patients, 50% have another defect, many have a bicuspid aortic valve, and 5% have berry aneurysms in the circle of Willis.

QUICK HIT

A quick differential diagnosis of neonatal shock is sepsis, obstructive cardiac defects (i.e., **coarctation of the aorta**), and adrenal insufficiency.

QUICK HIT

Prognosis is good if discovered early, although re-coarctation is a risk.

XIII. Patent Ductus Arteriosus

A. Definition: persistence of fetal connection between pulmonary artery and aorta
B. Cause/pathophysiology
  1. Failure of ductus to close normally after birth leads to L → R shunting, pulmonary overcirculation, and increased pulmonary artery pressure
  2. Increased incidence in prematurity, trisomy 21, maternal rubella
C. Clinical presentation
  1. Large ductus: age dependent (Table 1-4)
  2. Small ductus: systolic murmur, asymptomatic to mild activity intolerance
D. Testing
  1. CXR: increased vascular markings, cardiomegaly, interstitial edema
  2. Echo: gold standard of diagnosis
E. Therapy
  1. Indomethacin: for uncomplicated PDA in preterm neonates
  2. Surgical ligation: secondary option for uncomplicated PDA in preterm, term infants, and children; first option for complicated PDA
  3. Catheter device closure: uncomplicated PDA in child

XIV. Coarctation of the Aorta

A. Definition: narrowing in aorta causing obstruction to flow
B. Pathophysiology
  1. Increased afterload on heart causes LVH
  2. Upper body hypertensive, whereas lower body/GI tract hypoxic or ischemic
C. Clinical presentation: age of presentation depends on severity/collaterals
  1. Critical coarctation: neonatal presentation, *blood flow to lower body dependent on ductus arteriosus → heart failure/shock with decreased femoral pulses*
  2. Mild coarctation: may present at any age, even in adulthood
    a. Fatigue, poor growth
    b. Systolic murmur, decreased femoral pulses, hypertension
D. Testing
  1. Extremity blood pressures
  2. Echo: primary imaging test but can be limited
  3. Cardiac magnetic resonance imaging (MRI)/computed tomography (CT): best test to determine full anatomy of arch
E. Therapy
  1. Critical coarctation in neonates: *start PGE_1 immediately for ductal patency*
  2. Surgical repair

TABLE 1-4 Clinical Presentation and Progression of Patients with a Large Patent Ductus Arteriosus

Age Range	Neonate/Infant	Childhood	Adolescent	Adult
History	Poor feeding, poor weight gain	Activity intolerance and poor growth	Activity intolerance, poor growth, differential cyanosis	Activity intolerance, cyanosis, Eisenmenger
Murmur	Systolic or continuous	Continuous "machinery"	Systolic only or no murmur	Soft systolic murmur/no murmur
Respiratory	Tachypnea	Tachypnea/dyspnea	Dyspnea	Dyspnea, orthopnea
Pulses	Bounding	Bounding	Normal/slightly increased	Normal

Pulmonary hypertension ——→ Pulmonary vascular disease develops

XV. Hypertrophic Obstructive Cardiomyopathy

A. Characteristics
1. Definition: inappropriately hypertrophied, nondilated LV in absence of another disease process that can cause hypertrophy
2. Epidemiology: occurs in 0.2% of population (1/500)
3. Primarily genetic: list of genetic mutations associated with HOCM is long and continues to expand

B. Clinical features
1. History: can be 1 of 3 general clinical presentations
   a. Asymptomatic: most often in pediatric population but may change course during puberty; thought to be secondary to rapid somatic growth
   b. Heart failure: usually in 3rd–4th decade but can present at any age
   c. Arrhythmias: usually ventricular in origin, syncope or sudden death/aborted sudden death, palpitations
2. Physical exam findings: may be normal in patients without obstruction
   a. Obstruction: double apical impulse (due to atrial systole), medium pitch systolic murmur
   b. No obstruction: increased apical impulse, soft systolic murmur
   c. Heart failure: rales on lung auscultation

C. Diagnosis
1. Laboratory findings: genetic testing is available but cannot rule out a diagnosis of HOCM
2. Imaging findings
   a. CXR: cardiomegaly, increased pulmonary markings
   b. Echo: increased wall thickness and mass estimate
   c. Cardiac MRI: more sensitive study for wall thickness, more accurate myocardial mass measurement, adds ability for myocardial characterization
3. ECG findings: abnormal in 90%–95%, but patterns vary significantly among HOCM types

D. Treatment
1. Asymptomatic patients: longitudinal follow-up, no therapy
2. Heart failure symptoms
   a. Medical therapy (calcium channel blockers, β-blockers, angiotensin-converting enzyme [ACE] inhibitors)
   b. Septal myectomy if symptoms are refractory to medical therapy and obstruction present at rest or with provocation (i.e., exercise or stress test)
3. Arrhythmias/aborted sudden cardiac death: implantable cardioverter-defibrillator (ICD)
4. Infants with metabolic disease that causes HOCM should have underlying condition treated; if heart failure occurs, medical management as described previously
5. Prognosis
   a. Estimated mortality rate at 1% per year in overall HOCM population and ~2% per year in children with HOCM
   b. Family members and asymptomatic patients: ECG and Echo screening yearly during pubertal years and every 3–5 years as adults

XVI. Aortic Stenosis

A. Definitions
1. Left-sided obstruction due to aortic abnormality
   a. Valve abnormality most common (bicuspid, unicuspid/dysplastic)
   b. Subaortic stenosis
   c. Supravalvar stenosis

B. Cause/pathophysiology
1. Limited flow across LV outflow tract causes diminished cardiac output
2. Can lead to LVH and LV dysfunction
3. Abnormal valve can also have insufficiency

QUICK HIT

Most common cause of sudden cardiac death in young athletes; however, only a fraction of patients with HOCM are at risk for sudden death.

QUICK HIT

Sudden death results from chronic thickening of myocardium:
- Possibility of sudden outflow tract obstruction, which can lead to sudden poor coronary perfusion and arrhythmias
- Possibility of microscopic changes in myocardial tissue, which can cause arrhythmias

QUICK HIT

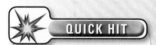

The murmur associated with HOCM varies depending on preload and afterload. Maneuvers such as squatting or hand grip will decrease the murmur, whereas standing and Valsalva will accentuate it.

QUICK HIT

Preparticipation athletic screening is controversial; current guidelines only call for a good history and physical exam. ECG and echo are proposed as possible screening tools, but false positives in healthy individuals may result in further unnecessary cardiac testing.

QUICK HIT

HOCM in infants as a result of insulin-dependent diabetic mothers is reversible over time. Generally, supportive care is the only necessary treatment.

C. Clinical presentation
  1. Critical AS: presents in neonatal period with poor LV function, poor cardiac output, acidosis, shock
  2. Less severe forms present with progressive fatigue and heart failure
  3. Cardiac exam findings
    a. **Systolic ejection click**
    b. Systolic ejection murmur along right upper sternal border
    c. If aortic insufficiency, may have early high-frequency diastolic murmur
  4. Rarely patients may have syncope or sudden cardiac death

D. Testing
  1. CXR: may have cardiomegaly, dilated aortic root
  2. Echo: quantify gradient and assess valve morphology

E. Therapy
  1. Balloon valvuloplasty or surgical valvotomy
  2. Eventually may need valve replacement

XVII. Pulmonary Stenosis

A. Definitions
  1. Right-sided obstructive lesion
    a. Valvar stenosis most common (~90%)
    b. Subvalvar: associated with TOF and double-outlet RV
    c. Supravalvar: pulmonary artery narrowing

B. Pathophysiology
  1. Limited flow across RV outflow tract limits blood flow to lungs → RV hypertrophy and dysfunction, decreased cardiac output
  2. Abnormal valve can also have insufficiency

C. Clinical presentation
  1. Critical PS: presents in newborns with cyanosis and RV dysfunction
  2. Less severe forms present with fatigue and exercise intolerance
  3. Cardiac exam: **systolic ejection click**, systolic ejection murmur at left upper sternal border, prominent RV impulse, **fixed widely split S2**

D. Testing: Echo to evaluate pulmonary valve morphology and gradient, RVH

E. Therapy
  1. Critical PS: *may require PGE_1 infusion to provide systemic blood flow*
  2. If asymptomatic and mild, can be followed; usually not progressive
  3. Moderate to severe: usually progressive, requiring balloon valvuloplasty (preferred), surgical valvotomy, or valve replacement

XVIII. Congestive Heart Failure

A. General characteristics
  1. Causes
    a. Structural heart disease most common in infancy (Table 1-5)
    b. Myocardial dysfunction (hereditary or acquired)
  2. Genetics: depends on etiology; *dilated cardiomyopathy is hereditary in up to 50% of cases*
  3. Risk factors: any congenital or acquired lesion that interferes with contractility
    a. CHD with significant L → R shunting
    b. CHD and/or acquired lesions that cause LVH
    c. Medications that cause myocardial injury
    d. Surgical procedures that create large aorto-pulmonary shunts (i.e., TOF repair or Fontan procedure)
    e. Diseases/medications that increase afterload
  4. Pathophysiology
    a. Systolic dysfunction: decreased contractility and decreased cardiac output → inadequate supply to meet body's metabolic demands
    b. Diastolic dysfunction: inability to fill ventricle with proper preload → pulmonary congestion ensues, causing tachypnea and dyspnea

QUICK HIT
About 25% of patients with Turner syndrome have aortic valve abnormalities, especially bicuspid aortic valve.

QUICK HIT
Patients with Marfan syndrome are also at higher risk of bicuspid aortic valve and aortic dissection.

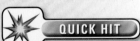

QUICK HIT
Critical AS may require PGE_1 infusion to provide systemic blood flow through PDA.

TABLE 1-5 Causes of Congestive Heart Failure Resulting from Congenital Heart Disease

Age of Onset	Congenital Heart Defect
Birth	Hypoplastic left heart syndrome (HLHS) Neonatal tachyarrhythmia (supraventricular tachycardia or atrial flutter) Volume overload lesions Severe tricuspid or pulmonary insufficiency (Ebstein anomaly)
First Week	Transposition of the great arteries (TGA) Patent ductus arteriosus (PDA) in small premature infants HLHS Total anomalous pulmonary venous return (TAPVR) Critical aortic stenosis (AS) or pulmonary stenosis (PS)
Weeks 1–4	Coarctation of the aorta (COA) Critical AS Anomalous left coronary artery from the pulmonary artery (ALCAPA) All other lesions listed above
Weeks 4–6	Endocardial cushion defect (ECD) with left to right shunt
6 weeks–4 months	Large left to right shunt lesions such as ventricular septal defect (VSD) and PDA

Adapted from Park MK. *Pediatric Cardiology for Practitioners*, 5th Edition, Table 27-1, Causes of Congestive Heart Failure Resulting from Congenital Heart Disease. New York: Mosby; 2008.

QUICK HIT

Supravalvar PS is associated with Noonan syndrome, Williams syndrome, and Alagille syndrome.

QUICK HIT

Peripheral pulmonary stenosis (PPS) can be a normal finding in newborns and young infants, due to turbulent flow through the pulmonary arteries. Exam reveals a soft systolic ejection murmur at the left upper sternal border radiating to the back and axillae. Infants usually outgrow this by age 6 months.

c. Large infusions of extrinsic volume (transfusions, rehydration solutions) can overdistend heart muscle, decreasing contractility
d. Compensatory mechanisms seek to enhance contractility
 i. Release of catecholamines results in increased heart rate
 ii. Increased renin → angiotensin II → myocardial hypertrophy
 iii. Eventual myocardial necrosis and fibrosis

B. Clinical features
1. Historical findings (symptoms)
 a. Poor feeding, poor weight gain
 b. Tachypnea, shortness of breath
 c. Diaphoresis
 d. Exercise intolerance
2. Physical exam findings: impaired cardiac function: tachycardia, gallop (S3, S4), weak pulses

C. Diagnosis
1. Differential diagnosis
 a. Underlying etiologies of CHF (Box 1-3)
 b. Pulmonary conditions that can mimic or exacerbate CHF
  i. Asthma
  ii. Pulmonary embolism
  iii. Pneumonia
  iv. Bronchiolitis
  v. Sleep apnea
  vi. Interstitial pulmonary disease
 c. Other conditions that can mimic or exacerbate CHF
  i. Atrial fibrillation and other supraventricular arrhythmias (SVAs)
  ii. Septic shock
  iii. Renal insufficiency/renal failure
  iv. Anemia

QUICK HIT

In CHF, the heart is unable to pump enough blood to the body to meet its needs, to dispose of systemic or pulmonary venous return adequately, or a combination of the two.

QUICK HIT

Left-sided heart failure leads to pulmonary congestion with tachypnea, dyspnea on exertion, orthopnea, wheezing, and crackles. Right-sided heart failure leads to venous congestion, leading to hepatomegaly, periorbital edema, and peripheral edema.

QUICK HIT

CHF should be considered in the differential diagnosis of patients with unexplained wheezing that is not responsive to bronchodilators.

BOX 1-3

Differential Diagnosis of Congestive Heart Failure in Children

Structural heart disease
Valvular heart disease
- Mitral regurgitation
- Aortic insufficiency
- Aortic stenosis
- Tricuspid regurgitation
- Pulmonic insufficiency

Chronic hypertension
Pulmonary hypertension
Genetic myocardial disease
- Cardiomyopathy
- Neuromuscular disorders (muscular dystrophies, myotonic dystrophy, Friedrich ataxia)
- Familial dilated cardiomyopathy
- Hypertrophic cardiomyopathy
- Storage diseases (Fabry, Gaucher, glycogen storage diseases, mucopolysaccharidoses)
- Hemochromatosis

Infectious myocardial disease
- Viral myocarditis
- Bacterial myocarditis
- Parasitic myocarditis (Chagas disease)

Myocardial ischemia/infarction
- Anomalous left coronary artery
- Kawasaki disease

Collagen vascular disease
- Acute rheumatic fever
- Systemic lupus erythematosus
- Polyarteritis nodosa
- Scleroderma
- Dermatomyositis
- Kawasaki disease

Granulomatous disease
- Wegener granulomatosis
- Giant cell arteritis
- Sarcoidosis

Metabolic/endocrine conditions
- Hypocalcemia
- Hyperparathyroidism
- Hyper- or hypothyroidism
- Severe acidosis
- Carcinoid syndrome
- Uremia

Nutritional deficiencies
- Thiamine deficiency
- Kwashiorkor
- Selenium deficiency

Severe anemia
Volume overload
- Renal failure
- Aggressive blood transfusion
- Overhydration

Arrhythmias
- Supraventricular tachycardia
- Atrial fibrillation

Medications/drugs/toxins
- Anthracyclines
- Cyclophosphamide
- Radiation
- Iron overload (chronic transfusion)
- Alcohol
- Cocaine
- Amphetamines

Other
- Endocardial fibroelastosis
- Cardiac transplant rejection
- Amyloidosis

2. Laboratory findings: *no single test is specific for CHF*
   a. Increased levels of B-type natriuretic peptide (BNP) (also called "brain natriuretic peptide")
3. Radiology findings: CXR shows **cardiomegaly**, **pulmonary edema/congestion**
4. ECG: may have left axis deviation, LAE, LVH with strain pattern, and left bundle branch block
5. Echo
   a. Enlarged ventricular chambers
   b. Impaired LV systolic function
   c. Impaired diastolic function
   d. Decreased fractional shortening or ejection fraction
6. Cardiac catheterization
   a. May be needed for biopsy to identify underlying cause
   b. Allows accurate assessment of pressures in various chambers

D. Treatment
1. Therapy
   a. Eliminate or treat underlying cause if possible (hypertension, arrhythmias, CHD)

b. Treat precipitating or contributing factors (infection, anemia, fever)
c. Treat symptoms of CHF
i. Diuretics (first line)
(a) Loop diuretics preferred (furosemide)
(b) Spironolactone may be added to prevent hypokalemia
ii. Afterload reduction
(a) Preferred: mixed vasodilators (ACE inhibitors)
(b) Arteriolar vasodilators (hydralazine)
(c) Venodilators (nitroglycerine, isosorbide dinitrate)
iii. Inotropic agents
(a) Digoxin
(b) Dopamine, dobutamine, epinephrine if severely ill
d. General measures
i. Keep infants/children in semi-upright position
ii. Supplemental oxygen/intubation if respiratory distress is severe
iii. Optimize nutrition
iv. Salt restriction in older children (<0.5 g/day)
6. Duration of therapy/prognosis: dependent on etiology, response to therapy, comorbidities, and general health of patient
a. For patients with CHD, surgical palliation or repair indicated if no improvement with medical management
b. Cardiac transplant if deterioration despite medical management
7. Prevention
a. Early surgical repair if lesion amenable, before irreversible myocardial and pulmonary dysfunction occurs
b. Good control of underlying conditions and comorbidities
c. Avoidance of cardiotoxic medications

QUICK HIT

Complications of diuretic treatment: electrolyte abnormalities and dehydration (hypokalemia, hypochloremic alkalosis, hyponatremia, increased blood urea nitrogen [BUN] and creatinine).

QUICK HIT

Digoxin toxicity can lead to rhythm disturbances, including prolonged PR interval; varying heart block; profound bradycardia (especially in infants); SA block; SVA; and, less commonly, VTs. Avoid hypokalemia and hypomagnesemia, which may worsen symptoms.

XIX. Infective Endocarditis (IE)

A. Characteristics
1. Definition: microbial infection of endothelial layer of heart
2. Epidemiology: 0.3/100,000 children per year with ~11% mortality; *incidence is increasing*
3. Cause: most common is bacterial
4. Risk factors
a. Children, adolescents: postrepair CHD
b. Neonates: indwelling catheters in neonatal intensive care unit (NICU)
c. Indwelling foreign material/patches/heart valves
d. Intravenous (IV) drug/central lines abuse
5. Pathophysiology
a. α-Hemolytic *Streptococcus*: subacute process
b. *Staphylococcus aureus*: acute process, patient appears toxic, damage to heart structures common, abscess formation
c. Coagulase-negative *Staphylococcus*: indolent course
d. Fungal: acute course, high embolization rate, highest mortality rate
e. Gram-negative rods: subacute course, emboli more common
6. Emboli: can be sterile or infectious, thrombus and immune complexes are implicated in embolic phenomenon; *kidney is most common site*

B. Clinical features
1. History: nonspecific myalgias, arthralgias, fatigue
2. Physical exam findings
a. Toxic appearing with more acute infections
b. New heart murmur
c. Neurologic findings (20%): due to infarct, abscess, or meningitis
d. **Osler nodes**: small/tender/raised nodes on pads of fingers/toes
e. **Janeway lesions**: flat erythematous lesions on palms and soles
f. **Roth spots**: eye finding, retinal hemorrhages with pale centers
g. Petechiae, **splinter hemorrhages**

QUICK HIT

Most common underlying diagnosis that predisposes to IE in the United States and developed countries is postrepair CHD. Rheumatic heart disease is still common worldwide and predisposes to IE.

QUICK HIT

IE development: Damage to the endothelium → nonbacterial thrombus formation → transient bacteremia (occurring all the time in everyone) → adherence of bacteria to thrombus → proliferation of bacteria within the thrombus

MNEMONIC

Gram-negative rods that cause endocarditis are called the **"HACEK"** organisms:
H = *Haemophilus parainfluenzae*
A = *Aggregatibacter* species
C = *Cardiobacterium hominis*
E = *Eikenella corrodens*
K = *Kingella kingae*

> **QUICK HIT**
> Fever (most common) is commonly the only presenting historical symptom.

> **QUICK HIT**
> Diagnosis is difficult in neonates, who may not mount a fever or present with signs of sepsis.

> **QUICK HIT**
> Embolic phenomena are more common in neonates, with higher rates of focal neurologic signs, meningitis, and osteomyelitis.

> **QUICK HIT**
> Biofilms produced by bacteria on synthetic foreign material make it difficult to clear the infection. Often removal of the material or very prolonged course of antibiotic therapy is required.

> **QUICK HIT**
> Antibiotic prophylaxis for dental procedures is only recommended in patients at high risk of adverse outcomes, including patients with previous infective endocarditis, prosthetic heart valves, or unrepaired congenital heart disease.

> **QUICK HIT**
> Among young patients with sudden cardiac death, 4%–15% have a coronary abnormality (second most common after cardiomyopathy).

C. Diagnosis
   1. Laboratory findings: *large-volume blood cultures are positive in 90%–95% of patients with IE*; rest considered "culture-negative IE" and diagnosed by clinical history or Echo
   2. Radiology findings: Echo: evaluate for valve disease, prosthetic valve dehiscence, patch integrity; false negatives are common

D. Treatment
   1. Antimicrobial coverage of offending organism
   2. Complications
      a. **Focal** or **diffuse glomerulonephritis**
      b. Embolization: left heart IE predisposes to embolization
      c. Abscess formation from septic embolization
      d. Immune complex deposition
   3. Duration/prognosis: more indolent organisms (α-hemolytic *Streptococcus*, coagulase-negative *Staphylococcus*) require longer treatment
   4. Prevention: prophylaxis in moderate- to high-risk groups is advised (patients with heart transplants, history of infectious endocarditis, prosthetic valves, and subset of patients with shunts or patches)

XX. Coronary Artery Disease (CAD) in Children

A. Definitions
   1. Acquired CAD: secondary to another disease process
   2. Congenital CAD: abnormal origins or pathways

B. Cause/pathophysiology
   1. Kawasaki disease: most common vasculitis in children, boys > girls, Asian
   2. Other acquired coronary disease: familial hypercholesterolemia, polyarteritis nodosa, Takayasu arteritis, and systemic lupus erythematosus
   3. Congenital coronary abnormalities: anomalous left coronary artery from the pulmonary artery (ALCAPA)

XXI. Myocarditis

A. Definitions: inflammatory infiltrate of myocardium with necrosis and/or degeneration of adjacent myocytes not typical of ischemia

B. Causes/pathophysiology
   1. Viral etiology is most common (especially Coxsackie virus)
   2. Less common causes: bacterial infections (Lyme disease, *Rickettsia*), protozoal (toxoplasmosis, Chagas disease, malaria), fungal infection, acute rheumatic fever, Kawasaki disease, hypersensitivity, collagen vascular disease, drugs, toxins

C. Clinical presentation: some patients may be asymptomatic
   1. Viral prodrome, flu-like symptoms, malaise, irritability, gastroenteritis
   2. CHF: dyspnea, poor appetite, exercise intolerance, hepatomegaly
      a. Gallop S3, S4 may be present
      b. If severe, regurgitant murmurs can be heard
   3. Dysrhythmias: VT, 1st-, 2nd-, or 3rd-degree heart block
   4. Pericarditis with pericardial friction rub may also be present

D. Testing
   1. CXR: Cardiomegaly +/− pulmonary vascular congestion
   2. ECG: tachycardia, *low-voltage QRS complexes with low-voltage or inverted T waves*, wide Q waves and ST-segment changes
   3. Echo: dilated and dysfunctional LV with segmental wall motion abnormalities
   4. Viral serology/culture/polymerase chain reaction may be helpful

E. Therapy
   1. Supportive therapy: rest, inotropes, and afterload reduction
   2. Immune modulation: intravenous immunoglobulin (IVIG) is sometimes used, but efficacy is not established
   3. Arrhythmia management: antiarrhythmics, pacemaker if necessary
   4. Ventricular assist device/heart transplantation

BOX 1-4

Etiologies of Pericarditis

Viral: Coxsackie virus, echovirus, adenovirus
Bacterial: *Staphylococcus aureus* most common
Tuberculosis: from direct spread
Drug induced (hydralazine, procainamide, INH)
Radiation exposure
Postpericardiotomy syndrome (can occur weeks after surgery)
Rheumatic fever
Kawasaki disease
Connective tissue disease (systemic lupus erythematosus, juvenile rheumatoid arthritis)
Malignancy (primary and secondary)
Uremia
Hypothyroidism (myxedematous pericardial disease, bradycardia present)

QUICK HIT

Persistent elevated heart rate without an explanation is a sensitive sign of myocarditis.

QUICK HIT

Have high clinical suspicion for myocarditis in a new case of heart failure, ventricular arrhythmia, or conduction block in a young child or infant.

QUICK HIT

Mortality rates for myocarditis are 10%–25% in children and up to 75% in infants (especially with Coxsackie B virus).

QUICK HIT

Normal amount of pericardial fluid is ~30 mL in an adult.

QUICK HIT

Pulsus paradoxus is an exaggeration of the normal decrease in systolic blood pressure (SBP) with inspiration. Decrease in SBP <10 mm Hg is normal; decrease in SBP >10 mm Hg is consistent with tamponade.

XXII. Pericarditis

A. Definition: inflammation of the serosal tissue surrounding heart
B. Cause/pathophysiology: inflammatory reaction causes irritation and increased fluid production in pericardial space (Box 1-4)
C. Clinical Presentation
   1. History: low-grade fever, fatigue, chest pain that worsens with lying flat and *improves with leaning forward*, shortness of breath with lying flat
   2. Physical: friction rub
D. Testing
   1. CXR: cardiomegaly
   2. ECG
      a. **Diffusely low voltages**: insulation from fluid
      b. Electrical alternans: cyclic variation of QRS due to wide swings of heart in large sac of fluid
   3. Echo
   4. Pericardial fluid drainage: diagnostic and therapeutic
E. Therapy
   1. Treat underlying cause
   2. Nonsteroidal anti-inflammatory drugs (NSAIDs) if inflammatory cause
   3. Pericardial fluid drainage: for diagnosis, tamponade/rapidly evolving effusion
   4. Duration/prognosis: can be acute, chronic, or recurrent; etiology dependent

XXIII. Cardiomyopathy *(Figure 1-7)*

A. Definition
   1. Disease of myocardium
   2. Hypertrophic, dilated, restrictive, or combination

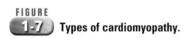

FIGURE 1-7 **Types of cardiomyopathy.**

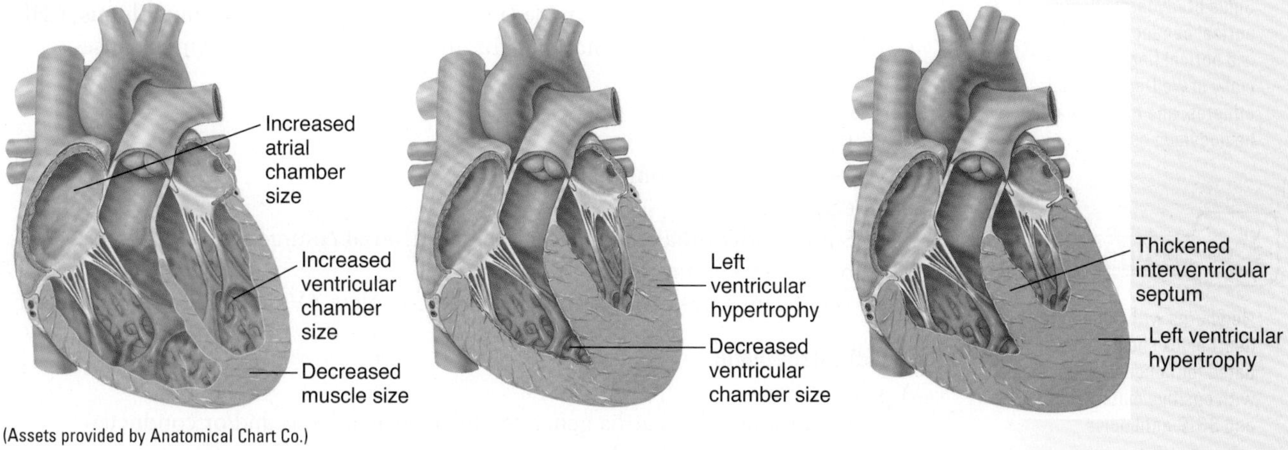

(Assets provided by Anatomical Chart Co.)

BOX 1-5

Primary Cardiomyopathies

Genetic	Acquired
Hypertrophic cardiomyopathy	Myocarditis
Arrhythmogenic right ventricular cardiomyopathy	Stress-provoked "tako-tsubo"
Left ventricular noncompaction cardiomyopathy	Peripartum
Metabolic storage diseases	Tachycardia induced
Conduction defects	Infant of diabetic mother
Mitochondrial disorders	
Ion channel disorders	

QUICK HIT

Tamponade findings include tachycardia, pulses paradoxus, muffled heart sounds, and jugular venous distention.

QUICK HIT

ECG findings of **PR depression** and **ST elevation** are seen in 80% of patients with pericarditis.

QUICK HIT

Dilated cardiomyopathy is the most common type of myocardial disease in children.

QUICK HIT

Sinus bradycardia has normal conduction and is a normal finding, especially in well-conditioned athletes, and has normal hemodynamics.

QUICK HIT

Newborns with congenital heart block should be evaluated for congenital lupus, with positive maternal SS-A and SS-B antibodies.

B. Cause/pathophysiology
   1. Heterogeneous group of disorders with multiple etiologies and phenotypes
   2. Most are genetic; also acquired forms (Box 1-5)

C. Clinical presentation: varies with type of cardiomyopathy
   1. *Sudden death or aborted sudden death due to unstable VT or ventricular fibrillation (VF)*
   2. CHF: poor feeding/growth, dyspnea, activity intolerance, tachycardia, edema
   3. Arrhythmia: stable VT

D. Testing
   1. CXR: cardiomegaly +/− pulmonary edema
   2. ECG: usually nonspecific
   3. Echo: ventricular hypertrophy +/− dilation, decreased shortening fraction
   4. Further testing depending on etiology
      a. Cardiac catheterization/biopsy: including skeletal muscle biopsy
      b. Cardiac MRI
      c. Genetic testing

E. Therapy: mostly supportive; depends on type of cardiomyopathy
   1. Afterload reduction: ACE inhibitors
   2. Neurohormonal blockade: β-blockers (selective and nonselective), angiotensin receptor antagonists, spironolactone
   3. Antiarrhythmics if necessary

XXIV. Bradycardia

A. Definitions: heart rate <100 bpm for infants or <60 for young children or <50 for older children and adults

B. Cause/pathophysiology
   1. Slowing at sinus node; may have junctional and/or ventricular escape beats
      a. Medications (β-blockers, digoxin, etc.)
      b. Increased vagal tone, increased ICP
   2. Slowing or blockage at AV node (Figure 1-8): congenital (**congenital lupus**, CHD)

C. Clinical presentation: palpitations, dizziness, syncope (usually sinus pauses >3 seconds)

D. Testing
   1. ECG
   2. 24-hour Holter monitor

E. Therapy
   1. Sinus bradycardia and isolated premature atrial contractions (PACs) are benign and do not require therapy
   2. Significant sinus node dysfunction and complete AV block require pacemaker

XXV. Tachyarrhythmia

A. Characteristics
   1. Definitions: tachycardia generated by abnormal focus and/or conducted through abnormal pathway

FIGURE 1-8 **Types of atrioventricular block.**

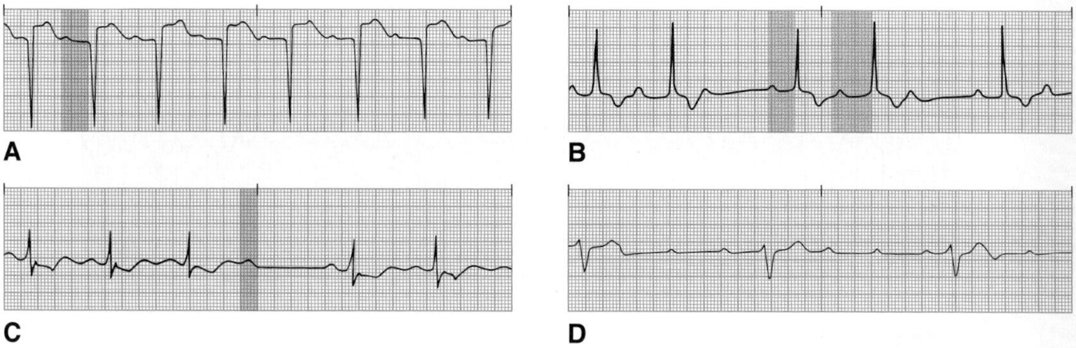

A. First-degree block, with prolonged PR >200 ms but ventricular rate unaffected. B. Second-degree block Mobitz type I with progressively longer PR until a beat is dropped. C. Second-degree block Mobitz type II with constant PR but occasional beats not conducted. D. Third-degree (complete) block with no AV nodal conduction and escape beats. (From Springhouse. *ECG Facts Made Incredibly Easy.* 2nd ed. Ambler: Wolters Kluwer Health; 2010.)

2. Cause
   a. SVT: generated proximal to AV node, usually in atria
      i. Atrial tachycardias
      ii. Intra-atrial re-entrant tachycardia (IART)
         (a) Atrial flutter
         (b) Atrial fibrillation
      iii. Orthodromic re-entrant tachycardia (ORT) and WPW
   b. Junctional tachycardia is generated close to or within the AV node
   c. Ventricular rhythms are generated distal to AV node
      i. Accelerated ventricular rhythm (AVR) <20% faster than normal sinus rate and does not result in hemodynamic instability
      ii. VT is faster than AVR and can result in hemodynamic instability
3. Risk factors
   a. Electrolyte abnormalities: hypokalemia, hypomagnesemia, hypercalcemia
   b. CHD
   c. Previous heart surgery
   d. Myocardial disease
4. Pathophysiology
   a. Atrial tachycardias are generated by an ectopic atrial focus
      i. Can have multiple foci
      ii. Can result from viral infection
      iii. *Conduction through AV node may be variable, leading to irregular rhythm*
   b. IART is result of re-entrant circuits within atria
   c. Junctional tachycardia usually iatrogenic after cardiac surgery
   d. VT and VF
      i. Can be exacerbated by electrolyte abnormalities
      ii. Can result from toxic ingestion
      iii. Seen in myocardial disease, CHD

B. Clinical features
   1. Historical findings: palpitations, dizziness, syncope
   2. Physical exam findings
      a. SVT/atrial tachycardia: may have regular or irregular rhythm
      b. If hemodynamically significant, will have poor pulses and perfusion

C. Diagnosis
   1. Differential diagnosis
      a. Sinus tachycardia
      b. Hyperthyroidism
      c. Premature ventricular beats
   2. Laboratory findings: evaluate for electrolyte abnormalities (Ca^{++}, Mg^{++}, K^{+})

QUICK HIT

Re-entrant tachycardia is associated with an accessory pathway, which conducts retrograde from the ventricle to the atria then down the AV node and back up the pathway, creating a cycle.

QUICK HIT

WPW is a specific type of re-entrant tachycardia in which the accessory pathway is capable of conducting both antegrade and retrograde, which can lead to VT or fibrillation.

QUICK HIT

After the first 24 hours of life, the T wave in V_6 should always be upright/not flat.

FIGURE 1-9 Tachyarrhythmias

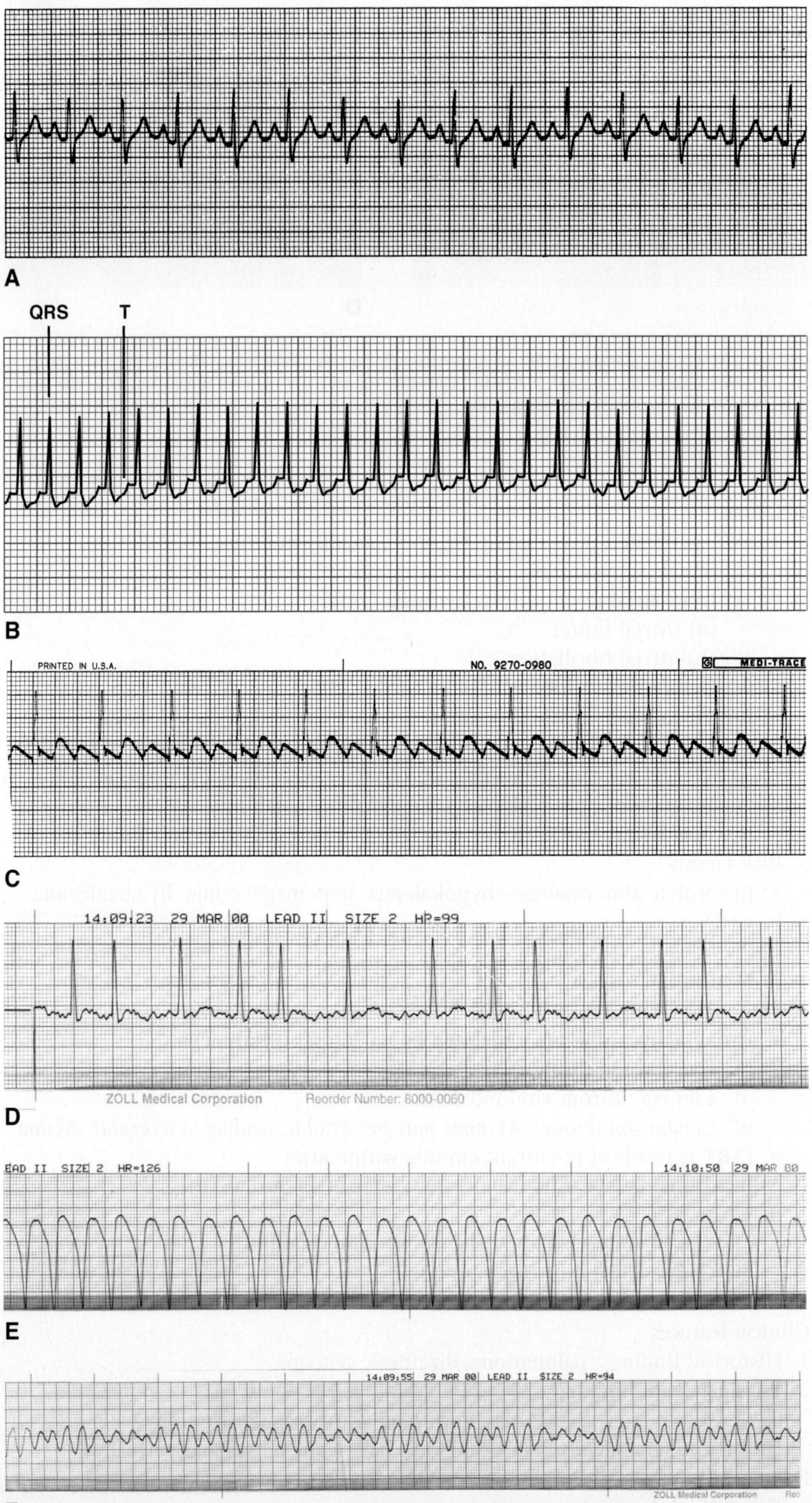

A. Sinus tachycardia. Note P waves before each QRS. **B.** SVT. Note rapid rate and lack of variability. **C.** Atrial flutter with 2:1 conduction. **D.** Atrial fibrillation. **E.** Ventricular tachycardia. Note regular wide complex QRS. **F.** Ventricular fibrillation.

(**A**: From Nettina SM. The *Lippincott Manual of Nursing Practice.* 7th ed. Philadelphia: Lippincott Williams & Wilkins; 2001. **B**: From Bickley LS, Szilagyi P. *Bates' Guide to Physical Examination and History Taking.* 8th ed. Philadelphia: Lippincott Williams & Wilkins; 2003. C: From Smeltzer SC, Bare BG. *Textbook of Medical-Surgical Nursing.* 9th ed. Philadelphia: Lippincott Williams & Wilkins; 2000.)

3. ECG (Figure 1-9)
   a. Atrial tachycardias: ectopic focus (P wave with varying morphologies, aberrant axis)
   b. Atrial flutter: sawtooth pattern with variable conduction
   c. Atrial fibrillation: disorganized with indistinguishable P waves and variable narrow QRS depending on conduction
   d. ORT: absent or retrograde P waves
   e. WPW: delta waves (may be transient), short PR (Figure 1-10)
   f. Junctional tachycardia: can also have absent or retrograde P waves and AV dissociation, can be hard to distinguish from ORT
   g. VT: rate >120, regular, wide complex, absent, or dissociated P waves
   h. VF: disorganized with no discernible QRS
   i. Torsade de pointes: sine-wave twisting irregular wide complex
4. Echo: may be needed to rule out cardiomyopathy, structural abnormalities

D. Treatment
1. Therapy
   a. Atrial tachycardia: control AV conduction and ventricular rate
      i. β-Blockers
      ii. Digoxin
      iii. Flecainide
   b. ORT: slow or block conduction at AV node
      i. Synchronized cardioversion if unstable
      ii. If stable: vagal maneuvers, β-blockers, adenosine
   c. IART: synchronized cardioversion, overdrive pacing
   d. Junctional tachycardia: avoid triggers (minimize inotropes, cooling measures for fever), pharmacologic intervention

QUICK HIT

Atrial and junctional rhythms are usually narrow complex in nature; ventricular rhythms are usually wide complex.

QUICK HIT

Paroxysmal SVT can often be distinguished from sinus tachycardia by its higher rate (usually >220 bpm in infants or >180 bpm in children), lack of beat-to-beat variability, sudden onset, and absent or abnormal P waves.

QUICK HIT

Most common form of irregular heart rhythm is sinus arrhythmia

FIGURE 1-10 ECG characteristics of Wolff-Parkinson-White.

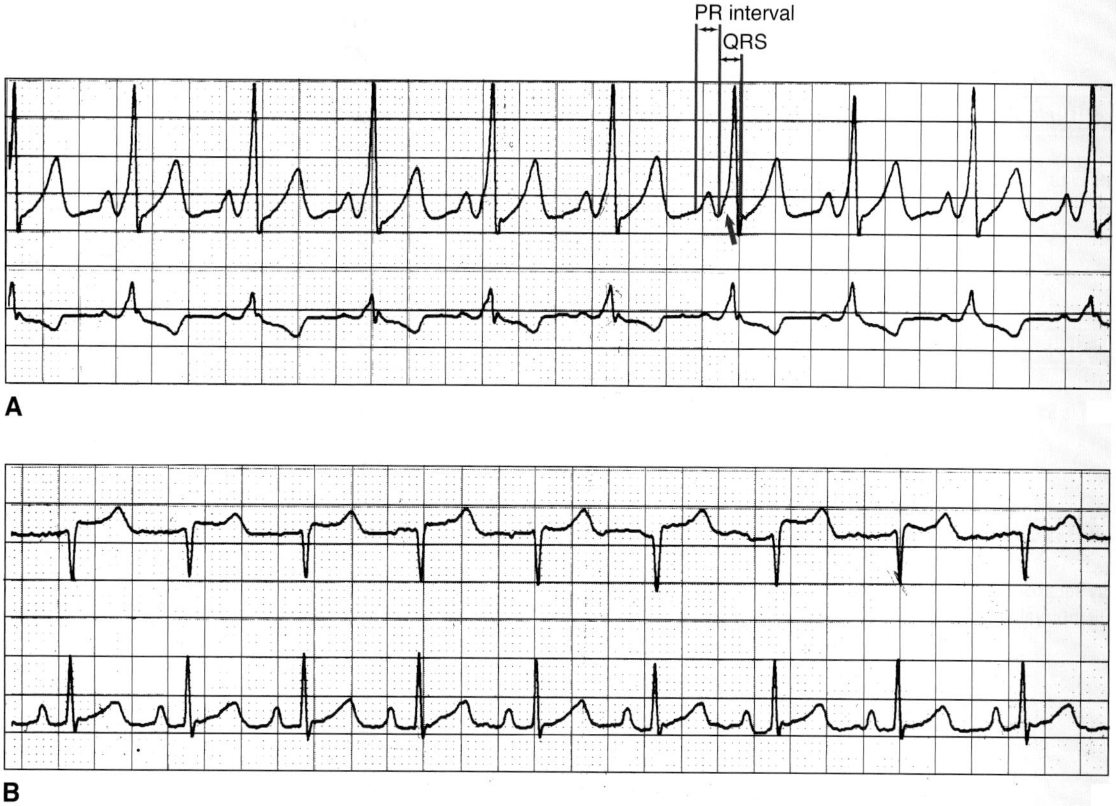

Note the short PR interval, slurred initial upstroke of the QRS complex (delta wave, at the *arrow*), and prolonged QRS duration. Upper lead II, lower lead V_1. (ECG strips courtesy of Linda Ardini and Catherine Berkmeyer, Inova Fairfax Hospital, Falls Church, VA.)

e. VT/VF
i. If stable/well-perfused: lidocaine, amiodarone
ii. For VT with pulses: synchronized cardioversion
iii. For VF or pulseless VT: unsynchronized defibrillation

QUICK HIT

Every other beat = **bigeminy**; every 3rd beat = **trigeminy**

XXVI. Premature Ventricular Contractions (PVCs) and Irregular Heart Beats

A. Cause/pathophysiology
1. PACs occur when atrial impulse other than sinus node occurs earlier than sinus node and may conduct through AV node
2. PVCs occur when ventricle is excited before normal sinus node

B. Testing
1. ECG; 24-hour Holter monitor
2. Evaluate for electrolyte disturbances

C. Therapy: isolated PACs or PVCs are benign

QUICK HIT

Sinus arrhythmia is normal variation with respiration and is benign. It occurs due to increased vagal tone during expiration, which decreases the heart rate, which then increases again during inspiration.

XXVII. Long QT Syndromes

A. Definition: QTc longer than normal for age

B. Cause/pathophysiology
1. At least 10 genotypes with multiple mutations and variable phenotype
2. Acquired forms due to medications (macrolides, antipsychotics)

C. Clinical presentation
1. Dizziness, syncope especially with exertion or emotional stress
2. May have chest pain, palpitations, or bradycardia
3. Some forms associated with sensorineural deafness (Jervell-Lange-Nielsen)

QUICK HIT

Clinical presentation may be asymptomatic or involve complaints of palpitations.

D. Testing
1. ECG findings: prolonged QTc for age
2. Assess for electrolyte abnormalities
3. Genetic testing, audiologic testing if indicated

QUICK HIT

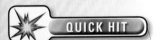

The QT varies by HR, so a calculated QTc must be performed.

E. Therapy
1. β-Blockers
2. ICD for high-risk patients
3. Avoidance of drugs that may prolong QT

QUICK HIT

Relatives of patients with long QT should be evaluated with ECG.

QUICK HIT

Risk for sudden death is 5%.

QUICK HIT

QTc = QT divided by square root of preceding RR interval.

2 Diseases of the Pulmonary System

SYMPTOM SPECIFIC

I. Approach to Wheeze

A. Background information

1. Wheeze: musical high-pitched noise, mainly in expiration
2. Common complaint in childhood
3. Impaired airflow due to narrowing of airway in lower respiratory tract
4. Differential diagnosis (Table 2-1)

TABLE 2-1 **Differential Diagnosis of Wheeze by Age**

Age	Differential Diagnosis
Infant (12 months and younger)	Bronchiolitis* Bronchopulmonary dysplasia* Foreign body aspiration† Aspiration syndromes Inherited disorders (example: cystic fibrosis, immunodeficiency states) Anatomic anomalies of the airway, such as: Laryngotracheobronchomalacia† Tracheoesophageal fistula Vascular ring or sling† Airway hemangioma† Laryngeal web†
Preschool age (1–4 years)	Viral-induced wheeze* Asthma* Foreign body aspiration† Community-acquired pneumonia Inherited disorders (example: cystic fibrosis, immunodeficiency states)
School age (5–12 years)	Asthma* Vocal cord dysfunction† Community-acquired pneumonia Inherited disorders (example: cystic fibrosis, immunodeficiency states)
Adolescence (13–18 years)	Asthma* Vocal cord dysfunction*† Hypersensitivity pneumonitis
Consideration at any age but uncommon	Pulmonary edema from congestive heart failure Tuberculosis External mass compressing the airway

*More common causes.

†May present or usually presents with stridor not wheeze.

QUICK HIT

Wheezing that begins at birth or in early infancy suggests a congenital or anatomic disease.

QUICK HIT

Keep a high index of suspicion for foreign body aspiration (FBA) in a toddler with acute new-onset wheezing.

QUICK HIT

Asthma, allergic rhinitis, and atopic dermatitis are known as the *allergic triad*.

QUICK HIT

Generally, **stridor** is caused by a narrowing of the area *above* the thoracic inlet, whereas **wheeze** is caused by a narrowing *below* the thoracic inlet. Patients with narrowing near the thoracic inlet may have both.

B. Historical findings
  1. When did the wheeze begin?
  2. Is there a pattern of wheeze?
     a. Episodic versus persistent
     b. New onset versus recurrent. If recurrent, how many episodes?
  3. Are there associated triggers?
     a. Fever, rhinorrhea, and nasal congestion suggest viral upper respiratory infection (URI)
     b. Environmental irritants (e.g., tobacco smoke exposure) or seasonal allergens
     c. Exercise and activity, including feeding in infants
  4. What improves or worsens the wheeze?
     a. Response to albuterol (bronchodilators) or other medications
     b. In infants, ask about relationship of wheezing with feeding (may indicate reflux or very rarely an H-type tracheoesophageal fistula)
  5. Associated medical problems
     a. History of prematurity with bronchopulmonary dysplasia
     b. History of other cardiopulmonary diseases
     c. Difficulty with weight gain or frequent infections
     d. History of gastroesophageal reflux disease (GERD)
     e. History of atopy (atopic dermatitis, allergic rhinitis, food allergy)
  6. Family history of asthma or atopy

C. Physical exam findings
  1. Overall appearance and degree of respiratory distress (see Approach to Respiratory Distress, page 30)
  2. Respiratory exam
     a. Assess respiratory rate, accessory muscle use, and air movement
     b. Assess for upper versus lower airway noises
     c. Location (bilateral versus unilateral), character, and timing (inspiratory versus expiratory versus biphasic) of wheeze
     d. Ratio of inspiratory to expiratory phase
  3. Cardiovascular exam
     a. Assess heart rate and rhythm, pulses, and capillary refill
     b. Signs of congestive heart failure (CHF) include
        i. Displaced point of maximum impulse (PMI)
        ii. Hepatomegaly
        iii. Peripheral edema and jugular venous distention
  4. Signs of hydration status (moist mucous membranes, presence of tears)
  5. Other physical exam findings
     a. Allergic stigmata (associated with asthma)
     b. Evidence of chronic process such as failure to thrive or clubbing (may indicate significant underlying disease such as cystic fibrosis [CF])

D. Laboratory testing and radiologic imaging
  1. Laboratory evaluation
     a. Pulse oximetry to measure oxygen saturation
     b. Other laboratory evaluation dictated by history and physical
        i. Rapid viral antigen testing is usually not indicated because rarely changes management
        ii. Pulmonary function testing in patient age >5 years may be indicated in severe asthmatic or child when evaluating for another underlying disease (e.g., pulmonary fibrosis)
        iii. Allergy testing may be indicated to help remove environmental triggers of wheeze
  2. Radiographic imaging
     a. Plain radiographs
        i. Chest radiograph (CXR) (posteroanterior and lateral views) should be considered in patients with new-onset wheezing
        ii. A CXR is generally *not* indicated in known asthmatic with suspected asthma exacerbation

iii. Airway films (anteroposterior and lateral soft tissue neck radiograph) should be performed in any patient with stridor and concern for foreign body aspiration (FBA)
iv. CXR and bilateral lateral decubitus *or* inspiratory/expiratory films often indicated to help rule out foreign body in lungs

b. Other imaging (may be indicated in severe or persistent wheezing)
   i. Chest computed tomography (CT) to evaluate for bronchiectasis and other anatomic abnormalities
   ii. Barium swallow or magnetic resonance imaging (MRI) to evaluate for extrinsic airway compression

3. Commonly, diagnostic trial of inhaled albuterol
   a. May be of use diagnostically as well as therapeutically (if responsive to albuterol, suggestive of asthma)
   b. Evaluation and assessment of respiratory rate, accessory muscle use, air movement, oxygen saturations, air entry, and wheezing prior to and after trial are important
4. Further evaluation may be indicated in severe, recurrent, or chronic cases or as history and physical suggest
   a. Arterial blood gas (ABG)
   b. Direct laryngobronchoscopy if high index of suspicion for FBA or concern for structural or anatomic abnormalities

E. Treatment
   1. Initial treatment goals are "ABC's," correct hypoxemia, and ensure patient is in appropriate level of care
   2. Secondary therapy differs depending on etiology and associated findings

II. Approach to Chronic Cough

A. Differential diagnosis
   1. Consider causes of chronic cough when it has lasted >4–8 weeks (Box 2-1)
   2. Differential must be narrowed by history and physical before testing

B. Historical findings
   1. Timing
      a. Chronic cough following a witnessed choking episode indicates FBA, although most episodes are not witnessed
      b. Psychogenic or "habit" cough if symptoms cease while asleep or distracted; often follows URI
      c. Neonatal onset or recurrent cough may represent congenital airway malformation such as tracheoesophageal (TE) fistula or pulmonary sequestration
   2. Triggers
      a. Exacerbation in recumbent position suggests allergic rhinitis or GERD
      b. Exertion is common trigger not only in asthma but also in chronic infection or CF
      c. Cough after swallowing suggests chronic aspiration or TE fistula

BOX 2-1

Differential Diagnosis of Chronic Cough

Asthma	Cystic fibrosis
Allergic rhinitis	Primary ciliary dyskinesia
Chronic sinusitis	Tuberculosis
Gastroesophageal reflux	Fungal infection
Psychogenic cough	Parasitic infection
Atypical infection	Tracheoesophageal fistula
Pertussis	Tumor
Mycoplasma	Immunodeficiency
Foreign body aspiration	Congestive heart failure
Chronic aspiration	Rheumatologic conditions (rare)

QUICK HIT

Allergic stigmata include atopic dermatitis, allergic shiners, and Dennie lines (an accentuated line or lines below the lower eyelid).

QUICK HIT

Recurrent wheezing episodes that are responsive to bronchodilator therapy are suggestive of asthma.

QUICK HIT

The expiratory phase is generally prolonged in a patient with wheeze.

QUICK HIT

Clubbing indicates prolonged hypoxemia and would not be consistent with asthma.

QUICK HIT

A foreign body usually traps air in the affected portion of the lung. When the child lies on his side, the heart will normally push down on the lung. If a foreign body is present, the lung may not collapse normally.

QUICK HIT

Patients with asthma frequently desaturate just after getting albuterol. This is because of a transient ventilation/perfusion ($\dot{V}/\dot{Q}$) mismatch as nonperfused lung "opens up"; thus, perfused lung is transiently underventilated.

QUICK HIT

The "ABC's" (maintaining a stable airway and ensuring adequate breathing and circulation) are a critical component in caring for any patient and a common question on multiple choice tests (e.g., "The most important next step is . . .").

QUICK HIT

The peak age for FBA is between ages 1 and 3 years.

QUICK HIT

Peanuts and popcorn are the most commonly aspirated objects.

QUICK HIT

CF is a cause of poor weight gain in children.

QUICK HIT

Unlike adults, children with CHF are more likely to have wheezing than rhonchi on pulmonary exam.

QUICK HIT

In a child with an abnormal heart murmur, chronic cough is a sign of CHF until proven otherwise.

QUICK HIT

Sputum cultures are generally not helpful in young children due to their inability to expectorate a good sample. A notable exception is in the setting of CF.

3. Character of cough
    a. Paroxysmal cough with "whoop" in between is characteristic of pertussis
4. Environmental exposures
    a. Allergen, including animal dander, dust mites, and pollen
    b. Exposure to tuberculosis (TB)
    c. Travel to areas where fungal pneumonias are endemic such as histoplasmosis in Ohio River Valley
5. Associated symptoms
    a. Fever suggests primary or secondary infectious etiology
    b. Wheezing is classic symptom of asthma but may also indicate atypical infection, FBA, or CHF
    c. Hemoptysis is a sign of serious illness and may occur with pulmonary sequestration, FBA, or cavitary lesion such as TB
    d. Failure to thrive is classic symptom of CF
    e. Atopic dermatitis is associated with asthma

C. Physical exam findings
1. General appearance and growth parameters
2. Pulmonary
    a. Work of breathing (retractions, accessory muscle use, nasal flaring)
    b. Air entry
    c. Rhonchi
    d. Wheezing
        i. Scattered in asthma and other causes of inflammation in medium- to small-sized airways
        ii. Focal in large airway obstruction, such as FBA or tumor
3. Nasopharynx and oropharynx
    a. Boggy, erythematous nasal turbinates seen with allergic rhinitis
    b. Nasal polyps common in CF
4. Cardiac exam
5. Neurologic exam (hypotonia is risk factor for chronic aspiration)

D. Testing: workup, if any, should be specifically tailored to narrowed differential
1. Complete blood count (CBC): only sometimes informative; does not distinguish between viral and bacterial illness but may be obtained if concerns for systemic inflammatory disease or may indicate eosinophilia in asthma, allergic disease, or parasitic illness
2. Spirometry: in older child if asthma is suspected
3. Specific tests: for infectious etiologies (pertussis polymerase chain reaction [PCR], TB skin test, *Mycoplasma* titers)
4. Chloride sweat test if CF suspected
5. Imaging
    a. Chest radiograph
        i. Rarely confirms a diagnosis but can guide subsequent testing.
        ii. Location of lung findings will narrow differential (focal versus diffuse)
        iii. Evaluate for hilar adenopathy or mediastinal widening
        iv. Evaluate cardiac silhouette
    b. Chest CT: important for congenital anomalies, bronchiectasis
    c. Barium swallow study if chronic aspiration is suspected
    d. Electrocardiogram (ECG) and echocardiogram (Echo) if CHF suspected
6. Bronchoscopy
    a. Flexible: used to evaluate for congenital anomaly and obtain lavage for cultures or brushings for ciliary dyskinesia
    b. Rigid: preferred for FBA because allows for foreign body removal

III. Respiratory Distress

A. Differential diagnosis
1. Infection
    a. URI (e.g., cold, croup, tracheitis): inflammation of respiratory lining along with increased secretions **obstruct** airflow

b. Lower respiratory infection (LRI): such as bronchiolitis, pneumonia
   i. Causes congestion in small air spaces and subsequent collapse of alveoli, **impeding gas exchange** and resulting in hypoxia and respiratory distress
   ii. Lung infections may be bacterial, viral, or fungal
2. Asthma
   a. **Recurrent** bouts of bronchoconstriction and underlying inflammation of airways, resulting in **reversible** obstruction to airflow
   b. Most children will wheeze, but severe obstruction → "silent chest"
3. FBA
   a. Common in children of all ages; peaks at ages 12–24 months
   b. Infants: small household objects more commonly ingested once child is mobile (crawling = 6 months), but may be inserted by others (i.e., sibling toddler tries to "feed" baby)
   c. Young children: small foods (seeds, nuts, popcorn) and smooth foods (grapes, hot dogs) are most commonly aspirated
   d. May have witnessed coughing/choking episode followed by new-onset change in breath sounds (wheezing, stridor, or hoarseness)
   e. Consider FBA when breath sounds are focally abnormal
4. Tumors: symptoms progressive over time, but may mimic asthma, compressing airway to cause obstruction
5. Pneumonitis
   a. Parenchymal inflammation caused by noninfectious irritants, including volatile hydrocarbons (oils, paint thinner), dusts, powders, and aspirated liquids (vomiting, near drowning)
   b. Symptoms worsen over first 24–48 hours, due to surfactant washout and poor lung compliance
6. Metabolic disturbance: breath sounds will be normal
   a. Diabetic ketoacidosis (DKA): characteristic **Kussmaul breathing** that is rapid, deep, and labored; "air hunger" appearance
   b. Hypoglycemia (especially in newborns): may be tachypneic or bradypneic
   c. Inborn errors of metabolism: typically have tachypnea associated with metabolic acidosis

B. Historical findings
1. Onset ("My child was well until . . .")
2. Changes in exposures/routines?
3. Sentinel events (choking episode, swimming, bee sting)
4. Duration
5. Prior episodes (i.e., asthma) or other medical illnesses
6. Associated symptoms: cough, chest pain, orthopnea, dyspnea, drooling, change in voice

C. Physical examination findings
1. Inspection
   a. Rate of breathing
      i. Normal respiratory rate varies by age of child
      ii. Rate initially increased in respiratory distress
      iii. Terminal phase of distress is respiratory failure, marked by fatigue, alteration of consciousness, bradypnea, cyanosis, and then apnea
   b. Work of breathing
      i. Supraclavicular/subcostal/intercostal retractions
      ii. Engagement of abdominal musculature
      iii. Expression of panic or "air hunger" → lethargy
2. Palpation/percussion
   a. Crepitus under skin in pneumothorax/pneumomediastinum
   b. Dullness to percussion over fluid (pneumonia, effusions, hemothorax)
3. Auscultation
   a. Stridor
      i. Inspiratory harsh squeaking sound indicating extrathoracic airway obstruction
      ii. Croup is a common viral cause of stridor

QUICK HIT

If you cannot find an aortic arch on the left side of a chest x-ray, your patient may have a vascular sling.

QUICK HIT

A medication trial may be more appropriate than extensive testing. Examples include an inhaled bronchodilator for asthma in a child who does not cooperate with spirometry or an intranasal steroid for allergic rhinitis.

QUICK HIT

Many like to teach about epiglottitis as a cause of respiratory distress, with stridor, drooling, "tripoding," and fever. Since the HiB vaccine, this is rare to see in patients, but not on multiple choice tests!

QUICK HIT

It is uncommon for bacterial pneumonia to cause wheezing.

QUICK HIT

Foreign bodies most likely to settle in right-sided airways due to more vertical take-off from the trachea.

MNEMONIC

Tumors That Can Cause Wheeze: "L's and T's"
Lymphoma
Lipoma
Teratoma
Thymoma
Thyroid

b. Wheezing
   i. May be inspiratory, expiratory, or both
   ii. May be due to infection, inflammation, or obstruction
c. Rhonchi and rales
   i. Congestion in airways, heard primarily on inspiration
   ii. Rales = crackles = "high pitched" = small airways/alveoli: sound similar to Velcro detaching
   iii. Rhonchi = "coarse" = "low pitched" = bronchioles, bronchi, trachea
d. Bronchophony
   i. Normal for breath sounds to be softer toward peripheral lung tissue
   ii. Breath sounds or spoken words ("ninety-nine") are *louder* over areas of consolidation
e. Egophony ("EE" to "AY" change over areas of lung consolidation)

D. Laboratory testing and radiologic imaging
   1. CXR
      a. Lobar consolidation suggests bacterial pneumonia, but may be due to postobstructive atelectasis (foreign body, airway cyst, tumor, etc.)
      b. Diffuse infiltrates suggest pneumonitis, as from hypersensitivity, fungal, viral, or atypical bacterial
      c. Lack of infiltrates with hyperinflation (lungs occupying >9 rib spaces) and flattened diaphragms indicate obstructive process like asthma (Figure 2-1)
      d. Lateral films helpful to exclude mediastinal masses, define extra pulmonic effusions, aid with retrocardiac densities, and place lesions in anterior–posterior dimension
   2. Blood gas
      a. Hypoxemic respiratory failure defined as a partial pressure of oxygen in arterial blood (PaO_2) <60 mm Hg while on FiO_2 >0.6

QUICK HIT

Look for pneumothorax on CXR: "Stiff lungs pop."

QUICK HIT

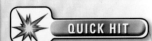

Fever may cause tachypnea in children.

QUICK HIT

Nasal flaring is a vestigial response to sensing airway resistance.

QUICK HIT

Percussion of lungs is helpful in diagnosis of effusions and pneumonia. Over fluid, the sound should be muted and less hollow sounding.

QUICK HIT

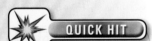

"Not all that wheezes is asthma."

QUICK HIT

A good trick is to hold the stethoscope in front of the child's nose. If the lungs sound similar, these may not be rhonchi, but rather transmitted upper airway sounds heard in the chest.

QUICK HIT

Grunting is an attempt to maintain positive end-expiratory pressure in alveoli, suggesting atelectasis, and is sign of significant distress.

FIGURE 2-1 **Asthma in a child. Hyperinflation is seen by inferiorly displaced and flattened diaphragms. This film also demonstrates peribronchial cuffing (*arrow*).**

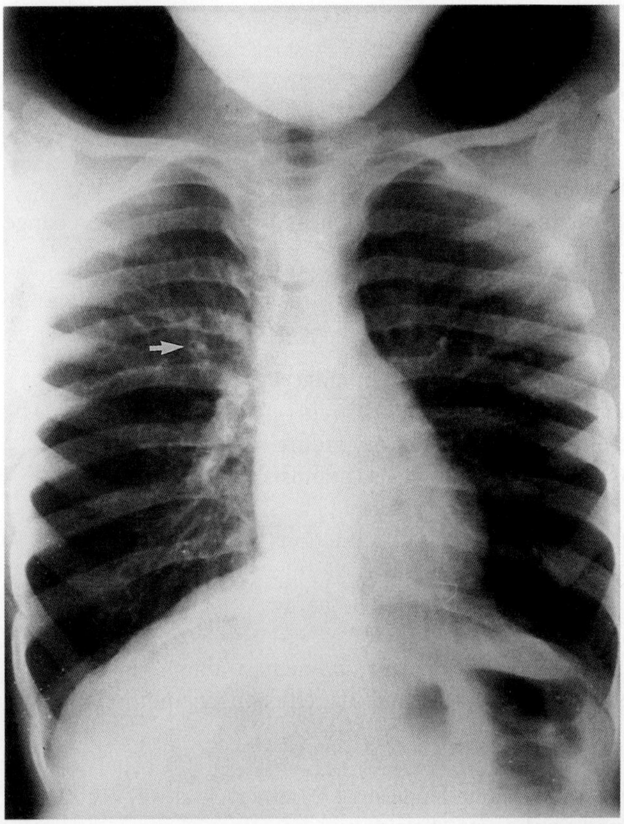

(From Daffner RH. *Clinical Radiology: The Essentials*. 3rd ed. Philadelphia: Lippincott Williams & Wilkins; 2007.)

b. Hypercarbic respiratory failure is defined as partial pressure of carbon dioxide in arterial blood ($PaCO_2$) >50 mm Hg
c. Respiratory failure is indication for intubation and mechanical ventilation
3. Blood culture
a. For pneumonia, only indicated for inpatients; very low yield in outpatient pneumonia; higher yield (about 10%) in patients with effusion
b. Most useful if obtained before starting antibiotics
4. White blood cell (WBC) count helpful only in extreme values; not routinely recommended unless ruling out another systemic illness
a. Elevation (>15,000 per high-power field) does not reliably distinguish between bacterial and viral pathogens
5. C-reactive protein (CRP) or erythrocyte sedimentation rate (ESR)
a. Sensitive but not specific seromarker of inflammation or infection
b. Not routinely indicated

E. Management
1. Open and maintain airway
a. "Head tilt–chin lift" maneuver to open airway
b. Secretions commonly obstruct airflow; have suction available
c. Foreign body with distress: urgent consultation for bronchoscopy
2. Breathing: assess for adequate ventilation (blowing off carbon dioxide [CO_2]) and oxygenation
a. Titrate oxygen to decrease distress and keep pulse oximeter >90%
3. Medications
a. Albuterol + oral prednisolone for asthma
b. Dexamethasone, 0.6 mg/kg oral (PO), intramuscular (IM), intravenous (IV) × 1 for croup
c. Racemic epinephrine, nebulized for moderate-to-severe croup
d. Antibiotics if bacterial illness likely
e. IV fluids if oral intake is poor or dehydrated

QUICK HIT

Routine CXR is not indicated in patients with asthma because areas of lung atelectasis may appear like bacterial pneumonia and inappropriate antibiotics may be administered.

QUICK HIT

For severe hypoxia, calculate the ratio of PaO_2:FiO_2. If a patient has a PaO_2 of 90 when on 30% O_2, the ratio is 90/0.3 = 270. Any level <300 is consistent with acute lung injury (ALI), and any level <200 is acute respiratory distress syndrome (ARDS).

QUICK HIT

Hypercarbia and sensation of lung collapse or consolidation are primary drivers of the sensation of "shortness of breath." A patient may be hypoxic and not even know it.

DISEASE SPECIFIC

IV. Diaphragmatic Hernia

A. Definition
1. Protrusion of abdominal contents through the diaphragm into thorax (Figure 2-2)
a. Herniated contents may include stomach, intestines, liver, and spleen
b. Bochdalek: most common (~90%), posterolateral chest wall, typically left sided (~90%), small/large intestines and intra-abdominal organs herniate into chest
i. Results from failure, at ~8 weeks gestational age, of pleuroperitoneal membrane to fuse to lateral chest wall
c. Morgagni type (2%–6%): anterior, retrosternal herniation
d. Hiatal hernia: stomach and/or intestines herniate through crux of diaphragm at esophageal hiatus
2. Prevalence
a. 1:4,000 live births
b. Female:male = 2:1
3. Survival
a. ~2/3
b. Spontaneous fetal demise in 7%–10%
c. Significant incidence of neurodevelopmental delay, chronic lung disease (CLD), and GERD

B. Pathophysiology
1. Abnormal thoracic contents → decreased lung inflation, pulmonary hypoplasia from insufficient blood flow and surfactant
2. Pulmonary artery musculature hypertrophy and pulmonary hypertension (HTN); left ventricular hypoplasia may be observed
3. Abnormalities persist even after surgical correction of hernia

QUICK HIT

Good rule to know: CRP has a quicker onset and quicker resolution than ESR in the face of transient inflammation.

QUICK HIT

Both congenital and traumatic herniation through the diaphragm are more likely to occur on the left side.

QUICK HIT

The presence of liver in the thorax is a poor prognostic indicator.

FIGURE 2-2 Congenital diaphragmatic hernia.

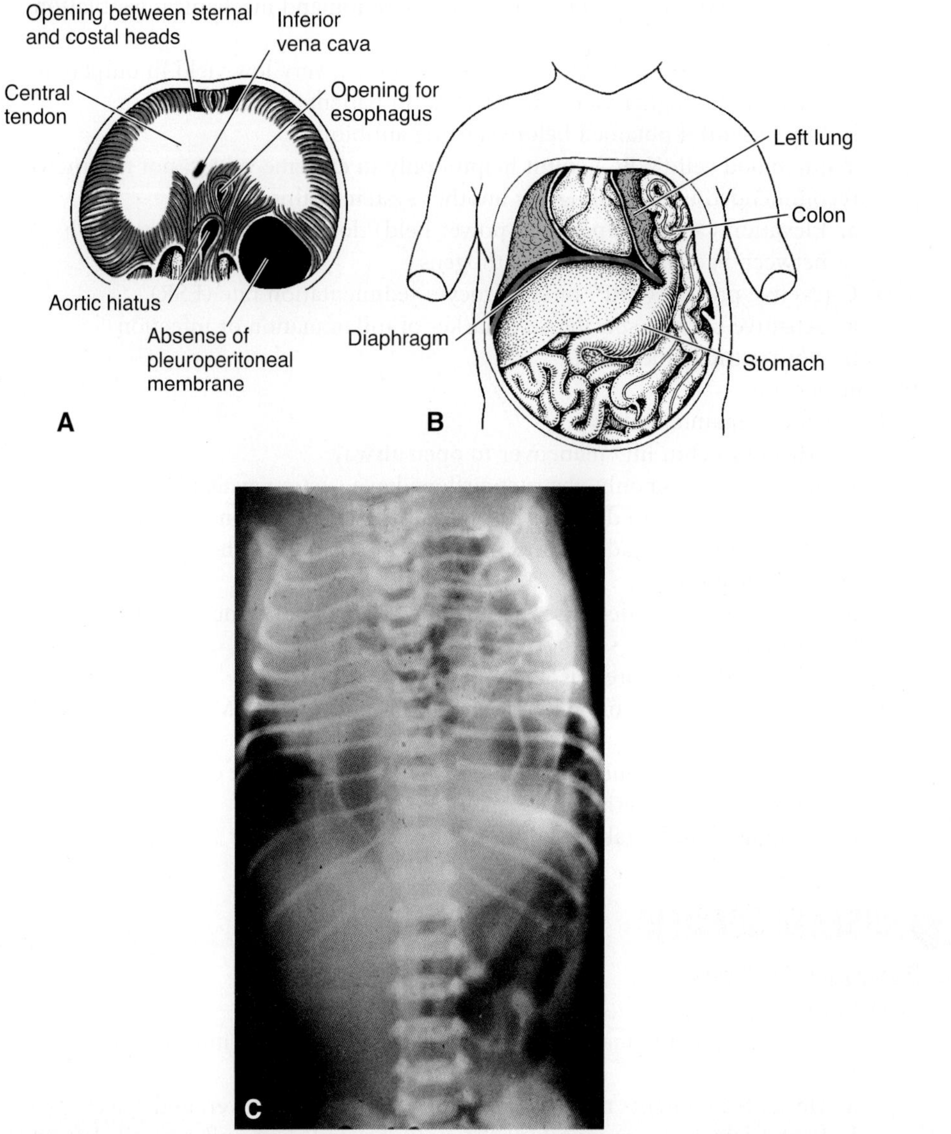

A. Abdominal surface of the diaphragm showing a large defect of the pleuroperitoneal membrane. **B.** Hernia of the intestinal loops and part of the stomach into the left pleural cavity. The heart and mediastinum are frequently pushed to the right and the left lung compressed. **C.** Radiograph of a newborn with a large defect in the left side of the diaphragm. Abdominal viscera have entered the thorax through the defect. (From Sadler T. *Langman's Medical Embryology.* 9th edition Image Bank. Baltimore: Lippincott Williams & Wilkins; 2003.)

QUICK HIT

Bowel sounds over the thorax are pathognomonic for diaphragm hernia.

QUICK HIT

Note that half of cases are diagnosed prenatally by fetal ultrasound, as early as 16 weeks of gestational age. Oligohydramnios is common.

C. Clinical presentation
  1. Physical exam findings
    a. Respiratory distress may be delayed 24–48 hours
    b. Scaphoid abdomen (i.e., sucked in)
    c. Large chest
  2. Associated anomalies in about 1/3 of cases can include
    a. Central nervous system (CNS) abnormalities
    b. Cardiovascular abnormalities
    c. Esophageal atresia
    d. Omphalocele
    e. Chromosomal abnormalities (e.g., trisomies 21 and 13, Turner syndrome)

D. Testing
  1. CXR: abdominal contents in thorax, displaced cardiac silhouette, small lungs

E. Therapy
1. Delivery room
a. Symptomatic infants with prenatal diagnosis are intubated at birth because bag-valve mask ventilation distends stomach and intestines, further compromising lung inflation
b. Severe pulmonary hypoplasia may require extracorporeal membrane oxygenation (ECMO, also known as *heart–lung bypass*) in babies >2 kg
2. Neonatal intensive care unit (NICU)
a. Echo for pulmonary vascular resistance and HTN
b. Exogenous surfactant is poorly supported by evidence
c. Surgical repair when stable and pulmonary HTN resolved, generally at least 48 hours old

> **QUICK HIT**
> Gore-Tex or porcine patch repair, versus native tissue repair, has higher incidence of recurrence.

V. Pulmonary Hypoplasia

A. Definition
1. Embryologic maldevelopment of pulmonary system resulting in incomplete growth of lung tissue
B. Cause/pathophysiology
1. Potter sequence
a. Initially described in infants with renal agenesis and oliguria; any condition resulting in oligohydramnios in fetus can lead to characteristic physical appearance and lung hypoplasia
b. Normal fetal lung development requires adequate space in thorax and movement of amniotic fluid into fetal lungs
c. Amniotic fluid is component of fetal lung fluid influencing development via growth factors

> **QUICK HIT**
> Development of pulmonary hypoplasia is an embryologic event. Timing of insult correlates with severity of disease, with earlier insults typically resulting in more severe disease.

C. Clinical presentation
1. Prenatal
a. Diminished maternal amniotic fluid levels
b. Diminished fetal movements
c. Excessive leakage of amniotic fluid <25 weeks' gestation
2. Postnatal
a. Respiratory
i. Apnea
ii. Severe respiratory distress at birth with diminished breath sounds
iii. Pneumothorax
iv. Bowel sounds heard overlying chest
b. Abdominal
i. Scaphoid abdomen
ii. Cystic renal mass, enlarged bladder
c. Other
i. Potter facies: flattened nose, hypertelorism, retrognathia, epicanthal folds, low-set ears
ii. Skeletal abnormalities

> **QUICK HIT**
> Prolonged leakage of amniotic fluid beginning at <25 weeks of gestation leads to oligohydramnios and resulting Potter sequence.

> **QUICK HIT**
> The fetal lung is an important source of amniotic fluid.

D. Testing
1. Prenatal ultrasound
2. CXR may demonstrate midline shift toward affected side, presence of bowel (congenital diaphragmatic hernia), congenital cystic adenomatous malformation (CCAM), or skeletal abnormalities
3. Bronchoscopy/MRI: definitive studies
E. Therapy
1. Prenatal therapy: amniotic infusions in patients with oligohydramnios
2. Postnatal therapy

> **QUICK HIT**
> Mortality rates are as high as 75%–95% depending on severity of hypoplasia. Patients with severe oligohydramnios have the worst outcomes.

VI. Congenital Cystic Adenomatous Malformation

A. Definition
1. Congenital malformation → 1 or more cysts within lung parenchyma
2. Most common congenital lung lesion (1–4 per 100,000 births)

B. Cause/pathophysiology
   1. Abnormal branching of developing lung creating 1 large cyst or multiple intercommunicating cysts
   2. Cystic tissue is dysplastic with adenomatous elements
   3. Leads to air trapping and harboring of infection
   4. In contrast to pulmonary sequestration, lesions are connected to bronchial tree and receive **pulmonary** circulation
C. Clinical presentation
   1. Single large cysts (>2 cm in diameter) are most common and often seen on prenatal ultrasound
   2. Small cysts may present later in childhood with recurrent pneumonia or pneumothorax from cyst rupture
D. Therapy
   1. Surgical resection of lobe
   2. Even if asymptomatic, resect within 1 year to prevent recurrent infections or malignancy

QUICK HIT

CCAMs are usually confined to single lobe.

QUICK HIT

Children with multiple cysts and other congenital anomalies have a poor prognosis.

VII. Congenital Lobar Emphysema

A. Definition: rare congenital malformation of lower respiratory tract resulting in **hyper**inflation of 1 or more lobes of lung
B. Cause/pathophysiology
   1. Abnormal embryologic development of lung tissue results in altered number and size of both airways and alveoli within lobe
   2. May be due to early obstruction, such as aberrant vessel, causing air trapping via ball-valve mechanism
C. Clinical presentation
   1. Presents between birth and age 6 months
   2. Tachypnea, dyspnea, +/− cyanosis
   3. Decreased breath sounds, wheezing, and **hyper**resonance to percussion
   4. Left upper lobe is most commonly involved

QUICK HIT

Not all cases of pulmonary emphysema are congenital. It may develop due to an obstruction from a mucous plug, foreign body, or tumor.

VIII. Right Middle Lobe Syndrome

A. Definition
   1. RMLS is persistent or recurrent atelectasis of right middle lobe caused most commonly by acute asthma exacerbation
   2. Atelectasis is incomplete expansion or complete collapse of segment or lobe of the lung, or can involve entire lung
B. Cause/pathophysiology: right middle lung is anatomically susceptible to atelectasis because of narrow diameter and acute takeoff angle of lobar bronchus
C. Clinical presentation
   1. If area of atelectasis is small, patient may be asymptomatic
   2. Most common symptoms include cough, wheezing, and sputum production
D. Testing
   1. Primarily, diagnosis made by posteroanterior and lateral chest radiograph (Figure 2-3)
   2. If atelectasis persists, consider high-resolution CT (HRCT) of chest to further define atelectasis and delineate anatomy
E. Therapy
   1. Treatment depends on etiology of atelectasis
   2. If patient has asthma, goal of therapy is to control underlying asthma
      a. Rescue medications such as inhaled albuterol for acute symptoms of wheezing, coughing, and increased work of breathing
      b. Controller medications such as inhaled corticosteroids for daily use
   3. Bronchoscopy has diagnostic and therapeutic roles
      a. May reveal foreign body or extrinsic/intrinsic compression of the airway
      b. Bronchoalveolar lavage (BAL) can reveal infectious agents and clear mucus plugging

QUICK HIT

In an acute asthma exacerbation, mucus plugging and compression from hyper-expanded right upper and lower lobes may contribute to RMLS.

FIGURE 2-3 Atelectasis, lobe, radiograph.

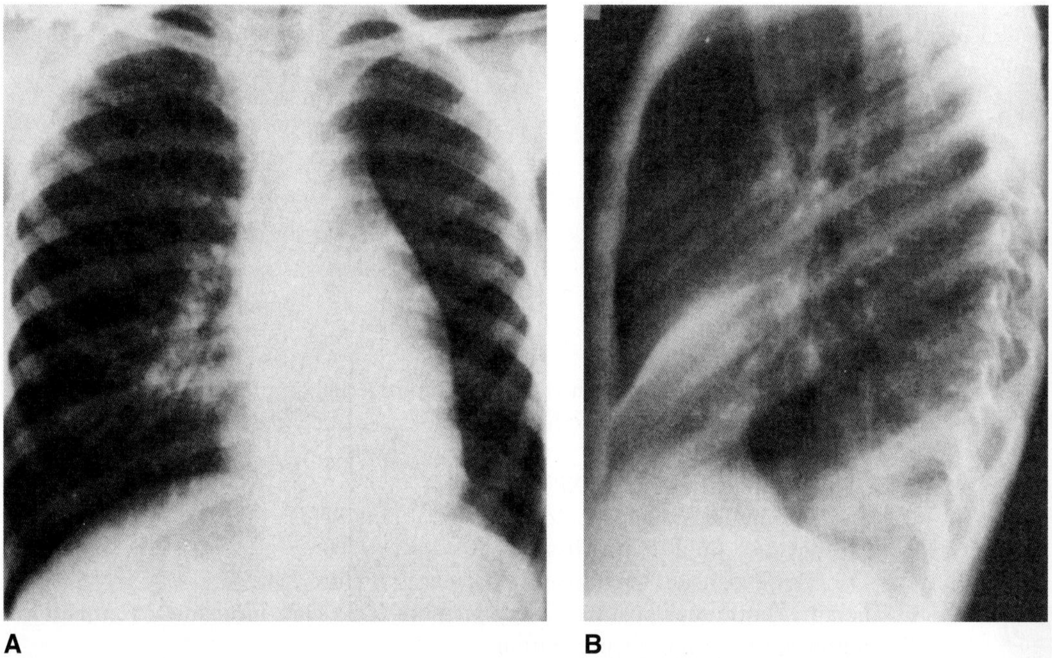

A. Chest radiograph of right middle lobe and left lower lobe atelectasis. Right middle lobe atelectasis seen as triangular density obliterating right cardiac silhouette. Left lower lobe atelectasis demonstrated as triangular-shaped area of density behind left cardiac silhouette. **B.** Right lobe atelectasis seen as linear area of density overlying cardiac silhouette. Left lower lobe atelectasis seen as area of density posteriorly and inferiorly, overlying vertebral bodies. (From LifeART images copyright © 2013 Lippincott Williams & Wilkins. All rights reserved.)

IX. Surfactant Deficiency

A. Definition: lack of pulmonary surfactant resulting in mild to severe respiratory compromise in neonatal period
B. Cause/pathophysiology
  1. Incidence varies, but inversely related to gestational age, as is severity
  2. Caused by deficiency of surfactant production from several mechanisms
  3. Lack of surfactant → increased surface tension → alveolar atelectasis at end expiration → greater force to expand alveoli and airways
  4. Symptoms exacerbated by increased chest wall compliance of premature infant
  5. Atelectatic lung is well perfused but not ventilated, causing hypoxemia
  6. Decreased lung compliance, increased work of breathing, and physiologic dead space combined with poor alveolar ventilation lead to hypercapnia
  7. Risk factors: prematurity, maternal diabetes, Cesarean delivery, asphyxia, cold stress, previously affected sibling
C. Clinical presentation
  1. Historical findings
    a. History of prematurity
    b. Intrapartum history, meconium, poor Apgar scores
    c. Associated inflammatory conditions (both maternal and neonatal)
  2. Physical exam findings
    a. Within minutes (rarely, hours) of birth, infant develops respiratory distress
    b. Breath sounds may be normal or decreased and have harsh tubular quality with fine crackles occasionally present
D. Testing
  1. Differential diagnosis (Box 2-2)
  2. Laboratory evaluation
    a. Ventilation/perfusion ($\dot{V}/\dot{Q}$) mismatch results in decreased PaO_2 and later increased $PaCO_2$ and metabolic acidosis on ABG

QUICK HIT

Surfactant deficiency is the leading cause of respiratory distress in the premature infant.

QUICK HIT

Surfactant is composed of phospholipids and proteins, which act to decrease surface tension.

QUICK HIT

The highest incidence is in premature males or white infants.

QUICK HIT

A late onset of tachypnea suggests other conditions.

BOX 2-2

Differential Diagnosis of Surfactant Deficiency

Transient tachypnea of the newborn
Neonatal pneumonia
Sepsis
Pulmonary hypoplasia
Meconium aspiration
Congenital heart disease
Congenital lung anomalies

b. Lecithin:sphingomyelin (L/S) ratio on maternal amniotic fluid estimates degree of surfactant production; ratio <2:1 likely results in surfactant deficiency
3. Radiographic findings (CXR)
   a. "Ground glass" appearance in bilateral lung fields
   b. Retained fluid in lung fissures
   c. Hypoexpansion with areas of atelectasis (Figure 2-4)

E. Therapy: continuous positive airway pressure (CPAP) or mechanical ventilation
F. Complications/prognosis/prevention
1. Complications result from barotrauma or lack of surfactant/supportive care and may include pneumothorax
2. Prognosis variable
3. Prevention
   a. Primarily based on decreasing premature birth, allowing lung development to occur
   b. **Prenatal corticosteroids** in mothers prior to delivery of premature infants increase surfactant production and lung maturation

QUICK HIT

Exogenous surfactant should be given by endotracheal tube to decrease alveolar surface tension in patients with surfactant deficiency.

FIGURE 2-4 **This premature infant presented with grunting, retractions, and cyanosis after delivery. The diffuse reticular–granular opacification, air bronchograms, and decreased lung volumes in the chest radiograph film indicate respiratory distress syndrome.**

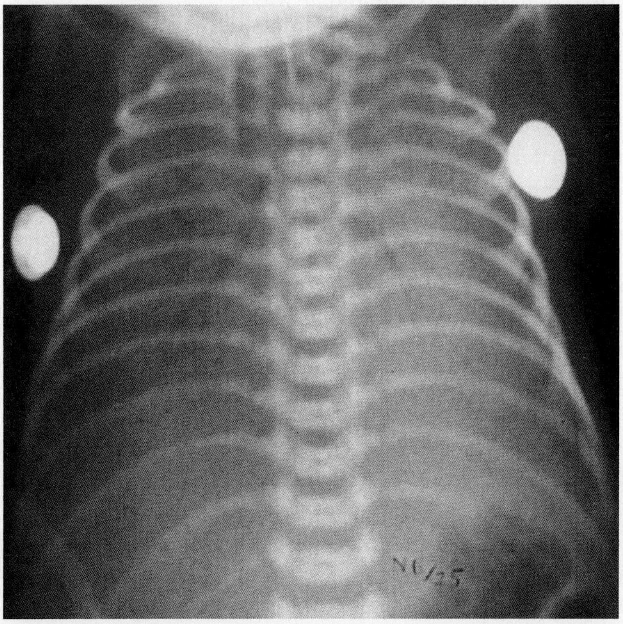

(From MacDonald MG, Seshia MMK, Mullett MD. *Avery's Neonatology Pathophysiology & Management of the Newborn.* 6th ed. Philadelphia: Lippincott Williams & Wilkins; 2005.)

X. Pulmonary Lobar Sequestration

A. Definition
   1. Rare congenital malformation of lower respiratory tract resulting in section of *nonfunctional* lung tissue
      a. *No* normal connection to bronchial tree; therefore, no gas exchange
      b. Lesions receive *systemic* rather than pulmonary blood flow
   2. Intralobar within a normal lung lobe or extralobar with its own visceral pleura
B. Cause/pathophysiology
   1. Abnormal development of lung bud early in embryologic development before separation of systemic and pulmonary circulations
   2. Pathogens can enter as result of rupture of infected material through an adjacent airway, and not easily cleared → recurrent pneumonia
C. Clinical presentation
   1. Varying presentation based on location of lesion
   2. Physical exam may reveal decreased breath sounds, dullness to percussion, and crackles, particularly if infection is present
D. Testing
   1. Ultrasound: pre- or postnatally
   2. Chest radiograph: uniform density often indistinguishable from pneumonia
   3. Chest CT with angiography or MRI/magnetic resonance angiogram (MRA) may identify aberrant systemic arterial blood flow
E. Therapy
   1. Definitive treatment is surgical resection
   2. Even if asymptomatic, resection of intralobar lesions to prevent recurrent infection

> **QUICK HIT**
> Ultrasound demonstration of aortic blood flow to the lesion is pathognomonic for a sequestered lobe.

XI. Aspiration Pneumonia

A. Characteristics: passage of foreign substances into lower airways, causing inflammation, obstruction to airflow, and/or alteration in normal gas-exchange barrier
   1. Cause
      a. Abnormal muscle tone or swallowing function (e.g., muscular dystrophy or cerebral palsy)
      b. Altered mental status (e.g., due to intoxication or trauma)
      c. Exposure to general anesthesia
      d. GERD/vomiting
B. Clinical features
   1. Historical findings (Box 2-3)
      a. Symptoms present within 1–2 hours of event, usually worsen over 24–48 hours
      b. FBA: abrupt onset of symptoms after choking event
   2. Physical exam findings
      a. Respiratory distress
      b. Cough (especially if productive of purulent sputum or blood)
      c. Evidence of lower airway involvement
         i. Tachypnea
         ii. Fever (common even in noninfectious pneumonitis)
         iii. Wheezing and/or crackles
         iv. Hypoxia/cyanosis

> **QUICK HIT**
> Aspiration pneumonitis is noninfectious inflammation of the bronchi and lung parenchyma in response to exposure to foreign substances, food, airborne particles, liquids, vomitus, or saliva.

> **QUICK HIT**
> Swallowing dysfunction with aspiration is the most common cause of recurrent pneumonia in children.

BOX 2-3

Important Historical Questions

1. Was a choking event observed? What was the child doing or eating?
2. When was aspiration?
3. Are there any associated symptoms?
   a. Fever: Indicates aspiration event occurred at least several hours, if not days, earlier, or that events happen chronically
   b. Change in mental status may indicate hypoxia or intoxication

C. Diagnosis
1. Laboratory findings are generally unhelpful in well-appearing patients with aspiration pneumonia
2. Radiology findings: CXR
a. Upright to reveal focal atelectasis (i.e., postobstructive), diffuse pneumonitis, pneumothorax, or radiopaque foreign body
b. Lateral to determine patency of tracheal air column, precise location of pneumonias

D. Therapy
1. Support "ABC's": high inspiratory pressures (CPAP or intubation) may be needed due to poor compliance of lungs
2. Supplemental oxygen

QUICK HIT

Other findings: test of swallowing function (oral–pharyngeal motility study by barium swallow) assesses whether thickened fluids or gastrostomy are necessary for safe feeding in the future.

QUICK HIT

Some children will respond to a diet with thickened liquids, whereas children with severe aspiration may require life-long G-tube feeding.

QUICK HIT

Antibiotic coverage for aspiration pneumonia targets oral flora. Clindamycin and ampicillin/sulbactam are good choices.

XII. Cystic Fibrosis

A. Characteristics
1. Definition: complex, multisystem genetic disorder characterized by progressive respiratory, gastrointestinal (GI), hepatobiliary, and reproductive disease and markedly shortened life expectancy
2. Epidemiology
a. Approximately 4% of whites in United States are carriers of CF gene mutation, but can occur in all ethnic groups
b. ~50% CF diagnoses are made before age 6 months; 75% by age 2 years
3. Genetics: autosomal recessive disorder
a. No clear relationship between type of mutation and clinical course
4. Pathophysiology
a. Cystic fibrosis transmembrane conductance regulator (CFTR) protein is complex chloride channel with additional regulatory properties found in all exocrine tissues
b. Abnormal transport/regulation of chloride ions → viscous secretions
c. Primarily affects lung, pancreas, liver, intestine, and reproductive tract
d. Pulmonary disease
i. Thick airway secretions, infection, and altered inflammatory response
ii. Recurrent infections → chronic inflammation → destroys medium and small airways and parenchyma → bronchiectatic changes on CXR
iii. Chronic bacterial colonization of airway
(a) *Staphylococcus aureus*, increasingly methicillin-resistant (MRSA) type
(b) *Haemophilus influenza*
(c) *Pseudomonas aeruginosa* (forms a "biofilm")
(d) *Burkholderia cepacia* (forms a "biofilm")
(i) Less common colonization, but more significant
(ii) Associated with worse lung function and poor outcome
(iii) Requires strict isolation from other CF patients if found
(e) Spontaneous pneumothorax (recurrent, but rare) from small airway plugging, air trapping, and bleb formation
(f) Pulmonary hemorrhage (due to inflammation and airway erosion)
e. Pancreatic disease
i. Thickened secretions can lead to duct obstruction, inadequate release of lipase and other enzymes, and subsequent autodigestion of pancreas
ii. Acute or chronic pancreatitis can occur
iii. Poor exocrine function leads to intestinal protein and fat malabsorption
(a) Malnutrition, inadequate caloric absorption
(b) Fat-soluble vitamin (A, D, E, K) deficiency
iv. Poor endocrine function can lead to cystic fibrosis–related diabetes (CFRD)
f. Intestinal disease
i. Thickened intestinal secretions → complete/partial intestinal obstruction
ii. Meconium ileus of newborn is almost diagnostic of CF
iii. Distal intestinal obstruction syndrome (DIOS) similar to meconium ileus, but in an older child and associated with unrecognized or undertreated pancreatic insufficiency

QUICK HIT

CF is the most common lethal inherited disorder in Caucasians.

QUICK HIT

CF is caused by a mutation of the cystic fibrosis transmembrane conductance regulator gene (CFTR) on chromosome 7.

QUICK HIT

Over 1,500 different CFTR gene mutations have been described, but about 70% of cases are ΔF508, 3 base-pair deletion→ absence of phenylalanine residue at codon 508.

BOX 2-4

Initial Presentation of Patients with Cystic Fibrosis

1. Meconium ileus in infancy (about 20%)
2. Asymptomatic, but abnormal newborn screen
3. Recurrent or persistent respiratory infections
4. Symptoms of pancreatic insufficiency, steatorrhea, generalized edema
5. Failure to thrive
6. Positive family history

g. Hepatobiliary disease
   i. Often asymptomatic, focal **biliary cirrhosis** is most common
   ii. Thickened, inspissated biliary secretions that decrease flow and increase concentration of bile
   iii. Can develop abnormal bile duct proliferation, gallstones
   iv. Presents with elevated liver transaminases and/or hepatosplenomegaly
   v. Rarely can develop hepatic dysfunction, portal HTN, cirrhosis, or even liver failure

B. Clinical features
   1. Patients present variously (Box 2-4)
   2. Pulmonary disease
      a. Historical findings: symptoms include persistent and productive cough, dyspnea, tachypnea, increased sputum production, anorexia, and fatigue
      b. Physical exam findings of pulmonary disease (Box 2-5)
   3. Upper airway disease: sinusitis and sinus polyps are very common and recurrent
   4. Pancreatic disease
      a. History of frequent, greasy, foul-smelling stools, cramping, flatulence, poor weight gain
      b. Physical exam findings of abdominal distention, vitamin deficiency, protein deficiency, failure to thrive
   5. Intestinal disease
      a. DIOS presents with progressive cramping abdominal pain (commonly right lower quadrant), distention, nausea, and/or vomiting.
      b. Rectal prolapse from constipation, chronic cough, malnutrition
      c. GERD is very common
         i. Worsened by chronic cough and lung hyperinflation
         ii. May contribute to respiratory symptoms

BOX 2-5

Physical Findings of Cystic Fibrosis Pulmonary Disease

1. Coarse crackles, focal or diffuse
2. Decreased air entry
3. Tachypnea
4. Use of accessory respiratory muscles
5. Air trapping/"barrel chest"
6. Digital clubbing
7. Hypoxemia
8. Exercise intolerance
9. Weight loss
10. Decreased pulmonary function on spirometry testing

QUICK HIT

Most patients are ultimately colonized with *Pseudomonas*, and it is almost impossible to eradicate.

QUICK HIT

Most patients with CF have some degree of progressive pancreatic involvement, commonly present from birth.

QUICK HIT

CFRD affects 8%–30% of patients; prevalence increases with age.

QUICK HIT

Meconium ileus is the presenting condition in 10%–20% of newborns with CF.

QUICK HIT

Rectal prolapse can be seen in infants and children with CF.

QUICK HIT

Ten percent of CF patients die of liver-related disease.

QUICK HIT

The main characteristic of CF is progressive, obstructive lung disease.

QUICK HIT

Consider CF in infant who fails to pass stool in first 48 hours.

6. Other clinical involvement
   a. Females may experience difficulty with conception due to nutritional insufficiency, but fertility in females may be unaffected
   b. Pregnancy complicated by respiratory/nutrition issues, but outcomes can be good, especially if lung function is adequate
   c. Poor bone mineralization is common
   d. Venous thrombosis and nephrolithiasis occur occasionally

C. Diagnosis
1. Newborn screening
   a. Most states test for immunoreactive trypsinogen (IRT)
      i. IRT = pancreatic enzyme with normally low blood level
      ii. Elevated levels suggest pancreatic dysfunction
      iii. Elevated IRT triggers either a repeat IRT or DNA test
   b. Newborn screening is approximately 95% sensitive (5% false-negative rate)
   c. Confirmatory sweat chloride test should be performed on infants at risk
2. Sweat test
   a. Should only be done at experienced centers
   b. Values >60 mEq/L considered positive for CF if patient is age >6 months (>30 mEq/L if age <6 months)
   c. Alternately, DNA analysis showing 2 CFTR mutations is diagnostic
   d. Nasal potential difference testing can help distinguish cases for which prior testing does not provide definitive diagnosis
   e. Indications for sweat chloride outside neonatal period (Box 2-6)
3. Other studies
   a. CXR can appear essentially normal for years, but eventually will show evidence of mucus plugging, hyperinflation, and bronchiectasis
   b. Pulmonary function tests (PFTs) show an obstructive pattern with prolonged forced expiratory volume in 1 second (FEV_1) and high residual volume; later can show low tidal volume and total lung capacity

D. Treatment
1. Respiratory therapy
   a. Includes adequate treatment of nutrition, glycemic control, and psychosocial issues
   b. Antibiotic therapy
      i. Recommended for all pulmonary exacerbations
      ii. Directed treatment toward suspected colonizing organisms
      iii. Unlikely to eradicate bacteria, but goal is to suppress
      iv. Long-term, continuous antibiotic use
         (a) Inhaled antipseudomonal therapy (e.g., tobramycin) on an every-other-month basis

QUICK HIT

In CF patients with suspected DIOS, other causes of acute abdomen, such as appendicitis, volvulus, and intussusception, must nevertheless be considered.

QUICK HIT

Infertility is nearly universal in male CF patients due to absent vas deferens, although spermatogenesis can be normal.

QUICK HIT

CF screening is part of all state newborn screening programs.

QUICK HIT

The sweat chloride test is the gold standard for diagnosis of CF.

QUICK HIT

When treating an acute CF respiratory exacerbation, base antibiotic therapy on the results of previous sputum or bronchoalveolar lavage cultures, if available.

QUICK HIT

Azithromycin provides benefit through its anti-inflammatory effects.

BOX 2-6

When to Consider Testing for Cystic Fibrosis

1. Recurrent episodes of cough
2. Recurrent pneumonia
3. Persistent or recurrent sinusitis
4. Unexplained poor weight gain or failure to thrive
5. Nasal polyps
6. Rectal prolapse
7. Family history of cystic fibrosis
8. Metabolic alkalosis during dehydration from chloride loss in sweat
9. Fat-soluble vitamin deficiency
10. Clubbing on exam
11. Bronchiectasis seen on imaging
12. Pulmonary *Pseudomonas* infection

c. Mechanical airway clearance
   i. To loosen and mobilize thickened, inspissated airway secretions
   ii. Mechanical methods
      (a) Postural drainage
      (b) Manual or mechanical chest percussive therapy
      (c) Cough-assist devices and cough techniques
      (d) Aerobic exercise
d. Inhaled medications
   i. Nebulized hypertonic (7%) saline to hydrate secretions
   ii. DNAse to cleave long strands of neutrophil DNA
   iii. Bronchodilator therapy
      (a) Most helpful in CF patients with asthma-like symptoms
      (b) Facilitates administration of other inhaled therapies
   iv. Inhaled corticosteroids are not consistently beneficial
e. Systemic corticosteroids can be used short-term for exacerbations, if reactive airway disease present
f. Chronic nonsteroidal anti-inflammatory drug (NSAID) use (e.g., ibuprofen)
g. Immunization against influenza annually and pneumococcus
h. Supplemental oxygen as needed for exacerbations or late-stage disease
i. Bilevel positive airway pressure (BiPAP) for chronic hypercarbia of late-stage disease
j. For pulmonary hemorrhage
   i. May require acute arterial embolization or surgical intervention
   ii. May require modification of pulmonary toilet (e.g., decreased chest physiotherapy)
   iii. Administer vitamin K (pancreatic insufficiency is a risk)
k. Lung transplantation
   i. Considered if patient has 5-year predicted survival without transplant of less than 30%
   ii. Always bilateral due to infection concerns
   iii. Five-year survival is around 60%–65%
   iv. May be contraindicated if patient colonized with *B. cepacia*

2. Sinus therapy for sinus/upper airway disease: systemic antibiotics; nasal steroids; and, occasionally, surgery
3. Pancreatic disease therapy
   a. Supplementation with fat-soluble vitamins ("ADEK")
   b. Insulin and oral hypoglycemic agents for reasonable glycemic control
4. Intestinal disease therapy
   a. DIOS usually nonsurgical; can be treated by laxatives, enemas, or bowel clean-out
   b. Rectal prolapse: manual reduction, prevent constipation
   c. GERD: H_2 blockers, proton pump inhibitors
5. Hepatobiliary disease therapy
   a. Some patients benefit from ursodeoxycholic acid
   b. Abdominal ultrasound/upper GI endoscopy if labs persistently abnormal
   c. Doppler analysis to look for portal HTN
   d. If liver disease progresses to liver failure, transplantation
6. Prognosis
   a. CF causes significant morbidity, requires aggressive and time-consuming treatment regimens, and has universally premature mortality
   b. Educational, career, and reproductive counseling is mandatory at all stages of life for newly diagnosed patients
   c. Optimal treatment is at CF foundation–certified treatment centers
      i. Close involvement with primary care physician
      ii. Pulmonologists, gastroenterologists, and other specialists
      iii. Key support personnel trained in CF disease, such as dieticians, social workers, genetic counselors, etc.

QUICK HIT

Long-term use of systemic corticosteroids leads to risks that outweigh any benefit.

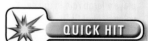

QUICK HIT

Pancreatic enzyme replacement therapy is required in nearly all patients.

QUICK HIT

Medium-chain triglycerides do not require pancreatic enzymes for digestion and, thus, are the preferred fat source for patients with CF.

QUICK HIT

Liver function tests should be performed annually.

QUICK HIT

Life expectancy of patients with CF has dramatically improved in the last 2 decades and is now close to age 40 years with proper treatment.

7. Prevention: early diagnosis seems to lead to better outcomes
   a. Early nutritional support improves lung function and brain development
   b. Treatment costs are lower in patients diagnosed earlier
   c. Allows for earlier referrals to CF centers

XIII. Chronic Lung Disease of Prematurity

QUICK HIT

CLD is also referred to as bronchopulmonary dysplasia (BPD).

QUICK HIT

CLD is more common in white boys.

QUICK HIT

Emergent respiratory support in the neonatal period plays a large role in the development of CLD.

QUICK HIT

Infants with CLD are 1.5 times as likely to be hospitalized with bronchiolitis.

QUICK HIT

Primary treatment for CLD is aimed at prevention via limiting mechanical ventilation, allowing for permissive hypercarbia, optimizing nutrition, and using anti-inflammatory medications/diuretics as needed.

A. Characteristics
1. Definition
   a. Chronic pulmonary disease starting as neonatal respiratory disorder from premature lungs and worsened by subsequent iatrogenic respiratory support in perinatal period
   b. Defined as oxygen requirement >28 days or at 36 weeks postmenstrual age in the premature infant with characteristic radiographic, clinical, and pathologic findings
2. Epidemiology
   a. Incidence varies; inversely related to gestational age
   b. More common in patients with previous surfactant deficiency
   c. Severity ranges from mild to lethal
3. Risk factors
   a. Prematurity
   b. Hyperoxia
   c. Prolonged mechanical ventilation
   d. Other pulmonary disease (e.g., air leak, pulmonary edema, meconium aspiration, pneumothorax, pneumonia)
   e. Poor nutrition/low birth weight
4. Pathophysiology
   a. Multifactorial and not completely understood
   b. Underlying genetic influence
   c. Hyperoxia and barotrauma in perinatal period play key role: oxygen free radical damage and inability to repair at cellular level → interstitial fibrosis

B. Clinical features
1. Historical findings
   a. Prematurity, persistent oxygen requirement, and prolonged need for mechanical ventilation
   b. Commonly, history of acute barotrauma and positive pressure ventilation at birth
   c. Severe or prolonged course with viral respiratory illness
2. Physical exam findings
   a. Tachypnea and retractions with occasional bilateral scattered crackles
   b. May be cushingoid from long-term corticosteroid therapy in severe cases

C. Diagnosis
1. Clinical and historical diagnosis, includes degree of oxygen requirement, duration of oxygen need
2. Laboratory findings
   a. Hypoxia and hypercarbia on blood gas analysis
   b. High serum bicarbonate, as compensation for chronic respiratory acidosis
   c. If on diuretics, contraction alkalosis, hypochloremia, and hypokalemia
3. Radiology findings
   a. CXR: diffuse haziness reflecting atelectasis, inflammation, or edema
   b. Typical radiographs show decreased lung volumes and occasional air trapping (Figure 2-5)

D. Treatment
1. Therapy
   a. Diuretics used to decrease fluid overload despite lack of evidence for long-term benefit; can be used in cases of acute pulmonary edema for older children
   b. Corticosteroids
      i. May decrease inflammation and need for mechanical ventilation but have increased risk of neurologic complications

FIGURE 2-5 **Typical chest radiograph of a 1-month-old infant with evolving bronchopulmonary dysplasia. The bilateral hazy appearance represents inflammatory exudate, edema, and atelectasis.**

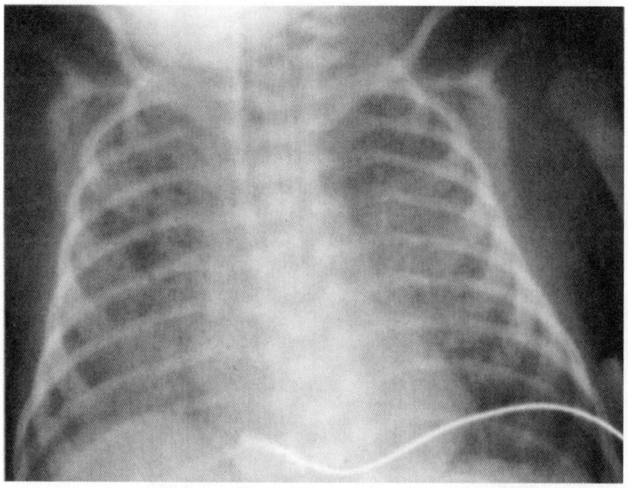

(From MacDonald MG, Seshia MMK, Mullett MD. *Avery's Neonatology Pathophysiology & Management of the Newborn.* 6th ed. Philadelphia: Lippincott Williams & Wilkins; 2005.)

ii. Not routinely recommended; not beneficial in infants hospitalized with bronchiolitis
iii. Inhaled corticosteroids may play role in long-term management

c. β-Agonist
   i. Used in acute situations of bronchospasm (usually age >5 years)
   ii. Not routinely recommended except in case of severe CLD or if concomitant reactive airway disease is suspected
   iii. Rarely beneficial in affected patients hospitalized with bronchiolitis

2. Complications (long term)
   a. Asthma
   b. Pulmonary HTN, CHF, systemic venous congestion
   c. Recurrent/worsened pulmonary infections
   d. Poor neurodevelopmental outcome
3. Monthly prophylaxis with monoclonal antibodies against respiratory syncytial virus (RSV) during bronchiolitis season depending on age, generally first 2 years of life

> **QUICK HIT**
> Asthma is very common in children born prematurely with CLD.

> **QUICK HIT**
> Monoclonal RSV antibodies are expensive and only minimally helpful in reducing severity of disease. Therapy is limited to severely premature patients, patients with congenital heart disease, and patients with CLD.

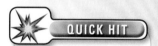

XIV. Primary Ciliary Dyskinesia

A. Definition/physiology
   1. Cilia: hair-like projections from epithelial surfaces to lumen of airways, nasal passages, sinuses, and cerebral ventricles; form motile element of sperm
   2. Respiratory cilia mobilize mucus and prevent stasis and bacterial overgrowth (Figure 2-6)

B. Cause/pathophysiology
   1. Primary ciliary dyskinesia results from mutations in proteins resulting in abnormal ciliary structure and function
   2. Prevalence: 1:16,000 live births for primary ciliary dyskinesia; 50% of primary ciliary dyskinesia patients have Kartagener syndrome
   3. Inheritance: generally autosomal recessive, although X-linked and autosomal dominant variants exist

C. Clinical presentation
   1. Chronic sinusitis, serous otitis media, productive cough, male infertility, persistent otorrhea even after tympanostomy tubes are placed
   2. 20% have nasal polyps or clubbing of digits
   3. Course variably severe; all have some respiratory distress at birth; some patients elude diagnosis until adulthood

FIGURE 2-6 Respiratory mucosa.

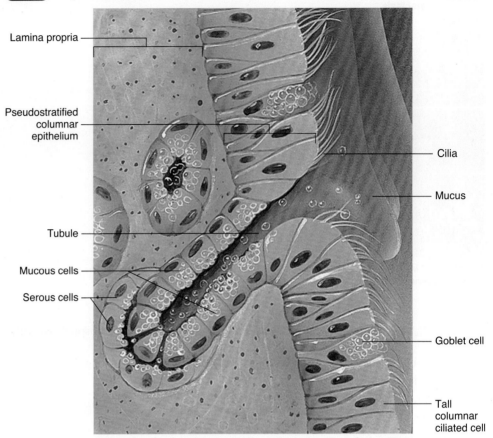

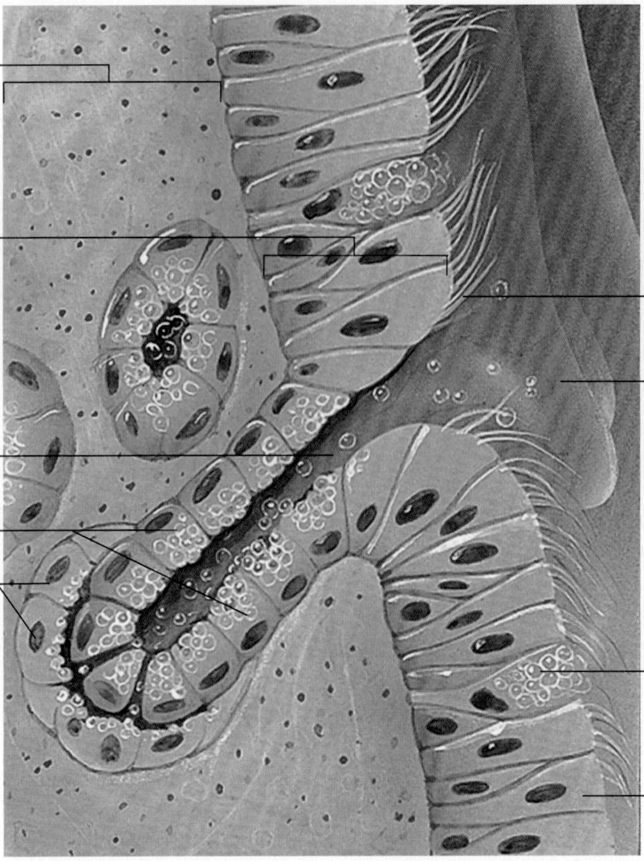

4. Kartagener syndrome: primary ciliary dyskinesia + situs inversus
5. Differential diagnosis
   a. CF: much more severe, progressive lung disease
   b. Primary immunodeficiency: screen with immunoglobulin levels
   c. Acquired ciliary dysfunction: smoking

D. Testing
1. CXR: may show situs inversus, hyperinflation, peribronchial thickening, atelectasis, and/or pneumonia
2. Chest CT sometimes indicated; may reveal bronchiectasis
3. PFTs show obstructive pattern
4. Gold standard electron microscopic evaluation of cilia (from nasal or bronchial specimens) demonstrating abnormal architecture (lack of dynein arms, abnormal microtubular pattern, disoriented cilia, etc.)
5. Immunoglobulins G, A, M, E to rule out immunodeficiency (should be normal)
6. Sweat chloride testing to rule out CF (should be normal)

E. Therapy
1. Chest physiotherapy to mobilize secretions
2. Antibiotics targeting growth in sputum cultures
3. Placement of tympanostomy tubes to preserve hearing
4. Avoidance of pulmonary irritants
5. Genetic counseling may be indicated
6. Prognosis: normal life span is possible with adequate treatment

QUICK HIT

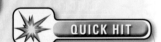

Half of patients with primary ciliary dyskinesia have situs inversus and, therefore, Kartagener syndrome, because organ rotation is random when unaided by ciliary action. Conversely, only 25% of patients with situs inversus have primary ciliary dyskinesia.

XV. Pulmonary Embolism (PE)

A. Definition
1. Blockage of the main pulmonary artery or one of its branches by varying materials generated elsewhere in body

B. Cause/pathophysiology
   1. Rarely seen in children; increasing incidence with improvement in treatment of more serious diseases and increased use of central lines
   2. Severity varies from asymptomatic to lethal; however, typically less severe than in adults, with 5× lower mortality rate
   3. Pathophysiology
      a. Most PEs originate as deep vein thrombosis, usually lower extremity, but also from pelvis, kidneys, upper extremities, or right side of heart
      b. Thrombus formation results from combination of host factors (i.e., Virchow triad = hypercoagulable state, stasis, and endothelial injury)

C. Clinical presentation
   1. History
      a. History of sudden-onset complaints of **pleuritic chest pain** or difficulty breathing
      b. 50% have cough, and ~30% have hemoptysis
   2. Physical exam
      a. Massive PE: rare in children but presents with cyanosis and signs of pulmonary HTN, right ventricular failure, or CHF, such as a loud pulmonary component of the second heart sound; right ventricular lift; distended neck veins; hypotension; heart murmurs and gallops; and peripheral edema
      b. In nonmassive PE, 50% will have tachypnea; tachycardia is common; crackles and friction rubs are rarely heard
      c. Lung sounds vary from diminished or absent breath sounds, to acute onset of wheezing, to normal lung findings

D. Testing
   1. Laboratory evaluation
      a. Routine laboratory tests (CBC, CRP, ESR) are not helpful
      b. ABG values show hypoxemia about 50% of the time, from $\dot{V}/\dot{Q}$ mismatch, intrapulmonary and intracardiac shunts, and decreased cardiac output; $PaCO_2$ often decreased due to hyperventilation
      c. D-dimer levels are highly sensitive but not specific, and may be elevated from generalized inflammation such as infection
   2. Imaging studies
      a. CXR: nonspecific, but may show atelectasis
      b. $\dot{V}/\dot{Q}$ scan: highly specific in terms of diagnostic accuracy when combined with high clinical likelihood
      c. Angiography: considered "gold standard" for diagnosis; however, has increased risk of morbidity/mortality
      d. Spiral CT
         i. Most common diagnostic technique due to ease and availability, equivalent in accuracy to $\dot{V}/\dot{Q}$ scan in ruling out PE
         ii. Radiation concerns may weigh against use in questionable cases

E. Therapy
   1. Anticoagulation: once stabilization of patient has occurred unless specifically contraindicated
      a. Initially low-molecular-weight heparin (LMWH) subcutaneously
      b. Long-term therapy depends on cause and future risk
   2. Thrombolytic therapy in clinically unstable patient with confirmed PE
   3. Inferior vena cava filters not indicated in pediatrics
   4. Embolectomy only in severe cases in which thrombolysis is ineffective or contraindicated

XVI. Allergic Bronchopulmonary Aspergillosis

A. Definition
   1. Hypersensitivity lung disease that occurs when *Aspergillus* colonizes bronchioles in patients with asthma or cystic fibrosis (CF)
   2. Affects 1%–2% asthmatic patients and 7%–9% CF patients

QUICK HIT

PE is exceedingly rare in children. If PE is found, an underlying cause should be sought.

MNEMONIC

Risk Factors for Pulmonary Embolism (The 3 I's & 3 O's)
Indwelling central line
Immobilization
Inherited disorders of hypercoagulation
Obesity
Oral contraceptive pills
Orthopedic surgery

QUICK HIT

Much like in adults, PEs can be the result of multiple causes including thrombi, air, tumor, or fat.

QUICK HIT

The majority of children found to have PE have symptoms that mimic other pediatric respiratory diseases, requiring a high index of suspicion for timely diagnosis.

QUICK HIT

If your patient has a normal D-dimer, the likelihood of PE is very low, and high radiation imaging likely is not indicated.

QUICK HIT

Initial therapy should be focused on resuscitation and stabilization of patient in whom PE is suspected.

QUICK HIT

Aspergillus species are ubiquitous molds that grow on decaying vegetation and in the soil and are transmitted primarily by inhalation of spores.

QUICK HIT

The first step when there is clinical concern for ABPA in a patient with asthma is a skin allergy prick test to *Aspergillus*.

QUICK HIT

Tobacco smoking significantly accelerates and worsens lung disease in A1AT deficiency.

QUICK HIT

Adenovirus is the leading pediatric etiology of postinfectious BO.

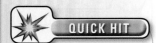

B. Cause/pathophysiology
1. In patients with asthma and CF, chronic bronchial colonization by *Aspergillus* causes an IgG- and IgE-mediated immune response with resultant inflammation, bronchial obstruction, and mucoid impaction
2. Pathologically, bronchial samples show eosinophilic pneumonia, mucoid impaction, and bronchocentric granulomatosis; *Aspergillus* species may also be seen on microscopy within bronchial lumen

C. Clinical presentation
1. Recurrent exacerbations in patient with asthma or CF with symptoms such as cough, wheeze, low-grade fever, and expectoration of brown mucus plugs; exacerbations commonly recur soon after stopping steroids
2. Needs high level of suspicion because acute symptoms are similar to exacerbations of asthma or CF
3. Long-term consequences of untreated ABPA include bronchiectasis, fibrosis, and respiratory compromise

D. Diagnostic testing
1. Can be diagnostically challenging to differentiate underlying asthma or CF from ABPA but important as correct diagnosis determines therapy
2. Criteria include allergy skin prick with immediate reactivity to *Aspergillus*, elevated total serum IgE >1,000 IU/mL, chest radiograph infiltrates, and peripheral blood eosinophilia.

E. Therapy
1. Treatment of choice is combination of systemic steroids and itraconazole
2. Prolonged steroid taper (3–6 months) to avoid relapse while monitoring with serum IgE levels and chest radiographs

XVII. α_1-Antitrypsin Deficiency

A. Definitions
1. Autosomal codominant genetic disorder causing reduced levels or abnormal forms of the enzyme α_1-antitrypsin (A1AT)
2. Occurs in about 1 in 3,000–5,000 people; more common in Caucasians

B. Cause/pathophysiology
1. A1AT is a protease inhibitor, particularly inhibiting elastase from neutrophils
2. Too little normal A1AT leads to unregulated destruction of elastin
3. Particularly important in lung where destruction of elastin leads to alveolar septal destruction and airspace enlargement (emphysema)
4. Abnormally formed A1AT cannot leave hepatocytes where it is made and leads to liver damage and chronic liver disease

C. Clinical presentation
1. Lung symptoms arise in early adulthood: dyspnea, chronic cough, wheeze
2. Often presents in infancy or early childhood with prolonged jaundice or hepatitis without another cause being found
3. Usually will have abnormal liver function tests or elevated transaminases early in life or may rapidly develop hepatic failure in childhood
4. With age, increased risk of developing advanced liver disease, cirrhosis, portal HTN, necrotizing panniculitis, or even hepatocellular carcinoma

XVIII. Bronchiolitis Obliterans

A. Definitions
1. Rare form of chronic obstructive fibrosing lung disease that results from obstruction/obliteration of the bronchioles and smaller airways
2. Develops after an insult to lower respiratory tract, most commonly seen in children after severe lower respiratory tract infection or as complication of lung or bone marrow transplantation

B. Cause/pathophysiology
1. Etiology is incompletely understood but related to an initial insult to small airways that results in dysfunction of epithelial cells or local necrosis
2. Pathologically characterized by obstruction and/or obliteration of small airways by inflammatory and fibrous tissue

3. Has been associated with connective tissue diseases, toxic fume inhalation, hypersensitivity pneumonitis, drugs (e.g., penicillamine), and Stevens-Johnson syndrome, but etiology is unknown in 1/3 of cases

C. Clinical presentation
1. In nontransplant patients, initial symptoms are similar to viral lower respiratory tract illness: fever, dyspnea, and cough
2. Symptoms progress to hypoxemia, tachypnea, wheezing, and crackles on exam that persist at least 60 days after initial insult

XIX. Children's Interstitial Lung Disease (chILD)

A. Characteristics
1. Group of rare conditions of lung parenchyma interfering with gas exchange
2. Share similar clinical features, radiologic picture, physiologic response, or pathologic appearance
3. Etiology: prevalence of about 3–4 cases per million children

B. Cause/pathophysiology
1. When cause of chILD is known, disorders can be grouped by primary pulmonary disorders and those secondary to systemic illness
2. Many forms are idiopathic and are grouped by histology or clinical picture
3. Some forms are specific to infants

C. Clinical features
1. Historical findings: common in child, but nonspecific
   a. Chronic cough
   b. Failure to thrive (suggests long-standing, advanced disease)
   c. Exercise intolerance
   d. Respiratory distress not responding to therapy
2. Physical exam findings
   a. Tachypnea, rales, retractions, dyspnea, wheezing
   b. Hypoxemia
   c. Abnormal cardiac exam (augmented P2, right-sided gallop) may suggest pulmonary HTN or cor pulmonale and indicate advanced disease
   d. Cyanosis and digital clubbing also indicate late-stage chILD
   e. Extrapulmonary findings that might suggest systemic illness
      i. Skin lesions (sarcoid, dermatomyositis, neurofibromatosis, etc.)
      ii. Eye changes (systemic lupus erythematosus, other vasculitis, etc.)
      iii. Lymphadenopathy (sarcoid, lymphoma, carcinomatosis, etc.)
      iv. Hepatosplenomegaly (Langerhans cell histiocytosis, amyloid)

D. Diagnosis
1. Differential diagnosis
   a. Extremely large number of diagnostic possibilities
   b. Infection, particularly in an immunocompromised host
   c. Aspiration from GERD, dysphagia/hypotonia, anatomic abnormalities
   d. Congestive heart disease
   e. Pulmonary vascular/lymphatic abnormalities or vasculitis
2. Laboratory findings
   a. Specific testing for underlying diseases may be indicated
   b. Viral or bacterial antibody titers (*Mycoplasma*, pertussis, etc.)
   c. Immune deficiency workup abnormalities, including HIV
3. Radiology findings
   a. CXR shows diffuse pulmonary infiltrates
   b. HRCT for disease location, severity, extent
      i. Classically shows ground glass opacities
      ii. Septal thickening, areas of hyperlucency, cysts, consolidation
4. Other findings
   a. PFTs: restrictive pattern, reduced forced vital capacity (FVC) and FEV_1
   b. ECG/Echo can show signs of pulmonary HTN
   c. Lung biopsy: most reliable diagnostic modality, guided by HRCT results

QUICK HIT
The chronic phase of chILD may last weeks to months with recurrent symptoms.

QUICK HIT
Most cases of chILD are diagnosed in the first year of life.

QUICK HIT
Thorough history is the key, particularly regarding feeding, environmental exposures, infection, and family histories.

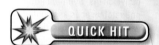

QUICK HIT
Routine labs are usually not helpful in diagnosis but can pick up underlying anemia, renal or hepatic disease, or hint at an immunodeficiency.

QUICK HIT
Oxygen saturation monitoring is normal with mild disease and low during sleep or exercise with moderate disease; chronic hypoxemia at rest occurs with advanced disease.

QUICK HIT
Biopsy is best by video-assisted thoracoscopy; transbronchial biopsy has limited usefulness in pediatric chILD.

QUICK HIT

Increased disease severity (i.e., more hypoxemia, lower activity tolerance, and pulmonary HTN) is associated with decreased survival. Overall, about 2/3 survive past 5 years.

QUICK HIT

All patients with chILD should be referred to a pediatric pulmonologist.

QUICK HIT

Spontaneous, primary pneumothoraces are most commonly due to ruptured subpleural blebs in the upper lobes of tall, thin males.

QUICK HIT

Small, asymptomatic pneumothoraces occur in 1%–2% of live births. Symptomatic pneumothoraces associated with meconium aspiration or positive pressure ventilation are much less common.

QUICK HIT

Pleuritic pain is sharp and stabbing in character, commonly with radiation to the ipsilateral shoulder.

d. BAL can be helpful in identifying certain conditions, but routine use in pediatric chILD is questionable

E. Treatment
1. Supportive care
2. Specific pharmacologic therapy
a. Some disorders and systemic disease causes have specific treatments
b. Corticosteroids are cornerstone of treatment for most types
c. Other immunosuppressive medications may be employed (e.g., hydroxychloroquine, cyclophosphamide, azathioprine, methotrexate)

XX. Pneumothorax

A. Characteristics
1. Accumulation of air between visceral and parietal pleura
a. Negative space is created as chest wall expands; air enters chest cavity and lung collapses
b. Subsequent hypoventilation and $\dot{V}/\dot{Q}$ mismatch
2. Spontaneous: rupture of visceral pleura
a. Primary: *no* underlying lung disease
b. Secondary: associated with underlying lung disease (Table 2-2)
3. Traumatic: rupture of visceral or parietal pleura
a. Penetrating or blunt trauma to lung, pleura, esophagus, or trachea
b. Iatrogenic: mechanical ventilation, bronchoscopy, central line placement, chest tube placement/removal
4. Pathophysiology
a. Simple: equalization of intrapleural and atmospheric pressures leading to partial lung collapse
b. Tension: 1-way valve through which air continues to enter, but cannot leave; intrapleural pressure is higher than atmospheric pressure, leading to increasing positive pressure in pleural space and progressive lung compression

B. Clinical features
1. Historical findings: abrupt onset with severity depending on degree of lung collapse
a. Small simple: asymptomatic +/− pleuritic chest pain
b. Large simple: sudden dyspnea and pleuritic chest pain
c. Tension: increasing dyspnea; altered mental status and other symptoms of shock may develop
d. Ask about symptoms of possibly causative underlying illness
i. Chronic or recurrent respiratory symptoms
ii. History of FBA or sudden choking episode
iii. History of extreme flexibility (i.e., Ehlers-Danlos syndrome)

TABLE 2-2 **Etiologies of Spontaneous Secondary Pneumothorax**

Congenital lung disease	Congenital cystic adenomatous malformation Congenital lobar emphysema
Increased intrathoracic pressure	Asthma Bronchiolitis Foreign body aspiration Cystic fibrosis
Connective tissue disorders	Marfan syndrome Ehlers-Danlos syndrome
Infection	Lung abscess Pneumatocele Bronchopleural fistula

2. Physical exam
   a. Small simple: <20% of lung collapsed; rarely have detectible pulmonary exam abnormalities
   b. Large simple: >20% of lung collapsed
      i. Increased work of breathing and hypoxia
      ii. Asymmetric chest rise
      iii. Decreased breath sounds and hyperresonance to percussion over pneumothorax
   c. Tension: progressively increasing work of breathing and hypoxia
      i. Deviation of trachea and apical cardiac impulse to contralateral side
      ii. *Decreased venous return leads to decreased cardiac output with tachycardia and hypotension*
   d. Assess for stigmata of causative underlying illness
      i. Fever, rales, wheeze, or other respiratory symptoms
      ii. Physical exam findings for Marfan or Ehlers-Danlos syndrome
      iii. Clubbing, or other signs of chronic respiratory illness
   e. Transillumination may be performed in newborns; affected area will transilluminate more brightly

C. Diagnosis
1. Differential diagnosis
   a. Diaphragmatic hernia
   b. Lobar emphysema
   c. Cystic adenomatous malformation
   d. Pneumomediastinum
2. Radiologic findings
   a. Chest radiograph
      i. Hyperlucent region without lung markings (Figure 2-7).
      ii. Atelectasis of lung tissue
      iii. Flattening of diaphragm on ipsilateral side.
      iv. Deviation of trachea and mediastinum to contralateral side in case of tension pneumothorax (Figure 2-8)

D. Treatment
1. Therapy is based on size of pneumothorax, severity of respiratory distress, and presence or absence of underlying lung disease
   a. Simple and small (<20% of lung volume)
      i. Inpatient observation with repeat chest radiograph
      ii. Supplemental oxygen hastens reabsorption of intrapleural air
      iii. Usually resolves within 1 week

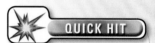

QUICK HIT

The chest radiograph should be taken with the patient in an upright position, if possible. If the patient is supine, air may layer anteriorly and not be detected as easily.

QUICK HIT

A CXR of a tension pneumothorax is an admission of a missed diagnosis. Needle decompression should be performed based on diagnosis by physical exam, and delay can result in significant morbidity/mortality.

FIGURE 2-7 **Chest radiograph demonstrating a small pneumothorax (<20% of lung collapsed) on the right.**

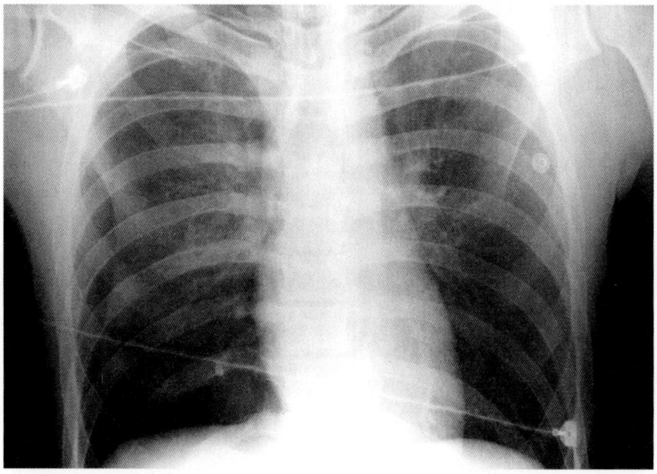

(From Harwood-Nuss A, Wolfson AB, Linden CH. *The Clinical Practice of Emergency Medicine*. 3rd ed. Philadelphia: Lippincott Williams & Wilkins; 2001.)

FIGURE 2-8 **Chest radiograph demonstrating a tension pneumothorax in a 5-year-old girl who was kicked in the chest by a horse.**

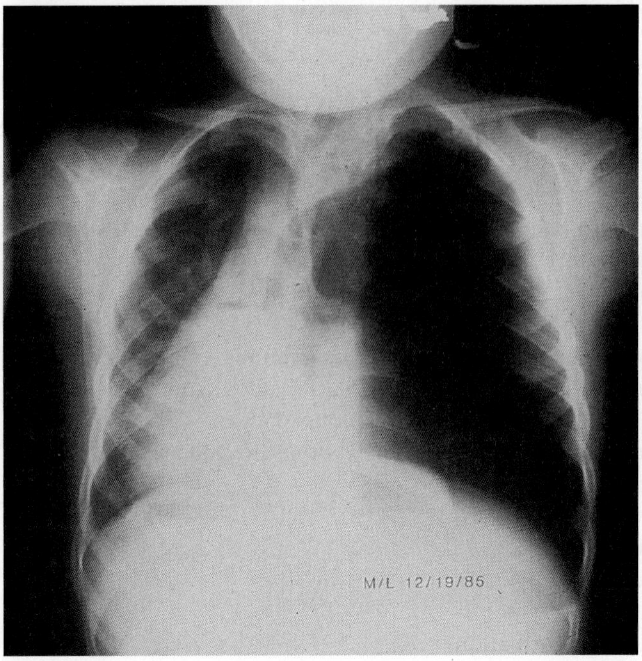

b. Tension or large
   i. Needle decompression: indicated for rapid decompensation or cardiopulmonary arrest
      (a) Insert large-bore angiocatheter into 2nd intercostal space at midclavicular line to aspirate air (Figure 2-9)
      (b) Should be followed by tube thoracostomy

FIGURE 2-9 **Needle decompression technique.**

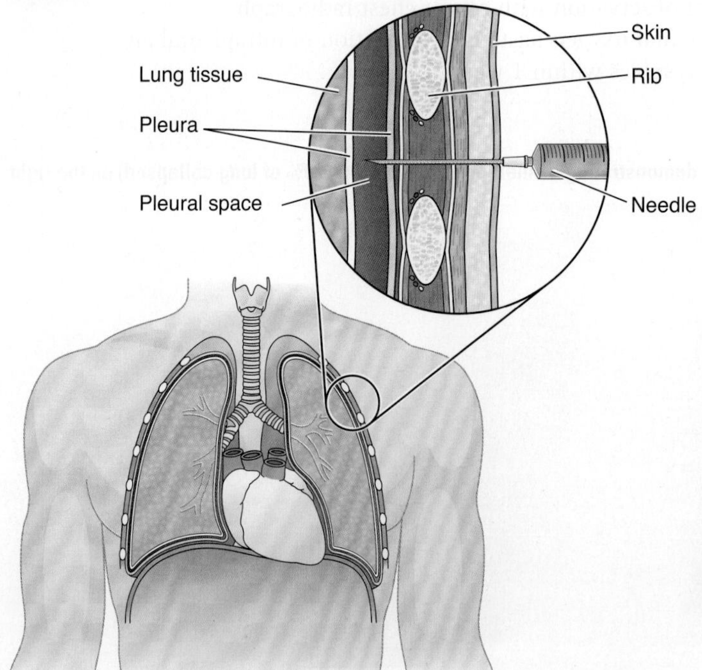

(From Cohen BJ. *Medical Terminology.* 4th ed. Philadelphia: Lippincott Williams & Wilkins; 2003.)

ii. Tube thoracostomy: insert chest tube into 5th intercostal space at midaxillary line
c. Intervention should *not* be delayed for confirmatory CXR in patient with evidence of pneumothorax on physical exam and respiratory distress or hemodynamic compromise
d. Surgical intervention may be required for persistent pneumothorax
2. Prevention: recurrence is common
a. Underlying lung disease, if present, should be addressed
b. Patients should avoid tobacco smoking, deep sea diving, and flying in unpressurized aircraft

3 Diseases of the Gastrointestinal System

SYMPTOM SPECIFIC

I. Acute Abdominal Pain

A. Background information
   1. Visceral/splanchnic pain
      a. Noxious stimuli affecting viscus or organ
      b. Tension, stretching, ischemia stimulate visceral nerve fibers
         i. Bilateral and unmyelinated fibers enter spinal cord at multiple levels
         ii. Pain is usually dull, poorly localized, and felt midline
            1. Foregut (lower esophagus and stomach): epigastric
            2. Midgut (small intestine): periumbilical
            3. Hindgut (large intestine): lower abdominal pain
   2. Parietal pain
      a. Noxious stimulation of parietal peritoneum
      b. Ischemia, inflammation, stretching of myelinated afferent fibers to dorsal root ganglion on same side and same dermatomal level as origination of pain
      c. Sharp, intense, localized
      d. Coughing or movement makes pain worse
   3. Referred pain
      a. Like parietal pain in remote areas, shared central pathways (supplied by same dermatome as affected organ)
      b. Achy and perceived near body surface
         i. Inflamed gallbladder T5, T10: scapular pain
         ii. Pneumonia T9: abdominal pain

B. Differential diagnosis (Box 3-1 and Figure 3-1)

C. Historical findings
   1. Location of pain (Figure 3-2)
   2. Timing, character, severity, duration, radiation
   3. Is the pain worse with movement?
   4. Is the patient vomiting? Is it bloody or bilious?
   5. Is the patient stooling normally? Is there blood in the stool?
   6. Is the pain relieved after a bowel movement or after vomiting?
   7. Any cough, shortness of breath, or chest pain?
   8. Any polyuria, dysuria, frequency, polydipsia, or unusual color of urine?
   9. Any associated joint pain or rash?

D. Pertinent physical exam findings
   1. General level of comfort and position of patient
   2. Vital signs
      a. Fever may indicate infectious etiology
      b. Tachypnea can result from pain but may also indicate respiratory infection or metabolic acidosis

> **QUICK HIT**
> Visceral pain is dull and poorly localized. Parietal pain is intense and localized.

> **QUICK HIT**
> Appendicitis begins as periumbilical pain that is poorly localized (visceral pain) and migrates to become RLQ pain (parietal pain).

> **QUICK HIT**
> There are many etiologies of acute abdominal pain that occur outside the GI system including pneumonia, streptococcal pharyngitis, and GU issues such as urinary tract infection, ectopic pregnancy, and ovarian torsion.

> **QUICK HIT**
> Previous abdominal surgery should alert the clinician to the possibility of small bowel obstruction caused by adhesions.

BOX 3-1

Differential Diagnosis for Acute Abdominal Pain

Gastrointestinal
Gastroenteritis
Appendicitis
Abdominal trauma
Peptic ulcer
Obstruction
Splenic infarct or rupture
Pancreatitis
Intussusception
Volvulus
Incarcerated hernia
Cholecystitis
Inflammatory bowel disease
Constipation

Metabolic
Diabetic ketoacidosis
Hyperglycemia

Pulmonary
Pneumonia
Pleurisy

Genitourinary
Urinary tract infection
Dysmenorrhea
Renal stones
Pelvic inflammatory disease
Threatened abortion/ectopic
Ovarian or testicular torsion
Endometriosis
Mittelschmerz

Heme
Sickle cell crisis
Henoch-Schönlein purpura
Hemolytic-uremic syndrome

Drugs/Toxins
Erythromycin
Salicylates
Lead poisoning/venoms

Miscellaneous
Colic
Functional pain
Pharyngitis

QUICK HIT

Because the abdominal exam of a toddler or young child can be challenging, watching the child move around the room, climb, walk, and interact with the parent prior to entering the room can provide useful information.

FIGURE 3-1 Evaluation of the child with abdominal pain.

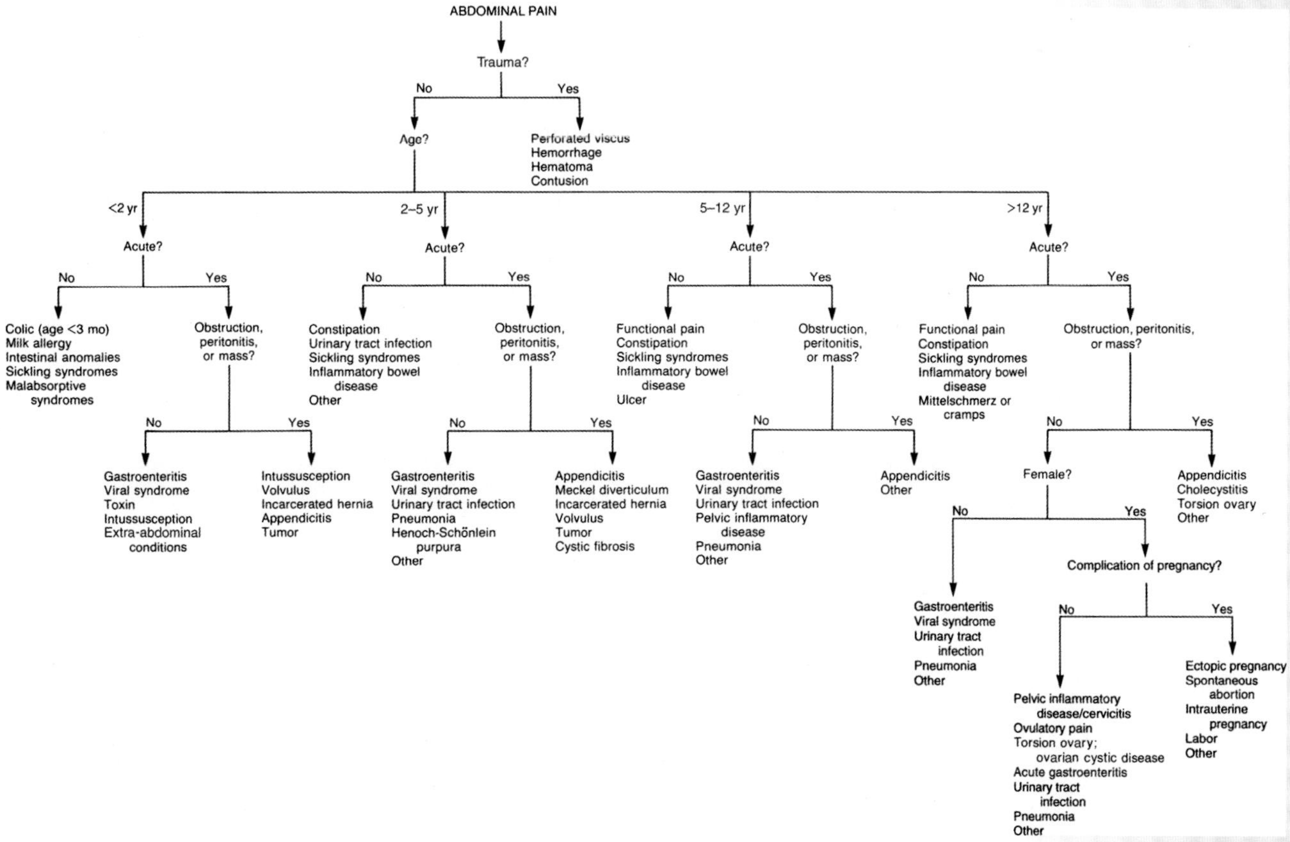

FIGURE 3-2 **Common sites of abdominal pain characteristic of various conditions.**

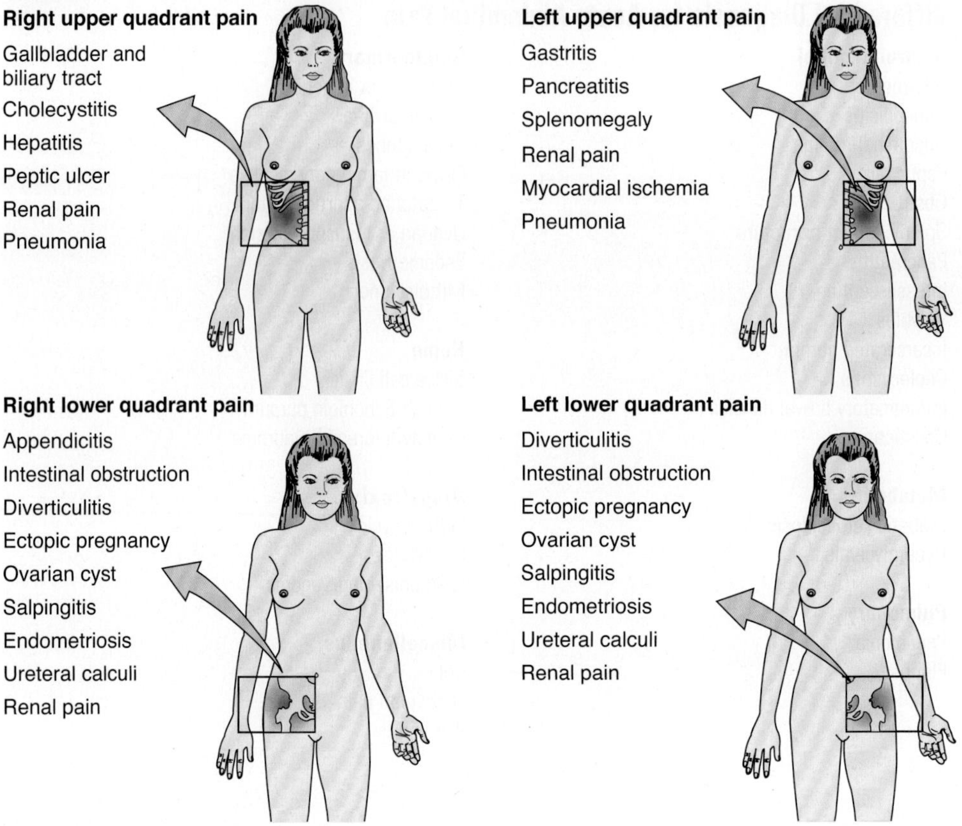

(From Willis MC. *Medical Terminology: A Programmed Learning Approach to the Language of Health Care*. Baltimore: Lippincott Williams & Wilkins; 2002.)

QUICK HIT

An immediate surgical consult is warranted for patients suspected of having peritonitis.

3. Abdominal exam
   a. Inspect: any signs of trauma or obvious masses, or asymmetry
   b. Auscultate: assess for bowel sounds in all 4 quadrants
   c. Palpate: assess for pain, guarding, rigidity, or signs of peritonitis (Box 3-2)
   d. Psoas sign: patient lies on left side, and examiner extends patient's right thigh while applying counter resistance to right hip; pain is elicited as inflamed retrocecal appendix comes in contact with stretched psoas muscle
   e. Obturator sign: patient lies on back with hip and knee flexed 90°; examiner moves lower leg laterally while applying resistance to lateral side of knee, resulting in internal rotation of femur; pain is elicited as inflamed appendix comes in contact with obturator internus muscle

BOX 3-2

Symptoms and Signs of Peritonitis

Symptoms
- Pain with movement
- Pain during bumpy car or ambulance ride

Signs
- Decreased or absent bowel sounds
- Involuntary guarding
- Rebound tenderness
- Rigid abdomen
- Tenderness while hopping up on and down on 1 leg

f. Murphy sign: patient inhales while examiner's fingers are wrapped under liver edge at bottom of rib cage; inspiration causes gallbladder to descend onto fingers, producing pain if gallbladder is inflamed
g. McBurney point: point on right side of abdomen 1/3 the distance from anterior superior iliac spine to navel; pain is elicited on palpitation
4. Rectal exam: look for fissures, skin tags, and fistulae, and, if indicated, assess for hard stool in vault and presence of blood
5. Genitourinary (GU) exam

E. Diagnostic workup
1. Laboratory evaluation as dictated by history and physical
a. Complete blood count (CBC)
b. Liver function tests (LFTs)
c. Amylase and lipase
d. Urinalysis
e. Urine pregnancy
f. Stool hemoccult
2. Radiologic imaging
a. Acute abdominal series
b. Ultrasonography
c. Upper gastrointestinal (GI) series can diagnose malrotation with midgut volvulus
d. Computed tomography (CT) scans
e. Chest x-ray (CXR) to assess for pneumonia, if indicated

QUICK HIT

In any menstruating female with abdominal pain, consider urine pregnancy test and pelvic exam.

QUICK HIT

Abdominal films may reveal signs of obstruction. The presence of free air is an indication for surgical evaluation.

QUICK HIT

Ultrasonography avoids the radiation associated with a CT scan and can be especially helpful in looking for gallstones, intussusception, ovarian cysts or torsion, and appendicitis.

II. Chronic Abdominal Pain

A. Background information
1. Classic definition of chronic or recurrent abdominal pain
a. Pain at least once per month for 3 consecutive months
b. Must interfere with routine, daily functioning
2. Estimated that ~50% of children will experience recurrent abdominal pain during childhood
3. Pain can be caused by an organic disease process or be functional in nature

B. Historical findings
1. Location of pain
a. Right upper quadrant (RUQ): liver or gallbladder
b. Left upper quadrant (LUQ): spleen
c. Right lower quadrant (RLQ): appendix or ovary
d. Left lower quadrant (LLQ): intestine or ovary
e. Epigastric: stomach or pancreas
f. Periumbilical: intestine
2. Does the pain radiate?
3. Are there exacerbating and alleviating factors?
4. Is the pain constant or episodic?
5. Historical red flags
a. Does the pain cause awakening from sleep?
b. Associated fevers?
c. Associated weight loss?
d. Any evidence of blood in the stool?
e. Emesis? If so, bile or blood stained?

C. Physical examination
1. Evaluation of growth parameters
2. Thorough abdominal examination, looking for tenderness, guarding, distension, and organomegaly

D. Differential diagnosis (Box 3-3)

E. Laboratory testing and radiologic imaging
1. Test should be ordered based on suspicion of diagnosis from history and physical examination
a. CBC: may reveal anemia, which can be seen with chronic disease or GI losses
b. Serum aminotransferases with total and direct bilirubin: can be abnormal in setting of cholelithiasis

QUICK HIT

Children with abdominal pain should receive the necessary analgesic medications to relieve their pain. The assessment can continue while relief is provided for the patient.

QUICK HIT

Functional abdominal pain implies that there is no identifiable organic etiology. It *does not* imply that the pain is fictitious or psychological.

QUICK HIT

Pancreatitis often causes back pain.

QUICK HIT

Any red flags that are elucidated by the history should prompt the physician to suspect a true organic cause for the child's pain and initiate an appropriate evaluation.

QUICK HIT

A proper evaluation of chronic abdominal pain must include assessment of all growth parameters. Organic disease may compromise weight, height, or both. Growth parameters typically remain normal in functional abdominal pain.

QUICK HIT

Abdominal examination should be used to determine if there are signs of an acute abdomen necessitating surgical intervention or hospitalization.

QUICK HIT

The level of dehydration helps determine the urgency of intervention.

QUICK HIT

Emesis from increased intracranial pressure tends to be recurrent and occurs after waking up in the morning.

QUICK HIT

Emesis in a neonate or small child without clear history or with change in mental status warrants workup for nonaccidental trauma.

BOX 3-3

Common Causes of Chronic Pain in Children by Anatomic Location

RUQ Pain
- Cholelithiasis
- Biliary dyskinesia
- Sphincter of Oddi dysfunction
- Musculoskeletal
- Functional abdominal pain

LLQ Pain
- Constipation
- Functional abdominal pain
- Irritable bowel syndrome
- Nephrolithiasis

LUQ Pain
- Gastritis
- *Helicobacter pylori* infection
- Celiac disease

Epigastric Pain
- Gastritis
- Esophagitis
- *Helicobacter pylori* infection
- Functional dyspepsia
- Celiac disease

RLQ Pain
- Appendiceal colic
- Constipation
- Irritable bowel syndrome
- Inflammatory bowel disease
- Functional abdominal pain
- Nephrolithiasis

Periumbilical Pain
- Functional abdominal pain
- Irritable bowel syndrome
- Constipation
- Celiac disease
- Inflammatory bowel disease
- Lactose intolerance

c. Albumin: hypoalbuminemia can suggest GI loss due to inflammation, decreased production by liver, or urinary losses in renal disease
d. Markers of inflammation (erythrocyte sedimentation rate [ESR] or C-reactive protein [CRP]): nonspecific, but are often elevated in inflammatory bowel disease (IBD)
e. Stool lactoferrin or fecal calprotectin: markers of intestinal inflammation
f. Stool *Helicobacter pylori* antigen
  i. Good sensitivity and specificity for active infection
  ii. False positives can occur if patient is taking proton pump inhibitors (PPIs)
g. Stool occult blood

2. Abdominal ultrasound
3. Abdominal x-ray: can provide information regarding stool burden

III. Approach to Vomiting

A. Background (Table 3-1)
  1. Definition
    a. Vomiting: forceful, coordinated expulsion of stomach (and sometimes intestinal) contents
    b. Regurgitation is effortless
  2. May be accompanied by nausea or retching

B. Historical findings
  1. Is the patient dehydrated?
  2. Is the emesis bilious, which could indicate intestinal obstruction?
  3. Is the emesis bloody, which could indicate a bleed from esophageal varices or a peptic ulcer?
  4. Are there any associated symptoms?
    a. Fever
    b. Headache
    c. Diarrhea
    d. Abdominal pain
    e. Altered mental status or lethargy
    f. Delayed menstrual cycle
    g. Rapid weight loss
  5. How long has the vomiting been going on?
    a. Acute
    b. Chronic: 3 or more episodes in 3 months
  6. What's the timing of vomiting in relation to feeds?
  7. Is the emesis recurrent, with asymptomatic periods between emesis?
  8. Detailed social history

TABLE 3-1 **Differential Diagnosis of Vomiting by Age**

Conditions	Characteristics	Associations
Birth to 6 months of age		
GERD	Emesis effortless <30 minutes after feedings Labs not required and/or normal Most infants grow out of condition	Poor growth in minority of cases Some present as ALTE Arching and discomfort during or after feedings
Pyloric stenosis	Projectile Around 4 weeks of age Healthy and hungry Visible peristalsis in epigastric area	1st born male child Hypochloremic metabolic alkalosis
Intestinal obstruction	Nonbilious: pyloric stenosis Bilious: ○ Malrotation with volvulus ○ Hirschsprung disease ○ Intestinal atresia ○ Intussusception (more common >6 months)	Malrotation: gastroschisis, diaphragmatic hernia, omphalocele, cardiac anomalies Hirschsprung: delayed meconium >48 hours Duodenal atresia: double-bubble sign on KUB, Down syndrome
Inborn errors of metabolism	Lethargy Poor feeding Acidosis Shock Seizure	CAH: hyperkalemic acidosis, hypotension, ambiguous genitalia in female infants Infants may have "fruity odors"
Shaken baby syndrome	May have other signs of abuse/trauma History not consistent with extent of illness	Retinal hemorrhage Multiple fractures of varying ages
Meningitis	Fever Bulging or tense anterior fontanelle	
UTI	Fever without a clear source	Uncircumcised male infant Congenital genitourinary anomalies
6 months to adolescence		
Acute gastroenteritis	+/− fever Sick contact	Diarrhea
Intussusception	6 months to 3 years Preceding URI Intermittent, colicky, with interval well periods Sausage-shaped abdominal mass in RLQ	Legs drawn up to abdomen Currant jelly stool (late finding) Meckel diverticulum
Meningitis	Inconsolable irritability Nuchal rigidity usually >18 months Absence of diarrhea	Purpuric rash in meningococcal disease
UTI	Fever without a clear source Dysuria, frequency, and urgency symptoms in verbal children	Uncircumcised male infant Congenial genitourinary anomalies
Appendicitis	Periumbilical, progressing to RLQ pain Tenderness at McBurney point	Perforation for delayed diagnosis Usually perforated at diagnosis <5 years of age
Pancreatitis	Epigastric pain radiating to the back Elevated amylase and lipase Etiology includes abdominal trauma	Cholecystitis
Hepatitis A	Often asymptomatic in young children Jaundice, acolic stool, and dark urine in older children	

(continued)

Diseases of the Gastrointestinal System

TABLE 3-1 **Differential Diagnosis of Vomiting by Age *(Continued)***

Conditions	Characteristics	Associations
Cholecystitis	(+) Murphy sign Sharp, colicky RUQ pain radiating to the back Worsened with fatty food	Underlying hemolysis: hemoglobinopathies, RBC membrane fragility
DKA	Polydipsia, polyphagia, and polyuria Hyperglycemia Weight loss	Fruity breath
CNS tumors	Recurrent morning emesis Absence of nausea	
Cyclic vomiting	School age Recurrent Well in the interim	Migraine
Munchausen by proxy	History of "doctor hopping" Extensive workup negative Symptoms exhibited only when caretaker is present	
Toxic ingestion	History often indicative	
Adolescents		
Peptic ulcer disease	Recurrent Epigastric	Psychosocial stressors *Helicobacter pylori* infections
Acute gastroenteritis	+/− fever Sick contact	Diarrhea
Pregnancy	Sexually active Tanner III and above	Menstruating female
Ovarian torsion	Intermittent, colicky pain, becoming more constant	
Bulimia	Distorted body image Psychosocial stressors	Large parotid glands, callus on knuckles, eroded enamels
Hepatitis A	Jaundice, acolic stool, and dark urine	
Hepatitis B	Jaundice, acolic stool, and dark urine	Sexual activities
Cholecystitis	(+) Murphy sign Sharp, colicky RUQ pain radiating to the back Worsened with fatty food	Female Obesity Underlying hemolysis
DKA	Polydipsia, polyphagia, and polyuria Hyperglycemia Weight loss	Fruity breath
Toxic ingestion	Psychosocial stressors Suicide ideation or attempt	
Migraine	Recurrent Phonophobia Photophobia Relieved by sleep (+) family history	+/− auras (+) family history Triggers
Pseudotumor cerebri	Elevated opening pressure	Vitamin A toxicity

ALTE, apparent life-threatening event; CAH, congenital adrenal hyperplasia; CNS, central nervous system; DKA, diabetic ketoacidosis; GERD, gastroesophageal reflux disease; RBC, red blood cell; RLQ, right lower quadrant; RUQ, right upper quadrant; URI, upper respiratory infection; UTI, urinary tract infection.

C. Pertinent physical exam findings
  1. Signs of dehydration
  2. Signs of peritonitis: "acute abdomen" (see Box 3-2)
  3. Complete exam is helpful to elucidate extra-abdominal etiologies of vomiting

D. Diagnostic workup
  1. Laboratory
    a. Electrolytes
      i. High blood urea nitrogen (BUN)/creatinine (Cr) ratio = dehydration
      ii. Decreased HCO_3^- = acidosis
        (a) Acute gastroenteritis (AGE) with excessive diarrhea
        (b) Inborn errors of metabolism
        (c) Metabolic acidosis in diabetic ketoacidosis (DKA)
    b. Urinalysis
    c. Lumbar puncture is indicated when there is concern for meningitis
    d. LFTs and amylase/lipase
    e. Pregnancy test in adolescent females
  2. Imaging studies
    a. Abdominal x-ray
      i. Absence of gas in rectum suggests obstruction
      ii. Upright or decubitus film required to visualize air–fluid levels characteristic of obstruction
    b. Upper GI with small bowel follow-through
      i. Visualizes intestinal anatomy, including constriction at terminal ileum to suggest IBD
    c. Ultrasound
    d. Abdominal CT

QUICK HIT

Presence of leukocyte esterase, elevated white blood cell (WBC) count on microscopy, and/or nitrite suggests UTI.

QUICK HIT

Abdominal x-ray is sometimes referred to as KUB (kidney, ureters, and bladder).

QUICK HIT

Upper GI without small bowel follow-through is sufficient to identify malrotation.

IV. Approach to Diarrhea

A. Definition
  1. By volume, >10 mL/kg/day of fluid lost through stools
  2. Leading cause of pediatric morbidity and mortality worldwide
  3. Caused by disturbed intestinal water absorption
    a. Secretory diarrhea: intestinal epithelial cells are actively secreting water and electrolytes due to secretagogue (e.g., cholera toxin)
    b. Osmotic diarrhea: ingested solutes are poorly absorbed either due to indigestible solute (e.g., sorbitol) or problem with small bowel mucosa (e.g., lactase deficiency)
    c. Motility disorders: increased motility leading to decreased transit time or decreased motility leading to bacterial overgrowth
    d. Decreased surface area (e.g., short bowel syndrome [SBS]) causing decreased solute absorption and decreased transit time

QUICK HIT

Per World Health Organization (WHO), diarrhea is defined as passage of 3 or more loose or watery stools per day.

QUICK HIT

The majority of diarrhea in developed countries is osmotic in nature.

TABLE 3-2 **Causes of Acute Diarrhea**

Etiology	Infants and Young Children	Older Children
Infectious	Viral gastroenteritis Bacterial enteritis *Clostridium difficile* Systemic infection (urinary tract infection, otitis media) Parasites	Viral gastroenteritis Bacterial enteritis *C. difficile* Food poisoning Parasites
Noninfectious	Antibiotic associated Hirschsprung toxic colitis Intussusception Neonatal opiate withdrawal Congenital adrenal hyperplasia	Antibiotic associated Appendicitis

Diseases of the Gastrointestinal System

TABLE 3-3 **Causes of Chronic Diarrhea**

Etiology	Infants and Young Children	Older Children
Infectious	Parasites Appendiceal abscess	Parasites Appendiceal abscess
Malabsorption	Postinfectious lactase deficiency Food protein intolerance Toddler's diarrhea Cystic fibrosis Celiac disease Shwachman-Diamond syndrome Disaccharidase deficiency Short bowel	Lactose intolerance Laxative abuse Celiac disease Disaccharidase deficiency Secretory neoplasms
Inflammatory	Eosinophilic gastroenteritis	Ulcerative colitis Crohn disease Eosinophilic gastroenteritis
Immunodeficiency	Severe combined immunodeficiency HIV enteropathy	HIV enteropathy
Endocrine	Adrenal insufficiency	Hyperthyroidism Hypoparathyroidism Adrenal insufficiency
Other	Intestinal lymphangiectasias Rare congenital bowel disorders Toxins	Encopresis (constipation) Irritable bowel syndrome Toxins

B. Differential diagnosis
   1. Acute: onset <2 weeks prior to presentation (Table 3-2)
      a. Most common etiology in all age groups is viral gastroenteritis
   2. Chronic: >2 weeks duration (Table 3-3)

C. Historical findings
   1. Presence of fever points to infectious etiology
   2. Blood or mucus in stools (bacterial enteritis or inflammation)
   3. Recent travel (parasites including *Giardia*)
   4. Recent antibiotic use (antibiotic-associated diarrhea or pseudomembranous colitis)
   5. Exposure to farm animals or reptiles (bacterial enteritis)

D. Physical examination findings
   1. Evaluate for dehydration
   2. Evaluate for other signs of systemic infection that could be causing diarrhea
   3. Careful abdominal exam to rule out appendicitis, peritoneal signs, distention, intra-abdominal mass
   4. Inspection of perianal area for fissures, fistulae, skin tags that may be suggestive of IBD

E. Laboratory testing
   1. Serum electrolytes indicated for all children with moderate to severe dehydration or prolonged course of diarrhea to rule out electrolyte abnormalities
   2. Stool bacterial cultures are indicated if blood or mucus in stools
   3. If suspicious of hemolytic-uremic syndrome, order specific culture for *Escherichia coli* O157:H7
      a. Evaluate renal function (BUN/Cr)
      b. CBC with smear to look for evidence of hemolysis, thrombocytopenia, and renal failure
   4. Stool for *Clostridium difficile* antigen testing or detection by polymerase chain reaction (PCR) if recent antibiotic exposure
   5. Can send stool rotavirus antigen to help distinguish from other causes
   6. Stool ova and parasite if international travel to endemic area
   7. Urinalysis to evaluate for urinary tract infection (UTI)

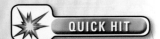

QUICK HIT

Toddler's diarrhea is a common phenomenon related to excessive fruit juice (sorbitol) ingestion by children ages 6 months to 3 years. Children are otherwise well appearing and gaining weight normally.

QUICK HIT

Fluid resuscitation with isotonic crystalloid solution should be initiated promptly in children with severe dehydration. For those with mild to moderate dehydration, oral rehydration may be attempted first.

QUICK HIT

E. coli O157:H7 is not detected by routine stool culture test, so it must be requested separately.

8. For chronic diarrhea associated with failure to thrive (FTT), consider testing for the following:
    a. Cystic fibrosis (CF): stool elastase, sweat test
    b. IBD: elevated inflammatory markers, ESR/CRP
    c. Malabsorption: stool-reducing substances, fecal fat
    d. Immunodeficiency: HIV, lymphocyte enumeration, immunoglobulin (Ig) profile

F. Endoscopy/colonoscopy: may be necessary for patients with chronic diarrhea and suspicion of IBD or malabsorption

V. Approach to Conjugated Hyperbilirubinemia

A. Definition of conjugated hyperbilirubinemia: >1 mg/dL if total bilirubin is <5 mg/dL or >20% of the total bilirubin

B. Differential diagnosis
1. Newborn (Box 3-4)
    a. Extrahepatic disorders
    b. Intrahepatic disorders
2. Older infants and children
    a. See list for differential in neonates

BOX 3-4

Differential Diagnosis of Conjugated Hyperbilirubinemia in the Newborn Period

Extrahepatic
- Biliary atresia
- Choledochal cyst
- Spontaneous perforation of the bile ducts
- Cystic fibrosis resulting in inspissated bile
- Neonatal sclerosing cholangitis
- Mass (stone, rhabdomyosarcoma, hepatoblastoma, neuroblastoma)

Intrahepatic
- Idiopathic neonatal hepatitis
- Hereditary syndromes of cholestasis
    - Alagille syndrome
    - Hereditary familial intrahepatic cholestasis
    - Progressive familial intrahepatic cholestasis
    - Neonatal Dubin-Johnson syndrome
    - Rotor
- Anatomic
    - Congenital hepatic fibrosis
- Metabolic disorders
    - α_1-Antitrypsin deficiency
    - Amino acid disorders (tyrosinemia)
    - Lipid disorders (Neiman-Pick disease, cholesterol ester storage disease, Wolman disease, Gaucher disease)
    - Carbohydrate disorders (galactosemia)
    - Peroxisomal disorders (Zellweger syndrome)
    - Disorders of bile acid metabolism
    - Disorders of bile acid transport
    - Urea cycle disorders (arginase deficiency)
- Infection
    - Bacterial
    - Viral
- Systemic disease causing cholestasis
    - Genetic (trisomy 17, trisomy 18, Down syndrome, Donahue syndrome)
    - Endocrine (hypothyroidism, hypopituitarism)
    - Cystic fibrosis
- Toxins
    - Drugs
    - Parenteral nutrition
- Vascular
    - Budd-Chiari syndrome, perinatal asphyxia, multiple hemangiomas, cardiac insufficiency

QUICK HIT

Any infant with jaundice at age 2 weeks should be evaluated for cholestasis with a conjugated or direct bilirubin.

QUICK HIT

Elevated conjugated bilirubin is *never* normal in a neonate!

QUICK HIT

Tests of synthetic function in liver include: prothrombin time (PT) with international normalized ratio (INR), partial thromboplastin time (PTT), coagulation factors, albumin, glucose, and ammonia.

> **QUICK HIT**
> FTT is multifactorial because both medical and psychosocial factors can contribute in an individual patient.

> **QUICK HIT**
> Endocrinopathies, such as hypothyroidism, may present with normal weight but poor linear growth.

> **QUICK HIT**
> Plotting of sequential points on an age- and gender-appropriate growth chart is essential. Remember to adjust for gestational age when plotting premature infants on a growth chart for weight until age 2 years.

> **QUICK HIT**
> Calculating and plotting body mass index typically begins at age 2 years. Prior to age 2 years, a weight-for-length ratio can be calculated and plotted.

> **QUICK HIT**
> Some patients, such as those with CF, may have multiple causes (e.g., excessive metabolic demands, malabsorption).

> **QUICK HIT**
> Ask about any events surrounding the time period when growth began to slow.

b. Also consider Wilson disease, Epstein-Barr virus (EBV), autoimmune hepatitis (AIH), cholecystitis, cholelithiasis, tumor (hepatic, biliary, pancreatic, peritoneal, duodenal), primary sclerosing cholangitis (PSC), veno-occlusive disease

C. Historical findings
1. Family history of liver disease, consanguinity, complications of pregnancy or delivery, infectious exposures (including congenital infections)
2. Jaundice, icterus, acholic stools, dark urine, vomiting, poor feeding, dietary history, weight gain
3. Lethargy, irritability, fever

D. Physical examination findings
1. Growth parameters
2. Vital signs: fever, signs of shock/sepsis (tachycardia, hypotension)
3. Skin: degree of jaundice, petechiae, purpura, or bruising, telangiectasia
4. Conjunctival icterus
5. Cardiac murmur or signs of heart failure
6. Abdominal exam: prominent abdominal vasculature, ascites, liver size and consistency, spleen size and consistency, abdominal mass

E. Laboratory testing
1. Total and direct/conjugated bilirubin, serum bile acids
2. Aspartate aminotransferase (AST), alanine aminotransferase (ALT), alkaline phosphatase (ALP), γ-glutamyl transpeptidase (GGT)
3. Tests of synthetic function
4. Specific investigations based on differential

F. Radiologic imaging and other
1. Abdominal ultrasound with Doppler: evaluate gallbladder, extrahepatic and intrahepatic bile ducts, mass, ascites, portal hypertension, triangular cord sign
2. Hepatobiliary scintigraphy (HIDA): evaluate for appropriate uptake and excretion of tracer
3. Cholangiogram (intraoperative, magnetic resonance, or endoscopic retrograde): definitive evaluation of intrahepatic and extrahepatic biliary tree
4. Liver biopsy: fibrosis, inflammation, bile duct proliferation, storage diseases (e.g., Niemann-Pick, Gaucher)

VI. Approach to Failure to Thrive

A. Definition: poor growth/growth failure when compared to peers on standardized growth chart
1. Objective measures used to identify children with FTT
   a. *Weight below 2nd percentile* for age and gender on more than 1 occasion
   b. *Weight <80% of ideal weight* for age
   c. *Crossing of 2 major percentile lines* over time beyond 6 months of age
2. Can affect weight, height, weight-for-height, and/or head circumference
3. Possible outcomes if untreated include short stature, secondary immune deficiency, and long-term effects on cognition and behavior
4. Classification system for causes of FTT is commonly employed (Table 3.4)
   a. *Inadequate intake or absorption*
   b. *Inefficient or defective use of calories*
   c. *Excessive metabolic demands*

B. History is most important component in evaluation of FTT
1. Prenatal/perinatal history
   a. Prematurity, intrauterine growth restriction (IUGR), low birth weight predispose to FTT
   b. Prenatal exposures (e.g., maternal infection, alcohol, maternal medications)
2. Growth and development history
   a. Has the child always been small?
   b. Did the child have normal growth and then slowly or suddenly "fall off the curve"?
   c. Has the child been meeting his/her developmental milestones at prior visits?

TABLE 3-4 **Causes of Failure to Thrive by Specialty**

Specialty	Examples
Ear, nose, and throat	Cleft palate/lip, oral motor dysfunction, dental caries, adenoidal hypertrophy, obstructive sleep apnea
Pulmonary	Bronchopulmonary dysplasia, cystic fibrosis, asthma
Cardiovascular	Congenital or acquired heart disease
Nutrition	Excessive juice consumption, inappropriate mixing of formula, insufficient maternal lactation, inappropriate feeding technique, inappropriate food for age, inadequate food quantity
Gastrointestinal	Celiac disease, inflammatory bowel disease, cystic fibrosis, food allergy, chronic constipation, Hirschsprung disease, gastroenteritis (i.e., bacterial, parasitic), gastroesophageal reflux, enzyme deficiency (i.e., disaccharidase deficiency), pancreatitis, intestinal obstruction (i.e., pyloric stenosis), short gut syndrome, hepatitis, chronic liver disease, biliary atresia
Renal	Renal tubular acidosis, urinary tract infection
Endocrine	Hyperthyroidism, hypothyroidism, adrenal insufficiency, diabetes mellitus
Hematology/oncology	Anemia (i.e., iron deficiency), malignancy
Neurology	Increased intracranial pressure (i.e., tumor, hydrocephalus), cerebral palsy, hypotonia, muscle weakness (i.e., myopathy), hypertonia, oral motor dysfunction
Infectious disease	Immunodeficiency (i.e., HIV), chronic infection
Rheumatology	Juvenile idiopathic arthritis
Genetic/metabolic	Genetic syndromes (i.e., chromosomal, teratogens), storage disorders (i.e., glycogen storage disorder), inborn errors of metabolism (i.e., galactosemia)
Psychosocial	Depression (patient or parent), anorexia nervosa, bulimia nervosa, neglect, economic hardship, Munchausen by proxy (i.e., ipecac administration), poor caregiver–child relationship, inadequate parental knowledge

3. Dietary and feeding history
   a. What is the child eating/drinking and how much?
   b. What is the setting at mealtimes?
      i. Distracting factors, including television
      ii. Duration of feedings: hurried, relaxed, prolonged
   c. Who feeds the child, and is there consistency among care providers?
   d. Does the child feed himself or herself? Is he or she developmentally able to?
   e. Does the child seem interested in eating?
      i. Decreased appetite seen with medications, chronic disease, excessive juice consumption
      ii. May stem from pain, including gastroesophageal reflux (GER), dental caries
      iii. Consider eating disorders in older children/teens
4. Review of systems
   a. Diarrhea
   b. Constipation
      i. Severe constipation leads to decreased appetite
      ii. Consider hypothyroidism, especially with poor linear growth
   c. Vomiting
      i. Arching behaviors seen with GER
   d. Cough or difficulty breathing
      i. Noisy/mouth breathing with adenoidal hypertrophy
      ii. Chronic lung disease increases metabolic demands

QUICK HIT

A 24- to 72-hour food diary is extremely helpful because parental recall is often inaccurate.

QUICK HIT

Inappropriate mixing of formula should be addressed due to altered caloric density and possible electrolyte disturbances.

QUICK HIT

Infants should breastfeed at least 8 times a day in the first 4 months of life.

QUICK HIT

Food avoidance behaviors (e.g., textures) may be seen in children with oral motor dysfunction, food allergies, or autism spectrum disorder.

QUICK HIT

Prolonged feeding times may indicate oral motor dysfunction.

QUICK HIT

Child autonomy can be a struggle; the child desires self-feeding while parents want to avoid a mess.

QUICK HIT

A common side effect of stimulant therapy in attention-deficit hyperactivity disorder is decreased appetite.

e. Frequent infections
   i. Consider immunodeficiency
   ii. Frequent pulmonary infections with CF
5. Family history, record parental and sibling heights
6. **Psychosocial factors** play significant role in FTT
   a. **Poverty**, young parental age, **parental depression/mental illness**, substance abuse, **marital problems** commonly seen with FTT
   b. Assess parental knowledge and beliefs about appropriate diets in children

C. Physical exam often reveals no obvious etiology for FTT
1. Look for signs of an underlying medical condition
2. Vitamin deficiencies due to malnutrition may have specific findings

D. Laboratory testing and radiologic imaging should be directed by history and physical exam
1. CBC to assess for anemia
2. Serum electrolytes, glucose, calcium, phosphorus, magnesium, albumin, total protein
3. Hepatic and renal function testing (i.e., liver enzymes, BUN/Cr)
4. Urinalysis and urine culture used to assess for chronic UTI or renal tubular acidosis
5. ESR and CRP assess for possible inflammatory disorder (e.g., IBD)
6. Tissue transglutaminase and/or anti-endomysial antibodies, total IgA to look for celiac disease
7. Growth hormone and thyroid testing reserved for those with poor linear growth

QUICK HIT

Celiac disease presents with chronic abdominal pain, poor growth, and diarrhea due to malabsorption. These children commonly, but not always, have abdominal protuberance and thin extremities.

QUICK HIT

Pyloric stenosis and gastric outlet obstruction (seen with eosinophilic gastritis) present with forceful emesis.

QUICK HIT

Frequent vomiting may be a sign of increased intracranial pressure due to hydrocephalus or tumor.

VII. Approach to Gastrointestinal Bleeding

A. Upper GI bleeding
1. Defined as bleeding *originating above ligament of Treitz*
2. Uncommon in children
3. Hematemesis: frank red blood indicates more rapid bleeding than "coffee ground" emesis (black grainy material)
4. Melena: black, tarry, foul-smelling stools
   a. At least 50–100 mL blood loss per 24 hours that may continue for 3–5 days

B. Lower GI bleeding
1. Defined as bleeding *originating distal to ligament of Treitz*
2. Hematochezia: bright red blood per rectum
3. Melena: black, tarry, foul-smelling stools; source is usually proximal to ileocecal valve

C. Differential diagnosis (Boxes 3-5 and 3-6)

QUICK HIT

Congenital heart disease often presents with respiratory complaints and tiring with feedings.

QUICK HIT

A history of frequent injuries may be a clue to poor supervision and neglect.

QUICK HIT

Calculating midparental height is helpful to determine genetic potential.

QUICK HIT

Less than 2% of FTT laboratory values are of diagnostic significance and can likely be predicted by the history and physical exam.

BOX 3-5

Causes of Upper Gastrointestinal Bleeding in Children by Age

Neonate
- Swallowed maternal blood
- Stress ulcers, gastritis
- Dietary protein intolerance (cow's milk, etc.)
- Acid peptic disease
- Trauma (nasogastric tube)
- Vitamin K deficiency (hemorrhagic disease of the newborn)
- Bleeding disorder/coagulopathy
- Duplication cysts
- Vascular malformations

Infants and Toddlers
- Dietary protein intolerance (cow's milk allergy)
- Gastritis
- Esophagitis
- Acid peptic disease
- Foreign body ingestion
- Mallory-Weiss tear
- Variceal bleeding
- Bleeding disorder/coagulopathy
- Bowel obstruction
- Duodenal or gastric webs
- Duplication cyst
- Vascular malformation

Children and Adolescents
- Gastritis
- Esophagitis
- Peptic ulcer disease
- Pill esophagitis/ulcers
- Mallory-Weiss tear
- Inflammatory bowel disease
- Foreign body/caustic ingestion
- Variceal bleeding
- Bleeding disorder/coagulopathy
- Bowel obstruction

BOX 3-6

Causes of Lower Gastrointestinal Bleeding in Children by Age

Neonate
- Swallowed maternal blood
- Dietary protein intolerance (cow's milk, etc.)
- Vitamin K deficiency (hemorrhagic disease of the newborn)
- Infectious enterocolitis
- Anorectal fissure
- Necrotizing enterocolitis
- Bleeding disorder/coagulopathy
- Hirschsprung disease with enterocolitis
- Malrotation with volvulus
- Vascular malformation

Infants and Toddlers
- Dietary protein intolerance (cow's milk)
- Infectious enterocolitis
- Anorectal fissure
- Hirschsprung disease with enterocolitis
- Malrotation with volvulus
- Ileocolic intussusception
- Bleeding disorder/coagulopathy
- Meckel diverticulum
- Vascular malformation

Children and Adolescents
- Anorectal fissure
- Hemorrhoids
- Infectious enterocolitis
- Juvenile polyps
- Allergic colitis
- Inflammatory bowel disease
- Meckel diverticulum
- Solitary rectal ulcer
- Bleeding disorder/coagulopathy
- Vasculitis (e.g., Henoch-Schönlein purpura)
- Hemolytic-uremic syndrome

D. Historical findings
1. Initial assessment
   a. Is the patient hemodynamically stable?
   b. Assess mental status, severity and characteristics of bleeding, coexisting disease
2. Is it really the patient's blood?
   a. Rule out swallowed maternal blood in newborn infants
   b. Ask about iron ingestion or red food/drink
3. Characteristics of bleeding
   a. Color (bright red, maroon, black, or "coffee ground"), volume, and duration of bleeding
   b. Consistency
      i. Hematochezia limited to outside of stool suggests anal or rectal origin
      ii. Hematochezia mixed through stool suggests colonic source
      iii. Mixed with mucus or loose stools suggests colitis
4. Additional history
   a. Associated GI symptoms (vomiting, diarrhea, pain)
   b. Associated systemic symptoms (fever, rash, dizziness, shortness of breath, jaundice, easy bleeding or bruising)
   c. Exposures: trauma, recent travel, ill contacts, contact with animals
   d. Medications: iron, nonsteroidal anti-inflammatory drugs (NSAIDs), warfarin, recent antibiotic use, corticosteroids
   e. Past medical history and family history of GI disorders, liver disease, bleeding problems/disorders

E. Physical exam findings
1. Skin: pallor, capillary refill, skin lesions (hemangioma, telangiectasia, ecchymoses, rash), jaundice
2. Head, eyes, ears, nose, throat: nasopharyngeal oozing, inflammation, tonsillar enlargement
3. Cardiovascular/respiratory: heart rate, pulse pressure, gallop rhythm, abnormal breath sounds
4. Abdominal exam: hepatomegaly, splenomegaly, tenderness, mass, ascites
5. Perineum/rectum: fissure, fistula, rash, induration, external hemorrhoids, vascular lesion, gross blood, melena, tender rectal exam

F. Testing
1. Laboratory testing
   a. Hemoccult or gastroccult to confirm the presence of blood (use correct test and beware of false positives (i.e., iron, red meat, cantaloupe, radishes, turnips, cauliflower, broccoli, and grapes have peroxidases)

QUICK HIT

Melena can be caused by upper or lower GI bleeding.

QUICK HIT

Is it really from the GI tract? Or could it be hemoptysis, swallowed blood from nasopharyngeal source (epistaxis, oral trauma), hematuria, menstrual blood, or bleeding from perineum?

QUICK HIT

"Currant jelly" suggests ischemic bowel lesions.

b. CBC (and repeated values to assess ongoing losses) with hemoglobin and hematocrit, platelet count, mean cell volume
c. Blood type and cross match
d. Coagulation studies
e. Chemistries: liver enzymes, albumin, BUN/Cr, ESR
f. Urinalysis
g. Apt-Downey test (for fetal versus maternal hemoglobin)
h. Stool studies (*C. difficile*, stool culture, ova and parasites, lactoferrin/calprotectin)

2. Nasogastric (NG) lavage: bright red blood or coffee grounds confirm GI or nasopharyngeal source; can assess whether blood loss is ongoing
3. Radiology/imaging studies
   a. Abdominal radiograph (obstruction, pneumatosis)
   b. Abdominal ultrasound (signs of liver disease/portal hypertension, varices, intussusception)
   c. Meckel scan
   d. Angiography (obscure or refractory bleeding; suspected arteriovenous malformation [AVM]; requires bleeding rate >0.5 mL/min)
4. Endoscopy/colonoscopy: for diagnosis and treatment
   a. Esophagogastroduodenoscopy (EGD)
      i. Preferred method for diagnosing and treating upper GI bleeding
      ii. Contraindicated if patient is unstable
      iii. Biopsies allow identification of inflammation and *H. pylori*
   b. Colonoscopy
      i. Preferred method for diagnosing and treating lower GI bleeding
      ii. Biopsies allow identification of inflammation

QUICK HIT

Colonoscopy is contraindicated if patient is unstable or if there is suspected obstruction or ischemia, fulminant colitis, toxic megacolon, suspected perforation or peritonitis, pneumatosis intestinalis, or suspected intussusceptions.

QUICK HIT

Appendicitis is a true surgical emergency that leads to serious complications without prompt treatment; untreated appendicitis leads to perforation, peritonitis, and abdominal abscess, usually within 72 hours.

QUICK HIT

Appendicitis is difficult to diagnose in children under age 5 years, in which the majority of cases present after perforation (>70%).

QUICK HIT

For most surgical causes of abdominal pain in children, including appendicitis, abdominal pain precedes emesis.

QUICK HIT

Significant pain in children often wakes them up from sleep or interferes with activities.

QUICK HIT

Children younger than 5 years old may not have classic symptoms; instead, they may present with fever, diarrhea, and fussiness.

DISEASE SPECIFIC

VIII. Appendicitis

A. General characteristics
1. Inflammation of appendix, an anatomic outpouching of cecum, usually in RLQ of abdomen
2. Most common childhood condition requiring emergency surgery
3. Incidence peaks in 2nd decade of life
4. Slightly higher incidence in boys
5. Usually starts with obstruction of the narrow outpouching, which results in its inflammation after overgrowth of gut flora within space
6. Appendiceal obstruction can be from fecalith, food particle, or tumor

B. Clinical features
1. Historical findings
   a. Classically include abdominal pain, fever, anorexia, and emesis
   b. Abdominal pain is initially vague periumbilical pain (splanchnic, visceral, or referred) progressing to RLQ pain over hours
   c. Include questions to assess hydration status; fluid resuscitation is often necessary
   d. History of sick contact is helpful with infectious etiology, such as AGE
   e. Obtain gynecologic and sexual history for adolescent female patients

C. Physical exam findings (Box 3-7)
1. Fever is almost always present, but usually not high grade
2. Dehydration is common feature, with resultant elevated heart rate
3. Patients with appendicitis, especially with peritonitis, guard their abdomen by splinting and avoiding any movement; pain is reported with movement of bed and ambulation
4. Tenderness with palpation classically at McBurney point, 2/3 way down straight line between umbilicus and anterior superior iliac spine (Figure 3-3)
5. Deeper palpation is required to elicit pain with inflamed appendix in retrocecal or pelvic position

BOX 3-7

Physical Exam Signs for Appendicitis

- Rovsing sign: RLQ pain (subjective) or tenderness (objective) with palpation of the LLQ
- Psoas sign: RLQ pain or tenderness when the right leg is hyperextended while applying counter resistance to the right hip (especially for retrocecal appendix)
- Obturator sign: RLQ pain or tenderness when the right hip is internally rotated (especially for pelvic appendix)

6. Rebound tenderness and Rovsing sign with peritonitis
7. Gynecologic exam and testicular exam for adolescents

D. Diagnosis
1. Appendicitis is clinical diagnosis supported by laboratory and imaging studies
   a. Clinical decision rules were developed to increase diagnostic certainty
2. Differential diagnosis
   a. Ranges from benign, self-limited conditions to serious surgical emergencies
   b. Gynecologic conditions, such as ovarian torsion or ectopic pregnancy, can mimic appendicitis in menstruating adolescents
3. Laboratory findings
   a. Elevated WBC with left shift (95%)
   b. Electrolytes may be abnormal in cases of dehydration
   c. High specific gravity or presence of ketones on urinalysis
   d. Sterile pyuria may be present
   e. Pregnancy test may indicate an ectopic pregnancy in adolescent females
4. Radiology findings (Figure 3-4)

E. Treatment
1. Therapy
   a. Surgical removal of inflamed appendix, either by laparoscopy or open laparotomy
   b. Surgical intervention must not be delayed
   c. Rehydration, including intravenous (IV) fluid resuscitation, is often required
   d. Perforation (~10%–20% in older children and adolescents) and abdominal abscess

FIGURE 3-3 **Appendicitis, location. Frontal view of female child's abdominal anatomy showing location of appendix; McBurney point is indicated as dot on dashed line drawn between anterior spine of ilium and the navel.**

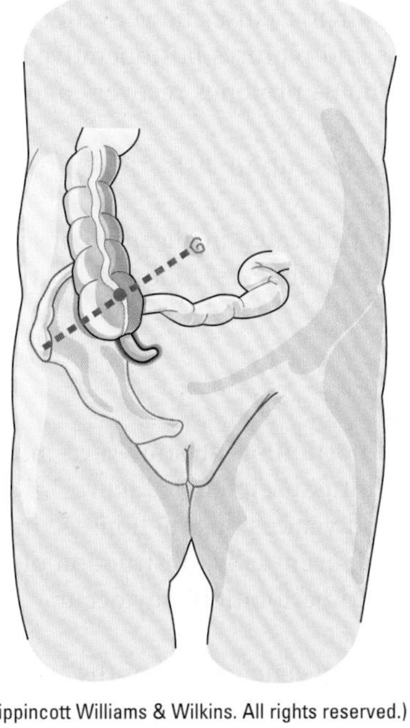

QUICK HIT

High fever, toxic appearance, signs of shock, WBC >15,000/mm^3, and elevated inflammatory markers suggest perforation and sepsis.

QUICK HIT

Children younger than 5 years old presenting with perforated appendix have high fever and symptoms of sepsis or shock.

QUICK HIT

A rectal exam can be helpful to diagnose an inflamed appendix in the retrocecal or pelvic position.

QUICK HIT

Sonogram or abdominal CT is useful in equivocal cases.

QUICK HIT

Narcotic pain medication should be used and will not prevent diagnosis from being made.

FIGURE 3-4 Abdominal film of an appendicolith (*A; open arrow*) in a gas-filled appendix (*closed arrow*).

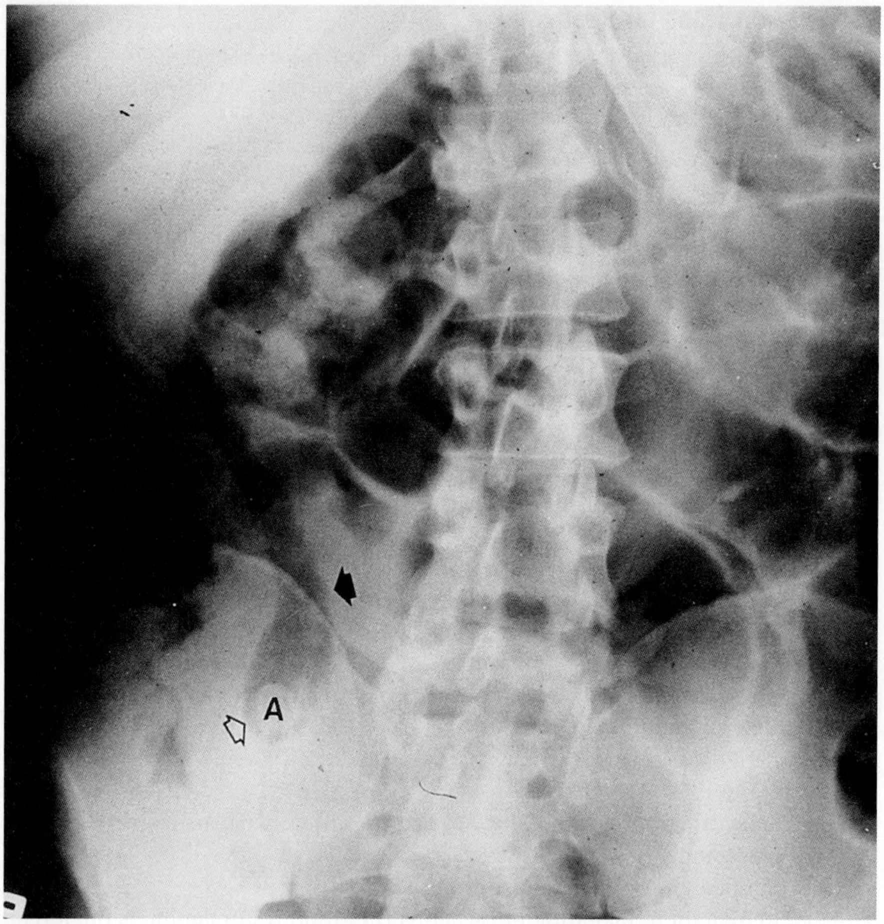

(From Daffner RH. *Clinical Radiology: The Essentials*. 3rd ed. Philadelphia: Lippincott Williams & Wilkins; 2007.)

2. Duration/prognosis
   a. Recovery is more rapid with laparoscopic appendectomy than with laparotomy
   b. Gangrenous appendicitis causes bowel wall compromise and microperforations and requires postoperative IV antibiotics
   c. Perforated appendicitis prolongs recovery and has highest rate of complications
      i. Abdominal abscess (up to 30%)
      ii. Persistent ileus
      iii. May be able to be treated medically (conservatively) with broad-spectrum antibiotics, followed by interval appendectomy; failure rate remains high (~30%–40%)

IX. Intussusception

A. General characteristics
1. Prolapse of proximal portion of intestine (i.e., intussusceptum) into distal portion of intestine (intussuscipiens) (Figure 3-5)
2. Mesentery dragged and venous obstruction occurs, resulting in edema; mucosal bleeding; and, eventually, obstruction of arterial flow as pressure increases; gangrene and perforation may occur
3. Epidemiology
   a. Most often occurs between ages 3 months and 6 years, with peak incidence in infants between ages 6 and 12 months

QUICK HIT

Most common location is near ileocecal junction (ileocolic intussusception).

FIGURE 3-5 **In this drawing of intussusception, note the telescoping of a portion of the bowel into the distal portion.**

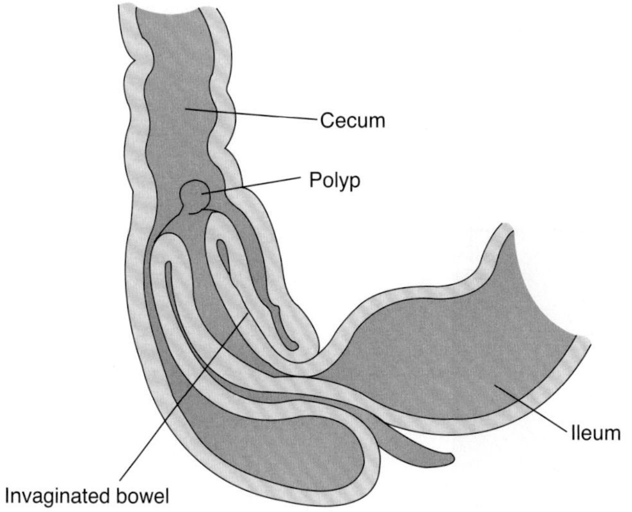

b. Older children tend to have "lead" point such as polyp, lymphoma, neurofibroma, Meckel diverticulum, hematoma with Henoch-Schönlein purpura (HSP), or inspissated stool with CF
c. Some evidence suggests there may be link with viral infections such as adenovirus

B. Clinical features
1. Historical findings
a. Sudden onset of severe paroxysmal colicky pain in previously well child
i. Classic pain lasts for 1–5 minutes, abates for 5–20 minutes, and recurs episodically
ii. Child may draw knees toward chest
2. Progressive fatigue and lethargy may ensue over hours
3. Vomiting is commonly present, is usually more frequent early in course, and may become bilious as obstruction progresses
4. Stools may appear normal initially, then decrease with little or no flatus; stools containing red blood and mucus may develop (i.e., "currant jelly" stool)
5. Physical exam findings
a. Abdominal exam may be normal or show abdominal distension
b. A slightly tender sausage-shaped mass may be palpable, usually in RUQ
c. Rectal exam may reveal gross blood, occult blood, foul-smelling stool, or "currant jelly" stool

C. Diagnosis
1. Laboratory findings: not helpful unless bowel is ischemic or necrotic, in which case acidosis may be present
2. Radiology findings
a. Plain films
i. Usually neither sensitive nor specific
ii. May see visible abdominal mass or abnormal distribution of gas or fecal contents, air–fluid levels
iii. "Target sign" to right of spine is occasionally seen and represents concentric circles of fat densities, surrounding or within the intussusception, alternating with layers of mucosa and muscle
b. Ultrasonography
i. "Bull's eye" or "coiled spring"
ii. Doppler may be helpful to identify bowel ischemia
iii. May help identify a lead point
c. CT is only helpful when other modalities are unrevealing
d. Enema: air, saline, or barium can be diagnostic and therapeutic (Figure 3-6)

QUICK HIT
Between episodes of pain, the child is commonly lethargic.

QUICK HIT
Ultrasonography is preferred modality because it can identify ileocolic to ileo-ileal intussusception.

QUICK HIT
The classic triad for intussusception is intermittent colicky abdominal pain, vomiting, and bloody stools.

QUICK HIT
Older children or children with nonileocecal intussusception need to be evaluated for polyp, lymphoma, Meckel diverticulum, and HSP.

QUICK HIT
A normal KUB or acute abdominal series does not rule out an intussusception. Further diagnostic imaging with ultrasound or air contrast enema is needed.

QUICK HIT
Other conditions may mimic aspects of intussusception or be associated with intussusceptions (e.g., gastroenteritis may have intermittent colicky pain and lethargy as dehydration ensues).

QUICK HIT
Air enemas are advantageous because they are easier to administer; have less radiation than fluoroscopy; and, if perforation occurs, are less dangerous than barium in the peritoneum.

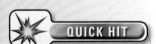

QUICK HIT

Up to 25% of pediatric cases of pancreatitis are idiopathic.

QUICK HIT

CF is an autosomal recessive disorder of the cystic fibrosis transmembrane conductance regulator (CFTR) gene, resulting in chronic sinopulmonary infection and pancreatic insufficiency.

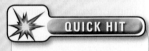

QUICK HIT

Ask about alcohol ingestion in teenage patients with pancreatitis.

QUICK HIT

Xanthomas suggest familial hyperlipidemia as an etiology for pancreatitis.

QUICK HIT

Remember, cholelithiasis can cause pancreatitis!

QUICK HIT

Elevated lipase levels are more specific than amylase levels. Elevated amylase may be of salivary, intestinal, or tubo-ovarian etiology.

QUICK HIT

Elevated serum calcium or lipids may indicate hyperparathyroidism or hyperlipidemia, respectively, as an etiology for pancreatitis.

FIGURE 3-6 **Ileocolic intussusception. Barium enema shows the intussusception as the filling defect within the hepatic flexure surrounded by spiral mucosal folds. Significant distended small bowel represents distal small bowel obstruction.**

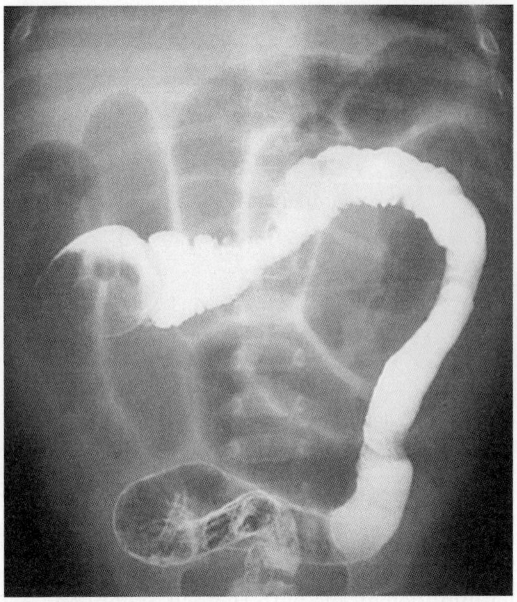

(From Fleisher GR, Ludwig S, Baskin MN. *Atlas of Pediatric Emergency Medicine.* Philadelphia: Lippincott Williams & Wilkins; 2004.)

D. Treatment
   1. Surgical treatment is indicated if there is concern of perforation, if patient is acutely ill, or if nonsurgical reduction was not successful
   2. Reduction by enema is highly successful; fluoroscopy is used to aid in visualization and confirmation of reduction
   3. Complications
      a. Main risk of radiologic reduction is bowel perforation
      b. Reduction may not be successful if lead point is present
   4. Prognosis
      a. Most infants recover if intussusception is reduced within 24 hours, but mortality rate rises rapidly as intussusception continues
      b. Recurrence possible after enema reduction or after surgery
      c. Patients should be observed in hospital after reduction for 12–24 hours because likelihood of recurrence is highest during this period

X. Pancreatitis

A. Characteristics
   1. Acute or chronic inflammatory process of pancreas
   2. Far more common in adults than children
   3. Multiple causes of pancreatitis in children
   4. Metabolic disorders and anatomic/mechanical anomalies increase risk
      a. Metabolic disorders
      b. Anatomic/mechanical anomalies
         i. Pancreas divisum: separate ductal systems of head and body of pancreas
         ii. Choledochal cyst: congenital dilation of biliary tree
         iii. Sphincter of Oddi dysfunction
   5. Pathogenesis involves premature activation of pancreatic enzymes → autodigestion and edema of pancreas → necrosis/hemorrhage in severe cases

B. Clinical features
   1. Severity of symptoms varies among individuals
      a. Upper or diffuse upper *abdominal pain*
         i. *Radiation to back*
         ii. Worsens with meals
      b. Nausea, vomiting, and fever

2. Physical exam should begin with assessment of vital signs
   a. Tachycardia due to pain, dehydration, or fever
   b. Hypotension occurs in severe cases
   c. Abdominal tenderness, especially in epigastric region
   d. Decreased bowel sounds due to peritoneal irritation and ileus
   e. Pseudocyst may present as palpable abdominal mass
   f. Abdominal distension may be due to ascites
   g. Hemorrhage may lead to abdominal wall ecchymoses
   h. Jaundice suggests biliary etiology

C. Diagnosis (refer to Acute Abdominal Pain, Chronic Abdominal Pain, and Approach to Vomiting for other causes of abdominal pain and vomiting)
1. Degree of laboratory abnormalities may vary based on severity
   a. Elevated amylase and lipase
   b. Elevated CRP correlates with severe disease
   c. Elevated ALP, GGT, ALT, and/or bilirubin indicate biliary etiology
   d. Poor prognosis if hypocalcemia, hyperglycemia, coagulopathy, or metabolic acidosis
2. Imaging modalities assist in diagnosis, complication assessment, and even treatment
   a. Abdominal ultrasound
      i. May be limited by overlying bowel
      ii. Useful to image biliary tree for possible etiology
      iii. Enlarged, hypoechoic pancreas with edema
      iv. Anechoic (black) areas represent pseudocyst formation
   b. Contrasted CT helps determine severity/necrosis
   c. Endoscopic retrograde cholangiopancreatography (ERCP) addresses obstructive causes of pancreatitis (e.g., stones, strictures)
      i. Pancreatitis is a complication of ERCP

D. Treatment depends on severity of acute episode
1. Acute uncomplicated pancreatitis
   a. *Pain control*
   b. *IV fluids* for rehydration and correction of electrolyte abnormalities
   c. PPI for acid suppression
   d. NPO (nothing by mouth) while vomiting and consider NG tube placement
      i. Reduced mortality, infection, need for surgery, and length of hospital stay with early enteral feedings
      ii. Nasojejunal tube feedings of high-protein, low-fat, semi-elemental formula if unable to tolerate feeds orally in timely fashion
      iii. Parenteral nutrition for patients unable to tolerate enteral feeds
2. Complications of pancreatitis
   a. **Pseudocysts** seen with acute or chronic pancreatitis
   b. Splenic vein thrombosis occurs in up to 19% of patients
   c. Sepsis, acute respiratory distress syndrome (ARDS), multiorgan failure
3. Duration/prognosis
   a. Uncomplicated cases resolve in 3–7 days
   b. Associated conditions affect prognosis when due to systemic disease or trauma
   c. Increased risk of pancreatic carcinoma in hereditary pancreatitis
4. Prevention
   a. Address any known etiologies
   b. Low-fat diet to prevent recurrent acute episodes

XI. Cholecystitis

A. Characteristics
1. Inflammation of gallbladder
2. More common with gallstones or biliary sludging (calculous)
3. Seen in children with predisposing risk factors (Box 3-8)

QUICK HIT

Bibasilar atelectasis, pleural effusions, and diaphragmatic elevation may be seen on chest radiography in children with pancreatitis.

QUICK HIT

Up to 50% of pediatric cases have no abnormalities on ultrasound.

QUICK HIT

Because pancreatitis may cause renal impairment, check creatinine prior to administering IV contrast.

QUICK HIT

Magnetic resonance cholangiopancreatography (MRCP) provides better imaging of ductal systems without ability to immediately treat.

QUICK HIT

Clinical picture should guide treatment, not serial amylase or lipase levels.

QUICK HIT

Restart liquid/soft diet as symptoms resolve and advance to low-fat diet as tolerated.

QUICK HIT

Infection with enteric gram-negative organisms may complicate necrotizing pancreatitis.

QUICK HIT

Drugs implicated in pancreatitis due to medications include valproic acid, furosemide, tetracycline, and opiates.

QUICK HIT

The most common type of gallstone is cholesterol stones.

QUICK HIT

RLL pneumonia can present with RUQ pain in children.

QUICK HIT

Perihepatitis (Fitz-Hugh-Curtis) caused by gonococcus should be included in the differential diagnosis of sexually active adolescents with RUQ pain and tenderness.

QUICK HIT

Ultrasonography has high specificity and can visualize stones and sludging. HIDA scan has high sensitivity to evaluate intestinal excretion of bile.

QUICK HIT

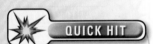

Constipation can be functional or organic. *Functional constipation* lacks evidence of a primary anatomic or biochemical cause and accounts for most constipation symptoms in children and infants outside the immediate neonatal period.

QUICK HIT

Children with encopresis may soil or leak daily but fail to evacuate the colon completely.

QUICK HIT

Organic causes can usually be excluded by thorough history and physical exam.

BOX 3-8

Predisposition Risk Factors of Gallstone Formation

- Age: adolescents
- Sex: female
- Obesity
- Pregnancy
- Hemolysis: hemoglobinopathies, red blood cell membrane fragility
- Infection: hemolytic-uremic syndrome, sepsis
- Others: total parenteral nutrition, ileal disease and resection, idiopathic

B. Clinical features
  1. Historical findings: classic cluster of symptoms in older children and adolescents (Box 3-9)
  2. Exam findings
     i. Fever and dehydration
     ii. RUQ tenderness with guarding
     iii. May have Murphy sign

C. Diagnosis
  1. Differential diagnosis
     a. Laboratory findings: demonstrate inflammation, obstructive cholestasis, and evidence of hepatocellular damage

D. Treatment
  1. Mostly medical management in acute stage
  2. Surgical removal
  3. Prevention of gallstone formation depends on predisposing factors

XII. Constipation and Fecal Incontinence

A. General characteristics
  1. **Constipation:** delay or difficulty in defecation
     a. Infants should pass meconium within 48 hours of birth
     b. Infants up to age 3 months pass 2–4 stools/day
     c. Stool frequency decreases to adult equivalent of ~1 stool/day by age 3–4 years
  2. **Fecal incontinence**: repeated passage of stool in inappropriate places by children who would be reasonably expected to have completed toilet training; soiling can be voluntary or involuntary
  3. Risk factors
     a. Dietary changes may result in constipation
     b. Behavior changes may enhance constipation
     c. Organic causes (Box 3-10)
  4. Pathophysiology
     a. Voluntary and involuntary muscle contractions involved in continence and stooling

BOX 3-9

Symptoms of Cholecystitis

- Abdominal pain
  - Acute
  - Sharp, colicky
  - Epigastric/RUQ
  - Radiating to the back
- Fever
- Nausea and vomiting
- Anorexia and bloating

BOX 3-10

Organic Causes of Constipation

Imperforate anus	Hypercalcemia
Anal stenosis	Hypokalemia
Pelvic mass	Diabetes mellitus
Meconium plug	Gluten enteropathy
Meconium ileus	Cystic fibrosis
Hirschsprung disease	Lead toxicity
Volvulus	Medication side effects (i.e., antacids, opiates, phenobarbital)
Botulism	
Spinal cord abnormalities	Developmental delay
Hypothyroidism	Sexual abuse

b. Child commonly has painful bowel movement and withholds stool
  i. Withholding stretches rectum and descending colon
  ii. Rectal sensation is decreased and even greater amount of stool is needed to cause urge to defecate
c. With chronic retention, internal sphincter dilates when external anal sphincter relaxes, and liquid stool leaks onto underwear (also referred to as *obstipation*)

B. Clinical features
1. Historical findings
  a. Birth history related to passage of meconium
  b. Frequency, consistency, and size of stools
  c. Pain with bowel movements
  d. Any associated findings such as fever, weight loss, or vomiting
  e. Dietary habits
  f. Medication history
  g. Toileting behavior (see Chapter 15)
2. Physical exam findings
  a. Abdominal exam: palpable stool in LLQ?
  b. Anal/rectal exam: position, anal wink, tone, distention or impaction, occult blood
  c. Skin: hair tufts or dimples, fissures
  d. Central nervous system (CNS): cremasteric reflexes, lower extremity tone, strength, and reflexes

C. Diagnosis
1. If organic cause is suspected, focused laboratory testing should be performed, such as electrolytes, thyroid function studies, lead level, sweat testing
2. Radiology findings: consider an abdominal film if history and physical are not diagnostic
3. Other studies
  i. Rectal biopsy, rectal manometry, barium enema may be helpful if considering Hirschsprung disease
  ii. Spinal x-rays or magnetic resonance imaging (MRI) scans are indicated if concern for spinal abnormality or neurologic impairment
  iii. Colon transit studies can be considered in patients who fail to respond to aggressive treatment of functional constipation

D. Treatment
1. Therapy in infants <1 year
  a. Osmotically active carbohydrates such as sorbitol-containing juices may be used
  b. Glycerin suppositories can be used intermittently
  c. Osmotic laxatives may be beneficial: lactulose, sorbitol, polyethylene glycol (Miralax)
  d. Stimulant laxatives are not recommended for use in infants

QUICK HIT

The goal of therapy is to disimpact and maintain a regular routine bowel movement, recommended to be the consistency of soft-serve ice cream.

QUICK HIT

Although dark corn syrup was recommended in the past, newer preparations often do not contain the glycoproteins converted to active particles in the colon.

QUICK HIT

Mineral oil is not recommended for infants or other children with GER because of the risk of pneumonitis if aspirated.

QUICK HIT

Miralax is becoming the first-line agent by many pediatricians in the treatment of constipation because of its ease of use and rare side effects.

QUICK HIT

It is important to review with caregivers the reason a laxative is being used and alleviate fears associated with laxative dependence.

QUICK HIT

The dose of the laxative should be increased every few days in order to achieve at least 1 soft bowel movement per day. If diarrhea occurs, the dose should be decreased.

QUICK HIT

A comprehensive program of behavior modification and maintenance therapy is usually necessary to achieve long-term success in functional constipation.

QUICK HIT

If a full-term infant has not passed meconium within the first 48 hours of life, Hirschsprung disease should be suspected.

QUICK HIT

Rectal suction biopsy is the gold standard for diagnosing Hirschsprung disease.

QUICK HIT

Infants with pyloric stenosis are described as "hungry vomiters," desiring to eat immediately following emesis.

2. Therapy in children
   a. Disimpaction methods
      i. Enemas: sodium phosphate, mineral oil, surfactant solution
      ii. Bisacodyl suppository may be used in older children
      iii. Oral or NG polyethylene glycol
      iv. Manual disimpaction may be necessary in extreme cases
   b. Maintenance therapy
      i. Balanced diet including whole grains, fruits, and vegetables
      ii. Osmotic laxatives
      iii. Stimulants (used less often)
      iv. Parental education to avoid reprimanding and punishing
      v. Behavior modification
         (a) Regular toilet sitting
         (b) Stool diaries
         (c) Reward system
3. Prognosis
   a. Adequate disimpaction and maintenance medication are key
   b. Discontinuing behavior regimen or medication regimen too early can lead to failure

XIII. Hirschsprung Disease (Congenital Aganglionic Megacolon)

A. Definition
   1. Congenital absence of ganglion cells in bowel wall
   2. Begins at anus and extends proximally
   3. Variable amount of bowel involvement
      a. 80% of cases limited to rectosigmoid colon
      b. 10%–15% with long segment disease (entire colon)
      c. 5% total bowel aganglionosis
B. Cause/pathophysiology
   1. Caused by failure of neural crest cell migration from proximal to distal bowel
   2. Usually sporadic
   3. Absence of submucosal and myenteric plexus causes inadequate relaxation of bowel wall leading to obstruction (Figure 3-7)
C. Clinical presentation
   1. Usually diagnosed in neonatal period due to failure to pass meconium, distended abdomen, emesis, or feeding intolerance
      a. Abdomen is usually tympanitic
      b. Rectal exam may cause explosive diarrhea/gas ("blast sign")
   2. In older infants, may present as chronic constipation, dilatation of proximal bowel, and FTT
   3. Rarely, stasis leads to bacterial proliferation and enterocolitis
D. Testing
   1. Rectal suction biopsy (gold standard): shows absence of ganglion cells
   2. Contrast enema: reveals "transition zone" between narrow aganglionic distal bowel and distended normal bowel above it
   3. Anorectal manometry: shows failure of internal anal sphincter relaxation when rectum is distended with balloon
E. Therapy
   1. Surgery is only therapy: resect aganglionic segment and "pull-through" normal bowel for anastomosis with anus
   2. Infants with enterocolitis or long-segment disease may have temporary ostomy followed by pull-through procedure at later date
   3. Most patients have normal bowel function after surgery, although constipation, fecal incontinence, or enterocolitis can recur

XIV. Pyloric Stenosis

A. General characteristics
   1. Hypertrophy of pylorus muscle resulting in gastric outlet obstruction
   2. Occurs in 1–3/1,000 live births

FIGURE 3-7 **Hirschsprung disease. The distal portion of the bowel lacks innervation. Because there is no relaxation in this narrowed segment, the bowel proximal to it is markedly distended.**

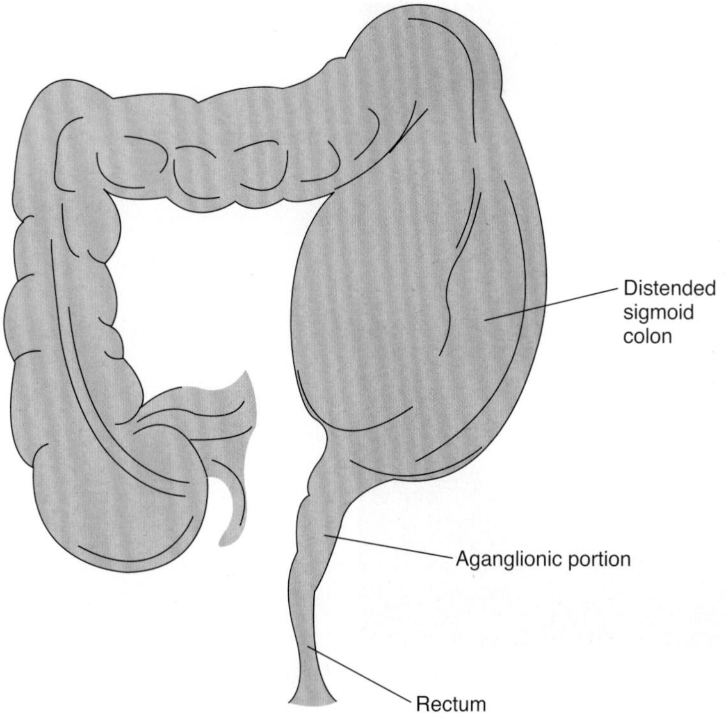

(From Pillitteri A. *Maternal and Child Nursing.* 4th ed. Philadelphia: Lippincott Williams & Wilkins; 2003.)

3. Cause is unknown; likely multifactorial (genetic and environmental)
4. Risk factors
   a. Firstborn male (30% of cases)
   b. Family history of pyloric stenosis
   c. Use of macrolide antibiotics during first 2 weeks of life

B. Clinical features
1. Historical findings: vomiting that is nonbilious, projectile, and postprandial
2. Physical exam findings
   a. Palpable "olive-like" mass in RUQ
   b. Peristaltic waves across abdomen from left to right prior to emesis
   c. Dehydration
   d. Jaundice

C. Diagnosis
1. Differential diagnosis: focused on disorders that cause vomiting
2. Laboratory findings
   a. Hypochloremic, hypokalemic metabolic alkalosis
3. Radiology findings (Figure 3-8): ultrasound confirms diagnosis in majority of cases

D. Treatment
1. Therapy
   a. Correct alkalosis (can cause postoperative apnea with anesthesia)
   b. Pyloromyotomy
      i. Longitudinal incision through pylorus to layer of submucosa
      ii. Can be performed laparoscopically
      iii. Feedings re-initiated 12–24 hours postoperatively

QUICK HIT

The "firsts of pyloric stenosis": 1st born, around 1st month, 1st correct electrolytes, emesis as 1st thing after feeding

QUICK HIT

Hypochloremic, hypokalemic metabolic alkalosis is the typical electrolyte abnormality in pyloric stenosis.

QUICK HIT

Classic laboratory and physical exam findings are less commonly seen now as greater awareness of pyloric stenosis and better imaging modalities have led to earlier diagnosis.

QUICK HIT

Correct any fluid or electrolyte abnormalities.

XV. Intestinal Atresias

A. Definition
1. Stenosis between 2 segments of bowel with or without separating web
2. Atresia with connecting fibrous band between 2 segments of bowel
3. Atresia resulting in 2 blind pouches of bowel ends

FIGURE 3-8 **Pyloric stenosis demonstrated by barium upper GI series showing pyloric channel narrowing (*N*) and elongation with antral shouldering (*arrows*).**

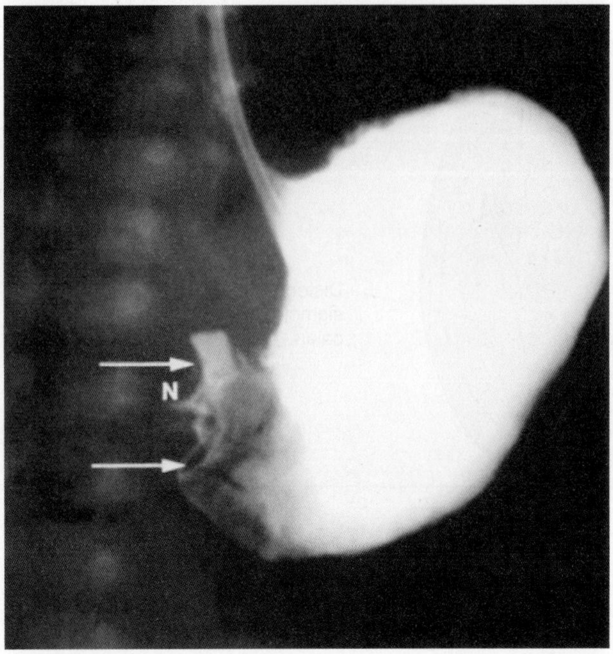

(From Mulholland MW, Lillemore ED, Doherty GM, et al. *Greenfield's Surgery Scientific Principles and Practice.* 4th ed. Philadelphia: Lippincott Williams & Wilkins; 2006.)

QUICK HIT

Intestinal atresia is the failure of hollow viscus organ to develop appropriately, resulting in spectrum of severity.

QUICK HIT

Atresia with 2 blind pouches is the most common, accounting for 50% of cases.

QUICK HIT

Severe, proximal atresias present earlier than distal or less severe stenoses.

QUICK HIT

Duodenal atresia is associated with trisomy 21 (Down syndrome).

QUICK HIT

Meconium peritonitis may appear as abdominal calcifications on x-ray.

B. Testing: evaluation includes review of maternal history, prenatal ultrasound findings, and physical exam findings
   1. Flat and upright and/or cross-table lateral abdominal radiographs
      a. Look for signs of obstruction, pneumoperitoneum, and/or meconium peritonitis
      b. Duodenal atresia: "**double bubble**" **sign** (Figure 3-9)
   2. Contrast studies
      a. Upper GI series may reveal malrotation with volvulus as cause for "double bubble"
      b. Contrast enema may reveal microcolon due to small bowel atresia or frank colonic atresia
C. Therapy: definitive correction requires surgical resection with anastomosis

FIGURE 3-9 **Double bubble of duodenal atresia.**

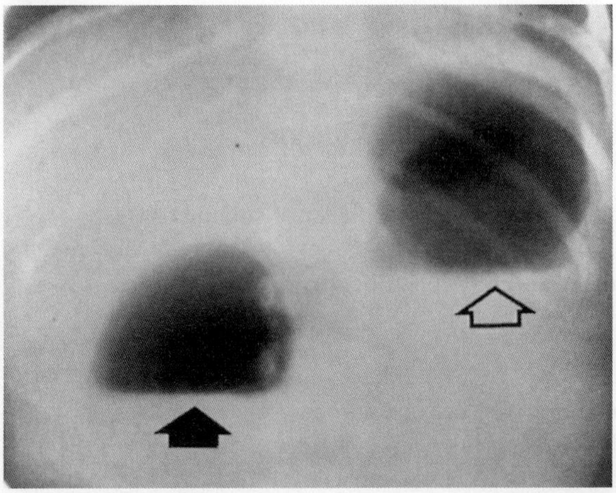

(From Eisenberg RL. *An Atlas of Differential Diagnosis.* 4th ed. Philadelphia: Lippincott Williams & Wilkins; 2003.)

XVI. Malrotation

A. Characteristics
  1. One of most common causes of intestinal obstruction in infancy
  2. Surgical emergency
  3. Most cases of symptomatic malrotation present as volvulus during infancy
  4. Close to 50% within 1st month of life
  5. ~90% within 1st year of life
  6. Result of incomplete rotation (3rd and final step) of gut during embryologic development
  7. Intestinal obstruction by 1 of 2 mechanisms (Figure 3-10)

B. Clinical features
  1. Historical findings
    a. Acute, forceful, bilious emesis
    b. Small bowel obstruction

QUICK HIT
May be asymptomatic: 1 in 500 found at autopsy of otherwise healthy patients

QUICK HIT
Symptomatic malrotation occurs in ~1 in 6,000 live births.

FIGURE 3-10 Malrotation with volvulus.

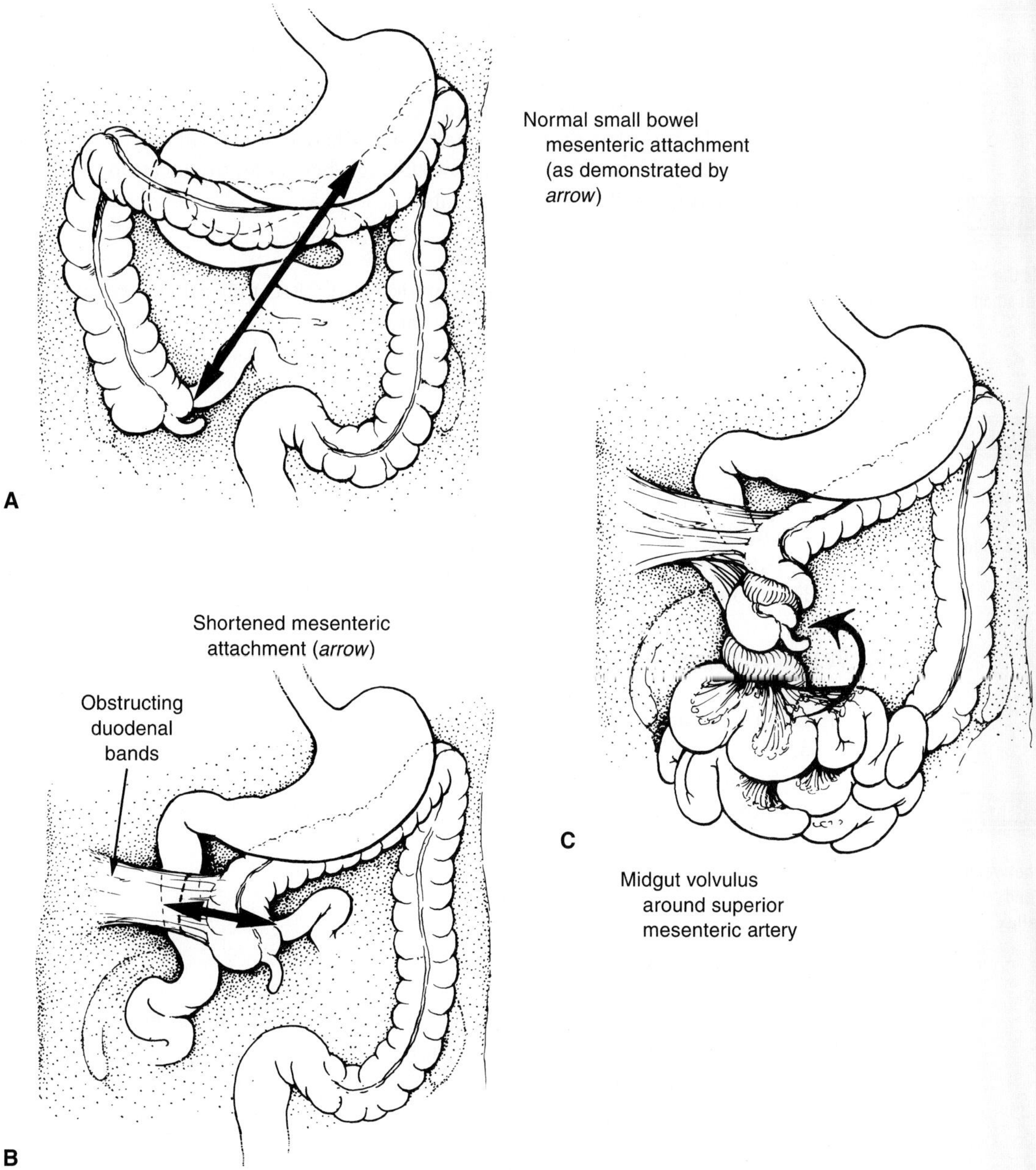

A. Normal small bowel mesenteric attachment (as demonstrated by the *arrow*). This prevents twisting of small bowel because of the broad fixation of the mesentery. **B.** Malrotation of colon with obstructing duodenal bands. **C.** Midgut volvulus around the superior mesenteric artery caused by the narrow base of the mesentery.

QUICK HIT

Ladd bands act like postoperative "adhesion" that can lead to small bowel obstruction.

QUICK HIT

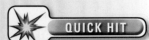

Bilious emesis, which indicates obstruction distal to the ligament of Treitz, requires emergent surgical evaluation.

QUICK HIT

Upright or decubitus films are required to visualize air–fluid levels.

QUICK HIT

Initial management is the same for all causes of small bowel obstruction.

QUICK HIT

Ladd procedure includes checking for small bowel viability and excision of Ladd bands.

QUICK HIT

Need to distinguish between *uncomplicated* GER and gastroesophageal reflux *disease* (GERD)

c. Early onset (<1st year of life)
d. Abdominal distention
e. Bloody diarrhea (late diagnosis)
f. Later onset (after 1st year of life)
i. May be asymptomatic
ii. Chronic, insidious
iii. FTT/anorexia/poor feeding
iv. Malabsorption
2. Physical exam findings
a. Signs of dehydration
b. Abdominal distention and diffuse abdominal tenderness
c. Shock or sepsis-like picture
d. Guaiac-positive stool to frank bloody stool

C. Diagnosis
1. Differential diagnosis of bilious emesis in infancy
2. Rule out other etiologies of small bowel obstruction
3. Requires surgical evaluation
4. Radiology findings
a. Studies will depend on patient stability
b. Plain film should include KUB and upright or decubitus abdominal x-ray
c. Distention loops of bowel with air–fluid levels
d. "Corkscrew" appearance on upper GI study with contrast
e. Can rule out other causes of small bowel obstruction in infancy
f. Upper GI with small bowel follow-through helps identify location of obstruction (only in stable patients)

D. Treatment
1. Medical
a. Stabilize patient with fluid resuscitation and correct electrolyte imbalances
b. NG tube to suction for bowel decompression
c. Broad-spectrum IV antibiotics for septic patients
2. Surgical
a. Ladd procedure
b. Resection of necrotic portion of small bowel
3. Complications
a. Necrotic bowel
b. Short bowel syndrome
c. Adhesions leading to subsequent small bowel obstruction
4. Duration/prognosis depends on time of diagnosis

XVII. Gastroesophageal Reflux

A. Characteristics
1. Definition: stomach contents leak backward into esophagus
a. Can be normal, physiologic process, particularly in young infants
b. Regurgitation is reflux to level of oropharynx
c. Indications of pathologic gastroesophageal reflux disease (GERD) in infants and children include
i. Esophagitis
ii. FTT
iii. Respiratory complications
iv. Pain/heartburn
2. Epidemiology
a. Up to 60% of young infants (age 0–6 months) regurgitate at least once a day
b. Only 5% still regurgitate at age 10–12 months
c. In older children and adolescents, 5%–8% report GERD symptoms, but only 1% are on treatment for it
3. Cause
a. Inappropriate relaxation of lower esophageal sphincter (i.e., not triggered by swallowing)

BOX 3-11

Symptoms of Gastroesophageal Reflux Disease

- Recurrent regurgitation or vomiting
- Weight loss or poor weight gain
- Irritability in infants
- Feeding refusal/anorexia
- Rumination (regurgitation followed by mastication and reswallowing)
- Heartburn/chest pain
- Hematemesis
- Dysphagia/odynophagia
- Recurrent pneumonia
- Recurrent wheezing or stridor
- Apparent life-threatening events

b. May be exacerbated by mucosal damage of lower esophagus from prolonged exposure to gastric acid
c. Esophageal peristalsis and diaphragm also important in preventing GER

4. Risk factors
   a. Neurologic impairment (cerebral palsy, Down syndrome)
   b. Obesity
   c. Esophageal abnormalities (esophageal atresia, congenital diaphragmatic hernia, achalasia)
   d. Chronic lung disease (including CF)
   e. Prematurity
5. Pathophysiology
   a. Esophagitis and pain result from exposure of esophageal epithelium to acidic refluxate
   b. Respiratory symptoms may result from regurgitation and aspiration or penetration of refluxate into airway
   c. FTT results when pain or vomiting prevents adequate caloric intake

B. Clinical features
1. Historical findings (Box 3-11)
2. Physical exam findings (Box 3-12)

C. Diagnosis
1. Differential diagnosis
   a. Symptoms in infant/nonverbal child are very nonspecific
   b. Older children with classic symptoms may be diagnosed clinically as in adults
2. Radiology findings
   a. Upper GI series (barium contrast study of upper GI tract)
      i. Poor sensitivity and specificity for GER
      ii. Helpful in ruling out anatomic abnormalities that cause vomiting

QUICK HIT

Infants with uncomplicated GER (those who feed well, gain weight, and do not have excessive irritability or breathing problems) are commonly called "happy spitters" and usually do not require intervention.

QUICK HIT

Sandifer syndrome describes the rare occurrence of opisthotonic posturing (severe arching of back and torsion of the neck) with GERD. It can be mistaken for seizure or tetanus.

QUICK HIT

The semi-upright positioning of an infant car seat can compress the stomach and actually exacerbates GER as compared to supine flat positioning.

QUICK HIT

Some infants with cow's milk protein allergy present with symptoms of GER.

BOX 3-12

Signs of Gastroesophageal Reflux Disease

- Wheezing
- Stridor
- Cough
- Hoarseness
- Pharyngeal inflammation
- Anemia
- Dental erosions
- Sandifer syndrome
- Apnea spells

QUICK HIT

Risks of acid suppression include increased rates of pneumonia, gastroenteritis, necrotizing enterocolitis (NEC), and candidemia.

QUICK HIT

Cow's milk protein intolerance differs from lactose intolerance. Primary lactase deficiency is rare in infants, although a secondary lactase deficiency may rarely occur after gastroenteritis due to temporary damage to the brush border.

QUICK HIT

Breastfeeding mothers can eliminate dairy from diet; may take 2 weeks for proteins to clear from breast milk.

QUICK HIT

Up to 50% of children with cow's milk protein intolerance will have a similar reaction to soy protein; therefore, soy formulas should be avoided in these patients.

QUICK HIT

Most children outgrow sensitivity within 1 year of diagnosis, with nearly all children tolerating cow's milk by age 2 years of age.

QUICK HIT

There is no evidence to suggest cow's milk protein intolerance predisposes to other GI disorders.

b. Nuclear scintigraphy: radiolabeled food or formula are introduced into stomach and scanned for evidence of GER or aspiration
   i. Poor sensitivity and specificity for GER
   ii. Helpful in evaluating for delayed gastric emptying

3. Esophageal pH monitoring (pH probe)
   a. Quantifies frequency and duration of acid in esophagus
   b. Can be combined with impedance monitoring to detect nonacidic GER
   c. Helpful in correlating nonspecific symptoms (e.g., stridor, apnea, irritability) with GER events
4. Endoscopy and biopsy: most reliable way to diagnose reflux esophagitis

D. Treatment
1. Therapy
   a. Education about feeding volumes: large-volume feedings promote regurgitation
   b. Pharmacologic therapy
      i. Acid suppression with histamine-2 receptor antagonists (H2RAs) or PPIs
         (a) Effectively increase gastric pH
         (b) PPIs more effective than H2RAs in adult studies
      ii. Prokinetic therapy: adverse effects outweigh benefits
      iii. Surgery: Nissen fundoplication, surgically wrap gastric antrum around distal esophagus
         (a) Reserved for children with chronic GERD that is not responsive to medical therapy
         (b) Most beneficial in children with respiratory complications
         (c) Symptom recurrence and complications are common
         (d) Unclear whether fundoplication or gastrostomy tube placement leads to better outcomes

XVIII. Cow's Milk Protein Intolerance (GI Food Allergy)

A. Characteristics
1. Several categories
   a. IgE-mediated immediate hypersensitivity reaction
   b. Eosinophilic esophagitis and gastroenteritis
   c. Food-protein–induced proctocolitis/enteropathy/enterocolitis
2. Cause: cow's milk–induced proctocolitis/enteropathy/enterocolitis is cell-mediated process
   a. Pathogenesis is poorly understood
   b. Large proteins present in cow's milk (casein and whey) trigger cell-mediated inflammatory response

B. Clinical features
1. Milk-protein–induced proctocolitis
   a. Blood-streaked stools
   b. Otherwise healthy-appearing infant (anemia is rare)
   c. 1st few months of life
2. Milk-protein–induced enteropathy
   a. FTT, diarrhea, and vomiting
   b. Abdominal distention
   c. More common in children fed whole milk prior to age 1 year
3. Milk-protein–induced enterocolitis
   a. Presents earlier (commonly within 2 weeks of birth) in infants fed with cow's milk formulas
   b. Severe vomiting, bloody diarrhea, and abdominal distention
   c. Failure to regain birth weight and dehydration
   d. Labs: hypoalbuminemia, leukocytosis, and heme-positive stools
   e. Infants may appear septic

C. Diagnosis
  1. No single laboratory test or study to confirm diagnosis
  2. Diagnosis usually made on basis of elimination diet followed by food challenge
    a. Symptoms resolve within days (proctitis) to weeks (enterocolitis) after complete elimination
    b. Formula-fed infants should be switched to protein hydrolysate– or amino acid–derived formula
D. Treatment
  1. Elimination of milk protein from diet
  2. Infants with enterocolitis may need to be NPO with IV fluids initially

XIX. Malabsorption

A. Background
  1. Carbohydrates, fats, and proteins undergo digestion by hydrolysis
  2. Malabsorption results when nutrients cannot be absorbed across intestinal epithelium
  3. Symptoms are nonspecific
  4. Diarrhea is common with carbohydrate, lipid, and protein malabsorption (Box 3-13)
B. Carbohydrate digestion
  1. Digestion of carbohydrates
    a. Mouth/oral cavity: saliva contains mucin and α-amylase, which initiate digestion
    b. Small intestine
      i. Pancreas secretes α-amylase into duodenum
      ii. Enterocyte disaccharides
        (a) Located in brush border at **villous tip**
        (b) Hydrolyze disaccharides to monosaccharides
        (c) *Hydrolysis of lactose leads to glucose and galactose*
    c. Absorption
      i. Glucose and galactose absorption is coupled with sodium absorption
      ii. Monosaccharides absorbed across basolateral membrane into circulation (GLUT2)
C. Fat digestion
  1. Triglycerides are main source of dietary fat
  2. Lipase and co-lipase important in lipid digestion
    a. Digestion begins with lingual and gastric lipase activity
    b. Pancreatic lipase and co-lipase contribute to digestion
    c. Digested triglycerides yield fatty acids and monoglycerides
    d. Fatty acids are hydrophobic and do not diffuse well across aqueous layer near enterocyte membrane
    e. Bile acids combine with fatty acids and form water soluble micelles
    f. Micelles deliver high concentration of lipids to enterocyte membrane
D. Protein digestion
  1. Begins in stomach with action of pepsin
  2. Most protein digestion occurs in duodenum through action of pancreatic proteases (trypsin, chymotrypsin, elastase)

BOX 3-13

Common Presenting Symptoms of Malabsorption

Diarrhea
Abdominal pain
Bloating
Poor weight gain
Failure to thrive
Dermatitis
Flatulence

QUICK HIT

Any process that damages the intestinal villi, such as infection, can lead to an acquired disaccharidase deficiency.

QUICK HIT

The most common cause of carbohydrate malabsorption is intestinal lactase deficiency.

QUICK HIT

Congenital lactase deficiency is rare and not a common cause of malabsorption in an infant.

QUICK HIT

Infants rely heavily of gastric and lingual activity because pancreatic lipase levels remain low until about age 2 years.

QUICK HIT

Short-chain and medium-chain fatty acids do not require micelles because they have adequate solubility and can diffuse across the aqueous layer.

QUICK HIT

Formulas with the majority of fat coming from medium-chain triglycerides are used to treat infants with cholestatic liver disease because these infants cannot secrete adequate amounts of bile acids into the duodenum for normal fat digestion.

QUICK HIT

Celiac disease is very common. Estimated prevalence is 1:300/1:80 in U.S./European children.

QUICK HIT

Classic presentation is malabsorption manifesting as diarrhea with vomiting, abdominal distention, and muscle wasting soon after being exposed to gluten between age 6 and 24 months.

QUICK HIT

Dermatitis herpetiformis is a celiac-associated skin condition presenting with pruritus and subepidermal blisters and erythematous papules, usually over extensor surfaces, but they can be generalized.

QUICK HIT

Serum antibodies in celiac disease include antigliadin antibody (AGA), antitissue transglutaminase (tTG), and anti-endomysial (EMA) IgA antibodies.

QUICK HIT

The total IgA level must be known to accurately interpret IgA-class celiac antibodies.

QUICK HIT

NEC accounts for the majority of pediatric short bowel syndrome.

BOX 3-14

Symptoms of Fat-Soluble Vitamin and Zinc Deficiency

- Vitamin A: night blindness, xerophthalmia, poor growth, susceptibility to respiratory and GI infections
- Vitamin D: rickets
- Vitamin E: hemolytic anemia, decreased deep tendon reflexes, ataxia, weakness and loss of proprioception
- Vitamin K: coagulopathy
- Zinc: diarrhea, skin rash, hair loss

3. Pancreatic enzymes are secreted in inactive form and then activated in duodenum; trypsinogen gets converted to trypsin by enterokinase
4. Absorbed through peptide/amino acid transporters

E. Vitamins and micronutrients
1. Fat-soluble vitamins (A, D, E, and K) will be malabsorbed with any condition causing fat malabsorption (Box 3-14)
2. Water-soluble vitamins and micronutrients are absorbed in the small intestine

F. Clinical features
1. Nonspecific symptoms such as diarrhea and bloating
2. Will often present with poor weight gain or FTT
3. Stools may look "greasy" in the setting of fat malabsorption (steatorrhea)
4. May be signs of specific micronutrient deficiency (Table 3-5)

G. Diagnosis
1. Stool studies
   a. Spot fecal fat: indicates fat malabsorption
   b. 72-hour fecal fat collection
      i. Quantitative assessment of fat malabsorption
      ii. Must know dietary fat intake to interpret results
   c. Fecal elastase: assesses pancreatic exocrine activity
   d. Stool pH: acidic pH will be seen in carbohydrate malabsorption
   e. Stool-reducing substances will be positive with carbohydrate malabsorption

H. Treatment
1. Approach should be to correct underlying cause
2. Supplemental vitamin and micronutrients

XX. Celiac Disease

A. Characteristics
1. T cell–mediated, inflammatory disorder of small intestine
2. Caused by ingested gluten found in wheat, rye, and barley
3. Susceptibility determined by genetics
   a. 75%–85% concordance for monozygotic twins

TABLE 3-5 Signs and Symptoms of Micronutrient Deficiency

Micronutrient	Signs/Symptoms of Deficiency
Vitamin A	Poor night vision, follicular hyperkeratosis
Vitamin D	Osteopenia, rickets
Vitamin E	Hyporeflexia, decreased vibratory and position sensing, ataxia
Vitamin K	Easy bruising, bleeding
Iron	Anemia, fatigue
Folic acid	Macrocytic anemia
Vitamin B_{12}	Macrocytic anemia, numbness and tingling in extremities
Zinc	Acrodermatitis enteropathica

BOX 3-15

Gastrointestinal Manifestations of Celiac Disease

Chronic diarrhea
Abdominal pain
Failure to thrive
Weight loss
Abdominal distention
Anorexia
Vomiting
Constipation

B. Clinical features
  1. Patients can present with GI symptoms and/or extraintestinal manifestations
    a. Younger children tend to have more abdominal and GI complaints (Box 3-15)
    b. Older children and adults tend to have more extraintestinal manifestations
  2. Silent or latent celiac disease can be present in high-risk patients
  3. Complications
    a. Protein, vitamin, and micronutrient malabsorption
    b. Short stature and osteoporosis
    c. Increased risk of intestinal lymphoma
C. Diagnosis
  1. Gold standard is histopathology: small bowel mucosal biopsies will reveal **villous blunting** and **increased intraepithelial lymphocytes**
  2. Serum antibodies
    a. Can identify symptomatic individuals who need biopsy
    b. Monitoring dietary compliance
D. Treatment: lifelong gluten-free diet; avoid wheat, rye, barley

XXI. Short Bowel Syndrome

A. Definitions
  1. Critical reduction in intestinal length
  2. Results from loss of intestinal length below minimal amount necessary to maintain normal digestion and absorption of nutrients and fluids required for maintenance
  3. Also defined as need for parenteral nutrition
B. Cause/pathophysiology
  1. Congenital anomalies (gastroschisis, malrotation with volvulus, atresias, omphalocele, or aganglionosis)
  2. Necrotizing enterocolitis (NEC) with bowel resection
  3. In older children: malrotation/volvulus, trauma, intra-abdominal neoplasia
C. Clinical presentation
  1. Anatomic considerations: impact of short bowel syndrome is not limited to length lost, but also to location of loss, and significantly affects intestinal adaptation
D. Complications
  1. Parenteral nutrition–associated cholestasis; can progress to chronic liver failure, necessitating liver transplant
  2. Catheter-related complications: sepsis (main cause of mortality in SBS), thrombus
  3. Other: gallstones, small bowel bacterial overgrowth, enterocolitis, bowel obstruction

XXII. Inflammatory Bowel Disease

A. IBD encompasses 2 disorders: **ulcerative colitis** (**UC**) and **Crohn disease** (**CD**)
  1. Both involve chronic inflammation of GI tract yet are pathologically distinct
    a. CD affects **any part of GI tract** from mouth to anus
    b. UC affects **colon only**

QUICK HIT

Short bowel syndrome is a loss of bowel length with inability to maintain electrolyte balance, adequate hydration, or appropriate weight and height growth without supplementation with parenteral fluids or nutrition.

QUICK HIT

The most common site of involvement in CD is the ileum.

QUICK HIT

"Backwash ileitis" may be seen with UC but otherwise is limited to the colon.

QUICK HIT

Dietary factors, including refined sugars, cow milk protein, and lack of breastfeeding, have been proposed but not established as risk factors.

QUICK HIT

Weight loss in IBD is multifactorial; anorexia, malabsorption, and food avoidance behaviors are seen.

QUICK HIT

Tenesmus, seen in UC, is the sensation of incomplete emptying after defecation.

2. **Bimodal peak** incidence of IBD between ages 15–25 years and ages 50–80 years
   a. Mean age of diagnosis in children in United States is 12.5 years
   b. 20% of pediatric cases diagnosed before 10 years
   c. Males > females in CD; equal in UC
   d. More prevalent in northern climates of United States, United Kingdom, and northern Europe
3. Precise cause is not understood but considered multifactorial
   a. Gut mucosal barrier dysfunction
   b. Dysregulated immune system responses to "normal" gut lumen antigens, including bacteria
4. Over 100 genes/loci identified in association with IBD
5. Risk factors identified that increase the risk of IBD
   a. **Jewish ancestry** is a significant risk factor
   b. **Smoking** increases risk of CD but decreases UC risk
   c. Appendectomy may be protective

B. Historical questions encompass intestinal and extraintestinal symptoms
1. **Abdominal pain**, **weight loss**, and **intermittent fevers** seen in UC and CD
   a. CD
      i. Crampy abdominal pain: diffuse or RLQ
      ii. Diarrhea: nonbloody, melanotic, or frank blood
      iii. **Perianal disease** is common
      iv. Recurrent **aphthous ulcers** are common
   b. UC
      i. Diffuse abdominal pain
      ii. **Bloody diarrhea**
      iii. Fecal urgency
      iv. **Tenesmus**
   c. Extraintestinal symptoms may precede abdominal complaints (Table 3-6)
   d. Asking about IBD in other family members is very important
2. Physical exam: should begin with assessment of vitals and growth trends
   a. Abdominal exam: tenderness with or without distension is common
      i. **Ileitis** may present as RLQ mass in CD
      ii. Perianal skin tags, fissures, fistulae seen with CD
   b. Extraintestinal manifestations (see Table 3-6)
      i. Eye pain or redness may indicate **uveitis**
      ii. Presence of aphthous ulcers suggests CD
      iii. **Arthritis** of large joints (knee, ankle, wrist, hip)
      iv. Skin rashes, including **erythema nodosum**, pyoderma gangrenosum
      v. Jaundice, scleral icterus seen with biliary involvement (i.e., **PSC**)
      vi. GU exam for Tanner staging may reveal **delayed puberty**

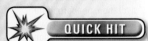

> **QUICK HIT**
> A positive family history of IBD is seen in up to 25% of patients.

> **QUICK HIT**
> A decrease in height velocity and poor weight gain often precede abdominal symptoms.

> **QUICK HIT**
> Abdominal tenderness is common in IBD, but the abdominal exam may be benign.

> **QUICK HIT**
> Morning back pain and/or stiffness are symptoms of spondylitis and sacroiliitis, which can be seen with IBD.

> **QUICK HIT**
> Enteral feedings can result in short-term remission by decreasing inflammation and hastening mucosal healing.

> **QUICK HIT**
> Erythema nodosum presents as red, warm, painful nodules typically found on the anterior lower leg. A well-defined ulcer with a deep red or purple border represents pyoderma gangrenosum.

> **QUICK HIT**
> Uveitis is seen in IBD and juvenile idiopathic arthritis. HLA-B27 positivity is associated with ankylosing spondylitis.

TABLE 3-6 Extraintestinal Manifestations of Inflammatory Bowel Disease

Organ System	Associated Findings
HEENT	Aphthous ulcers, uveitis, episcleritis
Cardiac	Pericarditis
Abdomen	Autoimmune hepatitis, pancreatitis, primary sclerosing cholangitis, cholangiocarcinoma
GU	Delayed puberty, perianal disease
Skin	Erythema nodosum, pyoderma gangrenosum
Musculoskeletal	Arthritis, ankylosing spondylitis, growth delay/failure, osteopenia/osteoporosis, digital clubbing

GU, genitourinary; HEENT, head, eyes, ears, nose, and throat.

C. Suspicion of IBD is based on history and physical and laboratory findings with definitive diagnosis by biopsy
   1. Laboratory testing
      a. **Iron deficiency anemia** and **elevated ESR, CRP** in 70%–75% of patients
      b. **Low albumin**, a marker of poor nutritional status, commonly seen
      c. Stool studies
         i. Culture for infectious enterocolitis
         ii. *C. difficile* toxin assay
         iii. **Fecal calprotectin**, **lactoferrin**: markers of gut inflammation
         iv. Fecal fat and α_1-antitrypsin seen with malabsorption
      d. Serology studies are not specific and recommended only in indeterminate cases
   2. Imaging
      a. Barium upper GI series may show fistulae, stenosis in CD
      b. CT may show bowel wall thickening, strictures, or abscesses
      c. MRI use increasing due to lack of radiation
   3. *Upper and lower endoscopy with biopsies are gold standard for diagnosis*
      a. CD and UC have characteristic gross and histologic findings
D. Treatment aims include remission, prevention of complications, and normal growth and development
   1. Medications
      a. **Corticosteroids**: IV or oral
         i. Used in acute flares with moderate-to-severe symptoms
         ii. Oral budesonide releases and treats in distal small bowel
      b. **5-Aminosalicylates**
         i. Used in mild-to-moderate UC
         ii. Uncertain mechanism of action
      c. Immunomodulators
         i. **Azathioprine** maintains remission in 75% of patients
         ii. **Methotrexate** used in patients who fail azathioprine
      d. **Infliximab** (monoclonal tumor necrosis factor [TNF]-α antibody) for induction and maintenance of remission
      e. Antibiotics
         i. Ciprofloxacin and metronidazole used for fistulae and pouchitis
         ii. Oral rifaximin improves abdominal pain and diarrhea
      f. Probiotics
         i. Help maintain remission if added to treatment regimen of UC
         ii. Help in prevention and treatment of pouchitis
   2. Nutritional considerations
      a. **Enteral feedings** are ideal if tolerated
      b. **Supplemental vitamins** may be necessary, especially in CD
      c. Parenteral nutrition needed in severe flares or to bridge during feed advancement
   3. Surgical management
      a. May be necessary in refractory disease, severe bleeding, perforation
      b. **Colectomy** with ileal pouch–anal anastomosis used in UC
      c. Segmental bowel resection (usually ileum) used in CD
      d. Perirectal disease in CD may require surgery
   4. Prognosis/complications
      a. Disease relapse occurs in >50% of patients within 2 years
      b. Adverse effects of therapies are common
      c. Delayed puberty and **lower final adult height** may occur
      d. Vitamin D deficiency and steroid use lead to **osteopenia/osteoporosis**
      e. **Toxic megacolon** more common in adults with severe UC
      f. Increased risk of **colorectal cancer**, especially in UC with pancolitis
      g. Increased risk of **cholangiocarcinoma** in patients with UC and associated PSC

QUICK HIT

A CBC may reveal microcytic anemia and elevated platelets in IBD. Fecal calprotectin and lactoferrin are elevated in IBD and infectious enterocolitis.

QUICK HIT

Fat-soluble vitamin, vitamin B_{12}, folic acid, and zinc deficiencies are a consequence of SBS.

QUICK HIT

Chronic steroid use may lead to poor growth, cushingoid facies, acne, hypertension, hyperglycemia, and adrenal suppression.

QUICK HIT

Consider stool testing for *Entamoeba histolytica* if there is a significant travel history.

QUICK HIT

Dual-energy x-ray absorptiometry scans assess bone mineral density in patients with poor growth and prolonged steroid use.

QUICK HIT

MRI has >90% sensitivity and specificity for detecting small bowel CD.

QUICK HIT

Colon cancer screening should begin 8 years after diagnosis of IBD.

MNEMONIC

Rule of "2s": 2% population, 2 feet from the ileocecal junction, 2 inches long

QUICK HIT

The diagnosis of Meckel diverticulum should be suspected in any infant or child who presents with painless rectal bleeding.

QUICK HIT

Fecal–oral transmission of hepatitis A occurs via direct contact or through contaminated water.

QUICK HIT

Reported incidence of hepatitis A in Unites States has been declining due to vaccination.

QUICK HIT

Symptoms of acute hepatitis A infection: fever, headache, malaise, anorexia, nausea, RUQ pain. HAV infection in infants and toddlers may be asymptomatic, thereby facilitating the spread of the virus to others.

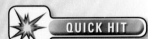

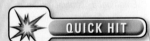

XXIII. Meckel Diverticulum

A. General characteristics
   1. Most common congenital malformation of GI tract
   2. Persistence of omphalomesenteric or vitelline duct, which connects yolk sac to gut of developing embryo

B. Clinical features
   1. Painless rectal bleeding that can be visible blood or melanotic stools
   2. Occasionally can cause bowel obstruction (serves as lead point for intussusception)

C. Diagnosis
   1. Patients may be anemic from blood loss
   2. A technetium-99m pertechnetate scan (Meckel scan) is study of choice
      a. Mucus-secreting cells take up pertechnetate

D. Treatment: surgical excision is treatment of choice

XXIV. Hepatitis A Virus (HAV)

A. General characteristics
   1. Single-stranded RNA virus
   2. Causes acute infection (no carrier state or chronic infection)

B. Clinical features
   1. Acute infection presents with nonspecific symptoms
   2. Physical examination may reveal tender hepatomegaly

C. Diagnosis (Table 3-7)

TABLE 3-7 Serologic Markers of Hepatitis Infection

Marker	Description	Significance
Hepatitis A virus (HAV)		
Anti-HAV IgM	IgM antibody to HAV	Current infection
Anti-HAV IgG	IgG antibody to HAV	Current or past infection
Hepatitis B virus (HBV)		
HBsAg	Hepatitis B surface antigen (viral surface protein)	Positive indicates infection
Anti-HBs IgG	Antibody produced in response to infection or vaccination	Positive indicates immunity or past infection
HBcAg	Viral core protein	Positive indicates past or current infection
Anti-HBc IgM	Antibody to core protein	Positive indicates acute infection
HBeAg	Viral protein present during active viral replication	Positive indicates active viral replication
Anti-HBe IgG	Antibody produced when HBeAg is no longer present	Positive indicates low to nondetectable levels of HBV DNA
HBV DNA	HBV viral DNA determined via polymerase chain reaction	Positive indicates active infection Provides a quantitative level of HBV DNA
Hepatitis C virus (HCV)		
Anti-HCV	Antibody to HCV	Positive indicates current or past infection May indicate maternal transfer of antibody in infants born to mothers with HCV
HCV RNA	HCV viral RNA determined via polymerase chain reaction	Positive indicates active infection

D. Treatment: supportive measures only
E. Immunoprophylaxis
  1. Serum immunoglobulin can be given before or after exposure
  2. Hepatitis A vaccine recommendations
    a. All children older than 1 year
    b. Persons traveling to endemic areas

XXV. Hepatitis B Virus (HBV)

A. General characteristics
  1. Double-stranded DNA virus
  2. Causes acute or chronic infection
  3. Transmission
    a. Percutaneous (needlestick, blood transfusion)
    b. Sexual
    c. Vertical (mother to offspring)
B. Clinical features
  1. Acute HBV
    a. Acute infection may lead to nonspecific symptoms
    b. Extrahepatic manifestations of infection occur
    c. Most cases of acute HBV infection resolve spontaneously
  2. Chronic HBV
    a. Commonly detected during screening of asymptomatic children born to mothers who are HBV positive
    b. Risk of developing chronic HBV varies by age, with younger children at higher risk than older children and adolescents
    c. Defined by presence of hepatitis B surface antigen (HBsAg) for >6 months
    d. Most children with perinatally acquired HBV remain in immunotolerant phase, which can last for decades; characterized by
      i. Normal to minimally elevated ALT and AST
      ii. High HBV DNA
      iii. Hepatitis B e antigen (HBeAg) positive
      iv. Minimal fibrosis on liver biopsy
C. Diagnosis: made by serologic markers (Table 3-8; also see Table 3-7)
D. Treatment: mainstays of therapy are interferon and lamivudine
E. Immunoprophylaxis
  1. Passive prophylaxis with hepatitis B immunoglobulin (HBIg)
    a. Indicated for single exposure (needlestick, sexual contact, perinatal exposure)
  2. Active prophylaxis with hepatitis B vaccine recommended for all infants as part of routine immunizations, given in 3 separate injections

XXVI. Hepatitis C Virus (HCV)

A. General characteristics
  1. Single-stranded RNA virus
  2. Causes acute or chronic infection

TABLE 3.8 Serologic Profile of Hepatitis B

HBsAg	Anti-HBc	Anti-HBs	Interpretation
+	+	–	• Infected • Chronic infection if HBsAg positive for >6 months
–	–	+	• Immune from vaccination
–	–	–	• Never infected • Should receive vaccination
–	+	+	• Resolved infection

QUICK HIT

No documented cases of infants acquiring HBV through breast milk.

QUICK HIT

Symptoms of acute hepatitis B: infection fever, anorexia, fatigue, malaise, nausea, jaundice. Asymptomatic presentations are more common in young children.

QUICK HIT

Extrahepatic manifestations of acute hepatitis B infection: migratory arthritis, maculopapular rash, urticarial rash, Gianotti-Crosti syndrome, angioedema

QUICK HIT

The risk of developing chronic HBV in the absence of adequate prophylaxis is inversely related to age. It is especially important to ensure that infants born to mothers who are HBsAg positive or whose status is unknown receive recommended prophylaxis within 12 hours of birth.

QUICK HIT

Most serious complication of chronic HBV is development of hepatocellular carcinoma (HCC).

QUICK HIT

The earliest to appear is HBsAg, and it typically presents before symptom onset.

3. Transmission
   a. Percutaneous (needlestick, blood transfusion)
   b. Sexual
   c. Vertical (mother to offspring)
4. Incidence has been declining over past 20 years

B. Clinical features
1. Acute HCV
   a. Majority of individuals are asymptomatic
   b. Nonspecific symptoms can be present similar to acute HAV or HBV
   c. Only 1/3 of patients will have jaundice
   d. Can be self-limited
2. Chronic HCV
   a. Perinatal transmission of HCV is 5%
   b. Perinatal transmission of HCV from mothers who are co-infected with HCV and HIV is 15%–20%
   c. Chronic inflammation leads to significant morbidity and mortality later in life due to development of cirrhosis and hepatocellular carcinoma (HCC)
   d. Reports of cirrhosis and HCC developing in children with aggressive disease

C. Diagnosis is made by serologic markers (see Table 3-7)

D. Treatment
1. Combination therapy with interferon and ribavirin
2. HCV genotype impacts effectiveness of therapy: genotype 1 associated with poorer response than genotypes 2 and 3

E. Immunoprophylaxis: does not exist

QUICK HIT

Chronic liver disease in adults from HCV is now the leading cause of liver transplantation.

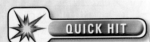

QUICK HIT

Perinatal transmission is the major route of acquiring HCV in children. Infants born to mothers with HCV may have positive antibodies due to passive maternal transfer. It is recommended to check antibodies at age 12–18 months when maternal antibodies are likely to have disappeared.

QUICK HIT

Detecting HCV RNA in infants born to mothers who have HCV can be helpful in establishing the diagnosis but should not be checked before age 2 months because there are known false positives. HCV RNA must be detected on 2 separate occasions, 6 months apart, to establish the diagnosis.

XXVII. Autoimmune Hepatitis

A. General characteristics
1. Chronic inflammatory hepatitis
2. Can be associated with autoimmune sclerosing cholangitis

B. Clinical features
1. Type 1 AIH more common and represents about 2/3 of cases
2. Predominance in girls (75%–80%)
3. Type 2 AIH tends to present at younger age
4. Both types associated with other autoimmune disorders

C. Diagnosis
1. Serologic markers
2. Liver biopsy

D. Treatment: requires immunosuppression

QUICK HIT

Types 1 and 2 AIH can present very similarly, and generally, one is not more severe than the other. The caveat is that type 2 can present with acute hepatic failure.

XXVIII. Biliary Atresia

A. Characteristics
1. Pathophysiology
   a. Normal development of biliary tree
   b. Perinatal insult (viral, toxic, or vascular) causes injury to bile duct mucosa
   c. Immunologic response/inflammatory infiltration and obstruction
   d. Ductular reaction with epithelial proliferation
   e. Progressive sclerosis, fibrosis, and obliteration of extrahepatic biliary ducts resulting in atresia within the first months of life
   f. Cholestasis leading to hepatocellular injury and secondary cirrhosis

B. Clinical features
1. Historical findings
   a. Healthy newborn, usually full term, initially normal weight gain
   b. May have brief perinatal jaundice but then "jaundice-free" period
   c. Progressive jaundice usually apparent by age 8 weeks
   d. Classically, acholic stools and dark urine

QUICK HIT

Biliary atresia is a progressive, sclerosing, inflammatory process of extrahepatic bile ducts causing complete biliary obstruction in first 3 months of life.

2. Physical exam findings
   a. Jaundice, scleral icterus
   b. Otherwise well appearing
   c. Soft hepatomegaly and may have mild splenomegaly

C. Diagnosis
1. Differential diagnosis (see Box 3-4 on conjugated hyperbilirubinemia)
2. Laboratory findings
   a. Total bilirubin 7–9 mg/dL
   b. Conjugated or direct bilirubin 3–6 mg/dL
   c. Markedly elevated GGT, ALP
   d. Mild to modest elevation of AST, ALT
   e. May have normal hemoglobin, albumin, and prothrombin time
3. Radiology findings
   a. Ultrasound to look for hepatomegaly, splenomegaly, or absent gallbladder
   b. HIDA
      i. Failure of tracer excretion into intestine suggests biliary atresia but is not diagnostic
      ii. Normal exam makes biliary atresia very unlikely
   c. Intraoperative cholangiogram: direct observation of biliary tree
4. Liver biopsy, diagnostic in up to 90% of cases: expanded portal tracts, edema, damaged and proliferated bile ducts, fibrosis and inflammation, canalicular and bile duct plugs

D. Treatment
1. Therapy
   a. Kasai portoenterostomy: roux-en-Y jejunostomy creating portoenterostomy connecting hilum of liver to loop of bowel; thereby directly draining bile from liver into intestine
   b. Liver transplantation: majority will require despite Kasai; however, not indicated as primary therapy, curative
2. Complications
   a. Failure to drain bile with Kasai portoenterostomy
   b. Ascending cholangitis
   c. Even with bile flow established and cholestasis improved, there is progressive fibrosis, cirrhosis, portal hypertension, and end-stage liver disease causing death or requiring transplantation
3. Duration/prognosis
   a. Results dramatically improved if identified and Kasai performed prior to 60 days of life
   b. Single most predictive factor is successful drainage of bile; if bilirubin returns to normal postoperatively, 90% 15-year survival reported
   c. Even with Kasai portoenterostomy, majority of patients will ultimately require liver transplantation (50% by age 2 years)

XXIV. Alagille Syndrome

A. Characteristics
1. Classic triad of cholestasis, peripheral pulmonic stenosis (PPS), and posterior embryotoxon
2. Dysmorphic facies: triangular facies, large forehead, wide nasal bridge and small pointed chin; eyes may be deep-set
3. Other features include butterfly vertebrae, growth and mental retardation, renal disease, pancreatic insufficiency, and vascular abnormalities
4. Genetics
   a. Autosomal dominant
   b. Defect on short arm of chromosome 20 (20p12)
   c. De novo mutations in 1/2 to 2/3 of cases
5. Pathophysiology: paucity of interlobular bile ducts (during hepatic architectural development) leading to cholestasis

QUICK HIT

Infants with biliary atresia are usually well grown and well appearing with jaundice and hepatomegaly.

QUICK HIT

It is useful to rule out a choledochal cyst, but a *normal ultrasound does not rule out biliary atresia*!

QUICK HIT

Biliary atresia is a time-sensitive diagnosis; if it is found and surgery performed prior to 60 days of life, outcome is significantly improved.

QUICK HIT

Biliary atresia is the most common indication for pediatric liver transplant.

QUICK HIT

While mostly benign, PPS murmur beyond 6 months warrants further investigation.

QUICK HIT

Persistent direct jaundice in the neonatal period in a baby with syndromic facies should prompt suspicion of Alagille syndrome.

QUICK HIT

Mild disease peaks at age 3–5 years and may resolve by age 10 years.

QUICK HIT

Patients with serious structural cardiac lesions have worst prognosis.

B. Diagnosis
   1. Need 3 of 5 features to make diagnosis plus evidence of cholestasis
   2. Definitive diagnosis requires liver biopsy
C. Treatment
   1. Mild disease
      a. Ursodeoxycholic acid to facilitate bile flow
      b. Diphenhydramine for pruritis
   2. Severe disease requires liver transplantation
   3. Optimized nutrition, including vitamin A, D, E, K, and zinc supplement
   4. Complications: multiple organs may be involved

4

Endocrine and Metabolic Diseases

SYMPTOM SPECIFIC

I. Approach to Short Stature

A. General characteristics
   1. Common clinical concern
   2. Symptom, not disease
   3. May be variant of normal growth but may indicate pathology
   4. Refers to height <2 standard deviations (SDs) or more below mean height for children of that sex, chronologic age, and ethnicity (below 3rd percentile)

B. Clinical features
   1. Historical findings
      a. History should be focused on assessing if this is short, healthy child or short child with pathology
      b. Important to elicit from birth history any risk factors predisposing to development of growth hormone (GH) deficiency or hypopituitarism
         i. Perinatal hypoxia (e.g., breech position, traumatic delivery)
         ii. Central nervous system (CNS) infection (e.g., meningitis)
      c. Elicit adequate dietary history to exclude malnutrition and poor weight gain as cause
   2. Historical questions
      a. Is the child developmentally normal or appropriate? Certain genetic syndromes with developmental delay are associated with short stature (e.g., Prader-Willi syndrome)
      b. Is the child growing appropriately for his genetic potential or family background? Determine the midparental target height of child using formula:
         i. Boys: (father's height [cm] + mother's height [cm] + 13 cm) ÷ 2
         ii. Girls: (father's height [cm] + mother's height [cm] − 13 cm) ÷ 2
   3. Review of systems should focus on systemic illness that may affect growth (e.g., Crohn disease, celiac disease, chronic kidney disease, anemia, hypothyroidism, Cushing syndrome)
   4. Physical exam findings
      a. May help elucidate cause of short stature or growth failure (goiter for hypothyroidism, midline defect and micropenis for hypopituitarism, central adiposity and cherubic/pudgy face for classic GH deficiency)
      b. Does child look dysmorphic (which may point to certain syndromes)?
         i. Turner syndrome: webbed neck, high arched palate, short 4th metacarpal, and shield chest
         ii. Russell-Silver syndrome: triangular face, relative macrocephaly, clinodactyly
      c. Proportionate short stature versus disproportionate short stature?

C. Diagnosis
   1. Differential diagnosis (Box 4-1)
   2. Physiology of growth

> **QUICK HIT**
> Growth velocity over a period of time (usually 6 months or 1 year) is more useful than a single height measurement. Always review growth chart to assess growth pattern over time.

> **QUICK HIT**
> Most children achieve an adult stature within approximately 10 cm or 4 inches of their target height.

> **QUICK HIT**
> Patients with classic GH deficiency have short stature, increased fat mass leading to a "chubby" or "cherubic" appearance, high-pitched voice, and bone age delay.

> **QUICK HIT**
> Conditions that cause disproportionate short stature include achondroplasia, hypochondroplasia, and Turner syndrome.

BOX 4-1

Differential Diagnosis of Short Stature

- Constitutional delay in growth and development
- Familial short stature
- Chromosomal abnormalities (Turner syndrome [45,X and other variants], trisomies 13, 18, 21)
- Skeletal dysplasia (achondroplasia, hypochondroplasia)
- Syndromes (Noonan, Russell-Silver, Prader-Willi syndromes)
- Systemic disorders
  - Gastrointestinal (celiac, Crohn disease, cystic fibrosis)
  - Cardiac (severe congenital heart defects)
  - Pulmonary (cystic fibrosis, asthma on chronic steroids)
  - Renal (chronic renal insufficiency, Fanconi syndrome)
- Nutritional (marasmus, kwashiorkor)
- Psychosocial growth retardation (child abuse/neglect)
- Endocrine
  - Hypothyroidism
  - Cushing syndrome
  - Growth hormone deficiency
  - Growth hormone insensitivity
  - Poorly controlled type 1 diabetes mellitus (Mauriac syndrome)
  - Pseudohypoparathyroidism (Albright hereditary osteodystrophy)
- Drugs (Glucocorticoids)

QUICK HIT

In the first year of life, thyroid hormone is a bigger mediator of growth than GH.

QUICK HIT

Bone age in children with constitutional delay in growth is usually delayed 2 or 3 years compared to chronologic age. The bone age in familial or genetic short stature is seldom delayed more than 1 year compared with chronologic age. In children with pathologic short stature (hypothyroidism, GH deficiency, or chronic disease), there may be marked bone age delay >2–3 years.

QUICK HIT

Chromosomal analysis or karyotype should be done in girls with unexplained cause of short stature.

3. Normal growth results from complex interaction of genetic, nutritional, environmental, psychosocial, and hormonal factors (GH, insulin-like growth factor 1 [IGF1], thyroid hormone, insulin, sex steroids, and glucocorticoids)
4. During normal childhood, growth involves an increase in length of bones
   a. Bone age x-ray assesses skeletal maturity
      i. Standard single view of left hand, fingers, and wrist
      ii. Appearance of representative epiphyseal centers is compared with age-appropriate published standards
   b. Bone age or skeletal age maturation is helpful in differentiating type of short stature
5. Laboratory tests to exclude pathologic causes of short stature
   a. Complete blood count (CBC) with differential
   b. Erythrocyte sedimentation rate (ESR), which is elevated in inflammation
   c. Thyroid function test (thyroid-stimulating hormone [TSH], free thyroxine [T_4] or total T_4)
   d. Electrolytes
   e. Tissue transglutaminase immunoglobulin (Ig) A Ab and total IgA level to identify celiac disease
   f. Serum IGF1 and IGFBP3 levels to screen for GH deficiency

D. Treatment
1. Depends on underlying etiology
2. Adequate nutrition or caloric intake in patients with malnutrition
3. Reassurance or counseling in patients with constitutional delay in growth and puberty; if psychosocial distress is present, consider short course of intramuscular (IM) long-acting testosterone for 4–6 months
4. Daily GH injections in children with GH deficiency

II. Approach to Precocious Puberty

A. Characteristics
1. Definitions: appearance of secondary sexual characteristics prior to lower limit of normal age of pubertal onset
   a. In boys, <9 years old
   b. In girls, <8 years old

2. Classified into 2 categories depending on source of hormonal production
   a. Central precocious puberty (CPP) or true precocious puberty (also known as *gonadotropin-dependent precocious puberty*)
      i. Results from activation of the hypothalamic–pituitary–gonadal axis
      ii. Elevated serum luteinizing hormone (LH) and follicle-stimulating hormone (FSH) with consequent elevation of serum testosterone or estradiol
   b. Peripheral: *also known as gonadotropin-independent precocious puberty (GIPP)*
      i. No activation of hypothalamic–pituitary axis
      ii. Gonadal (ovarian or testicular) steroid secretion is independent of gonadotropin-releasing hormone (GnRH) or could be iatrogenic exposure to gonadal steroids (low or normal serum LH, FSH with elevated serum testosterone, estradiol, or dehydroepiandrosterone sulfate [DHEAS])
3. CPP
   a. Girls: onset of **thelarche** (breast budding) <8 years old
   b. Boys: onset of testicular enlargement in boys <9 years old
   c. 5–10× more common in girls than in boys
   d. Occurs in 1/5,000 to 1/10,000 children
   e. Usually sporadic
   f. Most likely etiology depends on child's gender
      i. Most commonly identified CNS abnormality is **hypothalamic hamartoma** (i.e., congenital malformations consisting of heterotopic masses of normal neurons and glial cells, ectopically located at base of 3rd ventricle or tuber cinereum)
      ii. Other CNS causes include tumors (e.g., optic glioma, astrocytoma, craniopharyngioma) and cysts (e.g., arachnoid cyst)
4. Causes of peripheral precocious puberty/GIPP
   a. Ovarian cysts or tumors
   b. Testicular tumor (Leydig cell tumor)
   c. Adrenal tumors
   d. Congenital adrenal hyperplasia (CAH)
   e. Exogenous androgens or estrogens (topical testosterone gels/creams or estrogen-containing compounds [lavender or tea tree oils])
   f. Human chorionic gonadotropin (HCG)–secreting tumors, especially in boys (hepatoblastoma, CNS tumor, or mediastinal tumor in patients with Klinefelter syndrome)

B. Clinical features
1. History should focus on the points in Box 4-2
2. Physical findings should include
   a. Height measurement, weight, growth velocity/acceleration
   b. Papilledema (suggests increased intracranial pressure [ICP])
   c. Cranial nerve palsy (from CNS tumors)
   d. Café-au-lait spots
      i. McCune-Albright syndrome: irregular border coast of Maine–type
      ii. Neurofibromatosis: regular, smooth border coast of California–type
   e. Pubertal staging using Tanner method (for details on Tanner staging, see Approach to Delayed Puberty)

QUICK HIT

In girls, the most common cause of CPP is idiopathic (70%–90%), whereas in boys, identifiable CNS lesions account for 60%–94% of cases.

BOX 4-2

Key Questions for History in Precocious Puberty

- Age of onset of pubertal development: age of onset of thelarche, pubic hair development, growth spurt, and menarche
- Significant past medical history of central nervous system (CNS) abnormalities (neurofibromatosis, CNS radiation, CNS infection) that predisposes to central precocious puberty
- Review of systems: chronic headaches with blurred vision, vomiting, diplopia that suggest CNS tumors
- Exogenous exposure to androgens or estrogens (testosterone creams/gels or estrogen-containing oils/creams)
- Abdominal pain (ovarian mass/tumors)
- Rapid virilization (clitoromegaly, acne, pubic hair in girls—virilizing adrenal tumors)

C. Laboratory testing
  1. Children with CPP have pubertal or elevated levels of LH, serum testosterone, and estradiol
  2. Children with GIPP have low LH and FSH (prepubertal), and elevated serum testosterone or estradiol level

D. Radiology findings
  1. Bone age of left hand is advanced usually >2 SDs (>2 years above chronologic age)
  2. Pelvic ultrasound shows ovarian or uterine enlargement in girls with CPP
  3. In GIPP, labs should be ordered depending on etiology
    a. Serum HCG to detect HCG-secreting tumor (hepatoblastoma)
    b. Serum 17-hydroxyprogesterone (17-OHP) in 21-hydroxylase (21-OH) deficiency CAH
    c. Magnetic resonance imaging (MRI) of brain and pituitary gland may reveal CNS tumor or physiologic enlargement of pituitary gland

QUICK HIT

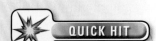

MRI of the brain and pituitary gland is indicated in all boys with CPP because incidence of CNS pathology is high. Unsuspected intracranial pathology has been reported in 40% of boys without neurologic findings.

E. Treatment
  1. Indications for treatment include poor height prognosis because premature closure of bone growth plates, early menarche, and psychosocial difficulties
  2. Administer long-acting GnRH agonist IM once every 4 weeks or subdermal implant that lasts 1–2 years
  3. Other GnRH agonist formulations are available that may be given IM every 3 months or via nasal spray or subcutaneously (subQ)
  4. GnRH agonist desensitizes pituitary to stimulatory effect of endogenous GnRH, leading to suppression of gonadotropin release, thereby stopping pubertal progression

QUICK HIT

The most important clinical criterion for GnRH agonist treatment is documented progression of pubertal development (growth acceleration and bone age maturation).

III. Approach to Delayed Puberty

A. General characteristics
  1. In boys, defined as lack of testicular enlargement by age 14 years (1st sign of puberty in boys)
  2. In girls, lack of thelarche by age 13 years
  3. 2.5% of healthy boys and girls have delayed puberty
  4. Pathophysiology grouped in 3 categories
    a. Constitutional delay
      i. 1/2 of cases (about 60% of boys and 30% of girls)
      ii. Usually family history of delayed puberty in parent or sibling
    b. Gonadotropin deficiency (hypogonadotropic hypogonadism)
    c. Primary gonadal failure (hypergonadotropic hypogonadism)
  5. Causes are summarized in Box 4-3

QUICK HIT

The most common cause of delayed puberty in children is constitutional delay.

BOX 4-3

Causes of Delayed Puberty

1. Constitutional delay in growth and puberty
2. Gonadotropin deficiency (hypogonadotropic hypogonadism)
  a. Isolated gonadotropin deficiency with anosmia (Kallmann syndrome)
  b. Functional gonadotropin deficiency (due to systemic illness, anorexia nervosa, excessive exercise)
  c. Multiple or combined pituitary hormone deficiency
    i. Congenital
    ii. Acquired (CNS lesions or tumor—craniopharyngioma)
3. Primary gonadal failure (hypergonadotropic hypogonadism)
  a. Klinefelter syndrome (47,XXY males or variants) in males and Turner syndrome (45,X and variants) in females
  b. Testicular irradiation for malignancies (tumors or leukemia)
  c. Chemotherapeutic/alkylating drugs toxic to gonads (ovaries and testes): cyclophosphamide, vinblastine, vincristine, cisplatin, etc.
  d. Total-body irradiation for malignancies
  e. Autoimmune ovarian failure

B. Clinical features
   1. Historical findings should focus on whether this is healthy, "late-blooming" child or child with pathology
   2. Key historical questions/assessments
      a. Family history of delayed puberty (age of menarche in mother and pubertal growth spurt in father)?
      b. Assess poor caloric intake or excessive exercise for anorexia nervosa
      c. History of radiation to CNS, testicles, ovaries?
      d. Surgery for bilateral cryptorchidism? (Suggests hypogonadotropic hypogonadism)
      e. History of chemotherapy for malignancies toxic to gonads (ovaries and testes)?
      f. Any systemic illness (e.g., Crohn disease, celiac disease, poorly controlled diabetes mellitus, severe hypothyroidism)?
      g. CNS signs and symptoms?
         i. Headaches, blurry vision, bitemporal hemianopsia suggest craniopharyngioma
         ii. Galactorrhea suggests prolactinoma
C. Physical exam should include height, weight, body mass index, arm span, and pubertal staging assessed by Tanner method (Figures 4-1 and 4-2)
   1. 1st sign of puberty in boys is testicular enlargement (>4 mL) usually at average age of 11.5 years
   2. 1st sign of puberty in girls is thelarche at average age of 10.5 years
D. Diagnosis
   1. Healthy child with unremarkable history or negative physical exam: LH and FSH, testosterone in boys, and serum estradiol in girls
   2. TSH, prolactin, CBC with differential, ESR, and C-reactive protein (CRP) should be considered, guided by child's history and physical exam

QUICK HIT

The average age of menarche in females is 12 years; menarche after age 14 years suggests delayed puberty.

QUICK HIT

The pubertal growth spurt in average maturing boys occurs between ages 13 and 14 years.

QUICK HIT

An arm span exceeding the standing height by more than 5 cm suggests eunochoidal body habitus and delayed epiphyseal closure secondary to hypogonadism.

QUICK HIT

Webbed neck, high-arched palate, short 4th metacarpal, and shield chest in a girl suggest Turner syndrome.

FIGURE 4-1 **The Tanner stages of female sexual maturity: breast and pubic hair development.**

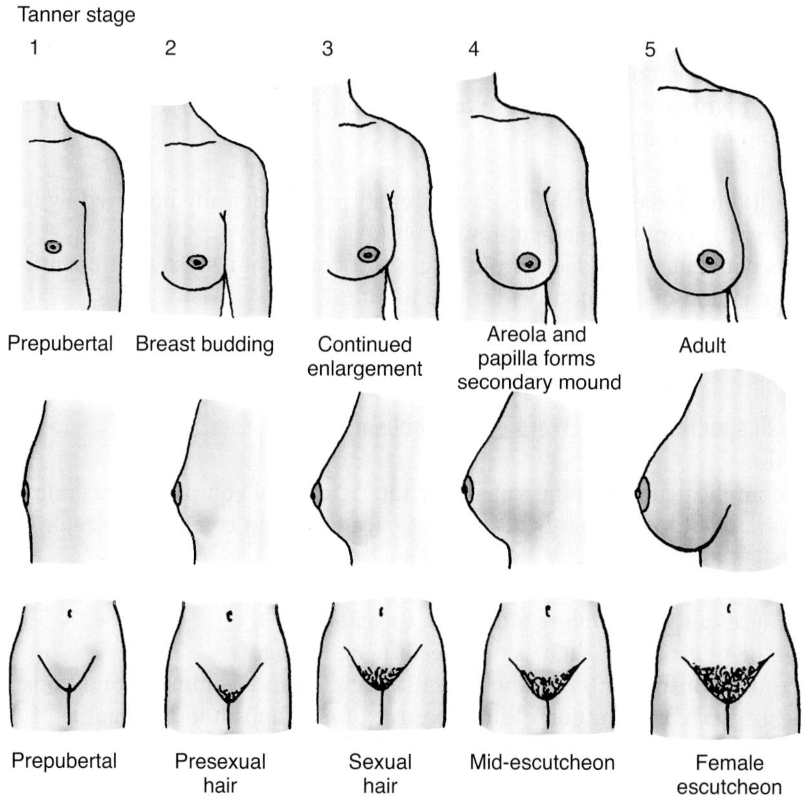

Endocrine and Metabolic Diseases

FIGURE 4-2 The Tanner stages of male sexual maturity.

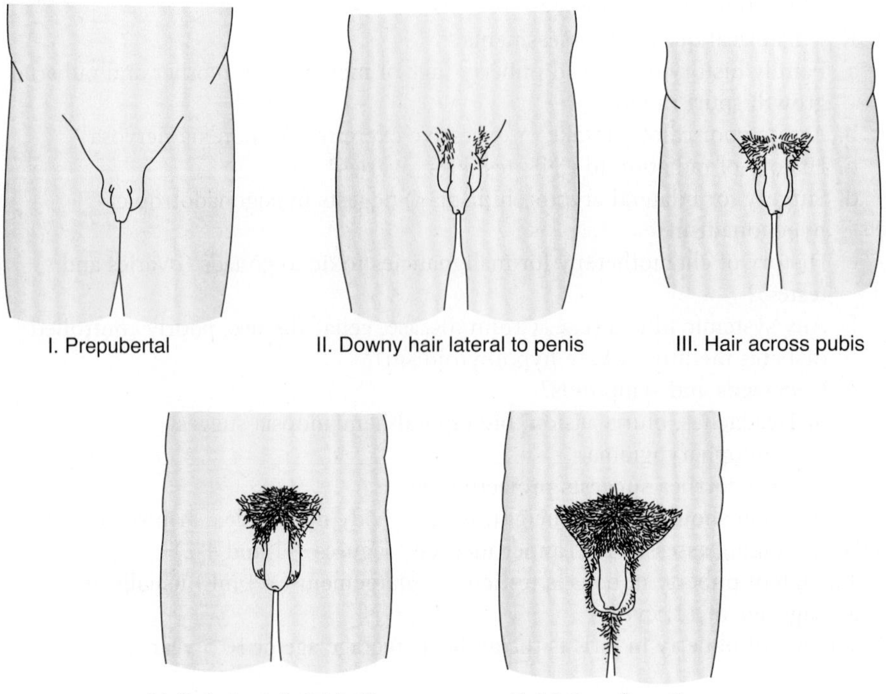

(From LifeART Nursing 1, CD-ROM. Baltimore: Lippincott Williams & Wilkins. NU118014.)

findings; check chromosomes if suspecting Turner syndrome or Klinefelter syndrome

3. Bone age x-ray (skeletal radiography) of wrist and hand in children with delayed puberty and short stature usually shows delay in bone maturation and is useful in assessing height prognosis
4. Other diagnostic imaging guided by etiology of delayed puberty (e.g., MRI of brain and pituitary gland for CNS tumors, such as craniopharyngiomas, and **Kallmann syndrome**

E. Treatment
1. Constitutional delay: in children who are not psychologically bothered by lack of puberty, reassurance and continued observation
2. In boys concerned with lack of puberty, short course of testosterone enanthate or cypionate in oil IM monthly for 4–6 months
3. In girls, short course of conjugated estrogen or micronized estradiol is an option, although long-term data on efficacy and outcome are limited

IV. Approach to Suspected Inborn Errors of Metabolism

A. Introduction
1. Rare, complicated conditions caused by interference of complex biochemical pathways resulting in energy defects, intoxications, and complex molecule defects
2. Symptoms
   a. Can present within hours after birth to years later
   b. Can be nonspecific, such as poor feeding and lethargy
   c. Because nonspecific symptoms are also seen in more common conditions like sepsis, consideration of inborn error of metabolism in differential of sick infant or child is crucial
3. Important to be familiar with common presentations and specific conditions

QUICK HIT

Bone age in children with constitutional delay in puberty is usually delayed by 2 or more years and usually matches the child's height age rather than chronologic age. Height age is the age at which the child's current height plots at the 50th percentile on the child's growth chart.

QUICK HIT

Kallmann syndrome is hypogonadotropic hypogonadism associated with anosmia or hyposmia. MRI findings include deficiency of the olfactory sulcus and rudimentary or absent olfactory bulbs and tracts.

QUICK HIT

Symptoms of hypoglycemia include sweating, pallor, irritability, and tremulousness.

QUICK HIT

Prompt recognition and reversal of hypoglycemia are necessary to prevent brain damage.

B. Clinical presentation
  1. Hypoglycemia
    a. Definition: serum glucose <50 mg/dL in infants and children, <40 mg/dL in neonates
    b. Signs and symptoms
      i. Neonates: poor feeding, seizure, coma
      ii. Older children: headache, lethargy
    c. Physical exam
      i. Growth parameters
      ii. Hepatomegaly with hypoglycemia, consider disorder of fatty acid oxidation or glycogen storage disease
      iii. Midline defects such as central incisor, cleft lip/palate, micropenis suggest hypopituitarism
    d. Differential diagnosis
      i. Carbohydrate metabolism disorders
      ii. Amino acid defects
      iii. Fatty acid oxidation defects
      iv. Hyperinsulinism (see Endocrine section)
        (a) Congenital hyperinsulinism
        (b) Insulinoma
      v. Hormone deficiencies
        (a) GH deficiency
        (b) Cortisol deficiency
      vi. Ketotic hypoglycemia
    e. Workup
      i. Most important step is to obtain critical sample prior to treating hypoglycemia
        (a) Blood: plasma glucose, insulin, C-peptide, cortisol, GH, free fatty acids, β-hydroxybutyrate, lactate, total and free carnitine, acylcarnitine profile, ammonia, plasma amino acid
        (b) Urine: ketones, reducing substances, urine organic acids
      ii. CBC with differential, urinalysis, arterial blood gas (ABG), and complete metabolic panel
      iii. Consider age of patient
      iv. Consider fed versus fasting state including length of fast
  2. Metabolic acidosis
    a. Definition: pH <7.3, HCO_3^- <15, often compensated by respiratory alkalosis with partial pressure of carbon dioxide (PCO_2) <30
    b. Signs and symptoms: altered mental status, vomiting, respiratory distress, anorexia, poor perfusion
    c. Differential diagnosis
      i. Ketones present
        (a) Hyperglycemia (diabetes, organic acidemias)
        (b) Normoglycemia (organic acidemias, respiratory chain disorders)
        (c) Hypoglycemia (gluconeogenesis defects, respiratory chain defects)
      ii. Ketones absent
        (a) High lactate (e.g., pyruvate dehydrogenase deficiency, fatty acid oxidation defects)
        (b) Normal lactate (e.g., renal tubular acidosis)
    d. Workup
      i. CBC with differential, urinalysis, ABG, and complete metabolic panel, glucose, and ammonia
      ii. Look for presence or absence of ketones
      iii. Lactate and pyruvate levels
        (a) Normal lactate: pyruvate suggests defects in pyruvate dehydrogenase or gluconeogenesis
        (b) Elevated lactate: pyruvate suggests pyruvate carboxylase deficiency, respiratory chain defects, or mitochondrial disorder

QUICK HIT

Short stature is associated with hypopituitarism and/or GH deficiency.

QUICK HIT

Transient hyperinsulinism in a neonate may be caused by maternal peripartum treatment with glucose or antihyperglycemic medications.

QUICK HIT

Ketotic hypoglycemia is a diagnosis of exclusion. Children often present in late infancy to early childhood (age 18 months–5 years) after prolonged fasting.

QUICK HIT

Infants with Beckwith-Wiedemann syndrome may present with hemihypertrophy and hypoglycemia.

QUICK HIT

In a toddler or older child with hypoglycemia, consider ingestion of β-blockers or hypoglycemic agents as a possible cause. Ask the family about medications in the home.

QUICK HIT

Hypoglycemia after prolonged fasting maybe associated with disorders of fatty acid oxidation and gluconeogenesis.

QUICK HIT

Most cases of metabolic acidosis due to an inborn error of metabolism have an increased anion gap.

3. Acute metabolic encephalopathy
   a. Definition: acute global cerebral dysfunction due to underlying metabolic condition, not structural brain abnormality
   b. Signs and symptoms: poor feeding, lethargy, vomiting, seizure, abnormal muscle tone, apnea, respiratory distress, coma
   c. Differential diagnosis
      i. Urea cycle defects
      ii. Organic acidemias
      iii. Fatty acid oxidation disorders
      iv. Maple syrup disease
      v. Nonketotic hyperglycinemia
      vi. Transient hyperammonemia of the newborn (THAN)
   d. Workup
      i. CBC with differential, urinalysis, ABG, and complete metabolic panel
      ii. Ammonia levels
      iii. Urine-reducing substances
      iv. Plasma/urine amino acids
      v. Urine organic acids
      vi. Lactate levels
      vii. Consider timing of symptoms

C. Treatment: for acute management of suspected inborn errors of metabolism
1. Airway, breathing, circulation (ABCs)
2. Intravenous (IV) hydration with D10 at 1.5–2× maintenance, increased glucose infusion rate to stop catabolic state
3. Treat acute hypoglycemia with 0.25–1 g/kg of D10–D25
4. Correct metabolic acidosis
   a. IV hydration
   b. If pH <7.0, consider slow correction with HCO_3^-
5. Eliminate potential toxic metabolites
   a. Nothing by mouth (NPO)
   b. For hyperammonemia
      i. Reduce protein intake
      ii. Alternate pathways for nitrogen excretion (e.g., Na^+ benzoate)
      iii. For severe cases, consider hemodialysis

QUICK HIT

In a newborn with tachypnea without evidence of respiratory infection, think metabolic acidosis. The infant may be blowing off CO_2 to compensate for acidosis.

QUICK HIT

The respiratory chain is a series of proteins in the mitochondrial wall that manufacture ATP through oxidative phosphorylation.

QUICK HIT

THAN is often seen in large, premature infants with pulmonary disease and hyperammonemia.

QUICK HIT

Any child with unexplained lethargy and vomiting should have ammonia levels checked.

DISEASE SPECIFIC

V. Type 1 Diabetes Mellitus (T1DM)

A. General characteristics
1. Definition: metabolic disorder of hyperglycemia resulting from absolute deficiency of insulin production and secretion from pancreas
2. Epidemiology
   a. Annual incidence in United States is 15 cases per 100,000 children
   b. Worldwide, incidence varies
      i. Highest: Finland, 35 cases per 100,000 children
      ii. Lowest: China and Venezuela, 1 case per 100,000 children
   c. Peak incidence in fall and winter
   d. Most common ages for diagnosis are 5–7 years and adolescence
   e. Increasing numbers of cases in younger age groups (age <5 years)
   f. No gender predilection
3. Cause
   a. Majority of cases due to T cell–mediated autoimmune destruction of insulin-producing pancreatic β cells
   b. Idiopathic
4. Genetics
   a. Strong association with certain human leukocyte antigen (HLA) and non-HLA alleles (e.g., HLA DR3 and DR4 convey 10-fold increased risk for developing T1DM)

QUICK HIT

In infants with coma secondary to hyperammonemia, the likelihood of neurologic impairment depends on the duration of neonatal hyperammonemic coma.

QUICK HIT

There is a higher incidence of T1DM in children born with congenital rubella and those who have had an enteroviral infection.

b. Risk of developing diabetes in first-degree relatives
   i. Identical twins: 50%
   ii. Nonidentical sibling: 5%–6% by age 20 years, 10% by age 60 years
   iii. Offspring: 5% if father is diabetic; 2%–3% if mother is diabetic
5. Risk factors
   a. Presence of high-risk alleles
   b. First-degree relative with T1DM
   c. Congenital rubella or acquired enteroviral infection
   d. Presence of other autoimmune diseases
6. Pathophysiology
   a. Immune-mediated destruction of pancreatic β cells leads to insulin deficiency
   b. Insulin deficiency leads to hyperglycemia, glucosuria, high serum ketones, and clinical symptoms

B. Clinical features
1. Symptoms
   a. Early stages
      i. Increased urination and thirst (the "poly's" = polyuria, polydipsia, polyphagia)
      ii. Weight loss (due to fat and protein catabolism)
      iii. Fatigue
   b. Progressive stages
      i. Abdominal pain and emesis (due to acidemia)
      ii. Shortness of breath (respiratory compensation for acidosis)
      iii. Confusion, stupor, or coma: due to cerebral edema
      iv. Death (from profound acidosis, hyperkalemia, cerebral edema)
2. Signs
   a. Early stages
      i. Asymptomatic
      ii. Weight loss/mild dehydration
   b. Progressive stages
      i. Polyuria despite marked dehydration
      ii. Tachycardia, tachypnea, poor skin turgor
      iii. Abnormal heart rhythm (due to hyperkalemia)
      iv. Delayed capillary refill
      v. Sweet or musty odor on breath (presence of ketones)
      vi. Abnormal mental status or confusion

C. Diagnosis
1. Differential diagnosis
   a. Urinary tract infection (UTI)
   b. Behavioral/psychogenic polydipsia
   c. Diabetes insipidus (DI)
   d. Stress hyperglycemia due to acute infection
2. Laboratory findings
   a. Random glucose >200 mg/dL with signs and symptoms of diabetes *or* glucose value >200 mg/dL, 2 hours post–glucose challenge *or* fasting glucose >126 mg/dL on 2 separate samples is diagnostic, or HbA1c >6.5%
   b. ~30% of new cases present in diabetic ketoacidosis (DKA) defined as
      i. Serum pH <7.3
      ii. Serum glucose >300 mg/dL
      iii. Serum bicarbonate <15 mEq/L
   c. Pseudohyponatremia (due to hyperglycemia) or hypernatremia in more advanced stages of dehydration
   d. Normal or elevated serum K^+ level
   e. Positive serum and urine ketones
   f. Elevated amylase and lipase: typically mild and transient
   g. Leukocytosis
   h. Low serum insulin and C-peptide levels
3. Radiologic findings: cerebral edema on computed tomography (CT) scan if performed

QUICK HIT

Autoantibodies can be measured in the serum of some patients months and even years before onset of clinical symptoms.

QUICK HIT

Autoimmune islet destruction is asymptomatic until >80% of β cells are destroyed.

QUICK HIT

Prior to the availability of insulin, T1DM was universally fatal within months of diagnosis.

QUICK HIT

The elevated or normal potassium levels found during DKA result from cellular H^+/K^+ exchange in the face of acidemia and may mask a significant systemic K^+ deficiency.

QUICK HIT

Peaked T waves on electrocardiogram (ECG) suggest hyperkalemia.

QUICK HIT

Cerebral edema may be seen on a CT scan in patients with ketoacidosis even when they have no clinical signs or symptoms. The utility of this finding is unknown.

QUICK HIT

Resolution of acidosis results in intracellular shifts of K^+, which can rapidly lower serum levels.

QUICK HIT

Adjust for fluid calculations of hypo- or hypernatremia carefully! For every 100 of glucose over normal, add 1.6 to the measured serum Na^+ to estimate what the Na^+ would be if the glucose were not contributing to osmolarity.

QUICK HIT

Bicarbonate therapy may worsen cerebral edema. It is *not* recommended unless there is life-threatening hemodynamic instability due to acidosis.

QUICK HIT

Treatment of DKA includes insulin to suppress ketone production and IV fluids to treat dehydration.

QUICK HIT

Cerebral edema is the most common cause of death in pediatric patients with DKA and may be worsened by overhydration and rapid correction of hyperglycemia.

QUICK HIT

A few months after diagnosis, many patients go through a transient "honeymoon" when they require less insulin (or even require none). It is critical for patients to understand that this is a *temporary* phenomenon and they are not cured of the disease.

D. Treatment
  1. Therapy
    a. Rehydration
      i. Calculations should assume 10% dehydration
      ii. Initial fluid is 0.9% normal saline (NS) due to presence of hyperosmolarity and risk of rapid cellular fluid shifts
      iii. Deficit is replaced gradually over 48–72 hours
      iv. Dextrose is added to IV fluids when serum glucose <300 mg/dL
      v. Bolus fluid therapy is reserved for hemodynamic instability
    b. Electrolyte therapy
      i. K^+ is withheld until serum levels are known
      ii. No K^+ is added to IV fluids until serum level is <5 mEq/L
      iii. Increasing amounts of K^+ are added as serum levels decrease
      iv. K^+ levels <2.5 mEq/L are treated aggressively, particularly if patient is still acidotic
      v. Pseudohyponatremia corrects with resolution of hyperglycemia
    c. Insulin
      i. Ketoacidosis is treated with IV insulin infusion
      ii. Start with insulin rate of 0.1 unit/kg/hr and titrate to maintain glucose reduction rate of 50–100 mg/dL/hr
      iii. In those without ketoacidosis or following resolution, begin subQ insulin administration with basal long-acting forms together with rapid-acting analog insulins
      iv. Choice of insulin based on medical, psychological, and social factors
      v. Initial dosing based on age and pubertal stage
  2. Complications
    a. Acute
      i. Cerebral edema
      ii. Hypokalemia
      iii. Hypoglycemia
    b. Chronic: due to poor glucose control
      i. Repeated episodes of ketoacidosis
      ii. Nephropathy and end-stage renal disease
      iii. Retinopathy and blindness
      iv. Extremity infections and amputations
      v. Peripheral neuropathy
      vi. Gastroparesis
  3. Prognosis
    a. Those with symptomatic cerebral edema may have residual neurologic deficits
    b. Overall prognosis is excellent with proper insulin therapy

VI. Type 2 Diabetes Mellitus (T2DM)

A. General characteristics
  1. Definition: metabolic disorder of hyperglycemia resulting from insufficient insulin secretion in face of insulin resistance
  2. Epidemiology
    a. Bimodal distribution with peak diagnosis between ages 10 and 18 years and between ages 50 and 55 years
    b. Overall prevalence among children in United States is 0.4%
    c. Prevalence among all cases of diabetes varies among ethnic groups
      i. Low: Caucasians (5%)
      ii. Moderate: Hispanics (20%); African Americans (33%)
      iii. High: Asian Pacific Islanders (40%); Native Americans (75%)
    d. Male-to-female ratio is approximately 1:5 among North Americans
  3. Cause: heterogeneous condition stemming from 2 main components
    a. Insulin resistance
      i. Peripheral insulin resistance (muscle and fat)
      ii. Hepatic insulin resistance (increased hepatic glucose production)
    b. Pancreatic β cell failure

4. Genetics
   a. Over 75% of diagnosed children have a 1st- or 2nd-degree relative with T2DM
   b. There is no HLA-specific association, but multiple genes have been implicated in pathogenesis
5. Risk factors
   a. Obesity
   b. Hispanic, African American, or Native American ethnicity
   c. Family history of T2DM
   d. Maternal gestational diabetes
   e. Large-for-gestational-age birth weight

QUICK HIT

Being premature or small for gestational age as an infant is a risk factor for developing adult-onset T2DM.

6. Pathophysiology
   a. Final common pathway is hyperglycemia due to an inability to sufficiently raise insulin secretion in response to insulin resistance
   b. Obesity carries an associated insulin resistance in muscle, fat, and liver
      i. Liver: Decreased downregulation of gluconeogenesis
      ii. Fat cells: Decreased fat storage, increased lipolysis and serum free fatty acids
      iii. Muscle cells: Decreased glucose uptake, increased protein catabolism and substrates for hepatic gluconeogenesis
   c. Excessive nutrient intake in obesity saturates fat cell stores
      i. Leptin resistance and decreased adiponectin levels ensue
      ii. Cellular changes and inflammation worsen insulin resistance
   d. Insulin resistance and compensatory elevated insulin secretion continue until β cell failure begins
   e. Hyperglycemia leads to lipotoxicity and increasing β cell failure
   f. Sufficient β cell failure leads to hyperglycemia and T2DM

QUICK HIT

Hyperglycemia causes downregulation of insulin transcription, and lipotoxicity from high serum free fatty acids causes decreased glucose-stimulated insulin secretion.

B. Clinical features
1. Symptoms
   a. Early stages
      i. Increased urination and thirst
      ii. Weight loss (due to fat and protein catabolism)
      iii. Blurry vision
   b. Progressive stages
      i. Irritability (due to hyperglycemia)
      ii. Abdominal pain and emesis (if acidemia is present)
      iii. Shortness of breath (response to acidosis)
      iv. Headache, confusion, stupor, or coma (due to cerebral edema)
      v. Death (from brainstem herniation or hemorrhage)
2. Signs
   a. Early stages
      i. Asymptomatic
      ii. Weight loss/mild dehydration
      iii. Acanthosis nigricans
   b. Late stages
      i. Polyuria despite marked dehydration
      ii. Tachycardia, tachypnea, poor skin turgor
      iii. Sweet or musty odor on breath (if acidosis is present)
      iv. Altered mental status
      v. Focal neurologic deficits (due to infarction or cerebral edema)

C. Diagnosis
1. Differential diagnosis
   a. UTI
   b. Behavioral/psychogenic polydipsia
   c. DI
   d. Stress hyperglycemia due to acute infection
2. Laboratory findings
   a. Random glucose >200 mg/dL with signs and symptoms of diabetes *or* glucose value >200 mg/dL 2 hours post–glucose challenge *or* fasting glucose >126 mg/dL on 2 separate samples is diagnostic, HbA1c >6.5%

> **QUICK HIT**
> To estimate the actual serum sodium in a patient with hyperglycemia, add 1.6 mmol/L to the serum sodium concentration for every 100 mg/dL glucose concentration above 100 mg/dL. Example: Measured Na = 130 mmol/L; serum glucose = 300 mg/dL Estimated serum sodium = (1.6 × 2) + 130 = 133.2 mmol/L

b. Approximately 30% of new cases present in DKA
c. Pseudohyponatremia
d. Normal or elevated serum K^+ level
e. Leukocytosis
f. Low or inappropriately normal insulin and C-peptide levels
g. ~10% of new cases present with hyperglycemic hyperosmolar state
h. Increased risk for cerebral edema, venous sinus thrombosis, and rhabdomyolysis

3. Other/radiologic findings
   a. Peaked T waves on electrocardiogram (ECG) due to hyperkalemia
   b. Cerebral edema on CT scan if performed

D. Treatment

1. Therapy of DKA similar as in T1DM
   a. Ketoacidosis is treated with IV insulin infusion
   b. Hyperglycemic hyperosmolar state may be treated without insulin and hydration alone until glucose is no longer decreasing
   c. Start with insulin rate of 0.1 unit/kg/hr and titrate to maintain glucose reduction rate of 50–100 mg/dL/hr
   d. In those without ketoacidosis or following resolution, begin subQ insulin administration with basal long-acting forms together with rapid-acting analog insulins
   e. Choice of insulin based on medical, psychological, and social factors
   f. Initial dosing is based on age and pubertal stage

> **QUICK HIT**
> Puberty induces a natural state of insulin resistance during which the insulin requirements are increased.

2. Oral agents
   a. Metformin
      i. Increases peripheral insulin sensitivity and decreases hepatic glucose production
      ii. Not used in acute setting
   b. Insulin secretagogues
      i. Increased risk of hypoglycemia
      ii. May cause weight gain
   c. Incretin mimetic agents
      i. Increase levels of glucagon-like peptide-1
      ii. Work through glucose-mediated insulin release
      iii. Result in weight loss and low risk of hypoglycemia
      iv. Not studied in children

> **QUICK HIT**
> Sulfonylureas are insulin secretagogues. They inactivate K^+ channels on β cells, resulting in easier depolarization and release of insulin.

> **QUICK HIT**
> Exenatide or liraglutide are incretin mimetics. Among other actions, they increase glucose-dependent insulin secretion and reduce glucagon secretion.

E. Complications

1. Acute
   a. Cerebral edema
   b. Hypokalemia
   c. Hypoglycemia
2. Chronic: due to poor glucose control
   a. Nephropathy and end-stage renal disease
   b. Retinopathy and blindness
   c. Extremity infections and amputations
   d. Peripheral neuropathy

F. Prognosis

1. Those with symptomatic cerebral edema may have residual deficits
2. Overall prognosis is excellent with proper medical therapy

> **QUICK HIT**
> A hyperglycemic hyperosmolar state confers a high risk of mortality (12%).

G. Prevention

1. Education about signs and symptoms of diabetes
2. Early diagnosis by testing those at risk
3. Aggressive measures to limit excessive weight gain and obesity

VII. Diabetes Insipidus

A. Definition

1. Unregulated free water diuresis resulting from ineffective production of or end-organ response to vasopressin (AVP, or ADH from former name antidiuretic hormone)

Endocrine and Metabolic Diseases

2. 2 forms
   a. Central: results from defective production or secretion of vasopressin from hypothalamus or posterior pituitary
   b. Nephrogenic: defective renal cell response to AVP

B. Causes
1. Central
   a. Developmental anomaly of hypothalamus or pituitary gland (septo-optic dysplasia)
   b. Direct injury to pituitary (tumors, trauma, or surgery)
   c. Infections (meningitis, encephalitis)
   d. Vascular injury/hemorrhage
   e. Inflammatory (Langerhans cell histiocytosis, Wegener granulomatosis)
   f. Genetic causes (familial DI, Wolfram syndrome)
   g. Idiopathic
2. Nephrogenic
   a. AVP2 receptor or aquaporin 2 water channel mutations
   b. Renal disease or malformations
   c. Medications

C. Clinical presentation: varies based on diagnosis and etiology; key historical questions summarized in Box 4-4
1. Central
   a. Main symptoms are polyuria and polydipsia
   b. Polyphagia may be seen with hypothalamic tumors
   c. May regress 3–5 days after surgery and present again following transient episode of syndrome of inappropriate antidiuretic hormone (SIADH) secretion; known as **triple-phase response**
2. Nephrogenic
   a. May present in 1st year of life as failure to thrive (FTT)
   b. Polyuria and polydipsia are main symptoms
   c. Familial forms may reveal other family members with same symptoms

QUICK HIT

Central diabetes insipidus may be the first and only sign of a brain tumor, so be aggressive in searching for an underlying cause.

QUICK HIT

Patients with concomitant cortisol deficiency may have their symptoms of DI unmasked only after cortisol replacement is initiated.

BOX 4-4

Key Historical Questions to Identify Causes of Diabetes Insipidus

1. Symptoms suggestive of craniopharyngioma or other central nervous system (CNS) mass
   a. Severe headaches
   b. Visual changes
   c. Decreased school performance
   d. Memory changes
   e. Increased hunger
   f. Decreased satiety
   g. Slow growth
2. Symptoms suggesting infiltrative disease
   a. Presence of systemic symptoms (fever, fatigue)
   b. Other organ system involvement (bone/joint pain, rash)
3. Medical history suggesting risk of vascular injury
   a. History of sickle cell disease
   b. Prior blood clots or hypercoagulable state
   c. Presence of patent ductus arteriosus (risk of embolus)
4. History suggesting neonatal/developmental causes
   a. Postpartum asphyxia: may lead to pituitary infarction and diabetes insipidus (DI)
   b. Hypoglycemia and micropenis at birth: may signal congenital hypopituitarism
   c. Midline cleft lip or palate: can be associated with midline anatomic defects
5. Medication use
   a. Lithium
   b. Demeclocycline
   c. Amphotericin
6. Other family members with similar symptoms of polyuria and polydipsia
   a. Autosomal dominant forms of familial central DI
   b. Autosomal or X-linked forms of nephrogenic DI

QUICK HIT

Patients with an intact thirst mechanism may hydrate well and have normal labs on a single analysis. With a high index of suspicion, a water deprivation test should be performed.

QUICK HIT

IV fluids should be limited to 1 L/m²/day in those also receiving IV AVP infusion to avoid the risk of hyponatremia and fluid overload.

D. Diagnosis and testing
   1. Confirmed upon finding of hyperosmolar serum (>300 mOsmol/kg) in presence of excessive and dilute urination (urine osmolarity <300 mOsmol/kg)
   2. Water deprivation test unmasks diagnosis in those with normal baseline labs
   3. Differential diagnosis of polyuria and polydipsia includes diabetes mellitus, primary polydipsia, and renal tubular defects
   4. Genetic testing for known mutations in familial forms and syndromes
   5. MRI of brain in confirmed central DI to identify potential underlying causes
      a. Posterior pituitary appears as "bright spot" on MRI images
      b. Absence of bright spot suggests ectopic posterior pituitary
E. Treatment
   1. Fluid hydration: oral route preferred for those who can tolerate it and are not severely dehydrated
   2. AVP: used subQ or IV in those unable to use oral or nasal route
   3. Desmopressin: synthetic AVP analog, available in oral or intranasal forms
      a. Intranasal form
         i. Advantages: rapid mucosal absorption, fast onset of action
         ii. Disadvantages: damage to nasal mucosa; cannot use in infants due to small nasal opening size
      b. Oral form
         i. Advantages: easy method of administration, can be crushed into solution to administer to infants
         ii. Disadvantages: slow onset of action with variable gastrointestinal (GI) absorption
   4. Goals of treatment
      a. Identify and treat any underlying cause
      b. Improve quality of life by reducing polyuria and thirst
      c. Maintain euvolemia and normal serum Na^+

VIII. Syndrome of Inappropriate Antidiuretic Hormone Secretion

A. Definition: inappropriate free water retention due to excessive secretion of antidiuretic hormone in presence of euvolemia and hyponatremia
B. Causes
   1. CNS disorders
      a. Intracranial tumors
      b. Infections (meningitis, encephalitis)
      c. Vascular injury/hemorrhage
      d. Surgical trauma
   2. Pulmonary disorders
      a. Asthma
      b. Cystic fibrosis (CF)
      c. Pulmonary malignancies
   3. Medications (tricyclic antidepressants [TCAs], amitriptyline: selective serotonin reuptake inhibitors [SSRIs], fluoxetine, omeprazole; angiotensin-converting enzyme [ACE] inhibitors)
   4. Other: inherited, idiopathic, gastroenteritis (usually presents as hyponatremia in face of high rate of hypotonic fluids)

QUICK HIT

Following intracranial surgery, SIADH may follow a 3- to 5-day initial period of DI. Excessive IV fluids following surgery coupled with SIADH can cause profound hyponatremia, pulmonary congestion, and cerebral edema.

C. Clinical presentation
   1. Patients are generally ill appearing due to underlying cause
      a. CNS lesions may present with headaches and focal signs
      b. Pulmonary diseases may present with dyspnea and chest pain
   2. Evaluation shows hyponatremia with no signs of dehydration
   3. Degree of hyponatremia may dictate mode of presentation
      a. Mild hyponatremia (Na^+ >125 mEq/L) is usually asymptomatic
      b. Severe hyponatremia (Na^+ <120 mEq/L) typically presents with lethargy, confusion, disorientation, ataxia, papilledema, or generalized seizures

Endocrine and Metabolic Diseases

D. Testing
1. Serum Na^+ <135 mEq/L and serum osmolality <280 mOsmol/kg
2. Inappropriately elevated urine osmolality (>100 mOsmol/kg), urine Na^+ concentration (>20 mEq/L), and fractional excretion of Na^+ (>1%)

E. Therapy
1. 3% hypertonic saline (4 mL/kg) as emergency therapy for seizures, raised ICP, or altered sensorium
2. Free water restriction to 1 L/m^2/day
3. Demeclocycline only in cases where water restriction is contraindicated (inhibits renal activity of ADH)
4. Treatment of underlying cause

IX. Hyperthyroidism

A. General characteristics
1. Commonly referred to as *hyperactive thyroid*
2. Graves is most common form in children (Box 4-5)
   a. Autoimmune disease, characterized by autoantibodies that stimulate TSH receptor
   b. More common in females

QUICK HIT

The elevated urinary Na^+ results from downregulation of aldosterone and upregulation of atrial natriuretic peptide secondary to volume expansion.

QUICK HIT

Fractional excretion of sodium = (Plasma Cr × Urine Na^+) / (Plasma Na × Urine Cr)

QUICK HIT

Serum Na^+ should be monitored carefully, with a maximum rise of 0.5 mEq/L/hr or 10–12 mEq/L/day.

BOX 4-5

Etiology of Hyperthyroidism

1. Graves disease
   Autoimmune disease characterized by autoantibodies that stimulate the thyroid-stimulating hormone (TSH) receptor and that result in autonomous excessive synthesis of thyroid hormone.
2. Hashitoxicosis
   Transient. Part of the clinical spectrum of autoimmune Hashimoto thyroiditis. Caused by autoantibodies that destroy thyroid follicular cells and release excessive thyroid hormone in the circulation.
3. Subacute thyroiditis
   Self-limiting inflammation of the thyroid, usually viral and associated with thyroid tenderness, that results in destruction of thyroid follicular cells and release of thyroid hormone in the circulation. Can be followed by a hypothyroid state and, eventually, by normal thyroid function.
4. Toxic nodule
   Autonomous thyroid nodule, usually benign, that results in excessive synthesis of thyroid hormone independent of TSH secretion.
5. Multinodular goiter
   Goiter characterized by multiple thyroid nodules that result in excessive synthesis of thyroid hormone independent of TSH secretion. Can be associated with certain genetic syndromes such as McCune-Albright.
6. Drugs
   Iodine excess
   Amiodarone: cardiovascular drug that can cause either hyperthyroidism or hypothyroidism due to its high iodine content and toxic effect on thyroid follicular cells resulting in destructive thyroiditis
   Lithium
   Interferon: used for the treatment of hepatitis C; causes thyroiditis
   Interleukin-2: used for the treatment of certain metastatic cancers and leukemia
7. TSH-producing pituitary adenoma
   Extremely rare
8. Radiation-induced thyroiditis
   Transient, caused by destruction of follicular thyroid cells and release of thyroid hormone
9. Selective pituitary thyroid resistance
   Rare. Resistance to the feedback effect of T_3 on TSH release. Presents with goiter and elevated T_4 and TSH concentrations.
10. Persistent congenital hyperthyroidism
   Rare. Caused by mutations in TSH receptor or GNAS leading to activation of TSH signaling. Can be associated with McCune-Albright syndrome.
11. Excessive thyroid hormone ingestion

QUICK HIT

Maternal Graves disease can cause either neonatal Graves due to transplacental transfer of antibodies, hypothyroidism due to maternal treatment with thionamides, or suppression of fetal TSH secretion by maternal hyperthyroidism.

QUICK HIT

Exophthalmos is pathognomonic of Graves disease.

QUICK HIT

Total T_4 includes a biologic active component, called free T_4, and a component bound to thyroid-binding globulin (TBG) and other proteins. Free T_4 by dialysis is the best way of assessing the free T_4 component.

QUICK HIT

"Free T_4 by dialysis" does not mean the patient is on dialysis. It is an ultrasensitive way of testing for free T_4.

QUICK HIT

The hallmark of hyperthyroidism is an elevated T_4, free T_4, and T_3 concentration along with a suppressed serum TSH level.

QUICK HIT

The presence of TSAs is specific for Graves disease. TSH binding–inhibiting immunoglobulins (TBIIs) are also present in Graves.

c. Can be associated with other autoimmune diseases, such as myasthenia gravis, T1DM, Addison disease, or vitiligo
d. Familial predisposition
   i. Neonatal Graves, caused by transplacental transfer of TSH receptor–stimulating antibodies (TSAs), is self-limiting and resolves over 6 months as maternal antibodies are cleared
   ii. Occurs in 1%–5% of neonates born to mothers with Graves disease

B. Clinical features
1. Historical findings (Table 4-1): questions should target all body systems and focus on disease duration and severity
2. Physical exam findings
   a. Vitals: tachycardia and hypertension present
   b. Systemic signs: warm, moist skin
   c. CNS findings: tongue fasciculations and tremor, which can be observed, especially with arms stretched up front with eyes closed
   d. Exophthalmos with lid lag and diffuse symmetrical thyroid with bruit suggest Graves disease, whereas an asymmetric thyroid suggests a nodule

C. Diagnosis
1. Laboratory measures are serum total T_4, triiodothyronine (T_3) uptake, free T_4, total T_3, and TSH
2. Radiology findings
   a. Radionuclide imaging: ^{125}I or ^{99m}Tc: radioisotope uptake; indicates activity of gland
   b. Increased radioisotope uptake is seen in hyperthyroidism caused by excessive thyroid hormone synthesis
      i. Homogeneously increased uptake is seen in Graves
      ii. Area of increased intensity (i.e., "hot" nodule) is seen with toxic nodule; remaining "healthy" thyroid tissue has decreased activity and, thus, will have suppressed radionuclide intake
   c. Decreased radioisotope uptake is seen in hyperthyroidism characterized by follicular thyroid cell destruction and release of thyroid hormone such as in thyroiditis

TABLE 4-1 Key Questions for History in Suspected Hyperthyroidism

History of Present Illness	
Symptom	**Relevant Questions**
Weight loss despite good appetite	How many pounds (kilograms)? Intentional or unintentional? Changes of appetite or activity during weight loss? Any associated gastrointestinal (GI) symptoms (nausea, vomiting, diarrhea, abdominal pain)?
Other systemic symptoms (feeling hot and sweaty)	Observations about using more clothes or blankets compared to peers or family members
Tachycardia (often perceived as a "funny feeling at the chest" or shortness of breath)	How long? Any difficulty breathing? Associated with activity or not?
Behavioral or neurologic symptoms (anxiety)	Any feelings of anxiety or irritability? Changes in school performance?
GI symptoms (diarrhea)	Any changes in bowel habits? Specify. Nausea or vomiting?
Family History	
Any family member with thyroid disease? How were they treated?	
Any family member with other autoimmune disease (diabetes, Addison, vitiligo)?	

3. Differential diagnosis
   a. Conditions that increased thyroid-binding globulin (TBG) concentrations may mimic some laboratory findings of hyperthyroidism
      i. Result in elevated total T_4
      ii. Biologic active free T_4 and T_3 levels are normal
      iii. TSH is not suppressed and in normal range
   b. Graves should be differentiated from Hashitoxicosis and subacute thyroiditis
      i. T_4 and T_3 concentrations are elevated, whereas TSH is suppressed in all 3 conditions
      ii. Diffuse symmetrical goiter can be present in all 3 conditions
      iii. Presence of antibodies and radioisotope uptake can help in differential: increased in Graves; decreased in Hashitoxicosis and subacute thyroiditis
   c. TSH α-subunit is elevated in TSH-secreting adenomas

D. Treatment
1. β-Blockers can be used to ameliorate the symptoms of hyperthyroidism
2. Medications that decrease thyroid synthesis
   a. Thionamides: methimazole, propylthiouracil (PTU), and carbimazole (not available in United States)
      i. Block thyroid hormone synthesis
      ii. Primarily used for hyperthyroidism caused by excessive thyroid secretion such as Graves
      iii. Goals of therapy in Graves are to normalize T_4 and TSH concentrations and achieve long-term remission
         (a) Remission rate ~30%
         (b) Larger goiter, male sex, and younger age are associated with higher risk for relapse
         (c) Permanent remission after relapse is unlikely; therefore, other therapy is recommended for children who relapsed after course of thionamides
      iv. Thionamides are considered 1st treatment option for Graves in children; however, increasing evidence indicates that radioactive iodine may be more appropriate as 1st treatment of choice
         (a) Methimazole is preferred compared to PTU because of concerns of irreversible hepatic toxicity with PTU
         (b) Thionamides are associated with many adverse effects, some of which can be life threatening
   b. Iodine
      i. Fastest onset of action
      ii. Blocks the synthesis and release of thyroid hormone and conversion of T_4 to T_3
      iii. Indications
         (a) Acute management of thyroid "storm," which represents degree of severe life-threatening thyrotoxicosis
         (b) Preparation for thyroid surgery, where manipulation of thyroid gland is expected to result in release of thyroid hormone in circulation
3. Radioactive iodine therapy
   a. Refers to intake of ^{131}I, which, when taken orally, accumulates in thyroid gland, causing its destruction
   b. Indications
      i. Graves disease, hyperthyroidism due to toxic nodule
      ii. Minimum age 5 years
   c. Side effects
      i. Radiation thyroiditis
         (a) Presents with recurrence or exacerbation of hyperthyroid symptoms
         (b) Occurs 2–3 weeks after treatment
      ii. Hypothyroidism; usually occurs 6–18 weeks after treatment
      iii. Inadequate control of hyperthyroidism, which may require 2nd dose
   d. Contraindications: pregnancy

QUICK HIT

Thyroglobulin and peroxidase antibodies, which are pathognomonic for autoimmune or Hashimoto thyroiditis, may also be present in Graves.

QUICK HIT

"Hashitoxicosis," or Hashimoto thyrotoxicosis, is a transient hyperthyroid state early in the onset of Hashimoto thyroiditis. The hyperthyroidism is usually self-limited and may resolve over a period of months.

QUICK HIT

There is a black box warning against PTU in children because of nonreversible hepatotoxicity.

QUICK HIT

There is no evidence that radioactive iodine therapy for hyperthyroidism causes cancer or fertility problems.

4. Surgery
    a. Indications: toxic nodule, Graves disease in very select cases that cannot be treated with medical therapy or radioactive iodine
    b. Total or subtotal thyroidectomy depending on indication
    c. Rates of postoperative hypothyroidism are proportionate to extent of thyroidectomy
    d. Patients should be rendered euthyroid prior to surgery to avoid postoperative thyroid storm

X. Hypothyroidism

A. General characteristics
1. Can be primary or secondary
    a. Primary far more common than secondary; involves abnormalities of thyroid itself
    b. Secondary: rare; due to decreased TSH secretion by pituitary or hypothalamic defect
2. Can be congenital or acquired
    a. Congenital
        i. Affects 1:2,000–4,000 newborns
        ii. Can be detected by newborn screening
        iii. Primary congenital hypothyroidism can be due to
            (a) Thyroid dysgenesis (i.e., aplasia or hypoplasia)
                (i) Sporadic
                (ii) Accounts for ~85% of congenital hypothyroidism
            (b) Dyshormonogenesis (i.e., involves enzymatic step in synthesis of T_4 or T_3); autosomal recessive disorder
    b. Acquired
        i. Much more common than congenital hypothyroidism
        ii. Acquired secondary hypothyroidism may occur with disorders that damage hypothalamic–pituitary areas such as tumors, infections, or trauma
3. Compensated or subclinical hypothyroidism refers to mildly elevated TSH in presence of normal total and free T_4 levels
4. Sick euthyroid or euthyroid syndrome refers to reduction of serum total T_3 or T_4 and elevation of reverse T_3 levels in patients with nonthyroidal illness
    a. Seen in patients with systemic illness, trauma, fever, starvation, and treatment with glucocorticoids
    b. May have protective metabolic effect
    c. Thyroid function recovers with resolution of acute illness so thyroid hormone treatment not needed

QUICK HIT

Congenital hypothyroidism of central etiology is usually associated with additional pituitary hormone deficiencies (panhypopituitarism) and certain brain structural defects (i.e., absence of corpus callosum) or syndromes (septo-optic dysplasia).

QUICK HIT

Hashimoto thyroiditis is the most common cause of hypothyroidism.

B. Diagnosis
1. Clinical features
    a. Signs and symptoms of acquired hypothyroidism commonly overlap with those of other disorders; therefore, easily missed (Table 4-2)

TABLE 4-2 Acquired Hypothyroidism: Signs, Symptoms, and Findings

Symptoms	Findings on Physical Exam	Questions to Ask
Decreased activity Fatigue Cold intolerance Constipation Dry skin and hair/hair loss Large fontanelle or delayed closure of the fontanelle	Goiter Linear growth deceleration in the face of good weight gain; high body mass index Delayed teeth eruption Coarse features, thickening and drying of the skin, hair loss with dry broken hair strands Delayed deep tendon reflexes Slowing down of mental and physical activity and metabolic rate Delayed puberty (precocious puberty in rare cases of severe hypothyroidism)	Ask for previous growth records Ask for changes in • school performance • sleeping habits • weight and height • bowel habits Ask for feeling cold or hot relative to others (use of blankets, extra clothing)

Endocrine and Metabolic Diseases

BOX 4-6

Congenital Hypothyroidism: Signs, Symptoms, and Findings on Physical Examination

- Constipation
- Decreased activity
- Large posterior and anterior fontanelle
- Prolonged jaundice (>7 days)
- Hoarse cry
- Coarse features
- Macroglossia
- Distended abdomen
- Umbilical hernia
- Hypotonia
- Goiter in case of dyshormonogenesis

b. Clinical symptoms of compensated or subclinical hypothyroidism are very mild

2. Physical exam findings (Box 4-6)
   a. Goiter and linear growth deceleration despite adequate weight gain are common findings on physical examination in acquired hypothyroidism
   b. Most newborns with congenital hypothyroidism lack abnormal findings on physical exam

C. Diagnosis
1. Differential diagnosis
   a. TBG deficiency: low total T_4 due to low TBG level with normal free T_4 and TSH
   b. Sick euthyroid syndrome needs to be considered in patients with illness and decreased total T_4 and T_3
   c. Congenital hypothyroidism detected by newborn screening must be differentiated from transient congenital hypothyroidism
2. Laboratory findings (Table 4-3)
   a. Hallmark of primary hypothyroidism is an elevated TSH concentration along with low total T_4 or free T_4 levels
   b. Positive thyroid antibodies establish diagnosis of autoimmune thyroiditis
3. Radiology findings
   a. Thyroid ultrasound
      i. Provides information about size, location, and structure of thyroid as well as presence of nodules
      ii. Indications: evaluation of thyroid nodules, goiter, and determining etiology of congenital hypothyroidism

QUICK HIT

Untreated congenital hypothyroidism causes severe developmental delay and short stature.

QUICK HIT

Normal thyroid function is critical for brain development in infants and children.

QUICK HIT

Prolonged neonatal jaundice can be symptom of congenital hypothyroidism.

QUICK HIT

Transient congenital hypothyroidism can be secondary to transplacental passage of TSH receptor–blocking antibodies in infants born to mothers with autoimmune disease or of antithyroid drugs given to mothers or iodine exposure.

TABLE 4-3 Laboratory Findings in Hypothyroidism

	Total T_4	Free T_4	TSH	Others
Primary	Decreased	Decreased	Elevated	Positive thyroid antibodies in autoimmune thyroiditis
Primary compensated	Normal	Normal	Mildly elevated	
Secondary	Decreased	Decreased	Low/normal/ mildly elevated	May be associated with other pituitary hormone deficiencies (i.e., GH, ACTH, LH, FSH)
Sick euthyroid syndrome	Decreased	Normal	Low/normal/ increased	Low T_3, increased reverse T_3
Thyroid-binding globulin (TBG) deficiency	Decreased	Normal	Normal	Decreased TBG concentrations

iii. Typical sonographic appearance of autoimmune thyroiditis is diffuse goiter with heterogeneous micronodular appearance due to lymphocyte infiltrates

b. Thyroid nuclear scan and imaging
  i. Provides information about size, location, and thyroid uptake
  ii. Indications: determining etiology of congenital hypothyroidism, although it does not affect its management
  iii. Radioisotopes: ^{99m}Tc or ^{123}I

D. Treatment
1. Oral levothyroxine (T_4) is treatment of choice
  a. T_4 is given orally once a day, usually in the morning 30 minutes before meal
  b. Goal of treatment is to normalize serum T_4 and TSH levels
2. Congenital hypothyroidism
  a. Goal of therapy is rapid replacement with adequate doses of T_4
  b. Starting dose is 10–15 mcg/kg/day or 37.5–50 mcg/day
3. Autoimmune thyroiditis
  a. T_4 treatment is started in case of hypothyroidism
  b. No need for therapy for children with positive thyroid antibodies and normal serum T_4 and TSH levels

QUICK HIT

Congenital hypothyroidism is the most common cause of preventable mental retardation. Treatment of congenital hypothyroidism should start as soon as possible (ideally within the first 3 weeks of life) to prevent developmental and cognitive defects.

XI. Congenital Adrenal Hyperplasia

A. Characteristics
1. Group of autosomal recessive disorders in which adrenal steroid synthesis is impaired
  a. Classic form: severe enzyme deficiency and prenatal onset of virilization
    i. Salt-wasting form
    ii. Simple virilizing form
  b. Nonclassic form: mild enzyme deficiency and postnatal onset of virilization
2. Worldwide incidence
  a. Classic 21-OH deficiency occurs in 1:15,000 to 1:16,000 live births of which ~75% are salt wasters
  b. Nonclassical CAH incidence is 1:1,000
3. Mutations in *CYP21A2* cause 21-OH deficiency CAH
4. Less common causes of CAH include other enzyme deficiencies such as deficiency of 11β-hydroxylase, 3β-hydroxysteroid dehydrogenase, and 17α-hydroxylase/17,20-lyase
5. Pathophysiology
  a. Deficient 21-OH enzyme activity leads to blockage of cortisol production pathway; thus accumulation of 17-OHP occurs; excess 17-OHP is shunted into intact androgen pathway (Figure 4-3)
  b. Because mineralocorticoid pathway requires minimal 21-OH activity, mineralocorticoid deficiency (salt wasting) is feature of most severe form of disease
  c. Low cortisol impairs negative feedback control of adrenocorticotropic hormone (ACTH) secretion from pituitary, leading to chronic stimulation of adrenal cortex by ACTH, resulting in adrenal hyperplasia

QUICK HIT

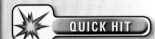

21-Hydroxylase (21-OH) deficiency accounts for >90% of all CAH cases.

QUICK HIT

Mineralocorticoids reclaim Na^+ and excrete K^+ in the collecting tubule of the kidney. Patients with mineralocorticoid deficiency have "salt wasting" and, on labs, have a low Na^+ and a high K^+.

B. Clinical features
1. Excess androgens cause virilization, which is hallmark of 21-OH deficiency CAH; if occurs prenatally, females have genital ambiguity as found in classic forms (Figure 4-4)
2. Aldosterone deficiency: salt-losing crisis presents within first 4 weeks
3. Skin hyperpigmentation: from excessive ACTH secretion
4. Hypoglycemia: as result of cortisol deficiency; not a constant finding
5. In salt-wasting disease, dehydration or shock can arise early and quickly, both from dehydration as result of Na^+ loss out of collecting tubule, and through decreased levels of cortisol

FIGURE 4-3 **The pathway of adrenal steroid synthesis.**

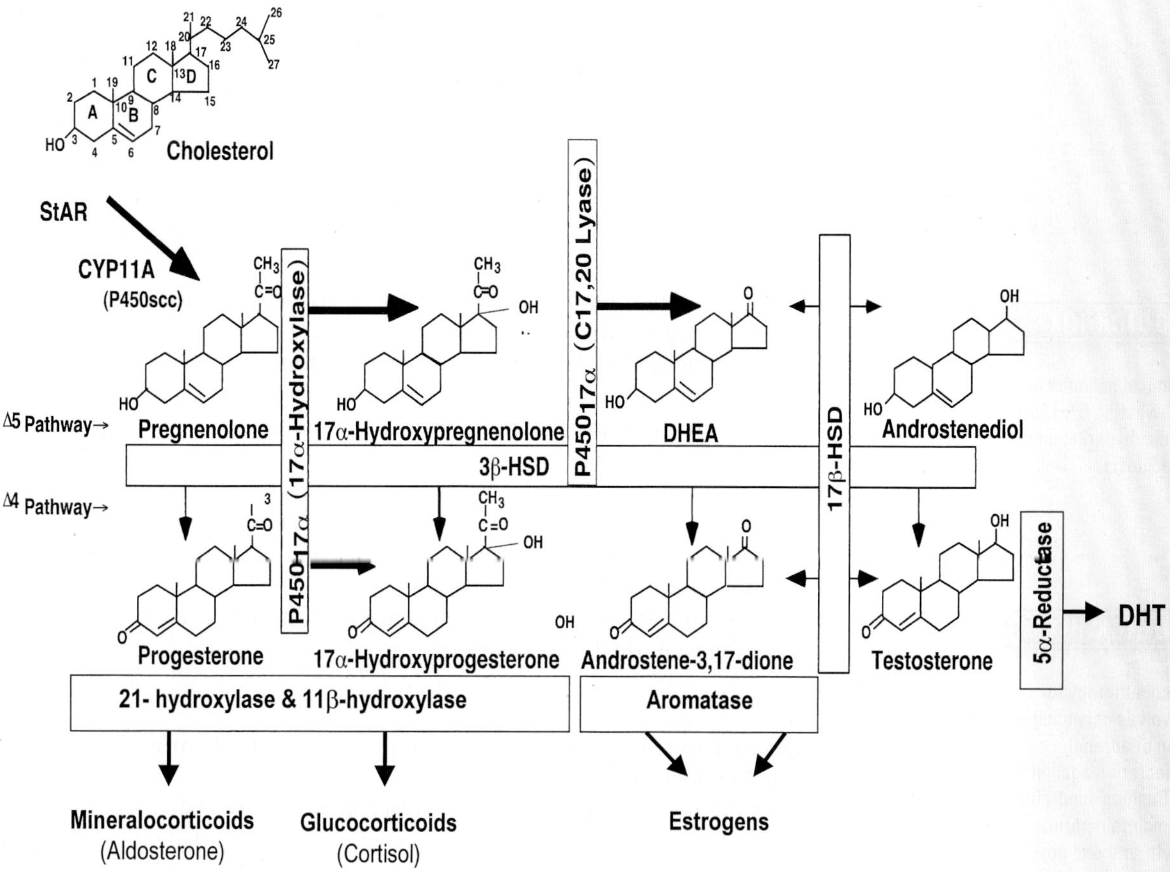

FIGURE 4-4 **Congenital adrenal hyperplasia.**

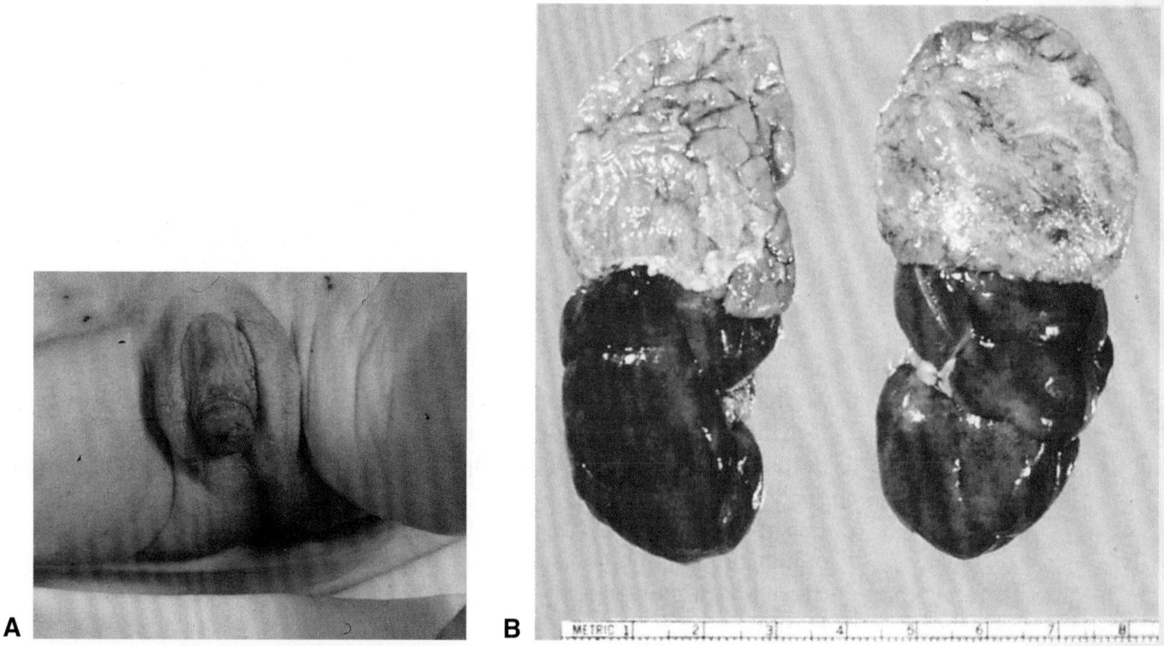

A. A female infant is markedly virilized with hypertrophy of the clitoris and partial fusion of labioscrotal folds. **B.** A 7-week-old male died of severe salt-wasting CAH. At autopsy, both adrenal glands were markedly enlarged. (**A:** Reprinted with permission from Rubin E. *Pathology.* 4th ed. Philadelphia: Lippincott Williams & Wilkins; 2005. **B:** From Rubin R, Strayer DS. *Rubin's Pathology: Clinicopathologic Foundations of Medicine.* 5th ed. Philadelphia: Lippincott Williams & Wilkins; 2008.)

C. Diagnosis
1. Differential diagnosis
   a. Virilization includes other forms of disorders of sexual differentiation (DSDs), adrenal or testicular hormone-secreting tumors, exogenous exposure to sex steroids
   b. Salt wasting
      i. Includes any form of CAH in which enzymatic blockages prevent adequate aldosterone production
      ii. Other causes of adrenal insufficiency (AI) or GI or renal salt loss should be considered
2. Laboratory findings
   a. Hormone findings: marked elevation of 17-OHP, androstenedione, and adrenal androgens in classical form
   b. For 21-OH deficiency CAH, molecular genetic testing of *CYP21A2* gene for panel of 9 common mutations and gene deletions detects ~80%–98% of disease-causing alleles in affected individuals and carriers
3. Radiology findings
   a. Pelvic ultrasound or MRI may be necessary in cases with ambiguous genitalia to identify Müllerian structure (ovaries and uterus)
   b. Bone age is important tool to gauge advanced body maturation in late-diagnosis cases and in treatment monitoring
4. Chromosome: females with 21-OH deficiency CAH have normal 46,XX karyotype; males have normal 46,XY karyotype

QUICK HIT

The biochemical hallmark of severe salt-wasting CAH is hyponatremic, hyperkalemic metabolic acidosis.

QUICK HIT

Glucocorticoid therapy for children involves balancing suppression of adrenal androgen secretion against iatrogenic Cushing syndrome in order to maintain normal linear growth rate and normal bone maturation.

D. Treatment
1. Therapy
   a. Imperative to make timely diagnosis to prevent effects of cortisol deficiency and mineralocorticoid deficiency
   b. Principally involves glucocorticoid replacement therapy, usually in form of hydrocortisone (10–15 mg/m^2/24 hr) given orally in 2–3 daily divided doses
   c. Treatment with fludrocortisone (0.05–0.3 mg/day orally) and NaCl (1–3 g/day added to formula or foods) is necessary in individuals with salt-wasting form of 21-OH deficiency CAH
   d. All newborn and early infant CAH patients should be treated as salt-wasting form
   e. Stress dose
      i. Glucocorticoid is increased during periods of stress (e.g., surgery, febrile illness, shock) in all individuals with classical 21-OH deficiency CAH and in nonclassical CAH whose adrenal function is suboptimal or iatrogenically suppressed
      ii. Typically, 2–3× normal dose is administered orally or by IM injection when oral intake is not tolerated
   f. Feminizing genitoplasty (urogenital sinus repair) in female with classical CAH may be necessary; however, clitoral recession and appropriate timing are subject to debate
2. Overtreatment with glucocorticoids can result in cushingoid features
   a. Commonly occurs when serum concentration of 17-OHP is reduced to physiologic range for age
   b. Acceptable range for serum concentration of 17-OHP in treated individual is higher (100–1,000 ng/dL) than normal
3. Appropriate treatment and follow-up allow CAH patients to have near-normal life
   a. Puberty: for majority of patients treated adequately from early life, onset of puberty in both girls and boys with classical 21-OH deficiency occurs at expected chronologic age
   b. Fertility
      i. Females: infertility may arise for various reasons, including anovulation, secondary polycystic ovarian syndrome, irregular menses, nonsuppressible serum progesterone levels, or inadequate introitus

ii. Males: if poorly treated, may have reduced sperm counts and low testosterone as result of small testes due to suppression of gonadotropins and sometimes intratesticular adrenal rests

4. Early detection: universal newborn screening of 17-OHP level is done in U.S. and many other countries to detect classical form before its presentation with potentially fatal adrenal crisis

QUICK HIT

Hyperandrogenism and chronic glucocorticoid replacement put CAH patients at higher risk for the development of metabolic syndrome (a constellation of obesity, elevated blood pressure, dyslipidemia, and impaired glucose metabolism) and cardiovascular disease.

XII. Approach to Ambiguous Genitalia

A. Background
1. Estimated to occur in 1 in 4,500 births
2. Incidences for most of disorders are unknown, except for 21-OH deficiency CAH (1:15,000)
3. Advances in molecular genetics, heightened ethical issue awareness, and patient advocacy concern led to revision of nomenclature to disorders of sex development
4. Disorders of sex development are defined as congenital conditions in which development of chromosomal, gonadal, and anatomical sex is atypical
5. Birth of child with ambiguous genitalia constitutes social emergency (Figure 4-5)

B. Differential diagnosis: classification of disorders of sex development is summarized in Table 4-4

C. Historical findings
1. Maternal history
   a. Medications that may virilize female fetus
   b. Symptoms of maternal virilization, suggestive of maternal androgen-producing tumor or placental aromatase deficiency
2. Family history
   a. Previous neonatal death, suggestive of unrecognized adrenal crisis due to 21-OH deficiency
   b. May help delineate recessive or X-linked disorders

D. Physical examination
1. Genital examination
   a. Palpable gonads are likely to be testes or have significant testicular tissue
   b. Degrees of genital virilization of external genitalia are classified into 5 Prader stages

FIGURE 4-5 **Ambiguous genitalia.**

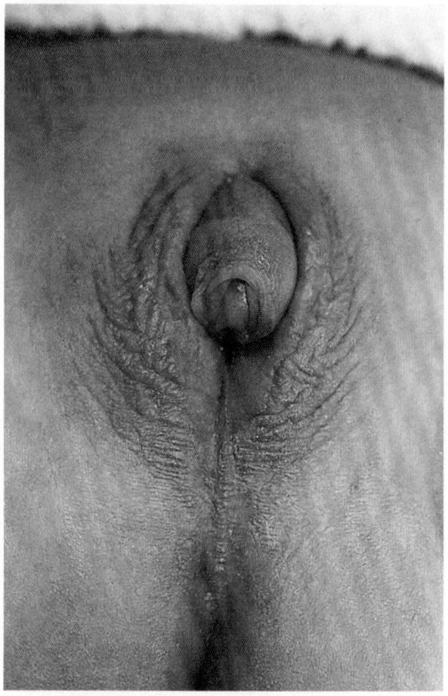

(Courtesy of T. Ernesto Figueroa.)

TABLE 4-4 Disorders of Sexual Development Classification

46,XY DSD	46,XX DSD
Disorders of Testicular Development	**Disorders of Ovarian Development**
1. Complete gonadal dysgenesis (Swyer syndrome) 2. Partial gonadal dysgenesis 3. Gonadal regression 4. Ovotesticular disorder of sexual development (DSD)	1. Ovotesticular DSD 2. Testicular DSD (e.g., SRY+) 3. Gonadal dysgenesis
Disorders in Androgen Synthesis or Action	**Androgen Excess**
1. Androgen biosynthesis defect (e.g., 17β-hydroxysteroid dehydrogenase deficiency, 5α-reductase deficiency, StAR mutations) 2. Defect in androgen action (e.g., complete or partial androgen insensitivity syndrome) 3. LH receptor defects (e.g., Leydig cell hypoplasia, aplasia) 4. Disorders of anti-müllerian hormone and receptor (persistent müllerian duct syndrome)	1. Fetal (e.g., 21-hydroxylase deficiency, 11β-hydroxylase deficiency) 2. Fetoplacental (aromatase deficiency, cytochrome P450 oxidoreductase deficiency) 3. Maternal (luteoma, exogenous, etc.)
Other	**Other**
1. Severe hypospadias 2. Cloacal exstrophy 3. Other syndromes	1. Cloacal exstrophy 2. Vaginal atresia 3. Müllerian, renal, cervicothoracic somite abnormalities (MURCS) 4. Other syndromes

QUICK HIT

Overall, the most common cause of ambiguous genitalia in the newborn is CAH.

2. Any associated dysmorphic features
3. Hyperpigmentation may be found in any forms of CAH
4. Absence of palpable gonads (testes) in newborn with ambiguous genitalia (clitoromegaly and labial fusion) is most likely baby with CAH
5. Although majority of *under*virilized XY infants remains unexplained, about 1/3 are related to androgen insensitivity syndrome (AIS)
6. Complete AIS (CAIS)
   a. Presents with discrepancy of chromosome 46,XY with normal female genitalia and inguinal hernia that contains testis
   b. Later in life, develop primary amenorrhea associated with reduced or absent pubic and axillary hair

E. Criteria that suggest disorders of sex development include
   1. Overt genital ambiguity
   2. Apparent female genitalia with enlarged clitoris, posterior labial fusion, or inguinal/labial mass
   3. Apparent male genitalia with bilateral undescended testes, micropenis, isolated perineal hypospadias, or mild hypospadias with undescended testis
   4. Family history of disorders of sex development such as CAIS
   5. Discordance between genital appearance and prenatal karyotype

F. Laboratory testing
   1. First-line investigations that results are generally available within 48 hours and provide sufficient information for working diagnosis
      a. Karyotyping with X- and Y-specific probe detection
      b. Measurement of 17-OHP, testosterone, gonadotropins, anti-Müllerian hormone, serum electrolytes
      c. Determination of internal anatomy by imaging (ultrasound or MRI)

2. Additional studies to guide diagnosis
    a. HCG and ACTH stimulation tests to assess testicular and adrenal steroid biosynthesis
    b. Urinary steroid analysis by gas chromatography and mass spectroscopy (GC-MS)
    c. Second-line imaging studies: urogenital sinogram or vaginoscope
    d. Biopsies of gonads
    e. Genetic analysis
        i. Some gene analyses are carried out in clinical service laboratories
        ii. However, current molecular diagnosis is limited by cost, accessibility, and quality control
        iii. Research laboratories provide genetic testing, including functional analysis, but may face restrictions on communicating result
    f. *SRY* gene mutation accounts for 20% of 46,XY with disorders of gonadal development, a subset of XY disorders of sex development

G. Management/treatment
1. Evaluation and long-term management are best carried out with experienced multidisciplinary team (endocrinologist, neonatologist, geneticist, surgeon, social worker, and psychologist)
2. Gender assignment must be avoided before expert evaluation
3. Open communication with patients and families is essential, and participation in decision making is encouraged
4. Patient and family concerns should be respected and addressed in strict confidence
5. Treatment of a child with CAH is discussed earlier in this chapter
6. When specific disorders of sex development diagnosis has been confirmed, therapy can be guided accordingly; issues to be discussed include gender of rearing, possible need for surgery, medical treatment, timely psychological counseling, and support

XIII. Cushing Syndrome

A. Definition: represents state of excessive circulating glucocorticoid concentration; rare in children

B. Classification
1. ACTH-dependent causes
    a. Cushing disease: pituitary adenoma secreting excessive ACTH
        i. Accounts for 75%–80% of cases
        ii. Tumor is almost always a microadenoma
    b. Ectopic ACTH syndrome
        i. Extremely rare in children but present in 15% of adults with Cushing disease
        ii. Responsible tumors are carcinoid tumors in bronchial, thymic, renal, or duodenum area as well as clear cell sarcoma and neuroendocrine tumors
2. ACTH-independent causes
    a. Supraphysiologic glucocorticoid treatment is most common cause
    b. Adrenocortical tumor (adenoma or carcinoma): more common in age <4 years
        i. Virilization is more common presentation (40%–50%) than combined Cushing syndrome plus virilization (~30%)
        ii. Isolated Cushing presentation is least common (3%–14%)
    c. Primary adrenocortical hyperplasia
        i. Primary pigmented nodular adrenocortical disease: rare, associated with multiple endocrine neoplasia (MEN) syndrome
        ii. Macronodular adrenal hyperplasia: rare
        iii. McCune-Albright syndrome
            (a) Activating mutation of Gsα subunit with triad of café-au-lait spots, precocious puberty, and polyostotic fibrous dysplasia
            (b) Can be associated with ACTH receptor activation and cortisol excess as well as other G protein hyperfunction (ACTH, LH, FSH, GH)

C. Clinical presentation
   1. Cushingoid appearance: facial change, plethora, weight gain together with poor growth
   2. Short stature in 40% of cases
   3. Virilization: premature pubic hair, acne, hirsutism, and irregular menstruation
   4. Other features are hypertension, emotional lability, fatigue
   5. Skin changes: violaceous striae (60%) and bruises (25%)

D. Testing
   1. Confirmation of Cushing syndrome
      a. 24-Hour urinary free cortisol (UFC)
      b. Serum cortisol samplings to assess circadian rhythmicity (morning, afternoon, and midnight)
      c. Low-dose dexamethasone suppression test at 0.5 mg (20 mcg/kg/day) orally every 6 hours and obtain serum cortisol at 24 and 48 hours
   2. Defining etiology of Cushing syndrome: ACTH dependent versus ACTH independent
      a. Basal ACTH level (undetectable in ACTH independent)
      b. Corticotropin-releasing hormone (CRH) test at 1 mcg/kg IV and assess significant rise in ACTH and cortisol in case of ACTH dependent
      c. Low-dose (20 mcg/kg/day or 0.5 mg orally every 6 hours; maximum dose 2 mg/day) versus high-dose dexamethasone suppression test (80 mcg/kg/day or 2 mg every 6 hours; maximum dose 8 mg/day); basal cortisol level and ACTH are obtained before and after 2 days of dexamethasone dose
         i. In exogenous obesity and other non-Cushing disorders, cortisol and ACTH levels are readily suppressed (cortisol <5 mcg/dL and ACTH <20 pg/mL)
         ii. In Cushing disease, cortisol and ACTH are not suppressed by low-dose but suppressed after high-dose dexamethasone
         iii. Adrenal adenoma, carcinoma, and ectopic ACTH syndrome are relatively insensitive to both low-dose and high-dose dexamethasone
   3. Radiologic investigations
      a. Pituitary imaging by MRI to evaluate suspected pituitary lesion for surgery
      b. Adrenal imaging for suspected lesion by CT or MRI scan
      c. Bilateral inferior petrosal sinus sampling for ACTH: highly specialized technique used to lateralize side of pituitary microadenoma and to exclude ectopic ACTH secretion

E. Treatment
   1. Adrenal lesion
      a. First line of treatment is surgical resection
      b. Important to supply stress dose of glucocorticoid because other adrenal gland may be suppressed
   2. Cushing disease
      a. Transsphenoidal surgery (TSS) for selective removal of pituitary adenoma is first-line therapy and is superior to bilateral adrenalectomy in which pituitary adenoma is left intact; adrenalectomy is reserved only for patients who cannot undergo TSS
      b. Pituitary radiation: children responded more rapidly to radiation than adults, and radiation can be used as second-line treatment
      c. Medical therapy: ketoconazole, metyrapone, and other adrenal-blocking agents may be used as palliative treatment before surgery or radiation

XIV. Addison Disease

A. Characteristics
   1. AI is categorized as primary or secondary and congenital or acquired
      a. In primary AI, combined deficiency of glucocorticoids, mineralocorticoids, and adrenal androgens

b. In secondary AI, lack of CRH secretion from hypothalamus and/or ACTH secretion from pituitary, resulting in hypofunction of adrenal cortex with mineralocorticoid function preserved

2. AI is uncommon in Western population
3. Causes of AI
   a. Primary
      i. Underdeveloped adrenals from transcription factor deficiencies: DAX-1 or SF-1 (steroidogenic factor 1)
      ii. Unresponsive to ACTH: isolated familial glucocorticoid deficiency or in association with achalasia and alacrima in triple A syndrome
      iii. Impaired steroidogenesis from adrenal enzyme deficiencies (all forms of CAH) and cholesterol synthesis defects (Smith-Lemli-Opitz syndrome and abetalipoproteinemia)
      iv. Adrenal destruction
         (a) Autoimmune process is most common cause of AI beyond infancy; may be isolated or occur in context of autoimmune polyendocrine syndrome (APS) with onset in childhood (type 1) or adulthood (type 2)
         (b) Infections, especially tuberculosis (TB) and meningococcal infection (bilateral hemorrhage, known as **Friderichsen-Waterhouse syndrome**)
            (i) Chronic fungal infections
            (ii) Virus: cytomegalovirus, HIV
         (c) Metabolic: adrenoleukodystrophy (ALD) is disorder of metabolism of long-chain fatty acids characterized by progressive neurologic dysfunction and primary AI, inherited in X-linked recessive mode
         (d) Infiltrative, especially hemochromatosis, histiocytosis, and sarcoidosis
         (e) Drugs: inhibition of cortisol production, especially from aminoglutethimide, etomidate, or ketoconazole
         (f) Adrenal hemorrhage: birth traumas related to difficult deliveries, sepsis, coagulopathy, traumatic shock, and ischemic disorders
   b. Secondary
      i. Underdeveloped hypothalamic–pituitary: septo-optic dysplasia, isolated hypothalamic–pituitary–adrenal (HPA) axis form or combined with other hypopituitarism
      ii. Iatrogenic suppression with exogenous glucocorticoids
      iii. Hypothalamic–pituitary destruction
         (a) Neoplasia
         (b) Radiation
         (c) Trauma
         (d) Surgery
         (e) Autoimmune hypophysitis
4. In congenital forms of both primary and secondary AI, genes have been identified
5. Signs and symptoms
   a. Can be nonspecific, and diagnosis may not be suspected early in course
   b. Delay in diagnosis can lead to life-threatening adrenal crisis and cardiovascular collapse
6. Adrenal glucocorticoids and mineralocorticoids play vital role in homeostasis
   a. Cortisol contributes to maintenance of normal blood pressure and blood glucose through several mechanisms
   b. Aldosterone is produced in zona glomerulosa and is controlled primarily by renin–angiotensin system and serum K^+. ACTH plays a minor role.
7. Primary action of aldosterone occurs at distal nephron, where it stimulates reabsorption of Na^+ and secretion of K^+ and hydrogen ions

B. Clinical features
1. Clinical presentation
   a. Acute AI
      i. Acute dehydration, low blood pressure, hypoglycemia, altered mental status
      ii. Orthostatic hypotension may be early presentation

QUICK HIT

Smith-Lemli-Opitz is autosomal recessive and results in a cellular inability to make cholesterols. It presents in early infancy with a variety of malformations including microcephaly; mental retardation; and malformations of the heart, lungs, kidneys, adrenal glands, GI tract, spine, extremities, and genitalia.

QUICK HIT

In the 1800s, TB was an important cause of Addison disease. Although less common in the United States, both TB and HIV are still common causes in the developing world.

QUICK HIT

ALD classically presents as ataxia, seizures, loss of motor milestones, and Addisonian crisis in boys between ages 4 and 10 years.

QUICK HIT

Infection and trauma may trigger acute presentation of adrenal insufficiency.

QUICK HIT

Hyperpigmentation of skin in susceptible areas such as gumline, knuckles, and scar tissues is an indication of chronic ACTH elevation.

QUICK HIT

Salt craving is a manifestation of adrenal insufficiency and chronic ACTH elevation.

QUICK HIT

Ambiguous genitalia can indicate CAH.

QUICK HIT

These patients are profoundly dehydrated. Rapid, early, and often-repeated boluses of normal saline are critical to a successful outcome.

iii. Commonly, there is concomitant illness that leads patient to become decompensated

b. Chronic AI
   i. Patients usually complain of chronic fatigue, anorexia, weight loss, drowsiness, recurrent abdominal pain, nausea, and vomiting
   ii. Some nonspecific symptoms overlap with depression or GI diseases

2. Clinical clues
   a. History of recent glucocorticoid usage suggests HPA axis suppression
   b. ACTH deficiency may be suspected when other hypopituitarism presentation is evident: short stature, micropenis, delayed puberty, secondary hypothyroidism, and DI

C. Diagnosis
1. Hyponatremia, hyperkalemia, and metabolic acidosis are common in primary AI due to aldosterone deficiency
2. Hypoglycemia is common finding in both primary and secondary AI
3. Hormonal findings
   a. Primary AI: markedly elevated plasma ACTH and inappropriately low cortisol
      i. If these are not evident, a standard 60-minute synthetic ACTH stimulation test (at 250 mcg or 15 mcg/kg) can be used to show inappropriate rise of cortisol
      ii. Aldosterone deficiency can be measured by aldosterone level in relation to renin
   b. Secondary AI: both ACTH and cortisol are low; low-dose ACTH (1 mcg) or ovine CRH test may be used as confirmatory test
4. Imaging studies
   a. Adrenal imaging (CT or MRI)
      i. Look for adrenal hemorrhage in cases of primary AI
      ii. Bilateral adrenal calcifications are pathognomonic for Wolman disease, a rare genetic cause of adrenal failure
   b. Imaging of pituitary–hypothalamic region (MRI)
      i. Obtained to rule out hypothalamic–pituitary mass lesions as etiology in cases of secondary AI
      ii. Hypothalamic causes of ACTH insufficiency include craniopharyngioma, pituitary adenoma, germinoma, and astrocytoma

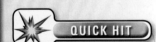

D. Treatment
1. Hemodynamically unstable patient due to adrenal crisis
   a. Critical sample
      i. After blood draw for critical sample for cortisol, electrolyte, glucose, and ACTH levels, plasma renin activity, and aldosterone level
      ii. Rapid restoration of intravascular volume with isotonic NaCl containing dextrose is needed
   b. Stress doses of glucocorticoid should be given simultaneously
      i. Hydrocortisone is the treatment of choice because of its mineralocorticoid activity
2. Maintenance treatment: required after the treatment of acute phase
   a. If mineralocorticoid deficiency is present, start fludrocortisone
   b. In 1st year of life, infants with primary AI are generally supplemented with 1–2 g of NaCl to ensure adequate Na^+ intake
3. Stress dose
   a. Because cortisol secretory rate increases substantially during physiologic stress, all patients with both primary and secondary AI should be educated to increase their glucocorticoid dose during stress to avoid adrenal crisis
   b. Recommendations vary between 2 and 10× maintenance dose or ~3× daily dose, divided into 3–4 doses
   c. In major surgery or sepsis, higher doses of hydrocortisone are required
   d. Family should be given injection kits of hydrocortisone for emergency use
   e. All patients with AI should wear Medic-Alert bracelet

XV. Benign Premature Thelarche

A. General characteristics
 1. Isolated breast development without other signs of sexual development (pubic hair, growth acceleration, nonestrogenized vaginal mucosa [bright red])
 2. May be unilateral or bilateral
 3. Usually occurs by age 2 years and rarely after age 4 years
 4. In some girls, breast development is present at birth and persists
 5. Breast enlargement usually regresses in a few months and in most girls by age 2–3 years
 6. In some girls, thelarche persists after age 3 years
 7. Usually sporadic
 8. Pathogenesis is unclear; plasma estradiol levels done by highly sensitive estrogen assays are slightly higher for age

B. Clinical characteristics
 1. History should focus on age of onset of breast enlargement and other associated pubertal signs (growth acceleration, vaginal bleeding, pubic hair development, axillary odor, clitoral enlargement)
 2. Exposure to estrogen-containing creams or oils should be explored
 3. Physical exam
  a. Should focus on presence of café-au-lait spots and fibrous dysplasia of bones (asymmetry or deformity), which may suggest McCune-Albright syndrome
  b. Pubertal signs, including pubic hair development and growth acceleration or growth spurt, indicate CPP
 4. Diagnosis
  a. Bone age should be considered if there is significant growth acceleration
  b. Serum LH, FSH, and estradiol concentrations are low and not diagnostic in typical premature thelarche
  c. Pelvic ultrasonography is rarely needed but may show some microcysts (<9 mm)
 5. Treatment: reassurance in most cases

QUICK HIT

McCune-Albright syndrome is characterized by triad of café-au-lait spots (irregularly shaped or Coast of Maine type), polyostotic fibrous dysplasia, and GnRH-independent sexual precocity.

QUICK HIT

Regression and recurrence of thelarche suggest functioning follicular cysts.

QUICK HIT

Most young girls ages 2–4 years with breast buds, normal growth, and Tanner 1 pubic hair require simple reassurance without any testing.

XVI. Hyperinsulinism

A. General characteristics
 1. Most common cause of persistent hypoglycemia in neonates and infants
 2. Must be diagnosed immediately to avoid risks of seizures and permanent brain damage
 3. Hyperinsulinism can lead to transient hypoglycemia or persistent hypoglycemia
 4. Causes
  a. Transient hyperinsulinism includes infants of diabetic mother or perinatal stress such as birth asphyxia
  b. Persistent hypoglycemia includes autosomal recessive and dominant defects of β cell insulin regulation and focal disease due to β cell adenomatosis
  c. Other causes of hyperinsulinism include Beckwith-Wiedemann syndrome (macroglossia, overgrowth, hemihypertrophy, umbilical hernia, ear pits)

B. Clinical characteristics: neonates can present with jitteriness, lethargy, poor feeding, tachycardia, pallor, and seizures

C. Diagnosis
 1. Plasma insulin levels are inappropriately elevated at time of hypoglycemia (blood glucose <50 mg/dL)
 2. In hyperinsulinism, lipolysis and ketogenesis are inhibited, causing low free fatty acid and β-hydroxybutyrate concentrations at time of hypoglycemia

D. Treatment
 1. First-line treatment for persistent prolonged hyperinsulinism is diazoxide; side effects of diazoxide include hypertrichosis and fluid retention
 2. Second-line treatment is octreotide, a long-acting analog of somatostatin that suppresses insulin release
 3. If a neonate fails diazoxide and octreotide, localization procedures and surgery (90%–95% pancreatectomy for diffuse disease or excision of focal adenoma) are next steps

XVII. Hypocalcemia

A. General characteristics
  1. Serum calcium homeostasis is maintained with narrow range by interplay that involves parathyroid hormone (PTH) and its receptor, vitamin D, and calcium-sensing receptor (CaSR)
  2. Serum phosphate and magnesium and presence of alkalosis can influence serum calcium concentrations
     a. Hyperphosphatemia lowers serum calcium concentration by binding to calcium and increasing tissue deposition, thereby removing calcium from circulation
     b. Hypomagnesemia decreases serum calcium concentration by impairing PTH release and causing end-organ resistance to PTH
     c. Alkalosis increases binding of ionized calcium to albumin, thereby decreasing serum calcium concentrations
  3. Serum calcium binds to serum proteins, especially albumin

QUICK HIT

Total serum calcium concentrations should be corrected for serum albumin levels by adding 0.8 mg/dL to the recorded calcium value for every 1 g/dL decrease in serum albumin.

B. Clinical features
  1. Historical findings: neonatal hypocalcemia can be divided into "early" if it occurs within 1st 72 hours of life and "late" if it occurs after 72 hours (Table 4-5)
     a. Questions related to early neonatal hypocalcemia focus on maternal illness, such as diabetes or hyperparathyroidism (HPT), or complications during birth, such as asphyxia or toxemia
     b. Questions related to late neonatal hypocalcemia focus on dietary phosphate intake (both formula or through IV fluids), family history of calcium abnormalities, or possible maternal vitamin D deficiency (i.e., prenatal vitamin D intake, exposure to sun)
     c. After neonatal period, questions should target family history of calcium abnormalities, factors that suggest vitamin D deficiency (i.e., sun exposure, dairy intake, and vitamin D supplementation), concurrent chronic or acute illness, and medical therapies
  2. Clinical features
     a. Mild hypocalcemia can remain asymptomatic
     b. Severe hypocalcemia can result in seizures, inspiratory stridor, tetany, and life-threatening arrhythmias
  3. Physical exam findings
     a. Facial dysmorphology or other somatic abnormalities may suggest specific syndrome
     b. Clinical signs of hypocalcemia include positive Chvostek sign and positive Trousseau sign (carpal pedal spasm) (Figure 4-6)

QUICK HIT

Breast milk has low vitamin D concentrations. Infants who are exclusively breastfed should be placed on vitamin D supplementation to avoid vitamin D deficiency.

TABLE 4-5 **Biochemical Presentation of the Most Common Causes of Hypocalcemia**

	Serum Phosphate	Serum Intact PTH	Serum 25-OH Vitamin D	Serum 1,25 Vitamin D	Other
Vitamin D deficiency	Low or normal	Elevated	Low	Varies (can be normal or high normal)	Elevated alkaline phosphatase; decreased urinary calcium (Ca) excretion
Hypoparathyroidism	Elevated	Low	Normal	Low	High normal urinary Ca excretion
Pseudohypoparathyroidism (also known as Albright hereditary osteodystrophy)	Elevated	Markedly elevated	Normal	Low	High normal urinary Ca excretion
Renal failure	Elevated	Elevated	Normal	Low	High normal urinary Ca excretion, decreased creatinine clearance
Calcium-sensing receptor (CaSR) disorders	High normal	Low/normal	Normal	Normal	Increased urinary Ca excretion

FIGURE 4-6 Clinical signs of hypocalcemia.

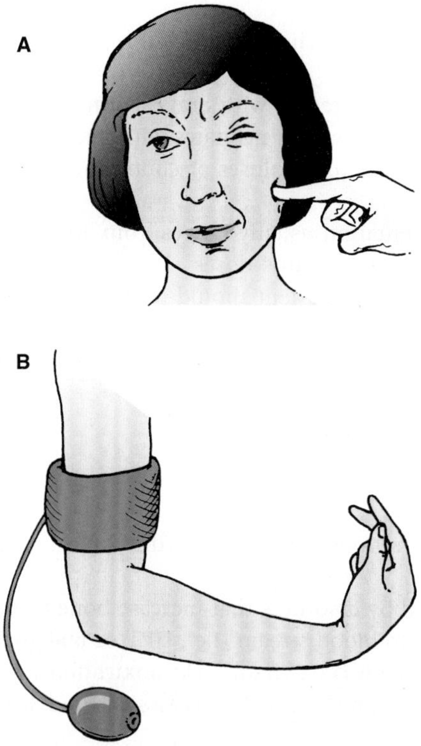

A. Chvostek sign refers to a unilateral spasm of the oris muscle that is initiated by a slight tap over the facial nerve anterior to the external auditory canal. It is a sign of tetany. **B.** Trousseau sign or carpal pedal spasm. It is a carpal spasm that occurs when the upper arm is compressed, as by a tourniquet or a blood pressure cuff. (From Nettina SM. *The Lippincott Manual of Nursing Practice.* 7th ed. Philadelphia: Lippincott, Williams & Wilkins; 2001.)

c. Presence of rachitic rosary, craniotabes, widening of wrists, and bowing of knees in an ambulating child is indicative of rickets
d. Presence of vitiligo or neuromas of oral mucosa in child or adolescent with acquired hypoparathyroidism is indicative of autoimmune polyglandular syndrome (APS)

C. Diagnosis
1. Differential diagnosis
   a. Vitamin D deficiency/rickets must be suspected in infants exclusively breastfed who do not receive vitamin D supplementation
   b. Differential of congenital hypoparathyroidism includes various syndromes such as DiGeorge syndrome (most common congenital syndrome associated with hypoparathyroidism)
2. Laboratory findings
   a. Laboratory evaluation is based on measurement of serum calcium, phosphate, alkaline phosphatase (ALP), intact PTH, 25-OH vitamin D, and urine calcium excretion
   b. Additional testing can be ordered as indicated by initial laboratory evaluation; diagnosis of DiGeorge syndrome is confirmed by presence of microdeletion of chromosome 22q11.2 as demonstrated by fluorescence in situ hybridization (FISH)
3. ECG: prolonged QT interval
4. Radiology
   a. Chest x-ray
      i. Absence of thymus in neonate with hypocalcemia is suggestive of DiGeorge syndrome
      ii. Rachitic rosary is indicative of rickets
   b. Wrist or knee x-ray: metaphyseal widening with cupping is indicative of rickets

QUICK HIT

Rickets is more common in breastfeeding infants whose mothers avoid sun exposure or who have increased skin melatonin.

QUICK HIT

DiGeorge syndrome is associated with characteristic facial features such as telecanthus and small palpebral fissures, upturned nose, and small mouth; cardiac defects, especially abnormalities of the outflow tract or aortic arch; and thymic hypoplasia, which may result in T-cell deficiency.

QUICK HIT

Telecanthus: space between eyes is wider than the width of 1 eye.

QUICK HIT

Serum 25-OH vitamin D concentrations reflect vitamin D stores. 25-OH vitamin D measurements are performed to determine vitamin D deficiency/rickets.

QUICK HIT

Markedly elevated serum alkaline phosphatase concentrations in a child with hypocalcemia suggest vitamin D deficiency.

c. Hand x-ray: short 4th metacarpal is typical of Albright osteodystrophy (pseudohypoparathyroidism)

D. Treatment
1. Should be directed against any underlying disease, if possible
2. Oral or IV calcium supplementation
a. Asymptomatic hypocalcemia can be treated with oral calcium
b. 10% calcium gluconate IV bolus is given in neonates with tetany or seizures because of hypocalcemia; repeat calcium boluses or continuous calcium infusion may be required
c. Daily dose of calcium supplementation usually ranges from 50 mg/kg to 100 mg/kg of elemental calcium divided in 4 doses
3. In addition to calcium supplementation, patient should receive vitamin D
a. Vitamin D deficiency/rickets
b. Calcitriol (1,25-dihydroxycholecalciferol, Rocaltrol) is recommended for treatment of hypoparathyroidism, renal failure, and pseudohypoparathyroidism

QUICK HIT

Ergocalciferol (vitamin D_2) or cholecalciferol (vitamin D_3) is the preferred form of vitamin D supplementation in nutritional rickets because it replenishes vitamin D stores.

XVIII. Hypercalcemia

A. General characteristics
1. Defined as serum calcium concentrations >10.5–11 mg/dL (2.64–2.75 mmol/L)
2. Increased serum calcium is caused by disorders that increase bone resorption and release of calcium from bone to blood stream (i.e., HPT or malignancy), increased calcium absorption from gut (i.e., vitamin D intoxication), or increased urinary calcium reabsorption (Figure 4-7; Tables 4-6 and 4-7)

B. Clinical features
1. Historical findings
a. Questions related to hypercalcemia in neonatal life and infancy focus on family history, maternal disorders, history of pregnancy and delivery, and feeding problems after birth
b. Questions related to hypercalcemia in childhood and adolescence focus on family history, medications, and determining symptoms indicative of hypercalcemia and their duration

FIGURE 4-7 **Algorithm of differential diagnosis of hypercalcemia based on intact parathyroid hormone (PTH) measurements.**

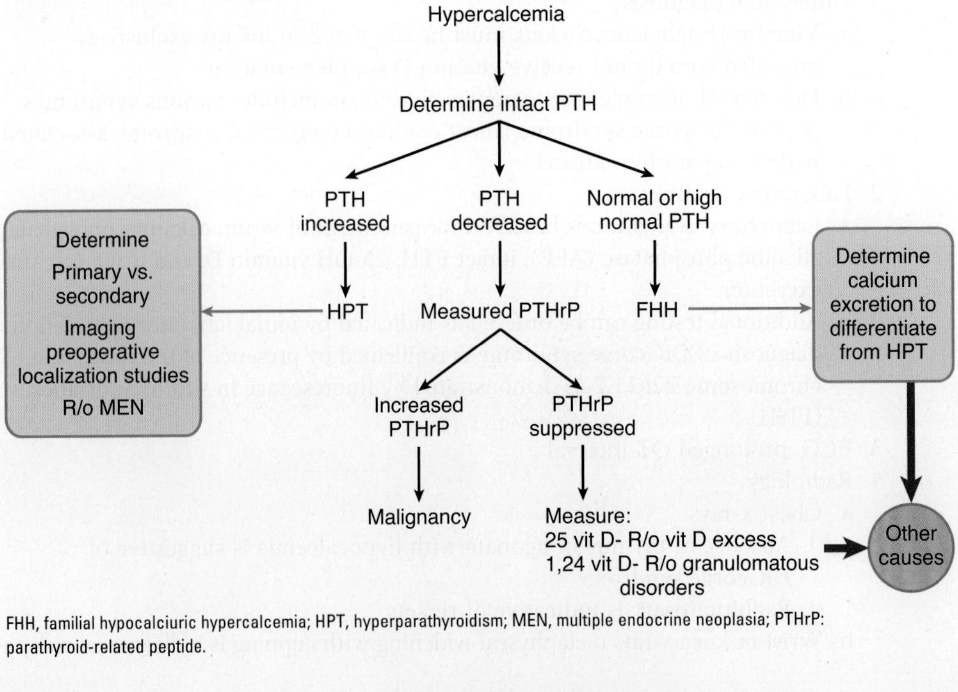

FHH, familial hypocalciuric hypercalcemia; HPT, hyperparathyroidism; MEN, multiple endocrine neoplasia; PTHrP: parathyroid-related peptide.

Endocrine and Metabolic Diseases

TABLE 4-6 **Causes of Hypercalcemia in Neonates and Infants**

Related to maternal conditions	Maternal hypocalcemia	• Results in fetal hypocalcemia and fetal parathyroid hyperplasia • Transient • Hypercalcemia moderate in severity
Familial/genetic disorders	William syndrome	• Deletion of contiguous genes at 7q11.2 • Hypercalcemia is present in 15% of children and usually resolves within 2–4 years of life • Additional abnormalities: elfin-like facies, supravalvular aortic stenosis and peripheral organ arterial stenosis, hypotonia, developmental delay
	Familial hypocalciuric hypercalcemia (FHH)	• Heterozygous inactivating mutations of *CaSR* gene • Autosomal dominant • Labs: mild hypercalcemia with hypocalciuria; parathyroid hormone (PTH) at high normal or mildly increased • Usually asymptomatic; requires no therapy
	Neonatal severe primary hyperparathyroidism (NSHPT)	• Homozygous inactivating mutations of *CaSR* gene • Usually autosomal recessive • Severe hypercalcemia; may be fatal • Serum PTH: markedly elevated • X-rays: rachitic changes with demineralization and fractures • Therapy: parathyroidectomy
	Jansen syndrome, or metaphyseal chondrodysplasia	• PTH receptor gain-of-function mutation that leads to autoactivation of the signaling as though PTH is present • Clinical signs: severe short stature with abnormal facies and irregular formation of the long bones resembling rickets • Hypercalcemia, hypophosphatemia, undetectable PTH levels, hypercalciuria
	Hypophosphatasia	• Rare inborn error of metabolism characterized by deficient activity of tissue-specific alkaline phosphatase • 4 forms: (1) perinatal: usually results in stillbirth; (2) infantile: frequently leads to death within 6 months; (3) childhood: mild; and (4) adult: mild • Low alkaline phosphatase and serum phosphate, hypercalcemia with hypercalciuria and nephrocalcinosis, skeletal demineralization
Miscellaneous	Subcutaneous fat necrosis	• Develops within 1–2 weeks after complicated delivery • Manifests with reddish or purple subcutaneous nodules at sites of pressure, such as back, buttocks, and thighs • Severe hypercalcemia with normal serum phosphate and alkaline phosphatase • Unclear etiology
	Hypophosphatemia	• Usually seen in low-birth-weight infants fed low-phosphate diet • Hypophosphatemia stimulates 1,25 vitamin D production, which leads to increased intestinal calcium absorption • PTH is suppressed and results in hypercalciuria

Endocrine and Metabolic Diseases

2. Physical exam findings
   a. No specific physical findings of hypercalcemia
   b. Findings may reflect system organ involvement caused by hypercalcemia
      i. Polyuria and poor appetite may result in dehydration: look for tachycardia, dry mucous membranes, and other signs of dehydration
      ii. Neurologic exam may document changes in sensorium and muscle weakness
      iii. Dysmorphic features and congenital abnormalities may reflect underlying genetic disorder

C. Diagnosis
1. Laboratory findings
   a. Serum calcium, serum phosphate, serum ALP, intact PTH, parathyroid-related peptide (PTHrP), 25-OH vitamin D, 1,25 vitamin D, and urinary calcium and creatinine

QUICK HIT

The symptoms of hypercalcemia can be remembered by "Stones, Bones, Groans, and Psychiatric Overtones." Stones: renal stones. Bones: pathologic fractures, osteoporosis. Groans: abdominal pain, constipation, vomiting. Psychiatric overtones: depression, memory loss, psychosis or delirium.

TABLE 4-7 **Causes of Hypercalcemia in Childhood**

Hyperparathyroidism (HPT)	Primary	• Hypercalcemia associated with elevated parathyroid hormone (PTH) levels • Single parathyroid adenoma or generalized parathyroid hyperplasia • Can occur as part of MEN1 or MEN2
	Secondary	• Renal failure: seen with prolonged disease • Can be the result of autonomous PTH overproduction (tertiary HPT)
Miscellaneous	Malignancy	• Seen with lymphoma/leukemia • Usually caused by parathyroid-related peptide (PTHrP) produced by the tumor, resulting in hypercalcemia and suppressed PTH levels
	Chronic granulomatous disease	• Usually caused by increased 1,25 vitamin D production
	Immobilization	• Caused by increased bone resorption • Hypercalcemia leads to PTH suppression and, therefore, hypercalciuria
Vitamins and medications	Vitamin D excess	• Vitamin D intoxication usually defined as 25-hydroxyvitamin D >150 ng/mL
	Vitamin A excess	• Increases bone resorption
	Thiazide diuretics	• Increase proximal renal tubule reabsorption
	Lithium	• Results in increased PTH levels
Endocrinopathies	Adrenal insufficiency	• Mild hypercalcemia • Caused by antagonistic effects of glucocorticoids on bone resorption and intestinal calcium absorption • Is associated with suppressed PTH levels
	Thyrotoxicosis	• Increased bone resorption

QUICK HIT

Spot test for hypercalciuria is the calcium:creatinine ratio (mg of urine Ca ÷ mg of urine creatinine). Normal value increases with age: 0–6 months < 0.8, 6–18 months < 0.6, 19 months to 6 years < 0.4, over 6 years < 0.2.

b. Calcium excretion can be determined by spot urine specimen or 24-hour urine collection
c. 25-OH vitamin D concentrations reflect vitamin D stores

2. Radiology: various imaging techniques are used for preoperative localization of parathyroid adenoma in case of primary HPT.
   a. Neck ultrasound
   b. Technetium-99m-sestamibi scan
      i. 12%–25% false-negative results in patients with primary HPT
      ii. Often unrevealing in patients with parathyroid hyperplasia or multiple parathyroid adenomas
   c. SPECT: sestamibi scintigraphy combined with single-photon emission computed tomography
      i. Provides 3-dimensional images
      ii. Has highest positive predictive value
3. Differential diagnosis
   a. Elevation of serum PTH concentrations in presence of high serum calcium is strongly suggestive of HPT
   b. Negative imaging does not rule out primary HPT
   c. Calcium excretion can help differentiate between HPT and familial hypocalciuric hypercalcemia (FHH): calcium excretion is high normal or increased in HPT and decreased in FHH
   d. Serum phosphate is low in HPT and hypercalcemia of malignancy
   e. Children with primary HPT need to be evaluated for possible MEN1 or MEN2A

D. Treatment

1. Acute management of hypercalcemia: aims to decrease serum calcium concentrations
   a. Patients with asymptomatic or mildly symptomatic (e.g., constipation) hypercalcemia (calcium <12 mg/dL [3 mmol/L]) do not require immediate treatment

b. Similarly, serum calcium of 12–14 mg/dL (3.0–3.5 mmol/L) may be well tolerated chronically and may not require immediate treatment
c. Severe hypercalcemia (serum calcium concentration >14 mg/dL [3.5 mmol/L]) or symptomatic hypercalcemia requires intervention.
i. Hydration IV
ii. Administration of diuretics such as furosemide
iii. Administration of medications that decrease serum calcium
(a) Calcitonin injections (efficacy limited to first 48 hours)
(i) Repeated doses lead to tachyphylaxis
(ii) Used in symptomatic patients with calcium >14 mg/L (3.5 mmol/L) to provide rapid reduction in serum calcium concentration
(b) Bisphosphonates: decrease serum calcium by decreasing bone resorption; pamidronate is most commonly used in children
(i) Serum calcium concentrations begin to decrease in 1–2 days; doses should not be repeated sooner than a minimum of 7 days to provide a more sustained effect on serum calcium.
(ii) Side effects may include flu-like symptoms (fever, arthralgias, myalgia, fatigue, bone pain) seen only with 1st infusion, ocular inflammation (uveitis), hypocalcemia, hypophosphatemia, impaired renal function, nephrotic syndrome, and osteonecrosis of the jaw (with prolonged use)
(c) Glucocorticoids are effective in treating hypercalcemia due to certain lymphomas, sarcoid, or other granulomatous diseases
(d) Dialysis
(i) Hemodialysis with little or no calcium in dialysis fluid and peritoneal dialysis are considered treatments of last resort
(ii) May be used in patients with severe malignancy-associated hypercalcemia and renal insufficiency or heart failure, in whom hydration cannot be safely administered
2. Treatment of underlying disorder: parathyroidectomy in case of HPT

QUICK HIT

MCAD is the most common fatty acid oxidation disorder. It has the mildest presentation with no cardiac or muscle involvement.

QUICK HIT

Measurement of an acylcarnitine profile checks levels of the various types of carnitine in the blood. This is abnormal in fatty acid oxidation disorders and can help identify which type is present.

XIX. Fatty Acid Oxidation Disorders

A. Characteristics
1. Definition: disorders in carnitine cycle, β-oxidation cycle, electron transfer chain, and ketone body synthesis that limit the ability to use fat as energy source during fasting and prolonged exercise
2. Epidemiology
a. Carnitine cycle defect <1:200,000
b. Medium-chain acyl-coenzyme A dehydrogenase deficiency (MCAD) ~1:15,000
3. Genetics: autosomal recessive inheritance
B. Clinical features: most present in early infancy as acute hypoketotic hypoglycemia coma
C. Treatment
1. Acute illness: IV glucose (D10 with saline at 1.0–1.5× maintenance) to suppress fatty acid oxidation and lipolysis
2. Long-term diet therapy: carbohydrate therapy at bedtime and avoidance of prolonged fasting (>12 hours overnight); consider continuous feedings and use of cornstarch at night

QUICK HIT

Mild hyperammonemia is often present in MCAD.

QUICK HIT

Because cornstarch must be broken down by pancreatic amylase into glucose, it provides a longer acting enteric availability of sugar, preventing hypoglycemia in these patients.

XX. Urea Cycle Defects

A. Characteristics
1. Definition: defects in main pathway for disposal of excess nitrogen as ammonium, resulting in ammonia toxicity
2. Epidemiology: ~1:30,000
3. Genetics: all urea cycle defects are autosomal recessive, except for ornithine transcarbamylase (OTC) deficiency, which is X linked

QUICK HIT

OTC deficiency is the most common urea cycle defect. Typical presentation is a male infant who is well at birth but refuses to feed and develops vomiting and encephalopathy.

B. Clinical features
   1. Urea cycle defects may present at any age
   2. Symptoms vary with age but include vomiting, tachypnea, apnea, FTT, developmental delay, and encephalopathy during acute stress period
C. Diagnosis: most important test is ammonia concentration with ammonia level usually >150 μmol/L during acute presentation
D. Treatment
   1. Emergency treatment involves discontinuing protein intake and administering glucose either orally or IV
   2. In severe cases, IV sodium benzoate, sodium phenylbutyrate, arginine hydrochloride, or dialysis
   3. Chronic treatment includes low-protein diet and alternative pathways for nitrogen excretion (sodium benzoate and sodium phenylbutyrate)

XXI. Disorders of Carbohydrate Metabolism

A. Characteristics
   1. Definition: autosomal recessive inborn errors of metabolism including glycogen degradation, galactose metabolism, and fructose metabolism
   2. Pathophysiology
      a. Glycogen storage diseases: enzymes defects of glycogen degradation, resulting in inability to produce glucose by liver and/or muscle
      b. Galactose metabolism
         i. Galactose is metabolized by galactokinase, galactose-1-phosphate uridyltransferase (GALT), and uridine diphosphate galactose 4′-epimerase
         ii. Deficiencies in these enzymes result in increased galactose and galactose-1-phosphate levels, which are reduced to galactitol and excreted in urine
      c. Hereditary fructose intolerance
         i. Inability of aldolase B to metabolize fructose-1-phosphate, resulting in accumulation of fructose-1-phosphate and decreased phosphate sources
         ii. Pyruvate and lactate levels are increased, causing metabolic acidosis

QUICK HIT

Fructose is found in honey, fruits, and vegetables. Glucose and fructose form the disaccharide sucrose, which is in many foods and drinks.

B. Clinical features
   1. Glycogen storage diseases
      a. Hepatic glycogen storage disease: short fasting hypoglycemia often associated with muscle weakness and, sometimes, hepatic cirrhosis
      b. Muscle glycogen storage disease: progressive muscle weakness; sometimes cardiomyopathy, fatigue, and exercise
   2. Galactose metabolism disorders
      a. Galactokinase deficiency: cataracts
      b. GALT deficiency
         i. Children with classical galactosemia are usually born with normal birth weight
         ii. After introduction of breast milk or cow's milk formula, failure to regain birth weight by age 2 weeks, refusal to feed, vomiting, lethargy, jaundice, *Escherichia coli* sepsis, hypoglycemia, cataracts, renal failure
      c. Hereditary fructose intolerance: symptoms only appear on exposure to fructose
         i. Abdominal pain, nausea, vomiting, hypoglycemia (severe), lethargy, seizure
         ii. If not diagnosed and fructose continues in diet, FTT, liver disease, bleeding tendency, and proximal renal tubulopathy

QUICK HIT

Infants with galactosemia are at increased risk for sepsis with *E. coli* and should receive early presumptive antibiotic coverage of *E. coli*.

C. Treatment
   1. Therapy
      a. Glycogen storage disease: mainstay is prevention of hypoglycemia (nasogastric tube feedings and uncooked cornstarch)
      b. Galactosemia
         i. Acute: discontinue feedings
         ii. Chronic: avoid dietary lactose and galactose
      c. Hereditary fructose intolerance (acute): reverse hypoglycemia, metabolic acidosis, and hypophosphatemia

XXII. Amino Acid Metabolism Defects

A. Characteristics
   1. Definition: autosomal recessive inborn errors of metabolism disrupting phenylalanine and tyrosine metabolism, resulting in toxic effects of these amino acids
   2. Epidemiology: common clinical conditions include phenylketonuria (PKU), homocystinuria, alkaptonuria, and hereditary tyrosinemia
   3. Pathophysiology: PKU caused by deficiency of phenylalanine hydroxylase, which catalyzes conversion of phenylalanine to tyrosine and results in elevated phenylalanine in tissues, plasma, and urine

B. Clinical features
   1. PKU: presents with developmental delay, infantile spasms, behavioral abnormalities, microcephaly, mental retardation, generalized seizures, and characteristic "mousy/musty" urine odor
   2. Physical exam findings in PKU: light pigmentation of eyes, hair, and eczema

C. Laboratory findings in PKU
   1. Neonatal screening: phenylalanine concentrations
   2. Confirmatory testing: plasma amino acid quantification
   3. DNA testing is available and useful to confirm diagnosis

D. Treatment
   1. Therapy: dietary treatment of phenylalanine-reduced formula and foods based on phenylalanine levels
   2. Prognosis
      a. PKU: early diagnosis and treatment are associated with better neurodevelopmental outcomes
      b. This is why states screen infants for PKU at birth

> **QUICK HIT**
> PKU is the most common inborn error of amino acid metabolism and occurs in 1:15,000 U.S. children.

> **QUICK HIT**
> Patients with homocystinuria are at increased risk for blood clots and embolism.

> **QUICK HIT**
> Mental retardation in patients with PKU can be prevented by avoiding phenylalanine-containing foods and drinks (e.g., diet soft drinks).

XXIII. Organic Acidemias

A. Characteristics
   1. Definition: inborn enzyme deficiencies in metabolism of branched-chain amino acids (leucine, isoleucine, and valine) resulting in accumulation of organic acids
   2. Epidemiology
      a. Maple syrup urine disease (MSUD): 1:150,000
      b. Propionic acidemia: 1:150,000
      c. Isovaleric acidemia: 1:150,000
      d. Methylmalonic acidemia: 1:100,000
   3. Genetics: autosomal recessive
   4. Pathophysiology
      a. Enzyme deficiencies in catabolism of branched-chain amino acid pathways result in accumulation of organic acids, causing toxic effects
      b. Acetyl coenzyme (CoA) and proprionyl CoA (end products of branched-chain amino acid pathway) are unable to enter citric acid cycle

B. Clinical features (Table 4-8) and treatment

> **QUICK HIT**
> MSUD is more common in the Amish and Mennonite populations of Pennsylvania.

> **QUICK HIT**
> Effects of organic acidemias usually occur during catabolic states (infection, stress, fasting). The brain, liver, and kidneys are the most commonly affected organs.

> **QUICK HIT**
> The most important diagnostic test in organic acidemia is the urine organic acids performed by GC-MS.

XXIV. Primary Lactic Acidosis

A. Characteristics: defect in assembly, structure, or function of complexes of respiratory chain *or* pyruvate dehydrogenase deficiency *or* pyruvate carboxylase deficiency, resulting in lactic acidosis

B. Diagnosis
   1. Differential diagnosis
      a. Organic acidemias
      b. Fatty acid oxidation defects
      c. Specific disorders of carbohydrate metabolism
   2. Laboratory findings
      a. ABG, complete metabolic profile, and liver function tests
      b. Lactate
      c. Pyruvate

TABLE 4-8 **Types of Organic Acidemias**

Condition	Enzyme Defect	Specific Features	Specific Treatment
Maple syrup urine disease	Branched-chain oxoreductase	Maple syrup–like odor Neonatal presentation: not severely dehydrated, slightly increased ammonia levels, normal lactate Cerebral edema, increased ICP, and chronic demyelination may occur if not treated in newborn period	Thiamine
Isovaleric acidemia	Isovaleryl CoA dehydrogenase	Sweaty feet odor Neonatal presentation: dehydration, hepatomegaly, metabolic acidosis ketonuria, elevated ammonia and lactate levels, glucose levels variable May develop alopecia, desquamation, corneal ulcers	Carnitine Glycine
Propionic acidemia	Propionyl CoA carboxylase	Neonatal presentation: dehydration, hepatomegaly, metabolic acidosis ketonuria, elevated ammonia and lactate levels, glucose levels variable May develop alopecia, desquamation, corneal ulcers Cardiomyopathy	Carnitine Metronidazole (reduces excretion of propionic acid metabolites)
Methylmalonic acidemia	Methylmalonic CoA mutase	Neonatal presentation: dehydration, hepatomegaly, metabolic acidosis ketonuria, elevated ammonia and lactate levels, glucose levels variable May develop alopecia, desquamation, corneal ulcers Cardiomyopathy Renal tubular acidosis and hyperuricemia	Vitamin B_{12} Carnitine Metronidazole

QUICK HIT

Ketones will be elevated in respiratory chain disorders.

QUICK HIT

Disorders of primary lactic acidosis have normal urine organic acids. If urine organic acids are positive, consider organic acidemias or fatty acid oxidation defects.

d. Lactate:pyruvate ratio
   i. Elevated in respiratory chain disorder and pyruvate carboxylase deficiency
   ii. Normal in pyruvate dehydrogenase deficiency
e. Urine ketones, plasma ketones
f. Blood glucose
g. Free fatty acids
h. Urine organic acids
i. Consider cerebrospinal fluid (CSF) studies and CSF lactate/pyruvate

3. Radiology
   a. MRI of brain for structural or degenerative abnormalities
   b. Magnetic resonance spectroscopy to detect lactate accumulation in specific areas
4. Other findings: affected tissue-specific enzyme activity is definitive diagnosis in respiratory chain disorders and pyruvate dehydrogenase deficiency

5 Neurologic Disorders

SYMPTOM SPECIFIC

I. Approach to Status Epilepticus

A. Characteristics
1. Definition: frequent, recurrent seizures without returning to baseline for >30 minutes
2. Types
   a. Generalized convulsive status epilepticus
   b. Nonconvulsive status epilepticus: focal or generalized electroencephalographic (EEG) activity, resulting in few convulsive clinical symptoms
3. Epidemiology
   a. About 1% of the population
   b. 16% of children with their 1st convulsive status epilepticus will have 2nd within 1 year
4. Pathophysiology
   a. Neurons involved undergo spontaneous paroxysmal depolarization with excitatory postsynaptic potentials and repetitive action potentials
   b. This likely causes spike or sharp wave, followed by hyperpolarization period, cause of aftergoing slow wave seen on EEG

B. Clinical features
1. Generalized convulsive status epilepticus
   a. After treatment initiation, nonconvulsive status epilepticus may occur so seizures are only seen in EEG
2. Focal status epilepticus
   a. Clinical presentation depends on cortical region involved
   b. Temporal and frontal status often cause confusional states

C. Differential diagnosis
1. Idiopathic
2. Structural causes
   a. Tumor
   b. Cortical dysplasia (focal, lobar, or hemispheric) including cortical tubers
   c. Cerebrovascular accidents
   d. Vascular lesions
3. Trauma
4. Inflammatory conditions
5. Central nervous system (CNS) infections
6. Progressive neurodegenerative or mitochondrial disease

D. Treatment
1. Laboratory studies
   a. Rule out an acute metabolic cause
      i. Chem 10 panel

> **QUICK HIT**
> Seizures lasting more than 5–10 minutes are unlikely to terminate on their own.

> **QUICK HIT**
> Frontal lobe status may cause bizarre, atypical movements or acts.

b. Targeted tests may be required based on patient's history
   i. Cerebrospinal fluid (CSF) culture if concerned for meningitis
   ii. Toxicology studies if suspicious for ingestion
   iii. Serum antiepileptic drug (AED) levels to verify effective levels
c. EEG: should be continued after convulsive episode ends to rule out nonconvulsive status epilepticus
d. Neuroimaging: to rule out structural lesion (magnetic resonance imaging [MRI] usually best)

2. Treatment
   a. Stabilization of airway, breathing, and circulation (ABCs) is 1st step
   b. Correct any metabolic derangements
   c. Benzodiazepines first-line medication to abort
3. Prognosis
   a. Overall morbidity and mortality are dependent on underlying cause, duration of status epilepticus, and age of child
   b. Prolonged status epilepticus may cause neuronal cell death

QUICK HIT

Benzodiazepines may cause respiratory depression, so continue to closely monitor your ABCs.

QUICK HIT

Increased ICP can decrease the cerebral perfusion pressure (CPP), which can compromise the blood supply to the brain and cause brain ischemia.

II. Increased Intracranial Pressure

A. Characteristics
1. Pathophysiology
   a. Brain is enclosed in fixed volume space (skull) with 3 components contributing to ICP: brain tissue, blood, and CSF
   b. Sum of 3 components is constant; change in volume in 1 component requires adjustment in another, or increased pressure results
   c. Normal ICP: 8–12 mm Hg
2. Causes: correlate with disruption of skull volume and/or protective mechanisms
   a. Head trauma/subdural hematoma
   b. Brain tumor or mass
   c. Hydrocephalus (congenital or acquired)
   d. Infection: meningitis/meningoencephalitis
   e. Hypoxemia/ischemia
   f. Severe hypertension
   g. Venous sinus thrombosis
   h. Pseudotumor cerebri (idiopathic intracranial hypertension)

QUICK HIT

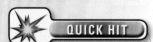

"Thunder clap" headache (one that reaches maximum intensity and severity in seconds to minutes) may be caused by venous sinus thrombosis or subarachnoid hemorrhages.

B. Clinical features
1. Historical findings: differ by age
   a. Neonate: poor feeding/vomiting, irritability, change in activity, seizures
   b. Children: headache that is worse in a.m., vomiting, vision changes, gait disturbance, altered mentation, seizures
2. Physical exam findings
   a. Neonate: macrocephaly, enlarging head circumference, full fontanelle, enlarged sutures, increased tone, hyperreflexia
   b. Children: increased head size, pupil changes, dilation, cranial nerve (CN) palsies (III, IV, and VI), ataxia
   c. Papilledema can confirm increased ICP but may be absent in acute presentations
   d. Decreased level of consciousness is worrisome sign
   e. **Setting sun sign**: downward gaze with visible sclera between iris and upper lid

QUICK HIT

Cushing triad indicates markedly increased intracranial pressure (hypertension, bradycardia, and irregular respirations).

QUICK HIT

A normal head CT does not rule out increased ICP. When a CT scan of the head is negative, a lumbar puncture with manometer to calculate the opening pressure can be performed.

C. Diagnosis
1. Urgent imaging with noncontrast head computed tomography (CT) scan can identify etiology (e.g., mass, intracranial hemorrhage) and increased ICP changes
   a. Increased ventricle size
   b. Edema
   c. Loss of gray and white matter differentiation
   d. Midline shift
2. Other diagnostics are directed by history/physical exam to find underlying cause

QUICK HIT

When increased ICP is suspected, head imaging should be performed prior to performing a lumbar puncture.

D. Treatment
  1. General measures
    a. ABCs
      i. Intubation with appropriate ventilation
        (a) Acute hyperventilation for refractory ICP
        (b) Sedation/muscle relaxation necessary to limit cerebral metabolism
      ii. Maintain adequate circulation
        (a) Fluid resuscitation with isotonic fluids
        (b) Vasopressors if needed for normotension
    b. Temperature control
    c. Avoid hyperthermia
    d. Elevate head of bed 15–30°
    e. Pain and seizure control
  2. Specific measures
    a. ICP monitoring/CSF drainage
    b. Osmotic diuretics: hypertonic (3%) saline or mannitol
    c. Corticosteroids: useful if underlying cause has inflammatory component (tumor/abscess)
    d. Barbiturate coma: for *refractory* ICP; decreases cerebral metabolism but causes hypotension

QUICK HIT

Increased ICP is a **medical emergency**! All initial treatment is aimed at stabilizing ICP and restoring cerebral perfusion pressure. *After* stabilization, the goal is to treat the underlying cause.

QUICK HIT

Some medications will increase ICP. Avoid ketamine (increases cerebral blood flow), hypotonic solutions (increase cerebral edema), and vasodilators in patients with increased ICP.

III. Approach to Headache

A. Background information
  1. Epidemiology and demographics
    a. Headaches are very common; increasing frequency with age
    b. Variability of clinical presentation by age
      i. Younger children may rock; hide; cry; regress; have behavioral concerns; have interference with ability to eat, sleep, and play
      ii. Older children are more able to perceive, localize, remember, and characterize pain

B. Differential diagnosis (Box 5-1)
  1. Primary headache disorders
    a. Migraine headaches
    b. Cluster headaches
    c. Tension headaches
  2. Secondary headaches
    a. ICP
    b. CNS infection
    c. Vasculitis
    d. Arteriovenous malformation
    e. Aneurysm
    f. Analgesic abuse and use (especially ibuprofen)

C. Historical findings: see Box 5-1
  1. Medication history
    a. Name, dose, frequency, effect of all medications
    b. Inquire if abruptly stopping medications after use in large amounts
  2. Thorough family history
  3. See Box 5-2 for history and physical exam clues
  4. **Headache diary** may be useful for families and/or patients

D. Physical examination findings (Box 5-2)
  1. Usually, exam will be normal in child with primary headache syndrome
  2. Patient affect and interaction with parents should be observed
  3. Neurologic exam to include
    a. Mental status and behavioral assessment
    b. CN function
    c. Motor strength
    d. Deep tendon reflexes
    e. Sensation

QUICK HIT

Most head injuries can be prevented with simple interventions (e.g., wearing a helmet while riding a bicycle).

QUICK HIT

Interviewing the patient is the most important component to making the proper diagnosis.

QUICK HIT

Family history is a significant risk factor for migraines.

BOX 5-1

Differential Diagnosis of Pediatric Headache

Vascular headache
Migraine type
Common
Classic
Complicated
Hypertension
Vasculitis
Cerebral aneurysm
Embolus or infarction
Cluster headache

Intracranial infections
Meningitis
Encephalitis
Intracranial abscess

Disorders of the head and neck
Eye strain (rare)
Glaucoma
Sinus infections
Streptococcal pharyngitis
Dental caries
Malocclusion
Temporomandibular joint dysfunction
Cranial neuralgias (rare in pediatrics)

Other causes
Systemic illness
Drugs
Poisoning
Hyperventilation
Hypoxia
Seizure, after seizure

Altered intracranial pressure
Increased pressure
Tumor
Intracranial hemorrhage/hematoma
Intracranial abscess
Cerebral edema
Hydrocephalus
Pseudotumor cerebri
Venous sinus thrombosis
Decreased pressure
After lumbar puncture

Trauma
Intracranial hemorrhage/hematoma
Posttraumatic, concussion
Muscle strain (whiplash)

Muscular headache
Tension
Muscle strain
Activity
Posture
Prolonged position

Psychogenic causes
Anxiety
Depression

BOX 5-2

Key Clues to Serious Headache

History
Headache worsening in severity and frequency
Nocturnal headache
Morning headache with vomiting
Severe pain at headache onset
Fixed location, occipital pain
Pain worse with Valsalva, recumbent position, or change in position
Change in previously established headache pattern
Headache in patients with ventriculoperitoneal shunts
Exposure to someone with meningitis or encephalitis
Neurologic symptoms or signs
Lethargy, confusion, irritability
Vomiting
Visual/sensory changes, weakness, ataxia
Headache *before* seizure
Migraine-type headache with seizure

Physical examination
Impaired mental status
Hypertension, especially if associated with bradycardia
Fever and ill appearance, especially with petechiae
Papilledema, retinal hemorrhage
Cranial bruit
Nuchal rigidity
Cranial nerve palsy
Strabismus, diplopia, decreased visual acuity or visual field deficits
Weakness, hyperreflexia, Babinski reflex
Ataxia, wide-based gait, positive Romberg sign
Neurocutaneous lesions
Macrocephaly

f. Cerebellar function
g. Optic fundoscopic examination

E. Laboratory testing and radiologic imaging
1. Laboratory testing rarely helpful in evaluation of childhood headache
2. Neuroimaging for suspicion of structural causes of secondary headache only
a. Indications for neuroimaging study with recurrent headache
i. Abnormal neurologic exam and/or seizures
ii. Complicated migraines or atypical migraine features
iii. Abrupt onset of severe headache
iv. Severe headache in child with underlying disease process that predisposes to intracranial pathology
b. Choice of imaging study
i. Head CT without contrast in emergent situations when hemorrhage or space-occupying lesion is suspected
ii. MRI usually preferred in nonemergent situations
3. Lumbar puncture with manometry (usually after neuroimaging)
a. For suspicion of intracranial infection, subarachnoid hemorrhage, or pseudotumor cerebri

QUICK HIT

Any abnormality on neurologic exam mandates an *urgent* evaluation.

IV. Approach to Ataxia

A. Background information
1. Ataxia: decreased coordination of voluntary movements
2. Differential diagnosis (Table 5-1)

B. Historical findings
1. Describe symptoms and acute or subacute onset
2. Associated nausea, vomiting, or headache suggests increased ICP
3. Fever suggests infectious process
4. Recent head or neck trauma (e.g., vertebral dissection, traumatic hemorrhage)
5. Recent upper respiratory infection (URI) symptoms or otitis media (e.g., labyrinthitis, abscess)
6. Mental status changes or seizures

C. Physical examination findings
1. Head, eyes, ears, nose, and throat (HEENT)
a. Meningismus
b. Papilledema or bulging fontanel = increased ICP
c. Mastoid tenderness, ear pain, or hearing loss

TABLE 5-1 **Differential Diagnosis of Ataxia**

Injury	Cerebral palsy, stroke, trauma, hypoxic injury
Neoplastic and paraneoplastic	Tumors of the cerebellum or brainstem, neuroblastoma with associated opsoclonus myoclonus syndrome
Degenerative and demyelinating	Ataxia telangiectasia, Friedreich ataxia, Wilson disease, spinocerebellar ataxias, multiple sclerosis, acute disseminated encephalomyelitis
Metabolic	Lipidoses, mitochondrial disorders, glutaric aciduria, vitamin deficiencies, lysosomal diseases, congenital disorders of glycosylation
Malformations	Joubert syndrome, Dandy-Walker malformation, Chiari malformation, vermian agenesis, cerebellar dysgenesis
Drug induced or toxic ingestions	Antiepileptic medications, antihistamines, barbiturates, lithium, alcohol, chemotherapy, heavy metal poisoning
Acute or paroxysmal	Acute cerebellar ataxias, episodic ataxias, electrolyte or glucose abnormalities, Miller-Fisher variant of Guillain-Barré syndrome, migraine variants
Infectious	Varicella and other viral illnesses

2. Neurologic exam
   a. Mental status
      i. Abnormal speech (dysarthria, abnormal modulation of prosody or tone)
      ii. Lethargy or altered mental status
   b. CNs
      i. Nystagmus or other abnormalities of extraocular movements
      ii. Opsoclonus myoclonus syndrome in neuroblastoma
   c. Motor exam
      i. Muscle weakness (either generalized or focal)
   d. Sensory exam: Romberg sign = test of proprioceptive sensory input
   e. Reflexes: absent deep tendon reflexes in Guillain-Barré syndrome (GBS) and its variants
   f. Cerebellar/coordination testing
   g. Gait exam

QUICK HIT

Opsoclonus-myoclonus-ataxia syndrome is associated with neuroblastoma.

QUICK HIT

Patients with cerebellar dysfunction will have difficulty maintaining balance with eyes open or closed.

D. Laboratory testing and radiologic imaging
1. Diagnostic workup
   a. Laboratory data
      i. Toxicology screen (serum and urine)
      ii. Metabolic testing
         (a) Liver function testing (LFT)
         (b) "Metabolic workup": ammonia, lactate, pyruvate, serum amino acids, and urine organic acids
      iii. Lumbar puncture if concern for infectious/postinfectious etiology
   b. Radiologic imaging
      i. MRI: superior visualization of posterior fossa
      ii. CT: rapid detection of hemorrhage, hydrocephalus, masses
   c. Electromyography (EMG) if considering GBS

QUICK HIT

Neuroimaging is warranted in any child with focal neurologic deficits, signs of increased ICP (papilledema or bulging anterior fontanel), or a history of trauma.

DISEASE SPECIFIC

V. Febrile Seizures

A. Most common cause of seizures and status epilepticus in childhood: familial inheritance
B. Clinical features
1. Historical findings
   a. Definition of simple febrile seizures
      i. Age 6 months to 6 years
      ii. Fever at the time of or immediately after the seizure
      iii. Occur in children without neurologic or significant developmental issues
      iv. Simple febrile seizures are typically brief, generalized, and limited to one episode
      v. Complex febrile seizures include any of the following deviations, which contribute additively to an increased risk of epilepsy later in life:
         (a) Duration > 15 minutes
         (b) Recurrence within 24 hours
         (c) Any seizure differing from a generalized convulsion (focal/staring/collapse, etc.)
      vi. Often there is a positive family history
   b. Elicit features that might identify fever source (e.g., URI or gastrointestinal [GI] symptoms, ill exposures, headache, throat pain)

C. Diagnosis
1. Differential diagnosis
   a. Most concerning possibility is meningitis/encephalitis as cause of seizure in context of febrile illness
   b. Lumbar puncture should be performed in children with clinical signs or symptoms concerning for meningitis

QUICK HIT

Febrile seizures occur in 2%–5% of children.

QUICK HIT

The primary reason for distinguishing simple from complex seizures is to predict the future risk of epilepsy.

QUICK HIT

Having a first-degree relative (sibling or parent) with febrile seizures increases the risk 4–5× that of the general population.

QUICK HIT

The rate of serious bacterial infection is not any higher in children with febrile seizures versus children with fever alone.

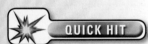

2. Further diagnostic evaluation
   a. EEG and MRI are *not* routinely indicated for simple febrile seizures
   b. Complex febrile seizures have no established parameters for further testing

D. Treatment
1. Seizures are typically self-limited; seizure medications generally unhelpful
2. Treat underlying cause of fever if indicated
3. Prognosis
   a. Outstanding prognosis
   b. Risk of recurrence 50% in children <1 year, 33% in children >1 year
   c. Simple: about 2% develop epilepsy (compared to 1% of the general population)
   d. Complex: increased risk of epilepsy with more complex features

QUICK HIT

Antipyretics do not reduce the risk of febrile seizures.

VI. Generalized Seizures

A. Characteristics
1. Definition: generalized, synchronous involvement of both cerebral hemispheres at onset, resulting in impairment of consciousness
   a. 6 generalized seizure types
      i. Generalized tonic-clonic
      ii. Absence
      iii. Myoclonic
      iv. Tonic
      v. Clonic
      vi. Atonic
   b. Generalized epilepsy syndromes (cluster of similar signs and symptoms in patient with epilepsy) may have combinations of seizure types
2. Epidemiology: epilepsy affects approximately 1% of persons age <20 years

B. Clinical features
1. Absence (typical)
   a. Child stares with vacant look, and tone is commonly preserved
   b. Abrupt onset of impairment of consciousness without prior warning with resumption of baseline activity immediately after seizure ends
   c. Commonly lasts <20 seconds and may be missed if child is not closely observed
   d. Accompanying features may include subtle clonic activity, especially of upper limbs, head, and neck area; eye blinking or rolling; automatisms; eyelid myoclonia; and subtle loss in tone without falls
   e. Usually develops in children with normal neurocognitive ability
2. Tonic-clonic
   a. Tonic phase
      i. Child simultaneously stiffens
      ii. Stiffening is often symmetric with flexion or extension of limbs and clenching of fist
      iii. Jaw is also clenched shut with eyes rolling upward
      iv. This phase often lasts <30 seconds
   b. Clonic phase
      i. Rhythmic jerking or convulsions of limbs, initially starting out fast and low in amplitude but gradually decreasing in frequency and increasing in amplitude of movements prior to its termination
      ii. Commonly associated with decreased respiratory effort
      iii. Urination during event is common, and biting cheek or sides of tongue may occur
      iv. Entire event rarely lasts >2 minutes
      v. Postictal period is continued: diffuse decrease in tone and drowsiness, then child very slowly regains consciousness
3. Myoclonic: rapid, lightening-like contraction of muscle or group of muscles
   a. May vary greatly in severity both in amplitude of movement and area involved
   b. Preservation of consciousness
4. Atonic: loss of some (head and neck) or all postural tone
5. Tonic: isolated tonic muscle contraction
6. Clonic: repetitive rhythmic jerking or convulsions

QUICK HIT

Recurrence risk of additional febrile seizures is 30% after 1 febrile seizure and 50% after 2 febrile seizures.

QUICK HIT

Children with prolonged febrile seizures are more likely to experience another prolonged febrile seizure if they recur.

QUICK HIT

In neonates and young children, seizures will appear differently than in older children and adults.

QUICK HIT

The EEG pattern in absence seizures is 3-Hz spike and wave.

QUICK HIT

Absence seizure may be induced by hyperventilation.

C. Physical exam findings
   1. Look for dysmorphic features
   2. Skin: birthmarks or neurocutaneous stigmata
   3. Complete neurologic exam: focal weakness suggests focal seizure with secondary generalization

D. Diagnosis
   1. Differential diagnosis
      a. Idiopathic (genetic)
      b. Symptomatic or presumed symptomatic (cryptogenic)
         i. Epilepsy with myoclonic astatic (atonic) seizures
         ii. Lennox-Gastaut syndrome
         iii. Progressive myoclonic epilepsies

E. Laboratory and other findings
   1. Screening labs for seizure medication side effects and levels (Table 5-2)
   2. CSF studies for metabolic or infectious disease

TABLE 5-2 **Common Antiepileptic Drugs**

Antiepileptic Drugs	Effective for Seizure Types	Required Monitoring	Side Effects
Carbamazepine	Partial seizures Generalized seizures	AED levels Complete blood count	Behavioral changes GI side effects Rash Stevens-Johnson syndrome (SJS) Bone marrow suppression Low serum sodium
Divalproex sodium	Generalized seizures Partial seizures	AED levels LFTs Amylase CBC, platelets	Fatal hepatic necrosis in young children (not used in age <2 years) Drowsiness Behavioral changes Nausea, vomiting Thrombocytopenia Leukopenia Pancreatitis
Ethosuximide	1st line for absence seizures	CBC, platelets	Drowsiness Behavioral changes Nausea, vomiting Aplastic anemia (rare) Lupus-like syndrome (rare)
Lamotrigine	Partial seizures Idiopathic generalized seizures Mixed seizure syndromes Lennox-Gastaut syndrome	AED levels	Rash, most common AED associated with SJS Nausea Dizziness and somnolence
Levetiracetam	Adjunct therapy for partial-onset seizures Adjunct therapy for myoclonic seizures Juvenile myoclonic epilepsy Primary generalized tonic-clonic seizures Idiopathic generalized epilepsy		Well tolerated Fatigue Dizziness
Phenytoin	Partial seizures Generalized seizures 2nd line agent for myoclonic and tonic-clonic seizures 2nd line agent for status epilepticus	AED levels	Gingival hypertrophy Body hair increase Lymphadenopathy Neurotoxic side effects with long-term use
Phenobarbital	Generalized seizures Partial seizures Not usually used long term due to sedating effects	AED levels	Sedation Behavioral changes Hyperactivity Rash, SJS
Topamax	Partial seizures Mixed seizure disorders Refractory generalized tonic-clonic convulsions Usually used as an adjunct therapy	CBC, platelets LFTs	Behavioral changes Decreased appetite, weight loss Metabolic acidosis Nephrolithiasis Impaired cognition

AED, antiepileptic drug; CBC, complete blood count; LFT, liver function test

3. EEG: may identify underlying seizure syndrome
4. Neuroimaging: MRI to rule out structural abnormality
5. Neuropsychological assessment: to determine level of cognitive function

F. Treatment
1. AED therapy
   a. ~60%–70% of children will be rendered seizure free after trying 1–3 AEDs
   b. AED selection based on seizure type (Table 5-2)
2. Surgical management: considered in patients refractory to AED, depending on localization, type, and frequency
3. Vagus nerve stimulator (VNS)
4. Ketogenic diet (mechanism is unclear but can be effective for refractory seizures)

G. Prognosis: idiopathic epilepsy: excellent prognosis for outgrowing or fully controlling with medication

QUICK HIT

The more recent International League Against Epilepsy classification uses "focal" to replace the prior terms "partial" or "localization related" to describe seizures originating from 1 cortical region.

VII. Focal (Partial) Seizures

A. Characteristics
1. Definition: epileptic seizure originating at onset from a cortical region in 1 hemisphere
2. Aura: distinctive warning preceding seizure
3. Clinical manifestations may include motor, sensory, autonomic, or psychic phenomenon, dependent on site of origin
4. Child may be fully aware of event (simple partial or focal), may have alteration of consciousness (complex partial or focal), or level of consciousness may be difficult to determine, especially in very young
5. Focal seizure may become more widespread

QUICK HIT

An aura is only experienced in individuals with focal seizures.

B. Clinical features
1. Medial temporal lobe epilepsy (MTLE)
   a. Auras may occur
   b. Often followed by cessation in movement and oral/alimentary automatisms (swallowing, pursing of lips, lip smacking, etc.) on ipsilateral side
   c. Dystonic posturing of contralateral upper extremity (UE) is often seen
2. Frontal lobe seizures: usually brief; characterized by excessive, sometimes bizarre but often stereotyped movement or tonic posturing; may cluster and have predilection for occurring during sleep
3. Parietal: somatosensory symptoms contralateral to side of seizure onset, or occasionally bilateral sensory symptoms may be experienced
4. Occipital
   a. Visual hallucinations (elementary, unformed)
   b. Sensation of ocular movement or double vision

QUICK HIT

Mesial temporal sclerosis is the most identified cause of symptomatic focal epilepsy.

C. Diagnosis
1. EEG: epileptiform activity or focal slowing may help identify area of seizure origin
2. Video EEG: video time-locked to EEG in order to capture, lateralize, and localize seizures
3. MRI: to rule out structural lesion

D. Treatment
1. AEDs
2. Definitive epilepsy surgery (e.g., topectomy, lobectomy, hemispherectomy)
3. Corpus callosotomy
4. Implanted device (e.g., VNS)
5. Ketogenic diet

VIII. Infantile Spasms

A. Characteristics
1. Generalized myoclonic or brief tonic flexion or occasionally extension of neck, trunk, and limbs (upper > lower)
2. Seizures may be clustered (90%) or individual, and usually occur while awake

QUICK HIT

The ketogenic diet mimics starvation by forcing the body to burn fat rather than carbohydrates.

3. Epidemiology
   a. Most begin between ages 3 and 7 months
   b. 85% begin before age 1 year
4. Causes
   a. Thorough evaluation for underlying cause will yield specific etiology in 70%–95% of cases
   b. Etiologies include congenital malformations, genetic syndromes, and diverse types of acquired brain injury

B. Clinical features
1. Historical findings
   a. Onset is frequently insidious and gradual and may be overlooked
   b. Clusters of spasms often cause distress and crying
   c. Occurrence of clusters of spasms often when awakening
2. Physical exam findings
   a. Often a normal neurologic exam
   b. Head circumference: microcephaly and macrocephaly may indicate cortical anomalies or poor brain growth
   c. Associated organ system anomalies or dysmorphic features may indicate chromosomal or syndromic etiology

C. Diagnosis
1. EEG findings: **hypsarrhythmia** (chaotic high-amplitude background with multifocal and generalized spikes)
2. MRI most useful for congenital or acquired structural lesions
3. Laboratory findings
   a. Metabolic evaluation (urine organic acids, serum and CSF amino acids, lactate, ammonia, and acylcarnitine profile)
   b. Genetics: start with karyotype, may progress to microarray; consider tuberous sclerosis testing

D. Treatment
1. Prompt effective therapy improves developmental outcome
2. Adrenocorticotropic hormone (ACTH) is first-line therapy

E. Prognosis
1. Mortality as high as 1/3 in 3 years
2. Most children eventually outgrow spasms, but majority develop other seizures types
3. Mental retardation (MR) in almost all patients; severe MR in 1/2 of cases

> **QUICK HIT**
>
> West syndrome describes a subset of infantile-onset patients who exhibit the triad of infantile spasms, an EEG showing hypsarrhythmia, and psychomotor retardation with or without developmental regression.

> **QUICK HIT**
>
> Children with symmetric cryptogenic spasms (normal development and examination) *with* hypsarrhythmia carry a good prognosis for full remission and normal developmental outcome.

> **QUICK HIT**
>
> CT scan may be useful in evaluating for calcifications, often associated with tuberous sclerosis.

> **QUICK HIT**
>
> Typical ACTH side effects include irritability, acne, weight gain, hypertension, and glucose intolerance.

IX. Benign Epilepsy with Centrotemporal Spikes (BECTS)

A. Definition
1. Also known as *benign rolandic epilepsy*
2. Presents with simple partial seizures with motor symptoms involving face
3. Typically begins in 2nd half of 1st decade of life in developmentally normal children
4. Seizures most commonly occur during sleep, often within 1st hour of falling asleep
5. Prognosis is excellent, with virtually all patients outgrowing their seizures by adolescence

B. Cause/pathophysiology
1. Genetic cause with low penetrance
2. Affects *region of facial and hand areas* of primary motor and sensory cortices, which explains clinical presentation

C. Clinical presentation
1. Seizures follow highly characteristic pattern
   a. Most commonly begin as **simple partial seizures**, with tingling paresthesias in lower face, in or around mouth, or unilaterally
   b. May develop clonic movements of mouth or inability to speak
   c. May spread into hand and arm on same side
   d. Can lead to secondarily generalized tonic-clonic seizure
2. Diurnal pattern: daytime seizures occur in <10% of patients
3. Age: typically occur in children ages 5–12 years

> **QUICK HIT**
>
> *Most seizures in BECTS occur during sleep*, often soon after sleep onset.

D. Testing
 1. EEG findings are very specific to this syndrome
 2. If all typical clinical and EEG features are present, brain imaging may not be required
E. Treatment
 1. Children with this syndrome "outgrow" their epilepsy
 2. *Severe developmental impairments do not occur*
 3. Treatment is optional

X. Migraine Headache

A. Characteristics
 1. Epidemiology
  a. Most common acute recurrent headache syndrome in childhood
  b. Disorder begins at age $<$20 years in 50%
 2. Genetics: no clear mode of inheritance, but often runs in families
 3. Risk factors
  a. Triggers
   i. Foods and chemicals, especially alcohol
   ii. Drugs
   iii. Environmental factors, such as bright lights or noise
   iv. Psychosocial factors such as emotional stress or fatigue
B. Clinical features
 1. Historical findings
  a. Symptoms vary with age
   i. Toddlers: episodes of pallor, decreased activity, and vomiting
   ii. Young children: often associated with nausea and vomiting and sensitivity to light and noise
   iii. Adolescence/adulthood: more typical gradual onset of pain that becomes throbbing when severity peaks
  b. Headache worsens with movement and activity
  c. Photophobia and phonophobia
  d. Lasts 1–72 hours
  e. Aura
   i. Less common in children; only 30% will have an aura
   ii. Usually visual spots, colored lights, or complex visual images
C. Diagnosis
 1. Clinical diagnosis requiring headache and associated symptoms
 2. Differential diagnosis (Box 5-3)
 3. Radiology findings: generally not helpful unless unusual symptoms indicating another problem (e.g., morning headache or headache waking from sleep)
D. Treatment
 1. Nonpharmacologic therapy
  a. Sleep, exercise, hydration
  b. Trial of food elimination based on triggers identified in headache diary
  c. Biofeedback
 2. Acute general treatment
  a. Analgesics
   i. Ibuprofen should be given early in course of migraine
   ii. Sumatriptan nasal spray approved for children age $>$12 years
  b. Other medications for acute migraines not responding to home management include promethazine, prochlorperazine, and others

BOX 5-3

Differential Diagnosis of Migraines

Chronic paroxysmal hemicranias
Cluster headache
Head injury
Intracranial hemorrhage
Migraine variants
Tension headache

QUICK HIT

Migraines are typically bitemporal in younger children and unitemporal in adolescence.

QUICK HIT

Complicated migraines may result in *temporary* neurologic deficits.

QUICK HIT

When a patient presents with a complicated migraine, a more thorough evaluation may be needed to rule out stroke, tumor, or infectious causes.

QUICK HIT

Status migrainosus occurs when a migraine lasts longer than 72 hours.

3. Chronic treatment/prophylaxis: if patient requires therapy for ≥3 migraines per week, preventive pharmacologic therapy may be considered

XI. Strokes

A. Characteristics
1. Definition/epidemiology
   a. Acute neurologic disturbance that lasts >24 hours secondary to disrupted blood supply
   b. Very rare in children
2. Cause: 3 broad categories
   a. Arteriopathy
   b. Cardioembolic
   c. Hematologic disorders (e.g., sickle cell diseases, prothrombotic conditions)

QUICK HIT

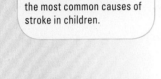

Congenital heart disease and sickle cell disease are the most common causes of stroke in children.

B. Clinical features
1. Historical findings
   a. Focal weakness; changes in vision, speech, sensation, or balance
   b. Neonatal stroke may present with seizures alone
2. Physical exam findings: hemiparesis is most common focal presentation
3. Radiology findings
   a. *MRI is test of choice*
      i. Better for early and small strokes
      ii. Magnetic resonance angiography (MRA) may be necessary to look for underlying vasculopathy
   b. CT may demonstrate larger ischemic stroke and exclude hemorrhage

QUICK HIT

A focal neurologic deficit in a child should be considered a stroke until proven otherwise.

C. Treatment
1. Therapy: emergency thrombolysis is poorly studied in children

XII. Guillain-Barré Syndrome

A. Characteristics
1. Definition: acute, progressive weakness
   a. Ascending pattern from legs to arms to CNs
   b. Progressive, over several days in most cases
   c. Can lead to respiratory weakness requiring aggressive supportive care, including mechanical ventilation
2. Cause
   a. Autoimmune inflammation of peripheral nerve roots, just as they exit spinal cord
   b. Inflammation principally affects myelin sheath surrounding nerve, although nerve axons may also be affected
   c. Preceding infection is present in most cases
      i. Diarrheal illness due to ***Campylobacter jejuni*** confers highest risk
      ii. *Mycoplasma pneumoniae* or viral respiratory illness
      iii. Recent vaccination is a very rare trigger

QUICK HIT

GBS is the most common cause of peripheral neuropathy. Symptoms will include hypotonia and diminished or absent reflexes.

B. Clinical features
1. **Ascending paralysis**
   a. In most patients, weakness begins in legs, then spreads upward
   b. However, proximal muscles (hips and shoulders) may be affected before distal muscles (hands and feet), even in classic ascending paralysis
   c. Weakness is symmetric between left and right
   d. Deep tendon reflexes are absent (may be a later finding)
   e. Weakness can progress to respiratory failure in just hours or over several weeks
2. Associated symptoms
   a. Pain, usually in limbs, is common
   b. **Autonomic dysfunction** can be dangerous
      i. Cardiac arrhythmias
      ii. Urinary retention
      iii. Gastroparesis
   c. Sensory loss is usually mild or absent

QUICK HIT

Areflexia is the physical finding most specific to disease of the peripheral nerves.

3. Diagnosis
   a. Variants of GBS
      i. Miller-Fisher syndrome
         (a) Weakness begins in CNs
         (b) Clinical triad of ataxia, areflexia, and ophthalmoplegia
   b. Differential diagnosis
      i. Cerebral lesions: more typically cause focal weakness, such as hemiparesis
      ii. Multifocal cerebral lesions, such as with acute disseminated encephalomyelitis (ADEM), may present similarly to GBS
      iii. Spinal lesions: often present with leg weakness, but sensory loss and urinary symptoms are usually more prominent, and deep tendon reflexes may be increased
      iv. Transverse myelitis
      v. Paraspinous abscess
      vi. Compressive lesion, tumor or traumatic
      vii. Poliomyelitis
         (a) Usually asymmetric weakness
         (b) Signs of systemic infection, fever, and CSF pleocytosis
      viii. Neuromuscular junction (NMJ) disorders
         (a) Myasthenia gravis (MG): usually slower in onset with prominent oculomotor symptoms and preserved reflexes
         (b) Infant botulism
         (c) Tick paralysis
      ix. Myositis

C. Diagnosis
   1. Nerve conduction studies
   2. MRI: enhancement of nerve roots
   3. Specific autoantibody testing is available
   4. With typical clinical presentation and CSF findings, other testing is usually not required

D. Treatment
   1. Medication
      a. *Corticosteroids are not useful* in treatment of GBS
      b. Intravenous immunoglobulin (IVIG) is mainstay of treatment: speeds recovery, slows progression
      c. Plasmapheresis is equally as effective as IVIG but is less commonly used in pediatric patients
   2. Supportive care
      a. Respiratory failure is main risk of GBS
         i. Negative inspiratory force (NIF) measurements are the most useful bedside screening tool
         ii. *Pulse oximetry is not effective* as screening tool because hypoxemia is very late finding in respiratory weakness if lung function is normal
         iii. Mechanical ventilation may be necessary for respiratory failure
   3. Prognosis
      a. >95% of children will make complete recovery
      b. Time to full recovery varies from days to as long as several months

QUICK HIT

Hallmark features of GBS are ascending weakness with areflexia.

QUICK HIT

Lumbar puncture in patients with GBS classically shows elevated protein and normal white blood cell (WBC) count in CSF called *albuminocytologic dissociation.*

XIII. Acute Disseminated Encephalomyelitis

A. Definition: brief (several weeks to months) but intense attack of inflammation in brain and spinal cord (and occasionally optic nerve) that causes damage to myelin sheath

B. Cause/pathophysiology
   1. Immune-mediated reactions against certain components of CNS
   2. Often preceded by viral infection, with an average latency period of 7–14 days
   3. May be a precursor of multiple sclerosis in some patients

C. Clinical features
  1. Symptoms: rapid-onset encephalitis-like symptoms
D. Diagnosis
  1. Radiologic testing: MRI is diagnostic for ADEM, symmetric gray matter involvement, and asymmetric white matter lesions
E. Treatment
  1. High-dose steroid is mainstay of therapy
  2. IVIG or plasmapheresis has also been used
F. Prognosis
  1. Patients with ADEM usually recover slowly, over 4–6 weeks
  2. At follow-up, ~60%–80% have no residual neurologic deficits

XIV. Spinal Muscular Atrophy (SMA)

A. Definition
  1. Autosomal recessive severe neuromuscular disease resulting in significant weakness
  2. Clinical types based on severity (I = severe; III = mild)
B. Cause/pathophysiology
  1. Caused by mutations in the survival motor neuron (SMN) gene
  2. Results in degeneration of anterior horn cells in spinal cord
C. Clinical presentation
  1. Progressive and symmetrical proximal weakness
  2. Lower motor neuron disease with absent deep tendon reflexes
  3. Muscle fasciculations of tongue
  4. Normal cognitive development
  5. Type I SMA (Werdnig-Hoffman disease)
    a. Severe generalized weakness and hypotonia from birth
    b. Presentation before age 6 months
    c. Most common genetic cause of infant death; death usually results from respiratory failure before age 2 years
    d. Respiratory support may prolong life, but its use in this regard is controversial
  6. Type II SMA
    a. Ability to sit but not stand or walk
    b. Presents between ages 6 and 18 months
    c. Will require respiratory and nutritional support
  7. Type III SMA
    a. Can walk independently initially but may lose this skill by age 10 years
    b. Presents after age 18 months
    c. Physical therapy and orthopedic follow-up are needed
D. Testing: *SMN1* gene deletion test
E. Therapy: no curative treatment, supportive care only

XV. Infant Botulism

A. Definition: acquired neuromuscular disease most commonly affecting infants age 1 week to 1 year
B. Cause/pathophysiology
  1. Due to ingestion of spores of *Clostridium botulinum* bacteria, which are typically found in dirt and dust, but also can contaminate honey
  2. Bacteria colonize and grow in immature colon and produce neurotoxin
  3. Neurotoxin blocks acetylcholine (ACh) release at presynaptic cleft in NMJ
  4. Result is cholinergic blockade of autonomic skeletal muscles and end organs
C. Clinical presentation
  1. Descending bulbar weakness: flat facial expression, weak cry, poor feeding with difficulty swallowing and drooling, sluggish pupils, and ptosis
  2. Skeletal muscle weakness: hypotonia and flaccid paralysis with progression to respiratory failure
  3. Lower motor neuron disease with absent deep tendon reflexes
D. Testing
  1. Isolation of toxin (or *C. botulinum*) in stool
  2. Confirmatory testing will take time; therapy should not be delayed for test results

QUICK HIT

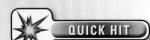

Muscle fasciculations are small muscle twitches or tremors that are a hallmark of anterior horn cell disease.

QUICK HIT

Weakness is decreased resistance to active movement; hypotonia is decreased resistance to passive movement.

QUICK HIT

Although honey is typically thought of as a risk factor, most cases of infant botulism are due to spores from dust and dirt.

QUICK HIT

Constipation is often the first sign of infant botulism.

QUICK HIT

Movements such as sucking and swallowing that require frequent neuromuscular transmission are notably affected due to fatigability with repetitive muscle use.

E. Therapy
   1. Botulism immunoglobulin (BabyBIG): prompt therapy decreases hospitalization and mechanical support
   2. 1/2 of patients will require mechanical ventilator support while awaiting resolution

XVI. Tick Paralysis

A. Definition: acute ataxia and ascending paralysis following female tick attachment, mating, and blood feeding
B. Caused by toxins in tick saliva that block axonal sodium channels, resulting in progressive weakness and even respiratory suppression
C. Therapy: removal of tick usually results in improvement within hours

XVII. Myasthenia Gravis

A. Definition: syndrome of chronic muscle weakness characterized by fatigability
B. Cause/pathophysiology: autoimmune; circulating antibodies bind to ACh receptors at NMJ
C. Clinical presentation
   1. Fatigable weakness; worsens with exertion
   2. Ocular muscles most affected, especially at disease onset
      a. **Ptosis**
      b. Weakness of extraocular muscles, causing diplopia
   3. Bulbar muscles are commonly affected: dysphagia and facial weakness
D. Testing
   1. ACh-receptor antibodies: many children with MG are seronegative
   2. Nerve conduction studies, Tensilon test
E. Treatment
   1. ACh-esterase inhibitors (pyridostigmine)
   2. Immunosuppression
      a. Prednisone is mainstay of chronic treatment
      b. IVIG and plasmapheresis are effective
      c. Thymectomy: not recommended for prepubertal children

XVIII. Duchenne Muscular Dystrophy

A. Characteristics
   1. Genetic disorder resulting in progressive degeneration of skeletal muscle
   2. Epidemiology
      a. Incidence of 1 in 3,500 male births
      b. High mutation rate: 1/3 of cases are due to new conditions
   3. Cause: mutation in *Xp21* gene resulting in deficiency of dystrophin protein
   4. Genetics: X-linked recessive: males affected, whereas females are carriers
B. Clinical features
   1. Historical findings
      a. Symptoms are usually not present until child starts walking, typically ~age 3 years
      b. Most common presenting symptoms are abnormal gait and walking/climbing difficulty
   2. Physical exam findings (signs)
      a. Symmetrical and proximal muscle weakness
      b. Pseudohypertrophy of calves
      c. Muscle wasting and contractures develop as weakness progresses
      d. Gowers maneuver (Figure 5-1)
C. Diagnosis
   1. Differential diagnosis (Box 5-4)
   2. Laboratory findings
      a. **Serum creatine kinase (CK)**
      b. Aldolase and LFTs may be elevated
      c. Diagnosis made by dystrophin gene testing

QUICK HIT

Aminoglycoside antibiotics should be avoided when infant botulism is suspected because they will potentiate the effects of the neurotoxin.

QUICK HIT

Ticks are often found on the scalp (using a fine-tooth comb may be helpful), because that is where they are most often hidden from sight.

QUICK HIT

Most patients present with ocular symptoms.

QUICK HIT

Proximal weakness is more often a sign of muscle disease, whereas distal weakness often signifies a neuropathy.

QUICK HIT

In Duchenne muscular dystrophy, CK may be elevated 50–200× above normal.

FIGURE 5-1 **A patient with muscular dystrophy showing wasting of the musculature in the shoulders and thighs; weakness and atrophy of the glutei cause difficulty in assuming the erect position, and the patient "climbs up on his thighs" (Gowers maneuver) in order to stand erect.**

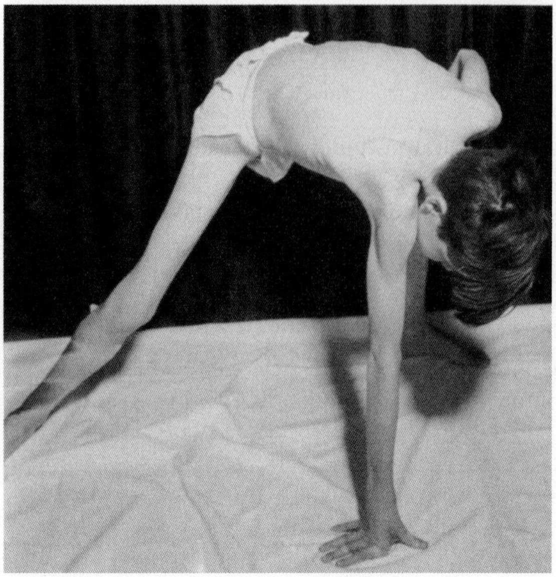

D. Treatment
   1. Therapy
      a. Glucocorticoids provide some increase in muscle strength and function
      b. Supportive care
   2. Complications
      a. Difficulty with respiratory infections due to restrictive lung disease
      b. Dilated cardiomyopathy and arrhythmias
   3. Duration/prognosis
      a. Course is progressive with loss of ambulation by age 7–13 years
      b. Early death from cardiorespiratory failure

XIX. Becker Muscular Dystrophy

A. Definition: milder phenotype of Duchenne muscular dystrophy
B. Cause/pathophysiology
   1. Mutation in *Xp21* gene resulting in semifunctional dystrophin protein
   2. X-linked recessive: males are affected; females are carriers
C. Clinical presentation
   1. Age of onset is typically later than in Duchenne but may be variable
   2. Weakness is milder, and course is more benign
      a. Ambulation usually continues into adolescence
      b. Very mild phenotypes may present with only muscle cramps after exercise

XX. Cerebral Palsy (CP)

A. Characteristics
   1. Definition: nonprogressive disorder of posture and movement caused by defect or insult to CNS early in development

BOX 5-4

Differential Diagnosis of Muscular Dystrophy

Duchenne muscular dystrophy
Becker muscular dystrophy
Limb girdle muscular dystrophy
Emery-Dreifuss disease/muscular dystrophy
Congenital muscular dystrophies
Congenital myopathies
Spinal muscular atrophy
Dermatomyositis
Acid maltase deficiency

2. Causes: antenatal factors
   a. Preterm delivery
   b. Low birth weight
   c. Infection/inflammation
   d. Multiple gestation
   e. Other pregnancy complications, particularly with potential birth asphyxia

B. Clinical features
1. Spasticity, ataxia, dystonia, and choreoathetosis are common
   a. Classification of spastic CP by anatomic distribution
      i. Spastic diplegia: bilateral spasticity with leg involvement > arm
      ii. Spastic hemiplegia: unilateral spasticity
      iii. Spastic quadriplegia: bilateral spasticity with arm involvement ≥ leg

C. Therapy
1. Intense physical therapy helps with improvement of motor skills
2. Botox injections block neuromuscular
3. For generalized spasticity, oral medications may be helpful, including benzodiazepines, dantrolene, and baclofen

QUICK HIT

Among extremely low gestational age newborns (i.e., gestational age <28 weeks), the prevalence of CP is 100-fold higher.

XXI. Mental Retardation

A. Characteristics
1. Definition
   a. Significantly impaired cognitive functioning
   b. Deficits in 2 or more adaptive behaviors
   c. Historically defined as an IQ score <70
2. Epidemiology: affects 2%–3% of population, either as isolated finding or as part of syndrome or broader disorder
3. Causes
   a. Multiple environmental, genetic, and social factors
   b. In 30%–50% of cases, etiology cannot be determined despite thorough evaluation
4. Classification: severity of MR can be classified based on IQ score (Table 5-3)

B. Diagnosis
1. Very detailed history and physical examination can help elicit possible cause
2. Other than IQ testing to define impairment, no testing is indicated other than to evaluate for underlying disorders

C. Therapy
1. Intense therapy to help with cognitive and social skills
2. More specific treatments may be directed toward underlying etiology

XXII. Tics and Tourette Syndrome

A. Characteristics
1. Definitions
   a. Tics: involuntary, repetitive, stereotyped movements or vocalizations that are brief and purposeless
      i. Motor and vocal tics can be simple or complex
      ii. Simple motor tics involve limited number of muscle groups
      iii. Complex motor tics involve several muscle groups

TABLE 5-3 **Classification of Mental Retardation**

Classification of Mental Retardation	IQ Score
Mild	50–55
Moderate	35–49
Severe	20–34
Profound	<20

QUICK HIT

Tics and Tourette syndrome are not separate disorders but rather a phenotypic spectrum of similar genetic traits with variable genetic expressions.

QUICK HIT

Tics are often worse during periods of anxiety and stress and decrease with motor activity such as sports.

QUICK HIT

A variety of neurologic insults may result in secondary tic disorders.

QUICK HIT

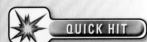

In the majority of children with tics and Tourette syndrome, associated symptoms and comorbidities may be more troublesome than tics.

QUICK HIT

Stimulants for ADHD may unmask tic disorders.

QUICK HIT

Infantile spasm is the most common seizure type in patients with TSC.

b. Tourette syndrome: multiple motor tics and at least 1 vocal tic (not necessarily concurrently)
c. Prevalence of all types of tics may be as high as 4.2%–6% of school-aged children

B. Clinical features
1. Historical findings
a. Mean age of onset of tics is ~6–7 years
b. Tics are involuntary
c. Simple motor tics involve blinking, grimacing, sudden jerking
d. Complex motor tic example: simultaneous abdominal tensing, upper body and arm jerking with head movements, and facial grimacing
e. Simple vocal tics involve throat clearing, coughing, etc.
f. Complex vocal tics include repeating words and uncontrollable obscenities (minority of cases of Tourette)

C. Diagnosis: differential diagnosis
1. Movement disorders
2. Tics are usually distinguishable
a. Can be suppressed for brief periods
b. Tend to persist during sleep
c. Waxing and waning course
3. Compulsions may be difficult to distinguish from complex motor tics

D. Treatment
1. Therapy
a. Supportive management
b. Pharmacotherapy: in cases in which tics are severe and interfere with function or cause stress or social embarrassment
i. Dopamine receptor–blocking agents (neuroleptics)
(a) Haloperidol and pimozide
(b) Frequent side effects limit use
2. Complications: up to 90% of patients with Tourette syndrome have comorbidities (e.g., attention-deficit hyperactivity disorder [ADHD], obsessive-compulsive disorder, learning disabilities)
3. Duration/prognosis
a. Transient tics completely resolve <1 year from onset
b. Up to 2/3 of children with tics have reduction or complete resolution before adulthood

XXIII. Neurocutaneous Syndromes

A. **Tuberous sclerosis complex** (TSC)
1. Genetics
a. Autosomal dominant inheritance with variable penetrance
b. 2/3 of cases are sporadic or new mutations
2. Clinical features
a. Neurologic
i. Seizures in up to 90%
ii. MR and developmental difficulties
b. Dermatologic
i. **Ash leaf spots**: hypopigmented macules
(a) Best seen under ultraviolet (UV) light (Wood's lamp)
(b) Present at birth in >90% cases
ii. Facial angiofibromas (**adenoma sebaceum**): seen in 75% of patients after age 3 years
iii. **Shagreen patch**: connective tissue nevi on lower back or flank
iv. **Ungual fibromas**: nodular lesions arising at nail bed
c. Cardiac **hamartomas** within muscular chamber walls
d. Other involvement of lungs, kidneys, retina
3. Diagnosis (Box 5-5)
4. Treatment: supportive

BOX 5-5

Diagnostic Criteria for Tuberous Sclerosis

Definite diagnosis requires 2 major features or 1 major feature plus 2 minor features.
Probable diagnosis requires 1 major plus 1 minor feature.
Possible diagnosis requires 1 major feature or 2 minor features.

Major features:	Minor features:
Cortical tubers	Bone cysts
Subependymal nodule	Multiple randomly distributed pits in dental enamel
Subependymal giant cell astrocytoma	Gingival fibroma
Cardiac rhabdomyomas, single or multiple	Multiple renal cysts
Facial angiofibromas or forehead plaque	Nonrenal hamartomas
Hypomelanotic macules (≥3)	Hamartomatous rectal polyps
Shagreen patch (connective tissue nevus)	"Confetti" skin lesions
Nontraumatic ungual or periungual fibromas	Retinal achromic patch
Multiple retinal nodule hamartomas	Cerebral white matter radial migration lines
Renal angiomyolipoma	
Lymph angiomyomatosis	

B. **Neurofibromatosis (NF)**
  1. Genetics: autosomal dominant with 50% due to new mutations, with variable penetrance
  2. Clinical features
    a. NF-1
      i. Skin lesions are most common manifestation
        (a) Café-au-lait spots: earliest, most common sign
        (b) Axillary freckling in >85%
        (c) Plexiform neurofibromas: soft tissue swellings under skin
      ii. Neurologic manifestations
        (a) 60% learning disability, 5% epilepsy
        (b) **Optic gliomas**, other tumors
        (c) At risk for hypertension, scoliosis, leukemia
    b. NF-2
      i. Acoustic neuromas, CNS schwannomas, other CNS tumors
      ii. Few or no café-au-lait spots
  3. Diagnosis
    a. NF-1 (Box 5-6)
    b. NF-2 diagnosis rests on findings of bilateral acoustic neuromas or vestibular schwannomas

QUICK HIT

Hearing loss is often 1st sign of acoustic neuroma in children with NF.

BOX 5-6

Diagnostic Criteria for Neurofibromatosis-1

2 or more of the following features are considered diagnostic:

- 6 café-au-lait spots larger than 5 mm in diameter in prepubertal children and larger than 15 mm in postpubertal children
- 2 or more neurofibromas (subcutaneous or intracutaneous) or 1 plexiform neurofibroma
- Freckling in the axillary or inguinal regions (≥3 freckles)
- Optic pathway glioma
- 2 or more iris hamartomas (Lisch nodules)
- Distinctive osseous lesion, such as sphenoid dysplasia or thinning of long bones
- A 1st-degree relative with NF-1

> **QUICK HIT**
> Almost all patients with myelomeningocele have CM-II, and most have obstructive hydrocephalus.

> **QUICK HIT**
> CM-I can present with a variety of manifestations related to elevated ICP, cranial neuropathy, brainstem compression, myelopathy, cerebellar dysfunction, and headache, as well as symptoms due to syringomyelia and scoliosis.

> **QUICK HIT**
> If myelomeningocele is present, think CM-II.

> **QUICK HIT**
> If posterior encephalocele is present, think CM-III.

> **QUICK HIT**
> Neurulation is the transformation of the neural tube into the CNS.

> **QUICK HIT**
> NTDs are among the most common birth defects.

> **QUICK HIT**
> Maternal serum AFP should be performed in all pregnant women at 15–20 weeks' gestation.

C. Sturge-Weber syndrome (SWS)
1. Definition: sporadic disorder characterized facial port-wine stain in ophthalmic distribution of trigeminal nerve and intracranial vascular anomalies
2. Clinical features
   a. Cutaneous angioma present at birth on upper eyelid and forehead
   b. Glaucoma in 70%
   c. Neurologic manifestations
3. Diagnosis: port-wine stain in appropriate distribution and neurologic symptoms
4. Treatment: anticonvulsants, aspirin as prophylaxis against stroke, laser therapy for face

XXIV. Chiari Malformation (CM)

A. Definitions
1. Congenital CNS anomaly with downward displacement of cerebellar structures into foramen magnum
2. 3 main types (I, II, III)
   a. Types are progressively more rare but more severe
   b. All managed by surgery if needed

XXV. Dandy-Walker Syndrome

A. Cystic dilatation of 4th ventricle and enlarged posterior fossa
B. Cause/pathophysiology: associated with chromosomal abnormalities, teratogen exposure
C. Clinical presentation
1. Macrocephaly: *hydrocephalus develops by age 3 months in 75% of patients*
2. Variable degrees of neurologic impairment, seizure

D. Therapy: shunt placement to divert flow of obstructed CSF

XXVI. Neural Tube Defects (NTDs)

A. Characteristics
1. Types
   a. **Anencephaly**: absence of forebrain and midbrain structures with preservation of hindbrain structures
   b. **Encephalocele**: midline skull defect with associated protrusion of brain and meninges
   c. **Myelomeningocele** (spina bifida): defect in vertebral formation with dorsal protrusion of neural tissue from the spinal cord and overlying meninges
   d. **Meningocele**: meninges protrude, no involvement of spinal cord
   e. **Spina bifida occulta**: incomplete fusion of vertebra without associated herniation of neural tissues or meninges
2. Risk factors: *folate deficiency is primary risk factor*

B. Clinical features
1. Historical findings
   a. Open NTDs are typically identified in utero or at delivery
   b. Closed NTDs may be identified later
      i. Weakness and/or sensory loss distal to lesion
      ii. Bladder or bowel dysfunction
      iii. Low back pain without neurologic deficit

C. Diagnosis
1. Laboratory findings
   a. Prenatal elevation of α-fetoprotein (AFP) seen in 70%–75% of open NTDs
2. Radiology findings
   a. May be identified via routine prenatal ultrasonography
   b. MRI or CT after birth

D. Treatment
1. Primary therapy is surgical repair, and ventriculoperitoneal (VP) shunt if needed for hydrocephalus

Neurologic Disorders

2. Complications
   a. Bowel and bladder dysfunction
   b. Mobility issues
   c. Muscle and joint dysfunction including spasticity, paralysis, joint contractures, scoliosis
   d. VP shunt complications
3. Duration/prognosis
   a. Anencephaly is incompatible with life
   b. Meningoceles may have little or no associated disability
   c. Other open NTDs give rise to wide range of disability
4. Prevention: prenatal supplementation of folic acid (1 mg daily) may reduce risk of developing NTDs

XXVII. Craniosynostosis

A. Definition: premature closure of cranial suture(s); not to be confused with simple positional plagiocephaly

B. Clinical presentation
1. Abnormal head shape with palpable bony ridge along affected sutures
2. Neurologic complications (e.g., hydrocephalus, increased ICP) rare, unless multiple sutures affected

C. Testing
1. Physical exam important to determine which sutures affected
2. CT is more helpful than plain films for identifying affected sutures, anatomy, and presence of hydrocephalus

D. Therapy: surgical repair requires multidisciplinary team

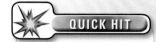

> **QUICK HIT**
>
> When craniosynostosis is caused by genetic syndromes, other facial features are commonly present, including hypertelorism, proptosis, midface hypoplasia, and prognathism.

> **QUICK HIT**
>
> A top-down view of the skull will reveal a parallelogram shape in cases of positional plagiocephaly.

XXVIII. Ataxia Telangiectasia (AT)

A. Cause/pathophysiology: autosomal recessive inheritance

B. Clinical presentation
1. Progressive ataxia, typically wheelchair dependent early in 2nd decade of life
2. Sensitivity to damage from ionizing radiation
3. Increased incidence of lymphoid and solid malignancies
4. Cellular and humoral immunodeficiency: repeated sinopulmonary infections
5. Telangiectasias on skin by middle childhood

C. Therapy
1. No effective treatment exists
2. Supportive therapy and monitoring for malignancy

> **QUICK HIT**
>
> AT is a neurocutaneous syndrome causing progressive ataxia, immunodeficiency, and ocular and cutaneous telangiectasias and an increased risk for malignancy.

XXIX. Friedreich Ataxia

A. Definition: autosomal recessive degenerative disorder characterized by progressive ataxia and neurologic dysfunction

B. Clinical presentation
1. Difficulty walking with progressive ataxia and gait dysfunction
2. Hearing and vision loss
3. Hypertrophic cardiomyopathy and diabetes mellitus

> **QUICK HIT**
>
> In Friedreich ataxia, the major symptoms are neurologic dysfunction, cardiac dysfunction, and diabetes.

6 Rheumatologic Disorders and Orthopedic Conditions

SYMPTOM SPECIFIC

I. Approach to Limp

A. Background information

1. Limp defined as abnormal, uneven, jerky, or laborious gait
2. Develops due to pain, neuromuscular weakness, deformity, or mechanical factors (Table 6-1)

TABLE 6-1 Differential Diagnosis of Limp

Due to Pain	Due to Mechanical Factors	Due to Neuromuscular Weakness
Infectious Causes Septic arthritis Osteomyelitis Lyme arthritis Discitis Pyomyositis Cellulitis and soft tissue abscesses Psoas abscess Appendicitis Pelvic inflammatory disease	**Developmental Causes** Developmental dysplasia of the hip Limb length discrepancies Clubfoot Congenital limb abnormalities	**Neurologic Causes** Peripheral neuropathy (e.g., Guillain-Barré syndrome) Charcot-Marie-Tooth disease Complex regional pain syndrome Cerebral palsy Meningitis Cerebellar lesions
Inflammatory Disorders Juvenile idiopathic arthritis Reactive arthritis Systemic lupus erythematosus Acute rheumatic fever	**Acquired Diseases** Blount disease Avascular necrosis (e.g., Legg-Calvé-Perthes disease) Slipped capital femoral epiphysis	**Congenital Causes** Myelomeningocele Tethered cord
Oncologic Causes Leukemia Benign bone tumors: Osteoblastoma, osteoid osteoma Malignant bone tumors: Ewing sarcoma, osteosarcoma Spinal cord tumors Neuroblastoma		**Muscular Causes** Dermatomyositis Viral myositis Myopathies Muscular dystrophy
Metabolic Causes Rickets		

(continued)

TABLE 6-1 Differential Diagnosis of Limp *(Continued)*

Due to Pain	Due to Mechanical Factors	Due to Neuromuscular Weakness
Trauma Fractures: Toddler's, child abuse Soft tissue injury Herniated disc Poorly fitting shoes Foreign body, splinters		
Overuse Injury Spondylolisthesis Stress fracture Osteochondritis dissecans Osgood-Schlatter disease Sever disease Chondromalacia patellae		
Hematologic Hemophilia and hemarthrosis Sickle cell disease (vaso-occlusive disease)		

B. Historical questions
1. Is there pain associated with the child's limp? (Table 6-2)
2. Was there a gradual or sudden onset of pain?
3. Is there any history of preceding trauma?
4. Are there any associated symptoms?
    a. Fever, weight loss, and night sweats: systemic symptoms that would increase likelihood of infectious, inflammatory, and oncologic causes
    b. Rash may be present in various infectious and rheumatologic causes
    c. Diarrhea, weight loss, and growth failure can occur in children with inflammatory bowel disease (IBD)

QUICK HIT

The abrupt onset of pain is more commonly associated with an acute injury or infection. A gradual onset can develop from a mechanical or inflammatory cause.

QUICK HIT

About 1/3 of cases of osteomyelitis are associated with a history of preceding trauma; therefore, a history of trauma does not rule out osteomyelitis.

TABLE 6-2 Associated Causes of Limp and Pain Characteristics

Type of Pain	Characteristics	Causes of Limp
Inflammatory pain	Morning stiffness Increase in pain after inactivity Pain improves during the day	Rheumatologic disorders Inflammatory conditions
Mechanical pain	Pain that worsens with activity Pain that is unable to disturb sleep	Overuse injuries
Bone pain	Constant, severe, and localized pain Not associated with changes due to activity	Infectious causes Traumatic injury, fractures Malignancy
Neuropathic pain	Worsens at bedtime Described as burning or shooting pain Allodynia is present	Neurologic causes Complex regional pain syndrome

QUICK HIT

While assessing gait, also look for signs of **ataxia** that could indicate a cerebellar cause mimicking limp.

QUICK HIT

Pathology in the hip will commonly present as referred pain in the knee or thigh. Pathology in the back may present with thigh or buttocks pain.

QUICK HIT

Acute rheumatic fever is associated with migratory polyarthritis.

C. Physical examination findings
 1. Evaluation of gait
  a. Normal gait is "smooth mechanical process that advances center of gravity with minimum expenditure of energy"
   i. **Swing phase**: time from foot leaving ground until next heel strike
   ii. **Stance phase**: occurs when heel strikes ground and ball of other foot leaves ground
  b. **Antalgic gait**: painful gait; in order to minimize pain, less time spent in stance phase of affected limb resulting in shorter stride
  c. **Nonantalgic gait**: develops when mechanical factor or neuromuscular weakness results in abnormal gait
   i. **Circumduction** gait: results from joint stiffness and/or spasticity; to improve limb clearance during swing phase, leg swings outward at hip
   ii. **Trendelenburg** gait: results when there is pelvic instability due to decreased muscle strength on 1 side of the pelvis; when both sides are involved, waddling gait is produced
   iii. **Steppage** gait: results from peripheral neurologic weakness in which foot slaps ground due to decreased ankle dorsiflexion
   iv. **Equinus** gait: occurs when patient toe-walks as opposed to normal heel-to-toe walking
 2. Musculoskeletal examination
  a. Observe child at rest to determine position of maximum comfort
   i. When children have inflammation in hip joint, they will keep their leg externally rotated and abducted at hip in attempt to minimize stretch of joint capsule and reduce pain
  b. Determine point of maximal tenderness; identification of single point of maximal tenderness suggests fracture or osteomyelitis
  c. Evaluate joints above and below area of concern so as not to miss causes of referred pain
  d. Assess distribution of joint involvement and evaluate for signs of inflammation, including warmth, swelling, and overlying erythema (Table 6-3)
  e. Look for any obvious limb deformities, including leg length discrepancy
 3. Neurologic exam
  a. Assess spine for any midline defects
  b. Perform stepwise evaluation of nervous system
 4. Skin exam
  a. Focus on presence of any signs of infection
  b. Evaluate soles of shoes and feet for indications of foreign body or improperly fitting shoes
  c. Purpura and petechiae may be seen with some inflammatory causes, including Henoch-Schönlein purpura (HSP), or with oncologic causes, including leukemia

TABLE 6-3 **Classification of Causes of Limp Based on Joint Involvement**

Monoarticular	Pauciarticular	Polyarticular
Trauma	Lyme disease	Polyarticular juvenile idiopathic arthritis
Hemarthroses	Psoriatic arthritis	Systemic lupus erythematosus
Septic arthritis	Oligoarticular juvenile idiopathic arthritis	Gonococcal arthritis
Lyme arthritis		Inflammatory bowel disease–associated arthritis
Tuberculosis arthritis		Serum sickness
		Acute rheumatic fever
		Reactive arthritis

5. Genitourinary (GU) exam
   a. Referred pain can also be present with GU causes, including inguinal hernia
   b. In adolescents, pelvic pathology may present with abnormal gait

D. Laboratory testing and radiologic imaging
1. Laboratory data
   a. Complete blood count (CBC)
      i. In infectious and inflammatory causes, the white blood cell count (WBC) will be elevated
      ii. Thrombocytosis may also be seen in infectious and rheumatologic causes due to platelets acting as an acute phase reactant
      iii. Cytopenias in all 3 cell lines can be seen in leukemia and systemic lupus erythematosus (SLE)
   b. Markers of inflammation
      i. In septic arthritis, the C-reactive protein (CRP) will peak within 2–3 days of onset of symptoms and normalize within 10 days with effective treatment
      ii. Erythrocyte sedimentation rate (ESR) will peak within 1 week of onset of symptoms and normalize within 3–4 weeks
   c. Synovial fluid: analysis shown in Table 6-4
   d. Other studies
      i. Lyme serologies if symptoms consistent with Lyme disease
      ii. Throat culture or antistreptolysin O and anti-DNase B titers should be performed when symptoms consistent with acute rheumatic fever are present
      iii. Coagulation profile should be sent when hemarthrosis is present and there is concern for a bleeding disorder
2. Radiologic imaging
   a. Plain films
      i. X-rays can highlight nonspecific symptoms, including soft tissue swelling, joint effusions, and osteopenia reactions, as well as fractures
      ii. Periosteal reaction can be seen 7–10 days after onset of symptoms in osteomyelitis
   b. Ultrasonography to identify joint effusions
      i. Hip ultrasound should be performed whenever there is high index of suspicion of hip pathology even if plain films are negative
   c. Magnetic resonance imaging (MRI) can show joints, soft tissue, cartilage, and medullary bone with high sensitivity and specificity

QUICK HIT

Right lower quadrant pain may masquerade as right hip pain, so careful examination of the abdomen is important to evaluate for appendicitis.

QUICK HIT

Blood culture will be positive in 30%–60% of patients with osteomyelitis and 40%–50% of patients with septic arthritis.

QUICK HIT

In septic arthritis, 50%–60% of patients will have positive cultures of synovial fluid.

QUICK HIT

Initial x-rays may be normal in stress fractures, toddler's fractures, osteomyelitis, and Legg-Calvé-Perthes (LCP) disease.

TABLE 6-4 **Evaluation of Synovial Fluid**

	WBC Count in Synovial Fluid	% Neutrophils
Normal	<500	<25%
Reactive arthritis	<15,000	<25% PMNs, mostly mononuclear cells
Tuberculosis arthritis	10,000–20,000	50%–60%
Lyme arthritis	2,000–100,000	Prominent PMNs, significant number of eosinophils
Juvenile idiopathic arthritis	5,000–60,000	Mostly neutrophils
Gonococcal arthritis	>50,000	
Bacterial septic arthritis	50,000–300,000	>75%–90%

PMNs, polymorphonuclear leukocytes; WBC, white blood cell.

d. Bone scan (technetium)
   i. Useful when unable to localize site of lesion based on history and physical exam
   ii. Images entire skeleton but with limited specificity; may be difficult to distinguish fractures from infection or bone metastases

II. Approach to Arthritis

A. Background information
   1. Arthritis is defined as joint swelling or presence of 2 or more of the following signs in 1 or more joints
      a. Limited range of motion (ROM)
      b. Tenderness or pain with motion
      c. Warmth
   2. Broad differential diagnosis for children with arthritis (Box 6-1)
   3. Arthritis can be categorized based on
      a. Duration of symptoms (acute versus chronic)
      b. Number of joints involved (monoarticular, oligoarticular, polyarticular)
      c. Joint distribution (peripheral, axial)
      d. Pattern of symptoms (migratory or additive)

B. Historical questions
   1. How long have the symptoms been present?
   2. What joints are involved?
   3. Are there any associated symptoms?
      a. Fever increases likelihood of infection or systemic autoimmune disease
      b. Rash may be present in various infectious and rheumatologic causes
      c. Gastrointestinal (GI) symptoms such as vomiting, diarrhea, or blood in stools may suggest IBD

C. Physical examination findings
   1. Musculoskeletal examination
      a. Assess each joint for signs of inflammation, including swelling, warmth, pain with movement, and decreased ROM
      b. Determine distribution of joint involvement
      c. Examine for **enthesitis** (i.e., inflammation at insertion at ligaments and tendons), most commonly involving Achilles tendon or plantar fascia
      d. Evaluate for leg length discrepancy
   2. Skin exam
      a. Many rheumatologic conditions have characteristic rashes
      b. The bull's-eye rash of Lyme disease is called **erythema migrans**
      c. **Erythema marginatum is seen in acute rheumatic fever** and appears as open or closed rings with sharp outer edges
   3. Ophthalmology exam

> **QUICK HIT**
> Chronic arthritis is defined as arthritis that has persisted for ≥6 weeks.

> **QUICK HIT**
> Children with systemic juvenile idiopathic arthritis (JIA) typically have very high fevers once or twice a day; at other times, the temperature is normal or subnormal.

> **QUICK HIT**
> Monoarticular joint pain and swelling have a broad differential diagnosis, including orthopedic abnormalities, infections, oncologic processes, and rheumatologic conditions.

> **QUICK HIT**
> Consider enthesitis-associated arthritis when children have sacroiliac joint involvement.

> **QUICK HIT**
> Children with oligoarticular JIA with asymmetric involvement of their lower extremities (LEs) may develop leg length discrepancies, with the involved leg growing longer.

> **QUICK HIT**
> Malar rashes can be seen in SLE and dermatomyositis.

BOX 6-1

Common Causes of Arthritis in Children

- Septic arthritis
- Lyme arthritis
- Viral infections
  - Parvovirus
  - Epstein-Barr virus
- Juvenile idiopathic arthritis
- Reactive arthritis
  - Postviral
  - Serum sickness
  - Rheumatic fever/poststreptococcal arthritis
- Systemic lupus erythematosus
- Dermatomyositis
- Vasculitis
  - Henoch-Schönlein purpura
  - Kawasaki
  - Granulomatosis with polyangiitis
  - Microscopic polyangiitis
- Arthritis associated with inflammatory bowel disease
- Behçet disease
- Sarcoid

D. Laboratory testing and radiologic imaging
   1. Laboratory data
      a. CBC
         i. WBC count and platelet count may be elevated in infectious and inflammatory causes of arthritis
         ii. Low WBCs, particularly lymphopenia, Coombs-positive anemia, and/or thrombocytopenia, are diagnostic criteria for SLE
      b. Markers of inflammation, ESR and CRP, may be elevated
      c. Blood cultures should be obtained in patients with suspected septic arthritis because they are positive ~50% of time
   2. Radiologic imaging
      a. Plain films
         i. X-rays to screen for bony abnormalities, such as fractures or periosteal reaction
         ii. Chronic arthritis can lead to joint space narrowing, periarticular osteopenia, and erosions
      b. Ultrasound
         i. Modality of choice for detecting hip effusions, which are commonly associated with infection or reactive arthritis (ReA)
      c. MRI: Helpful in confirming the diagnosis of synovitis or arthritis

III. Approach to Back Pain

A. Background information
   1. Very common; 50% of children will experience back pain prior to age 15 years
   2. Most common cause in children is muscular sprain and strain
   3. Back pain in children before the age 10 years is uncommon
   4. Back pain in adolescents is more closely related to adult back pain and is often mechanical in nature

B. Historical questions
   1. Did the pain begin suddenly or come on slowly over days, weeks, or months?
      a. Children may experience brief episodes of back pain related to strain from athletic activities or carrying heavy backpack
      b. Back pain that persists >4 weeks should be evaluated
   2. Is the pain worse at a particular time of day?
   3. Does the pain wake the child up from sleep?
   4. Are there certain positions that make the child feel better or worse?
   5. Are there associated neurologic symptoms?
      a. Symptoms of numbness, tingling, weakness, and urinary and bowel abnormalities suggest nerve or spinal cord abnormality
      b. **Cauda equina syndrome** is manifested as weakness of lower extremity (LE) muscles, urinary retention, fecal incontinence, and absence of ankle reflexes and is a *neurosurgical emergency*

C. Physical examination findings
   1. Evaluate posture and alignment of spine
   2. Observe transitional movements: how a patient moves from sitting to standing and laying to sitting
   3. Assess gait including toe- and heel-walking
   4. Neurologic assessment including strength, reflexes, and sensation
   5. Provocative maneuvers such as hyperextension

D. Laboratory testing and radiologic imaging
   1. Laboratory testing including CBC, ESR, and CRP can be used to screen for inflammatory conditions
   2. X-rays
      a. Include spine and pelvis to rule out fractures, dislocations, infection, and tumors
      b. Need oblique views
   3. MRI: needed if neurologic symptoms are present

QUICK HIT

Patients with systemic JIA typically have very high WBC and platelet counts.

QUICK HIT

Children with oligoarticular JIA typically have normal inflammatory markers.

QUICK HIT

Lyme arthritis most commonly involves 1 or both knees. It is relatively painless despite significant joint swelling. There are usually frequent relapses and remissions. In most cases, a tick bite is not remembered, and there may be no history of rash.

QUICK HIT

X-rays in acute arthritis are usually normal or may demonstrate soft tissue swelling; fluid in the joint may be appreciated, but exam is generally more sensitive (with exception of hips).

QUICK HIT

Back pain in young children warrants a thorough evaluation insofar as they are more likely to have a serious underlying disorder than are older children and adults.

QUICK HIT

Scheuermann disease is a form of juvenile **osteochondrosis** of the spine and is found mostly in teenagers. Patients have "wedge-shaped" vertebrae and present with lower and midlevel back pain and kyphosis.

E. Treatment
1. Urgent treatment needed for tumors, spinal cord abnormalities, intra-abdominal and intrathoracic abnormalities, and apophyseal ring fractures
2. Start with conservative treatment for muscle strain, overuse, stress fractures, disc herniations, Scheuermann disease
   a. Conservative treatment options include physical therapy, core fitness program, Pilates, yoga, and activity modification
   b. Nonsteroidal anti-inflammatory drugs (NSAIDs) can be used as needed
   c. All patients need follow-up appointment if pain is not improving
   d. Children can return to normal activities when they are pain free

QUICK HIT

Osteoid osteoma, a benign bone tumor that can involve the spine, typically is associated with increased pain at night.

QUICK HIT

If the pain is severe enough to interfere with the child's activities, it warrants further evaluation.

DISEASE SPECIFIC

IV. Spondylolysis and Spondylolisthesis

A. Background information
1. Both spondylolysis and spondylolisthesis are most common in patients ages 10–15 years who participate in hyperextension sports
2. Dull aching pain localized in lower back and exacerbated by activity

B. Spondylolysis
1. Stress fracture of pars interarticularis
2. Most commonly at L5 level
3. Thought to occur due to repetitive hyperextension of lumbar spine
4. Symptoms exaggerated with lumbar spine hyperextension and rotation
5. 5% of population has radiographic evidence of fracture
6. Prognosis is excellent with nonoperative management; surgery is rarely recommended

C. Spondylolisthesis
1. Forward slippage of 1 vertebra on its adjacent vertebra
2. Often due to displacement at site of stress fracture of pars interarticularis or dysplastic development of posterior elements of L5/S1

QUICK HIT

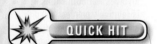

When neurologic symptoms accompany back pain, urgent evaluation and treatment are indicated.

QUICK HIT

Spondylolysis is the most common cause of structural back pain in children.

V. Juvenile Idiopathic Arthritis (JIA)

A. General characteristics
1. Pain, swelling, decreased ROM, stiffness in 1 or more joints for at least 6 weeks with onset before age 16 years
2. Other causes of arthritis must be ruled out, such as infection, injury, or other autoimmune disease
3. Classification (Table 6-5)
   a. Systemic
   b. Oligoarticular
   c. Polyarticular
   d. Enthesitis associated
   e. Psoriatic
   f. Undifferentiated
4. Most common rheumatologic condition in children
   a. Prevalence 1:1,000 children
   b. Incidence 1:7,000/year
   c. Female:male ratio = 5:1 oligoarticular, 3:1 polyarticular, 1:1 systemic
5. Cause is unknown
6. Genetics
   a. Multiple genes related to inflammation and immunity are likely involved
   b. Children with arthritis often have family members with history of autoimmune disease
   c. 1 in 100 chance that sibling of child with JIA will be affected
   d. 50% concordance with monozygotic twins

QUICK HIT

Spondylolysis can be considered a "grade 0" spondylolisthesis because it is the earliest change and can progress to spondylolisthesis if there is displacement at the site of fracture.

TABLE 6-5 **Classification of Juvenile Idiopathic Arthritis**

Type	Systemic JIA	Oligoarticular JIA	Polyarticular JIA	Enthesitis-Associated JIA
Frequency (% of total cases of JIA)	5%	30%	25%	25%
Number of joints affected	Any number	4 or fewer joints	5 or more joints	Any number
Types of joints affected	Large and small joints	Medium and large joints in asymmetric pattern	Small and large joints in symmetric pattern	Lower extremity, large joints, sacroiliac joints
Systemic features	High (39°–40°C) fever occurring 1–2× daily Evanescent salmon-pink macular rash prominent on pressure areas, especially when fever is present Enlarged liver and spleen Lymphadenopathy Inflammation of lining of heart and/or lungs Tendonitis Hepatitis	Asymptomatic uveitis	Low-grade fever, fatigue, rheumatoid nodules, anemia of chronic disease	Inflammation at tendinous insertion site, such as tibial tubercle or heel Symptomatic uveitis

JIA, juvenile idiopathic arthritis.

7. Pathophysiology
   a. Synovium is target organ for inflammation, results in proliferation of synovial tissue and secretion of increased amount of joint fluid
   b. Result is joint swelling, increased blood flow, and increased inflammatory cells within joint
   c. Persistent synovitis can result in permanent destruction of cartilage, underlying bone, and other surrounding joint structures such as ligaments and tendons

B. Clinical features
1. Historical findings
   a. Joint pain, joint swelling, and/or warmth
   b. Morning stiffness, stiffness after staying still for long periods (i.e., **gelling**)
   c. Limp
   d. Systemic manifestations: high fevers 1–2× per day, evanescent rash, chest pain
2. Physical examination findings
   a. Physical findings vary based on classification
   b. Joint swelling, warmth, and tenderness
   c. Loss of ROM and function
   d. Systemic findings: salmon-pink evanescent rash, lymphadenopathy, hepatosplenomegaly

C. Diagnosis
1. Differential diagnosis
   a. Diagnosis of exclusion: other conditions must be ruled out before settling on diagnosis
   b. Need to consider orthopedic, infectious, malignant, and other rheumatologic causes

QUICK HIT

In children with arthritis, 25% report no pain, and only swelling is observed.

QUICK HIT

Polyarticular JIA is divided into rheumatoid factor (RF) positive and RF negative. Children with RF-positive arthritis are at high risk for chronic, erosive arthritis equivalent to adult rheumatoid arthritis.

QUICK HIT

Timing of pain can help in distinguishing cause of pain. In inflammatory conditions, patients frequently have increased symptoms in the morning with associated stiffness. In contrast, patients with an orthopedic abnormality typically have increased symptoms later in the day and after activity.

QUICK HIT

Children with JIA rarely seek massage to alleviate symptoms. If massage alleviates symptoms, then **growing pains** should be suspected. Other characteristics of growing pains include poorly localized bilateral pain in the lower legs, pain occurring at night often waking the child from sleep, no objective signs of inflammation, and no daytime symptoms.

QUICK HIT

RF is a bad screening test for JIA. Most patients with JIA have a negative RF. It is a useful test for categorizing polyarticular disease.

QUICK HIT

Patients on **methotrexate** need CBC and liver function tests every 2–3 months to monitor for neutropenia and elevated transaminases.

QUICK HIT

Leg length discrepancy is most common in oligoarticular JIA because this form is more commonly asymmetric, affecting larger joints in children who are still growing. The leg with the affected joint(s) is thought to overgrow because of increased growth factors in these areas of increased blood flow.

QUICK HIT

Uveitis occurs in 20% of children with oligoarticular JIA. Risk factors include female gender, disease onset under 7 years, and positive ANA laboratory test.

QUICK HIT

Uveitis is asymptomatic and can cause blindness if untreated.

2. Laboratory findings
   a. No diagnostic test for JIA
   b. Elevated inflammatory markers such as WBC, platelets, ESR, and CRP may be seen
   c. Rheumatoid factor (RF) present in 5%–10% of children with JIA
   d. Positive antinuclear antibody (ANA) (>1:80)
      i. Associated with increased risk of uveitis
      ii. Often seen in polyarticular RF-positive arthritis
   e. Liver enzymes and coagulation screen may be abnormal in systemic JIA
   f. HLA-B27 antigen is associated with enthesitis-associated arthritis
3. Radiology findings
   a. Plain films
      i. Used primarily in early disease to exclude other conditions
      ii. Early-stage arthritis: soft tissue swelling and possibly periarticular osteoporosis
      iii. Late-stage arthritis: joint space narrowing and erosive changes
   b. MRI may demonstrate erosive change and joint damage earlier than standard x-ray films

D. Treatment
1. Objective is to treat inflammation, restore function, relieve pain, maintain joint motion, and prevent damage to cartilage and bone
2. Variety of medications are used to control inflammation
3. Complications
   a. Leg length discrepancy with involved limb growing longer
   b. Uveitis
      i. Routine ophthalmologic screening with a slit lamp is recommended; more frequent screening if ANA is positive
   c. Muscle atrophy
   d. Micrognathia (from temporomandibular joint [TMJ] involvement)
   e. Contractures
   f. Retardation of linear growth and pubertal delay
4. Prognosis
   a. Prognosis is variable depending on subtype of disease
      i. Children with oligoarticular JIA have highest rate of clinical remission
      ii. Children with RF-positive polyarticular JIA are least likely to go into remission and have highest risk for chronic, erosive arthritis that may continue into adulthood
      iii. Prognosis for children with systemic arthritis is determined by extent of arthritis, persistence of systemic symptoms beyond 6 months, and presence of thrombocytosis

VI. Reactive Arthritis

A. General characteristics
1. Autoimmune condition that develops in response to infection
2. Usually occurs after enteric or GU infections
   a. Common arthrogenic bacteria include *Chlamydia trachomatis*, *Yersinia*, *Salmonella*, *Shigella*, and *Campylobacter*
   b. May also develop after streptococcal infection; these patients are at increased risk of developing rheumatic heart disease with subsequent streptococcal infections
3. Typically self-limited condition, lasting for 1–4 weeks

B. Clinical features
1. Preceding symptomatic infection 1–4 weeks prior to onset of arthritis
2. Acute onset of arthritis that may be migratory
3. Classic triad: **can't see** (ocular inflammation), **can't pee** (urethritis), and **can't climb a tree** (arthritis), although ocular inflammation is rarely seen in children

C. Diagnosis
  1. Testing for causative agent
  2. HLA-B27 testing: prevalence of HLA-B27 in patients with ReA is up to 85%
  3. Rule out other potential causes such as active infection, acute rheumatic fever, SLE

D. Treatment
  1. NSAIDs are mainstay
  2. Steroids (either oral or intra-articular): can be helpful
  3. Treatment of active infections should follow standard practice
  4. Children with poststreptococcal arthritis warrant prophylactic antibiotics for at least 1 year to prevent recurrence of infection given increased risk for developing rheumatic heart disease

> **QUICK HIT**
> When the hip is involved, this form of ReA is often referred to as **transient synovitis of the hip**.

VII. Psoriatic Arthritis

A. General characteristics
  1. Defined as arthritis with psoriasis or arthritis with 2 of following
     a. **Dactylitis**
     b. Nail abnormalities (2 or more **nail pits** or **onycholysis**; Figure 6-1)
     c. Family history of psoriasis in 1st-degree relative

B. Clinical presentation
  1. Arthritis: typically asymmetric affecting both large and small joints
  2. Psoriasis: well-demarcated, erythematous, scaly lesions occurring over extensor surfaces of elbows, forearms, knees, and interphalangeal joints
  3. Enthesitis: inflammation at insertion of ligaments and tendons
  4. Dactylitis: 1/3 have distal interphalangeal (DIP) joint involvement and often have "**sausage digits**"
  5. Uveitis: usually asymptomatic, occurs in 15% of children
  6. Nail changes: nail pitting or onycholysis

> **QUICK HIT**
> Nail pits look as if someone has stuck a pin into the fingernail. They are strongly associated with psoriasis and sometimes develop prior to the characteristic skin changes.

> **QUICK HIT**
> Onycholysis is characterized by a spontaneous separation of the nail plate starting at the distal free margin and progressing proximally.

FIGURE 6-1 **Nail pits and onycholysis in a patient with psoriatic arthritis.**

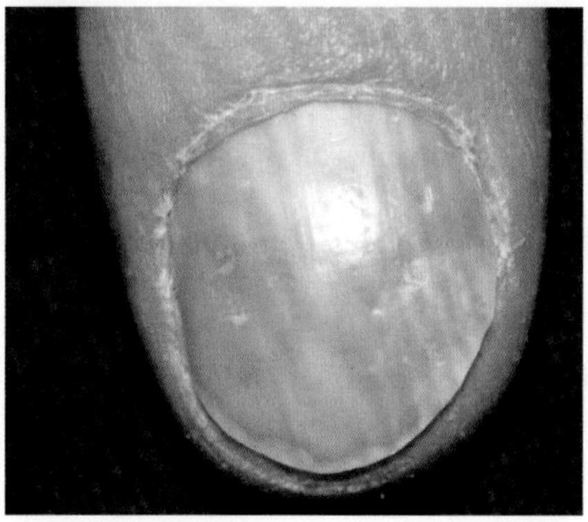

(From Goodheart HP. *Goodheart's Photoguide of Common Skin Disorders.* 2nd ed. Philadelphia: Lippincott Williams & Wilkins; 2003.)

VIII. Inflammatory Bowel Disease–Associated Arthritis

A. General characteristics
  1. Arthritis is common extraintestinal manifestation of IBD, occurring in up to 50% of patients
  2. Joint manifestations can precede GI symptoms
  3. Arthritis is more common in patients with active intestinal disease, particularly colonic involvement
  4. Children may present with involvement of sacroiliac joints and/or peripheral joints

IX. Juvenile Ankylosing Spondylitis

A. General characteristics
  1. Chronic inflammatory arthritis of peripheral and axial skeletons
  2. Commonly accompanied by enthesitis

3. Negative for RF and ANA (i.e., seronegative)
4. Strong correlation with **HLA-B27**
5. Arthritis of sacroiliac joint eventually develops in all patients
6. Onset usually in late childhood or adolescence
7. Male-to-female ratio of 7:1
8. Cause unknown but bacterial enteric or GU tract infections may trigger

X. Systemic Lupus Erythematosus

A. Characteristics
1. Multisystem inflammatory disease affecting joints, skin, kidneys, blood, central nervous system (CNS), and serosal linings
2. Immune complex disease in which antibody–antigen complexes are formed and deposit in involved tissues, leading to tissue damage through activation of leukocytes, neutrophils, and complement
3. Cause is unknown but thought to be related to environmental, genetic, and hormonal factors
4. Most commonly affects girls
5. Peak age of presentation in childhood is 9–15 years

> **QUICK HIT**
> Asians, African Americans, and Hispanics are more commonly affected than Caucasians.

B. Clinical features
1. Constitutional symptoms: fatigue, fever, weight loss
2. Cutaneous
   a. Malar rash: photosensitive "butterfly" rash on cheeks and nasal bridge but sparing nasolabial folds (Figure 6-2)
   b. Discoid rash: annular, scaly rash on scalp, face, and extremities that can lead to scarring
   c. Photosensitivity, alopecia, painless oral and/or nasal ulcers
3. Cardiopulmonary: pericarditis, Libman-Sacks endocarditis, myocarditis, **Raynaud phenomenon** (vasospasm in hands triggered by cold exposure), pleuritis, pleural effusion, pulmonary hypertension, pulmonary hemorrhage
4. Renal: proteinuria, hematuria, pyuria, hypertension, renal insufficiency
5. GI: pancreatitis, hepatitis, intestinal vasculitis, protein-losing enteropathy
6. Musculoskeletal: arthritis, myositis, avascular necrosis
7. CNS: stroke, psychosis, seizures, chorea, transverse myelitis, cranial neuropathies, depression
8. Hematologic: leukopenia (particularly lymphopenia), anemia, thrombocytopenia, thrombosis

C. Diagnosis
1. American College of Rheumatology has established criteria to aid in diagnosis
2. 4 of 11 criteria must be met to establish a diagnosis (Box 6-2)

FIGURE 6-2 Systemic lupus erythematosus.

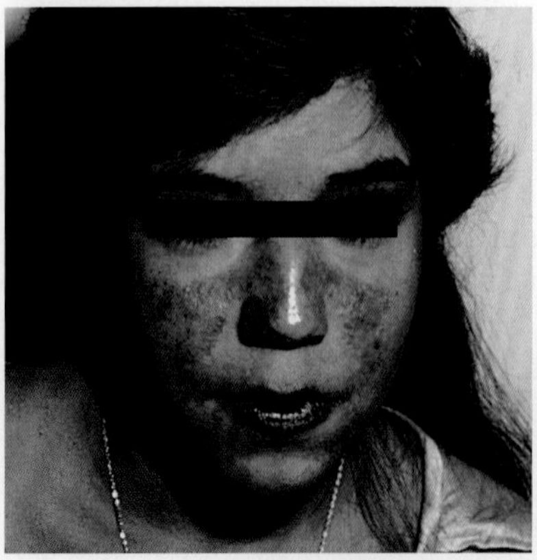

This young girl has the classic "butterfly" rash of lupus. (From Goodheart HP. *Goodheart's Photoguide of Common Skin Disorders.* 2nd ed. Philadelphia: Lippincott Williams & Wilkins; 2003.)

BOX 6-2

American College of Rheumatology Criteria for Diagnosis of Systemic Lupus Erythematosus

A patient has systemic lupus erythematosus (SLE) if 4 or more of the 11 criteria are present:
Mnemonic: "M.D., Please Offer All R.N.s A Holiday Immediately."

1. Malar rash
2. Discoid rash
3. Photosensitivity
4. Oral/nasal ulcerations (on the hard palate and/or nasal septum)
5. Arthritis
6. Renal abnormalities (proteinuria [>0.5 g/day or >3+] and/or cellular casts)
7. Neurologic abnormalities (seizures or psychosis)
8. Serositis (pericarditis and/or pleuritis)
9. ANA positive
10. Hematologic abnormalities (Coombs-positive anemia, leukopenia, lymphopenia, and/or thrombocytopenia)
11. Immune autoantibodies (anti–double-stranded DNA, anti-Smith, antiphospholipid antibodies)

3. Laboratory findings
    a. Leukopenia, anemia, and thrombocytopenia are common
    b. Electrolyte abnormalities, elevated kidney function tests, or hypoalbuminemia due to renal involvement
    c. ESR is usually elevated
    d. CRP is rarely elevated in SLE and warrants investigation for infection
    e. C3 and C4 are low with active disease due to complement consumption in process of clearing immune complexes
    f. ANA is positive in >95% of patients, usually with titers of 1:320 or higher
    g. Negative ANA virtually excludes SLE, but false positives are common
    h. Obtain testing for antiphospholipid antibodies because 50%–60% of pediatric SLE patients have these antibodies, which puts them at increased risk for arterial and venous thrombosis
4. Kidney biopsy is performed to classify histologic subtype of lupus nephritis; different subtypes have different prognosis

D. Treatment
1. Dependent on organ system involved
2. Mainstay is with oral prednisone (2 mg/kg/day) or intravenous (IV) methylprednisolone for significant organ involvement
3. Antimalarials such as hydroxychloroquine (5–7 mg/kg/day) can be used for skin manifestations, fatigue, arthritis, and antiphospholipid antibodies
4. NSAIDs help manage pleuritic chest pain, headaches, and arthritis
5. For persistent disease, mycophenolate mofetil, methotrexate, azathioprine, cyclophosphamide, or rituximab should be added
6. Presence of antiphospholipid antibodies should be treated with baby aspirin every day to prevent thrombosis
7. Sun precautions should be discussed because skin manifestations can be exacerbated by sun exposure

XI. Granulomatosis with Polyangiitis (Previously Known as Wegener Granulomatosis)

A. Definition
1. Autoimmune condition associated with inflammation of medium blood vessels of upper respiratory, lower respiratory, and renal systems
2. Rare disease
3. Etiology is unknown

B. Clinical presentation
1. Constitutional symptoms: fever, weight loss, malaise, and anorexia
2. Pulmonary: hemorrhage, pulmonary nodules, and cough
3. Renal involvement is common and includes hematuria, proteinuria, hypertension, and renal insufficiency

QUICK HIT

The Coombs test is positive in 15% of patients, but anemia can also be secondary to blood loss, kidney disease, or chronic disease (bone marrow suppression).

QUICK HIT

Anti-Smith and anti–double-stranded DNA are very specific for SLE. ANA is very sensitive.

QUICK HIT

Other diseases and illnesses to consider on the differential diagnosis for SLE are JIA, mixed connective tissue disease (MCTD), rheumatic fever, vasculitis, malignancies, and viral and bacterial infections.

QUICK HIT

The key predictors of mortality from SLE are *race, renal disease, and CNS disease.*

QUICK HIT

SLE is characterized by frequent exacerbations and remissions. The survival rate is >95% for 5 years and >85% for 10 years.

4. Upper respiratory: chronic otitis media, sinusitis, purulent or bloody nasal discharge, inflammatory trachea, saddle-nose deformity
5. High titer (anti-neutrophil cytoplasmic antibodies [c-ANCA]) and/or proteinase-3 antibodies in >80% of patients

XII. Goodpasture Syndrome

A. Definition: rare form of vasculitis that involves kidneys and lungs

B. Clinical presentation

1. Constitutional: fever, malaise, weight loss
2. Pulmonary: dry cough, **hemoptysis**, respiratory distress
3. Renal: edema, hypertension
4. Serum testing for anti–glomerular basement membrane (anti-GBM) antibodies diagnostic
5. Anti-GBM antibodies produce characteristic linear deposition along GBM that can be seen on immunofluorescent staining on pathology specimens in involved tissues

XIII. Scleroderma

A. Definitions

1. Characterized by presence of hard skin due to excessive production of collagen and extracellular matrix
2. 2 broad types
   a. Localized scleroderma: most common in children; does not develop into generalized form
   b. Systemic scleroderma: rare in children

B. Clinical presentation

1. Localized scleroderma
   a. Presents with thickened, tight skin with pigment changes in plaques (i.e., **morphea**) or **linear** distribution
   b. Does not have systemic involvement
   c. May cause abnormal growth of involved extremity or restricted joint movement

XIV. Henoch-Schönlein Purpura

A. Characteristics

1. Most common systemic vasculitic condition in children
2. Preceding viral, upper respiratory, or streptococcal infection in 80% of cases
3. Small vessel leukocytoclastic vasculitis with deposition of immunoglobulin A (IgA) primarily in kidneys and skin

B. Clinical features

1. Skin manifestations (100%): palpable purpura on LEs and buttocks (Figure 6-3)
   a. Significant edema of scalp, extremities, scrotum, and periorbital regions may occur
   b. Rash may lag behind other symptoms, making diagnosis more challenging

QUICK HIT

Patients with granulomatosis with polyangiitis commonly present with chronic otitis, chronic sinusitis, or pneumonia that is *unresponsive to antibiotics*.

QUICK HIT

A common late clinical sign is a saddle-nose deformity, which results from cartilage destruction.

QUICK HIT

Localized scleroderma involving the forehead is called **en coup de sabre**.

QUICK HIT

HSP is more common in *boys*, with peak occurrence between ages 3 and 15 years.

FIGURE 6-3 A patient with Henoch-Schönlein purpura.

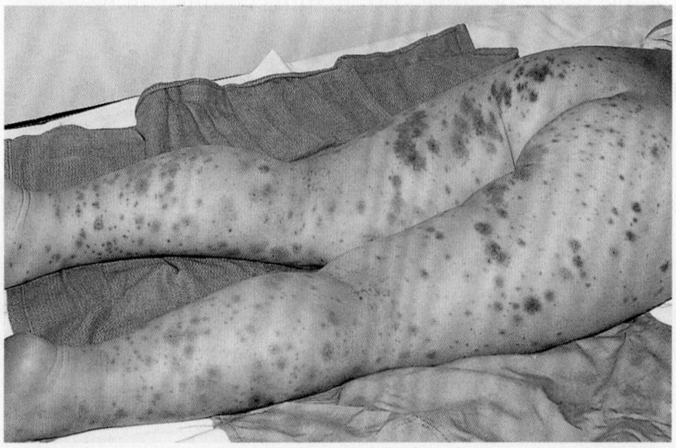

The lesions are well demarcated and slightly raised. (From Fleisher GR, Ludwig S, Baskin MN. *Atlas of Pediatric Emergency Medicine*. Philadelphia: Lippincott Williams & Wilkins; 2004.)

2. Arthritis (84%): migratory, transient, and oligoarticular
3. GI involvement (50%): abdominal pain, cramping, GI bleeding, intussusception (20%–30%)
   a. Intussusception is commonly limited to ileum (ileal–ileal)
   b. Makes ultrasound diagnostic modality of choice
4. Renal involvement (20%–50%): hematuria and proteinuria; renal insufficiency rare

C. Diagnosis
1. No diagnostic tests
2. ESR and CRP are typically elevated
3. Urinalyses should be monitored regularly for first 2–3 months after diagnosis to evaluate for renal involvement
4. Abdominal ultrasound for severe abdominal pain to detect intussusception

D. Treatment
1. Supportive therapy with hydration, rest, and pain management
2. Symptomatic therapy with acetaminophen or NSAIDs if abdominal and joint pain
3. Prednisone is for severe abdominal pain, intestinal hemorrhage; must be tapered over at least a few weeks to avoid rebound of symptoms
4. Typically have complete resolution within 1–2 months
5. Common to have at least 1 recurrence within 4 months after initial episode
6. Long-term sequelae of renal disease if severe kidney involvement or if hematuria lasts >6 months

QUICK HIT

In HSP, the most common joints affected are the hips, knees, and ankles.

QUICK HIT

The most common GI complication associated with HSP is **intussusception**.

QUICK HIT

Laboratory tests will show *normal or elevated platelet counts* in HSP.

XV. Kawasaki Disease

A. Characteristics
1. One of the most common forms of vasculitis in childhood (Box 6-3)
2. Peak incidence is between ages 6 and 11 months, with 80% occurring in patients age <5 years
3. Multisystem inflammatory condition of medium blood vessels
4. Usually self-limited with fever and acute inflammation lasting about 12–14 days if untreated

B. Clinical features (refer to diagnostic criteria in Box 6-3)
1. Constitutional: fever of 39–40°C for 5 or more days plus at least 4 of the following
   a. Eyes: bilateral limbic-sparing, nonpurulent conjunctivitis without discharge (90%) and photophobia
   b. Oral mucous membranes (90%): red, dry, cracked, swollen lips and/or a "strawberry" tongue
   c. Lymphadenopathy: unilateral cervical lymphadenopathy >1.5 cm in diameter
   d. Skin: maculopapular rash (70%–90%) (Figure 6-4A–D)
      i. Involves trunk, face, extremities, and diaper area
      ii. Once lesions heal, skin will peel at affected site
   e. Edema and/or erythema of hands and feet

C. Diagnosis
1. ESR, CRP, and WBCs are significantly elevated
2. Other findings: elevated liver function tests, normocytic anemia, thrombocytosis, sterile pyuria, and increased WBC count in cerebrospinal fluid (CSF) with negative bacterial and viral cultures

QUICK HIT

The fever associated with Kawasaki disease is unresponsive to antibiotics, and ibuprofen and acetaminophen provide minimal benefit.

QUICK HIT

Cardiovascular involvement is the most serious manifestation and consists of dilation of coronary arteries. Myocardial involvement is also possible.

BOX 6-3

Diagnostic Criteria for Kawasaki Disease

Mnemonic: "CRASH and burn"; 4 out of 5 criteria (CRASH), plus 5 or more days of fever (burn)

1. Conjunctivitis (usually bilateral, nonpurulent, and sparing the area around the iris ["limbic sparing"])
2. Rash (for the criteria, can have any appearance, and usually appearance is nonspecific)
3. Adenopathy (at least 1 cervical lymph node >1.5 cm in diameter)
4. Strawberry tongue, or any mucous membrane changes (often dry, swollen, or cracked lips)
5. Hand or feet changes (generally redness or swelling, later peeling)

FIGURE 6-4 Kawasaki disease.

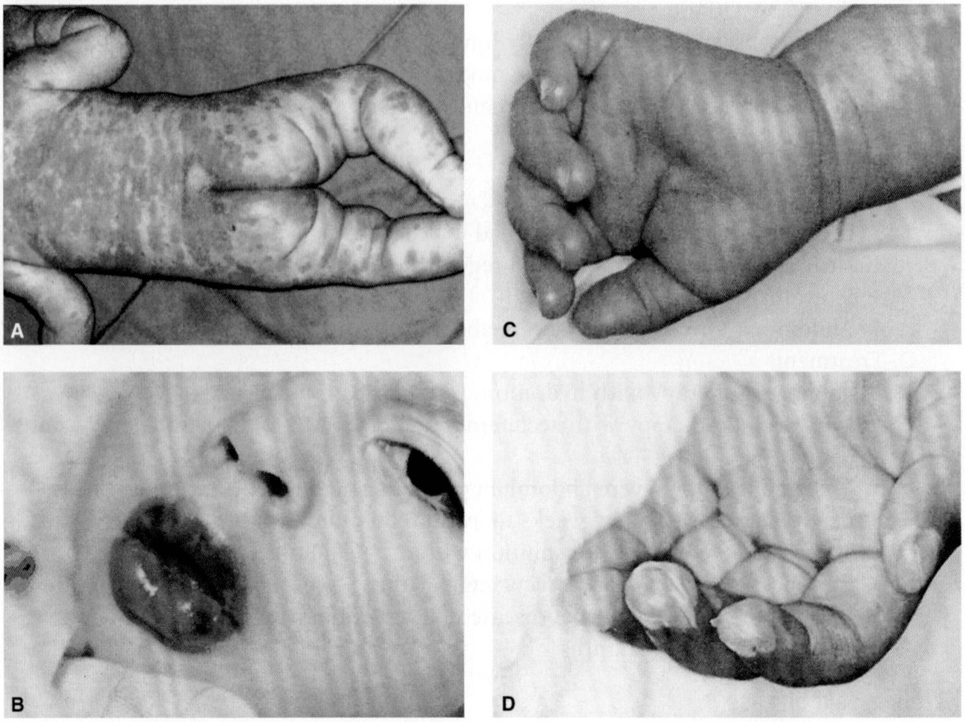

A. Rash of Kawasaki disease in a 7-month-old child on the 4th day of illness. **B.** Conjunctival injection and lip edema in a 2-year-old boy on the 6th day of illness. **C.** Erythema and edematous hand of a 1½-year-old girl on the 6th day of illness. **D.** Periungual desquamation in a 3-year-old child on the 12th day of illness. (From The Council on Cardiovascular Disease in Young, Committee on Rheumatic Fever, Endocarditis, and Kawasaki Disease. Diagnostic guidelines for Kawasaki disease. *Circulation.* 2001;103:335–336.)

3. Echo initially and then repeated in 2–6 weeks
4. Atypical Kawasaki disease
   a. Rare; known to exist only because children without all criteria have presented with coronary artery aneurysms
   b. Difficult diagnosis; requires 2 or more criteria, associated with supportive laboratory findings

D. Treatment
1. Standard treatment is IV immunoglobulin (IVIG) 2 g/kg as single infusion
2. Aspirin (80–100 mg/kg daily divided into 4 doses) should be initiated to prevent clot formation and decrease inflammation and then lowered to 3–5 mg/kg/day to aid with antiplatelet effects
3. Infants age <1 year old have a higher risk for coronary artery aneurysm because they lack typical features, thus delaying diagnosis

QUICK HIT

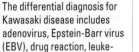

The differential diagnosis for Kawasaki disease includes adenovirus, Epstein-Barr virus (EBV), drug reaction, leukemia, sepsis, and systemic JIA.

QUICK HIT

Treatment is focused on preventing vascular inflammation and thrombosis.

QUICK HIT

Kawasaki disease is one of the *very few* instances where aspirin is given to children because antiplatelet and anti-inflammatory effects improve long-term outcomes.

XVI. Juvenile Dermatomyositis

A. Characteristics
1. Most common inflammatory muscle disease of childhood
2. Average age at onset is 7 years
3. Can affect pharyngeal and laryngeal muscle groups, retina, and GI tract
4. Autoimmune condition related to inflammation of small arteries and veins
   a. Proliferation of intima and thrombus formation
   b. End-organ destruction
   c. Subsequent calcinosis (soft tissue calcification) may follow inflammatory process in muscles and skin

B. Clinical features
1. Constitutional symptoms: anorexia, fatigue, fever, malaise, weight loss
2. Muscle weakness
   a. Proximal muscle weakness affecting neck, shoulders, and abdominal and pelvic muscles

QUICK HIT

Unlike adult-onset dermatomyositis, juvenile dermatomyositis is *not* associated with malignancy in children.

b. Commonly have positive Gowers sign (also sign for Duchenne muscular dystrophy, another cause of proximal muscle weakness)
c. Most comfortable with limbs in flexion leading to flexion contractures, and muscle atrophy may be present

3. Skin involvement
   a. Heliotrope rash (83%) with reddish purple hue on upper eyelids along with malar rash (42%)
   b. Gottron papules (91%): shiny, erythematous, scaly plaques on extension surface of elbows, knuckles, and knees
   c. Nail-bed telangiectasias (80%) and digital ulcerations may indicate worse prognosis
4. Arthritis: symmetric, nonerosive involvement
5. GI involvement
   a. Vasculitis can affect any part of GI tract
   b. Can impair absorption of nutrients and medications
   c. Can progress to ulceration with perforation

C. Diagnosis
1. Elevated muscle enzyme levels to confirm diagnosis; assess activity and monitor response to treatment (creatine phosphokinase [CPK] and aldolase)
2. ESR and CRP are usually normal
3. MRI, electromyography, and muscle biopsy can be ordered in equivocal cases
4. Other conditions to consider *if the rash is absent* include: muscular dystrophy, metabolic myopathies, viral infections, and other rheumatologic conditions

D. Treatment
1. Initial treatment with prednisone (begin with 2 mg/kg/day and slowly taper over 1–2 years) and methotrexate
2. If persistent disease or GI or pulmonary involvement: cyclosporine, mycophenolate, etanercept, or cyclophosphamide is added
3. For skin involvement, hydroxychloroquine and IVIG are helpful
4. Sun precautions should be discussed because skin rashes are photosensitive
5. Physical and occupational therapy should be initiated early in disease

XVII. Chronic Recurrent Multifocal Osteomyelitis (CRMO)

A. General characteristics
1. Inflammatory disease characterized by recurring episodes of pain and swelling over affected bones and radiologic and histologic changes suggestive of osteomyelitis with *negative infectious workup*
2. Cause is unknown
3. Some association with palmoplantar pustulosis, psoriasis, arthritis, sacroiliitis, IBD, and **Sweet syndrome** (neutrophil dermatosis)

B. Clinical presentation
1. Fever
2. Acute onset of multifocal bone pain
3. Periodic painful relapses and remissions
4. Most commonly affects tibia, ribs, clavicles, and vertebral bodies

C. Testing
1. Elevated ESR
2. Radiographic abnormalities characterized by bilateral, symmetrical radiolucent bone lesions with reactive sclerosis and soft tissue swelling
3. Biopsy necessary to exclude other possibilities such as infectious osteomyelitis and malignancy

D. Therapy
1. NSAIDs usually bring symptomatic relief
2. In more severe cases, other immunosuppressants such as corticosteroids, methotrexate, and tumor necrosis factor (TNF) inhibitors have been used

QUICK HIT

The hallmark of the disease is *muscle weakness* and a characteristic *rash*.

QUICK HIT

In patients with proximal muscle weakness, the presence of heliotropic rash and Gottron papules distinguishes dermatomyositis from muscular dystrophy.

QUICK HIT

Test for a Gowers sign by asking the patient to get up off the floor from a sitting position. A positive sign occurs when the patient has to use his or her hands to walk up his or her body and is an indicator of proximal muscle weakness.

QUICK HIT

Respiratory muscle weakness can lead to decreased ventilator capacity in the absence of respiratory symptoms. Respiratory muscle weakness can be assessed by measuring negative inspiratory flow.

QUICK HIT

Patients with laryngeal or pharyngeal muscle involvement are at risk of aspirating food and drink. A swallow study will help determine aspiration likelihood.

QUICK HIT

Sweet syndrome consists of fever, high WBC count, tender red skin lesions, and sometimes arthritis or eye findings. It is associated with a number of inflammatory conditions including cancer (especially acute myeloid leukemia) and autoimmune disease.

QUICK HIT

Consider CRMO in patients with osteomyelitis of the clavicle, ribs, or vertebrae. A bone scan may reveal multiple sites of involvement.

XVIII. Developmental Dysplasia of the Hip (DDH)

A. Characteristics
1. Results from partial or complete dislocation/subluxation of femoral head out of acetabulum
2. 1:1,000 live Caucasian births; less prevalent in African Americans
3. ~60% of unstable hips in newborns normalize spontaneously within 1st several weeks
4. In older child, dislocation becomes more fixed, resulting in bony changes to femoral head and acetabulum
5. Long-term complications: osteoarthritis, pain, abnormal gait, decreased agility, flexion contractures

B. Clinical features
1. Birth–3 months
   a. **Barlow maneuver**: causes hip to dislocate (hip is located, but dislocates with this maneuver where hip is slightly adducted and gently pushed posteriorly, causing "clunk" sensation)
   b. **Ortolani maneuver**: causes hip to reduce and "click" may be felt (hip is abducted while femur is gently lifted with fingers at greater trochanter) (Figure 6-5)
2. Older infant
   a. Limited abduction of hip (<70° from midline is positive finding)
   b. Leg length discrepancy
   c. Unequal knee heights when supine and knees are flexed (**Galeazzi sign**)
   d. Asymmetry of thigh folds
3. Walking child
   a. Leg length discrepancy
   b. Possible curvature of spine

FIGURE 6-5 Examination for developmental dysplasia of the hip.

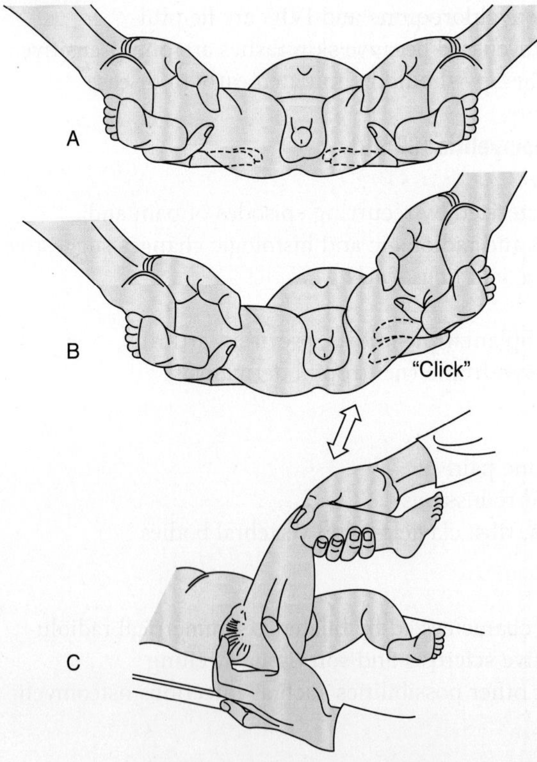

A. In the newborn, both hips can be equally fixed, abducted, and externally rotated without producing a "click." **B.** A diagnosis of congenital dislocation of the hip may be confirmed by Ortolani "click." **C.** Lateral view of Ortolani maneuver. (From Hoppenfeld S. *Physical Examination of the Spine and Extremities*. New York: Appleton-Century-Crofts; 1976.)

c. Abnormal gait (limp, asymmetric intoeing or outtoeing, unilateral toe walking; hyperlordosis if bilateral)

C. Diagnosis
1. In infant, diagnosis is primarily based on clinical exam but obtain good history including associated risk factors for DDH
   a. Breech delivery
   b. Family history of DDH
   c. Congenital muscular torticollis
   d. Oligohydramnios
   e. Primiparous or older mother
2. Ultrasound between ages 6 weeks and 4 months (<6 weeks yields high false-positive rates)
3. Age >4 months: obtain an anteroposterior (AP) and frog lateral pelvis x-ray

D. Treatment
1. Generally, the earlier the treatment, the better the prognosis
2. Birth–age 6 months: **Pavlik harness** (device that holds hips flexed at 100° and prevents adduction) with 90% success rate

> **QUICK HIT**
> Associated findings that also develop secondary to a cramped intrauterine environment include torticollis, metatarsus adductus, and clubfoot.

XIX. Talipes Equinovarus (Clubfoot)

A. General characteristics
1. Congenital, complex, fixed foot deformity comprising midfoot and forefoot adductus, equinovarus of hindfoot, and cavus of midfoot (high arch)
2. Generally idiopathic, but may be associated with other conditions such as arthrogryposis, spina bifida, or other neuromuscular diseases
3. Etiology is unknown but strong familial tendency even with distant relatives

B. Clinical presentation
1. Present at birth, and diagnosis is obvious
2. Clubfoot is rigid, as opposed to metatarsus adductus (MA), which can be passively corrected
3. Evaluate for underlying neurologic condition or syndrome

C. Therapy
1. Prompt referral to orthopedics to begin as soon as possible after birth
2. If left untreated, child would walk on side and top of foot
3. Initial treatment is nonoperative
4. Surgical treatment
   a. Initial surgical treatment is soft tissue release usually performed between ages 6 and 12 months
   b. If soft tissue releases fail, tendon transfers and/or bony procedures may be indicated usually after age 5 or 6 years

XX. Metatarsus Adductus

A. General characteristics
1. Foot deformity in which forefoot is turned inward or adducted
2. Most common foot deformity in newborn infant, occurring in 5 in 1,000 live births
3. Frequently bilateral (50%)
4. Increased incidence with positive family history
5. Cause is unknown but may be related to tight intrauterine “packaging”
6. Often associated with torticollis and DDH (10%)

B. Clinical presentation
1. Medial deviation of forefoot with normal hindfoot
2. Forefoot can be passively corrected to neutral
3. Ankle dorsiflexion and plantar flexion are normal

C. Therapy
1. Generally, no treatment is needed for flexible MA
2. Tends to self-correct by ages 12–18 months but may take as long as 3–4 years
3. Generally, the more flexible the forefoot, the faster the deformity resolves
4. Refer to orthopedics if fixed deformity, pain, or difficulty wearing shoes

QUICK HIT

Try making the child grab an offered popsicle with the affected arm outstretched after reduction. The pain is gone, but sometimes children are reluctant to try using the arm again.

QUICK HIT

If the child does not begin using his or her arm after the reduction, then radiographs are necessary to rule out fracture.

QUICK HIT

Congenital scoliosis often affects chest cage development with fused ribs leading to **thoracic insufficiency syndrome**, which is defined as an inability of the thorax to support normal respiration or lung growth.

QUICK HIT

The **Adams forward bend test** is the screening test used most often to screen for scoliosis. The child bends forward, dangling the arms, with the feet together and knees straight. Any imbalances in the rib cage or other deformities along the back can be a sign of scoliosis.

XXI. Subluxation of the Radial Head (Nursemaid's Elbow)

A. General characteristics
   1. Most common elbow injury in childhood between ages 1 and 4 years
   2. Sudden longitudinal traction on outstretched arm causes subluxation of radial head (usually caused by an adult pulling up on child's outstretched arm, such as when a child is swung by the arms or putting on a coat)
   3. Radial head is pulled distally, causing it to slip partially through annular ligament
   4. When traction is released, radial head recoils, trapping proximal portion of ligament between it and capitellum

B. Clinical presentation
   1. Child will not use arm and holds elbow in slightly flexed, pronated position
   2. Should not have joint swelling, deformity, point tenderness of elbow, joint erythema, or warmth

C. Therapy
   1. Closed reduction: performed by fully extending elbow, and then fully supinating and then flexing elbow with gentle pressure over radial head
   2. Usually a pop or click is felt as ligament snaps back into place
   3. Child should begin to use arm within 15–20 minutes

XXII. Scoliosis

A. General characteristics
   1. Condition in which spine is curved
   2. Classified as idiopathic, congenital, and neuromuscular
   3. If severe, cardiopulmonary function may be compromised

B. Clinical presentation
   1. May present with uneven musculature on 1 side of spine, rib, or scapular prominence or uneven hips or shoulders
   2. Children may have **trunk shift**, which is a shift of thoracic cage to right or left of midline at apex of scoliosis
   3. Test for degree of involvement using scoliometer, which is much like a carpenter's level; get x-ray for any value >7° (Figure 6-6)

FIGURE 6-6 Scoliosis checkup.

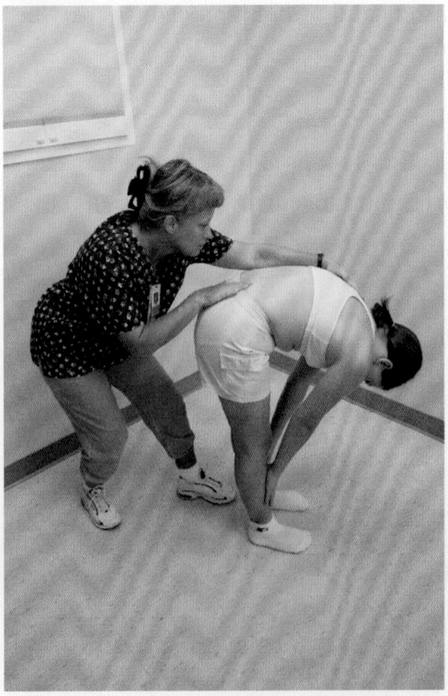

With the child bending over and touching her toes, the examiner checks for a curvature of the spinal column.

C. Testing
   1. Standard radiographic method for assessing curvature is measurement of **Cobb angle**
   2. If severe, consider MRI of entire spine (including base of brain) to evaluate for Chiari malformation or syrinx

D. Therapy
   1. Observation for mild scoliosis
   2. Refer to an orthopedist
      a. Scoliometer >7°, and Cobb angle unable to be obtained
      b. Cobb angle >20° in prepubescent child ages 12–14 years
      c. Any Cobb angle >30°
      d. Progression of Cobb angle by >5°
   3. Moderate forms are treated with casting or bracing
   4. Surgery is indicated if casting or bracing has failed or for severe curves

QUICK HIT

X-rays are indicated to assess the curvature and to rule out congenital abnormalities.

QUICK HIT

Scoliosis is commonly associated with a number of neuromuscular conditions, including cerebral palsy, muscular dystrophy, spinal muscular atrophy, Friedreich ataxia, and Charcot-Marie-Tooth disease and commonly requires surgical intervention.

XXIII. Legg-Calvé-Perthes (LCP) Disease

A. General characteristics
   1. Possibly develops from interruption of blood supply to variable area of femoral head, physis, and femoral neck
   2. Patients tend to be shorter in stature and have delay in skeletal maturation
   3. Most patients develop permanent deformity of femoral head and acetabulum

B. Clinical presentation
   1. Most common between ages 4 and 10 years
   2. Children often present with pain in groin, thigh, or knee and/or **Trendelenburg gait**
   3. On exam, patients have irritable hip, decreased ROM, and later may have leg length inequality

C. Testing: plain x-rays progress through 4 stages: joint widening, fragmentation, reossification, and healing/remodeling (Figure 6-7)

D. Therapy
   1. Conservative management includes rest, activity modification, NSAIDs, and physical therapy for ROM and strengthening
   2. Surgery may benefit children age >8 years with more severe forms

QUICK HIT

Trendelenburg gait: During the stance phase of the gait cycle, weakened abductor muscles allow the pelvis to tilt down on the contralateral side and, to compensate, the trunk lurches to the weakened side to attempt to maintain a level pelvis.

QUICK HIT

Most patients with LCP function well into the 4th or 5th decade of life before requiring a total hip arthroplasty.

XXIV. Slipped Capital Femoral Epiphysis (SCFE)

A. General characteristics
   1. Posterior and inferior slipping of capital femoral epiphysis from femoral neck through physis

FIGURE 6-7 **Legg-Calvé-Perthes disease of left hip. Epiphysis is narrowed and radiodense.**

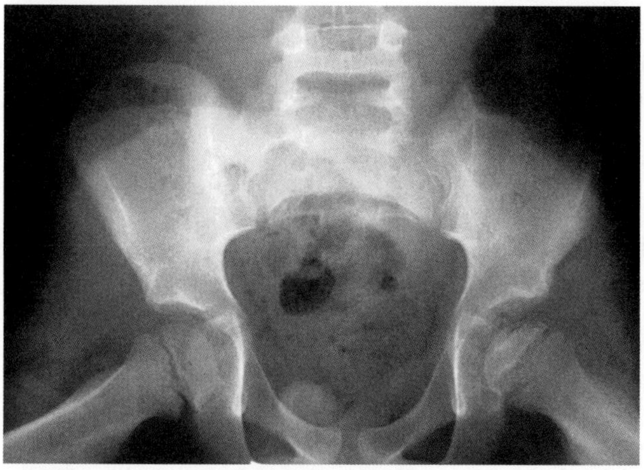

A subchondral fracture is also visible. (From Fleisher GR, Ludwig S, Baskin MN. *Atlas of Pediatric Emergency Medicine.* Philadelphia: Lippincott Williams & Wilkins; 2004.)

QUICK HIT

SCFE is the most common disorder affecting adolescent hips with incidence of 10 per 100,000 in the United States.

QUICK HIT

SCFE is bilateral in 20%–60% of cases, and it is more common in children age <10 years.

QUICK HIT

The name is a misnomer, because the epiphysis remains in normal position, whereas the remainder of the femur is displaced.

QUICK HIT

Appearance of the head of the femur in relation to the shaft looks like a scoop of ice cream falling off the ice cream cone.

QUICK HIT

Apophysitis is inflammation of an apophysis, an area of bony growth that occurs at a bone–tendon interface in skeletally immature patients.

FIGURE 6-8 Slipped capital femoral epiphysis of right hip.

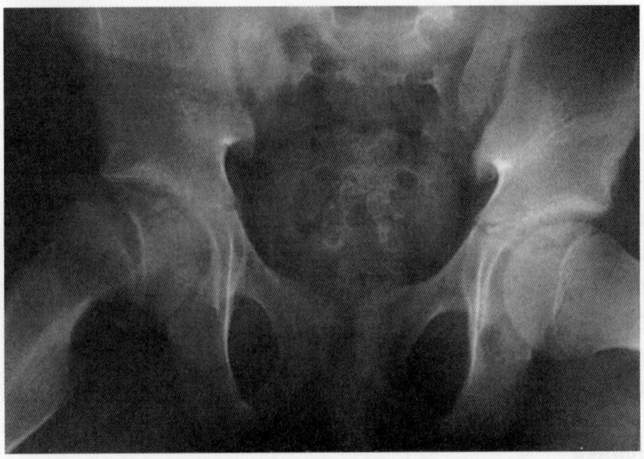

Epiphysis is displaced medially on the frog view.

2. Occurs due to increased mechanical forces through susceptible physis
3. Single greatest risk factor is obesity, with 75% of patients above 90th percentile

B. Clinical presentation
1. Males with peak age between 12 and 13 years
2. Presents with acute or chronic hip, thigh, or knee pain
3. Patients may have limp or inability to bear weight

C. Testing
1. Lateral and AP views of hip show displacement of metaphysis (Figure 6-8)
2. Line drawn along superior margin of femoral neck on AP film does not intersect epiphysis as it normally should
3. Consider endocrine evaluation to rule out predisposing conditions (e.g., serum thyroid-stimulating hormone, serum calcium, vitamin D levels)

D. Therapy: regarded as *orthopedic emergency* because further slippage may result in occlusion of blood supply and lead to avascular necrosis

XXV. Blount Disease

A. General characteristics
1. Disorder of medial aspect of proximal tibial physis that produces varus deformity of proximal tibia
2. Parents often report that child is walking with "bowed legs" or with their toes pointing in with or without pain

B. Clinical presentation
1. May have infantile, juvenile, or adolescent onset
2. Physical exam reveals **genu varum** (bowleggedness) and intoeing

C. Therapy
1. Bracing in child <3 years is used to achieve more normal joint and limb anatomy, thereby improving joint mechanics
2. Lowers chances of developing degenerative joint disease in involved joint as adult
3. If braces do not work, or if it is not diagnosed until child is older, surgery is usually required

XXVI. Osgood-Schlatter Syndrome

A. General characteristics
1. Represents painful traction **apophysitis** of tibial tubercle apophysis
2. Frequent cause of knee pain in children ages 10–15 years old, especially in those who participate in repetitive impact activities that involve running and jumping
3. Occurs because repetitive quadriceps contraction exerts force on apophysis during period of skeletal development when it is weakest link in kinetic chain, causing inflammation and subacute fracturing at apophysis

B. Clinical presentation
  1. May have a "bump" on anterior proximal tibia
  2. Pain is worse when starting physical activity, with high-intensity impact activities, after completion of play, and with sitting with knee bent for prolonged period
  3. Tenderness to palpation over tibial tubercle

C. Therapy
  1. Methods to decrease inflammatory response such as NSAIDs, elevation, ice, and activity modifications
  2. Physical therapy to address flexibility and strength issues thought to be cause of pain

QUICK HIT

Symptoms of Osgood-Schlatter disease can be prevented with treatment of associated issues, including hamstring stretching and hip and core strengthening.

XXVII. Patellofemoral Syndrome

A. General characteristics
  1. Refers to general pain involving patellofemoral joint or arising from anterior aspect of knee
  2. Very common cause of knee pain in adolescents and young adults
  3. Pain worsens with activity
  4. Risk factors include an active lifestyle, overweight, abnormal LE alignment
  5. Caused by abnormal forces between patella and femur that exceed tissues' mechanical strength, causing inflammation of involved and/or surrounding structures and resulting in pain

B. Clinical presentation
  1. Usually insidious onset of anterior knee pain, often described as behind patella
  2. Location of pain and tenderness is most diagnostic but may have **positive patellar grind testing**
     a. Examiner displaces patella inferiorly and then patient is asked to contract quadriceps against resistance from examiner
     b. Test is positive if patient's pain is reproduced

C. Therapy
  1. NSAIDs, ice, elevation, and activity modifications
  2. Physical therapy to address flexibility and strength issues

QUICK HIT

Excessive **femoral anteversion**, **external tibial torsion**, and **genu valgum** ("knock knees") contribute to the development of patellofemoral syndrome.

QUICK HIT

Pain is worse when starting physical activity, with jumping or running, with ascending and descending stairs, and with sitting with knees bent for prolonged periods.

QUICK HIT

Occasionally, a symptomatic synovial plica, small chondral lesion, or other minor structural anomalies may be missed and cause similar pain.

XXVIII. Osteogenesis Imperfecta (OI)

A. Characteristics
  1. Spectrum of disorders characterized by abnormal bone fragility
  2. Incidence of 1 in 20,000 children
  3. Caused by mutations in genes that code for type I collagen (*COL1A1* and *COL1A2*)
  4. Histologically, bone has decreased number of trabeculae and decreased cortical thickness with an increase in numbers of osteoblasts and osteoclasts
  5. Children have increased incidence of fractures, which heal at normal rate
  6. Most severe form of OI is fatal during perinatal period

B. Clinical features
  1. **Sillence classification** is used to characterize different types of OI (Table 6-6)
  2. Autosomal dominant inheritance or spontaneous mutation
  3. Differential diagnosis includes nonaccidental trauma

C. Diagnosis
  1. May have hypercalciuria
  2. Collagen synthesis analysis from skin biopsy using cultured dermal fibroblasts
  3. Prenatal DNA mutation analysis may be performed
  4. Imaging studies
     a. Mild forms show cortical thinning of long bones
     b. Severe forms may show beaded ribs, broad bones, and numerous fractures and long bone deformities
     c. Vertebral fractures are common

QUICK HIT

The structural defect in OI can be quantitative (production of normal collagen in decreased amount) or qualitative (production of abnormal collagen).

QUICK HIT

Dentinogenesis imperfecta is a condition that causes teeth to be discolored (most often blue-gray or yellow-brown) and translucent. Teeth are also weaker than normal, making them more prone to wear, breakage, and loss.

TABLE 6-6 Sillence Classification of Osteogenesis Imperfecta

Type I—mild	Low or low normal height Sclera can be blue or normal **Dentinogenesis imperfecta** may be present Reduced exercise tolerance and strength Fractures most common in infancy May have kyphoscoliosis or hearing loss
Type II—extremely severe	Often lethal Fractures occur in utero May have blue sclera May have small nose, micrognathia, or both Death is usually pulmonary injury from rib fractures or pulmonary hypoplasia or from CNS hemorrhages
Type III—severe	All have dentinogenesis imperfecta Sclera is variable In utero fractures are common Short limbs with progressive deformities Joint hyperlaxity Skull deformities Basilar invagination may occur and be lethal Vertigo Kyphoscoliosis and resultant pulmonary compromise are common Hypercalciuria in 1/3 of patients with no renal compromise
Type IV—undefined	No consensus on sclera color Dentinogenesis imperfecta may be present Fractures begin in utero or in infancy Long bone deformities occur

D. Treatment
1. Pamidronate
   a. Reduces incidence of fracture
   b. Increases bone mineral density
   c. Reduces pain
   d. Increases energy levels
2. Adequate daily calcium and vitamin D
3. Orthopedic surgery, when indicated
4. Genetic counseling
5. Physical and occupational therapy to improve joint mobility and strength

7 Diseases of the Renal and Genitourinary System

SYMPTOM SPECIFIC

I. Approach to Hematuria

A. Background information
  1. **Gross hematuria** occurs when blood is seen during voiding; **microscopic hematuria**, defined as presence of ≥5 red blood cells (RBCs) per high-power field (hpf), is seen only on urinalysis
  2. 0.5%–2% prevalence among school-aged children
  3. Morbidity and mortality depend on primary etiology but are generally good in asymptomatic isolated hematuria
  4. Differential diagnosis of red-colored urine (Table 7-1)
     a. Hematuria: broad
     b. Myoglobinuria: rhabdomyolysis
     c. Hemoglobinuria: hemolysis
     d. Drugs: pyridium and rifampin
     e. Dyes: aniline dyes in candies
     f. Metabolites: porphyrins, bilirubin, and tyrosinemia
     g. Foods: beets and blackberries
     h. Infant urate crystals: dehydration ("pink diaper syndrome")
     i. Infections: hemorrhagic cystitis, especially with adenovirus

B. Historical questions: careful history can help direct evaluation and workup
  1. Is the hematuria gross or microscopic? Are there clots? What color is the urine? (May help identify where hematuria originates along urinary tract)
  2. Has the patient had a recent sore throat, upper respiratory infection (URI), or skin infection?
  3. Are there other associated symptoms like fever, flank pain, abdominal pain, or burning with urination?
  4. Does the patient have a history of high blood pressure (BP)?
  5. Is there any personal or family history of renal disease, kidney stones, or deafness?
  6. Does the patient have any chronic medical problems (such as sickle cell disease or systemic lupus erythematosus [SLE])?
  7. Are there other associated physical complaints like joint pain or rash? (May suggest Henoch-Schönlein purpura [HSP] or rheumatologic etiologies)
  8. Is there any history of trauma?

C. Physical examination findings may be minimal depending on underlying cause
  1. Obtain vital signs, focusing on BP
  2. Skin exam
     a. Purpuric, nonblanching rash predominately on lower extremities (LEs) suggests HSP
     b. Malar facial rash suggests rheumatologic process like SLE

QUICK HIT

Most causes of microscopic hematuria in children are **transient** (fevers, exercise).

QUICK HIT

Clots in the urine are more likely from the bladder, not the kidney.

QUICK HIT

A recent URI or skin infection may point to disorders like acute postinfectious (post-streptococcal) glomerulonephritis or immunoglobulin A nephropathy.

QUICK HIT

Fever, flank pain, and dysuria would suggest pyelonephritis, cystitis, or urolithiasis.

QUICK HIT

Alport syndrome is usually X-linked but can be recessive or dominant and can present with hematuria and slowly progressive hearing loss in adolescence.

TABLE 7-1 **Differential Diagnosis of Pediatric Hematuria**

Location	Category	Disease	Key Points
Upper Urinary Tract	Isolated renal disease	Immunoglobulin A nephropathy Alport syndrome Postinfectious glomerulonephritis Focal segmental glomerulosclerosis Rapidly progressive glomerulonephritis Membranous nephropathy Thin membrane disease/benign familial hematuria	Originates from nephron
	Multisystem disease	Lupus nephritis Henoch-Schönlein purpura Wegener granulomatosis Polyarteritis nodosa Goodpasture syndrome Hemolytic-uremic syndrome Sickle cell disease HIV nephropathy	May be associated with cola-colored urine, RBC casts, or proteinuria depending on where in nephron it is originating
	Tubulointerstitial disease	Pyelonephritis Interstitial nephritis Papillary necrosis Acute tubular necrosis	
	Vascular	Arterial thrombosis Venous thrombosis Aneurysm Hemangioma Hemoglobinopathy	
	Anatomic	Hydronephrosis Polycystic kidney disease Multicystic dysplasia Tumor Trauma	
Lower Urinary Tract	Inflammation	Cystitis Urethritis Urolithiasis Trauma Coagulopathy Heavy exercise Bladder tumor Factitious syndrome	Originates from pelvocalyceal system, including the ureter, bladder, or urethra May be associated with gross hematuria that is bright red

QUICK HIT

Flank pain may indicate infection or urolithiasis.

QUICK HIT

Enlarged kidneys secondary to tumors, hydronephrosis, dysplasia, or cysts may present as abdominal masses.

QUICK HIT

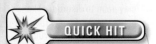

Wilms tumors will present with hematuria about 25% of the time.

QUICK HIT

Red urine with absence of RBCs on microscopic analysis is consistent with hemoglobinuria or myoglobinuria.

QUICK HIT

Microscopic hematuria can be transient, and repeat urinalysis in an asymptomatic patient is recommended before further invasive workup is necessary.

QUICK HIT

Presence of RBC casts is a hallmark of glomerular disease.

3. Abdominal exam
    a. Assess for flank pain
    b. Palpate for abdominal masses
4. Genitourinary (GU) exam may identify extraurinary cause for bleeding (i.e., anomaly, skin lesion, foreign body)

D. Diagnostic workup
1. Laboratory testing
    a. Urine dipstick
        i. Must confirm a heme-positive urine dipstick with microscopic urinalysis to assess for presence of RBCs
        ii. Presence of proteinuria may indicate more significant renal disease
        iii. Presence of leukocyte esterase, nitrites, or white blood cells (WBCs) may indicate infectious etiology; also send urine culture in these cases
        iv. RBC morphology differentiates between glomerular (abnormal morphology) and nonglomerular (normal morphology) causes

b. Urine electrolytes to assess urine calcium:creatinine ratio
c. Renal panel to assess electrolytes, blood urea nitrogen (BUN), and creatinine may be warranted to evaluate for intrinsic renal disease
d. Complete blood count (CBC) with differential may be warranted
   i. May suggest infection if WBC is elevated
   ii. Hemoglobin and hematocrit to assess extent of blood loss
e. C3 and C4 levels: low complement levels suggest poststreptococcal glomerulonephritis (PSGN), membranoproliferative glomerulonephritis (MPGN), or lupus nephritis
f. Other labs like antinuclear antibody (ANA), HIV, antistreptolysin O (ASO) titers, or others may be warranted depending on clinical scenario
g. Coagulation factors with personal or family history of bleeding disorder

2. Radiologic testing
   a. Renal and bladder ultrasound is first line and noninvasive
   b. Computed tomography (CT) scan is warranted when evaluating abdominal mass or in some cases of urolithiasis
   c. Voiding cystourethrogram (VCUG) is indicated with recurrent febrile urinary tract infections (UTIs), renal scarring, or hydroureter
   d. Cystoscopy is expensive, usually unnecessary, and requires anesthesia
3. Other testing
   a. Nephrology referral warranted in cases of persistent asymptomatic hematuria >1 year, nephritis, proteinuria, hypertension (HTN), renal insufficiency, urolithiasis, or positive family history of renal disease
   b. Kidney biopsy is rarely done but may be indicated for some children with persistent hematuria or hematuria associated with other complications

> **QUICK HIT**
> Elevated urine calcium: creatinine ratio suggests hypercalciuria and urolithiasis/stones.

> **QUICK HIT**
> Thrombocytopenia and hemolytic anemia may suggest hemolytic-uremic syndrome.

II. Approach to Proteinuria

A. Background information
1. Defined as detection of protein in urine
2. Finding isolated proteinuria is common in children, but persistent proteinuria and proteinuria >100 mg/m²/day reflects renal disease and warrants evaluation by a nephrologist
3. Roughly 10% of children have proteinuria detected on random urine dipstick, but only 0.1% will develop persistent proteinuria
4. Differential diagnosis is broad but can be divided into 3 main categories (Table 7-2)
   a. Benign isolated proteinuria that is transient or orthostatic
   b. Glomerular causes of persistent proteinuria
   c. Tubular causes of persistent proteinuria

B. Historical questions
1. Is there any history of fever, exercise, or stress? (Most common differential with these complaints would be transient proteinuria with known precipitant)
2. Is there a recent history of URI? (May point to disorders like acute PSGN or immunoglobulin A [IgA] nephropathy)
3. Does the patient have eyelid, face, or scrotal edema or unexplained weight gain? (Suggests nephrotic syndrome or significant glomerular disease)
4. Does the patient have high BP? (Potential sequela of kidney disease)
5. Is the urine red? (Suggests associated hematuria concerning for glomerulonephritis [GN])
6. Is there a personal or family history of kidney disease? (Suggests inherited disorders like Alport syndrome, polycystic kidney disease [PKD], Wilson disease, or other such inherited disorders)
7. Does the patient have any chronic medical problems? (Diabetes mellitus [DM], sickle cell, and SLE are associated with glomerular disease)
8. Are there other associated complaints like abdominal or joint pain or rash?

> **QUICK HIT**
> 3+ or 4+ urine protein or urine XX needs to be evaluated for proteinuria.

> **QUICK HIT**
> Neonates typically have higher urinary protein due to reduced reabsorption of filtered proteins.

TABLE 7-2 **Differential Diagnosis of Proteinuria in Children**

	Disease	Key Points
	Transient proteinuria	Caused by fever, seizures, stress, dehydration, exercise; protein ≤1–2+ on dipstick; self-resolving
	Orthostatic proteinuria	Most common cause in school-aged children; usually asymptomatic; diagnose with first morning void, in which protein should not be present; comorbidities absent
Glomerular Diseases	Minimal change disease Focal segmental glomerulosclerosis Mesangial proliferative glomerulonephritis Membranous nephropathy Membranoproliferative glomerulonephritis Amyloidosis Diabetic nephropathy Sickle cell nephropathy Acute postinfectious glomerulonephritis Immunoglobulin A nephropathy Henoch-Schönlein purpura Lupus nephritis Alport nephritis Secondary to infection (i.e., HIV, malaria)	High-grade fixed proteinuria with urine protein:creatinine ratio >1.0 OR proteinuria of any grade accompanied by hypertension, hematuria, edema, or renal dysfunction Nephrotic syndrome stems from glomerular disease and consists of nephrotic range proteinuria (>2 urine protein:creatinine ratio on first a.m. void) PLUS hypoalbuminemia, edema, and hyperlipidemia
Tubular Diseases	Cystinosis Wilson disease Lowe syndrome X-linked recessive nephrolithiasis Mitochondrial disorders Galactosemia Tubulointerstitial nephritis Heavy metal poisoning Acute tubular necrosis Renal dysplasia Polycystic kidney disease Secondary to obstructive uropathy Reflux nephropathy	Low-grade fixed proteinuria with urine protein:creatinine ratio <1.0 May be seen in acquired and inherited disorders

QUICK HIT

Edema is gravity dependent. In babies, it will be present in the face, whereas in adolescents, it will be seen in the feet or groin.

QUICK HIT

Abdominal pain + purpuric rash = HSP.

QUICK HIT

If protein is detected on dipstick, the patient is asymptomatic, and a repeat first-morning-void specimen is negative, orthostatic proteinuria is the most likely diagnosis.

QUICK HIT

Urine dipstick only detects albumin, but urine sulfosalicylic acid (SSA) detects all proteins.

C. Physical examination findings may be minimal depending on underlying cause, but thorough physical exam is important
   1. Skin exam
      a. Facial/periorbital edema occurs with nephrotic range proteinuria (Figure 7-1)

FIGURE 7-1 **Facial edema secondary to nephrotic range proteinuria.**

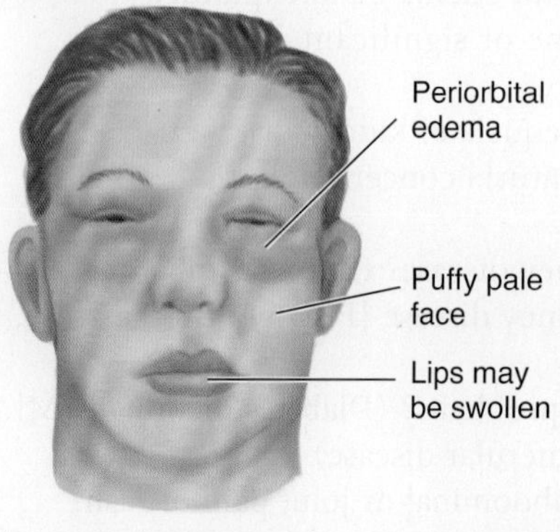

(From Bickley LS, Szilagyi P. *Bates' Guide to Physical Examination and History Taking.* 8th ed. Philadelphia: Lippincott Williams & Wilkins; 2003.)

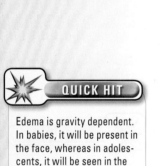

b. Purpuric, nonblanching rash predominately on LEs suggests HSP
c. Malar facial rash suggests rheumatologic process like SLE

2. Abdominal exam
   a. Examine for presence of abdominal ascites or abdominal pain
      i. Ascites suggests cirrhosis or nephrotic syndrome
      ii. Abdominal pain suggests HSP or infection
   b. Hepatomegaly occurs with Wilson disease, hepatitis, and cirrhosis
3. Musculoskeletal exam
   a. Joint pain or swelling may suggest HSP or SLE
   b. Extremity pain occurs with sickle cell disease with acute pain crisis
4. GU exam: evaluate for scrotal edema: suggests nephrotic range proteinuria

D. Diagnostic workup
1. Laboratory testing
   a. Urinalysis (Figure 7-2)
      i. Urine dipstick is good screening test: primarily detects albumin excretion and provides semiquantitative estimate of urinary protein
      ii. Measure spot urine protein:creatinine ratio
         (a) >0.2 is abnormal in kids age >2 years
         (b) >0.5 is abnormal in kids age 6–24 months
         (c) >2.0 is nephrotic range proteinuria
      iii. Presence of RBC casts is pathognomonic for GN
      iv. Presence of WBCs, nitrite, or leukocyte esterase suggests UTI
      v. Presence of glucose in urine suggests diabetic nephropathy or proximal tubular injury

QUICK HIT

Timed 24-hour urine protein collections are cumbersome with high noncompliance rates; for this reason, spot urine protein:creatinine ratios are commonly used.

QUICK HIT

If proteinuria is persistent or patient has other symptoms like HTN, obtain renal panel to assess electrolytes, BUN, creatinine, albumin, and cholesterol.

FIGURE 7-2 **Approach to asymptomatic proteinuria.**

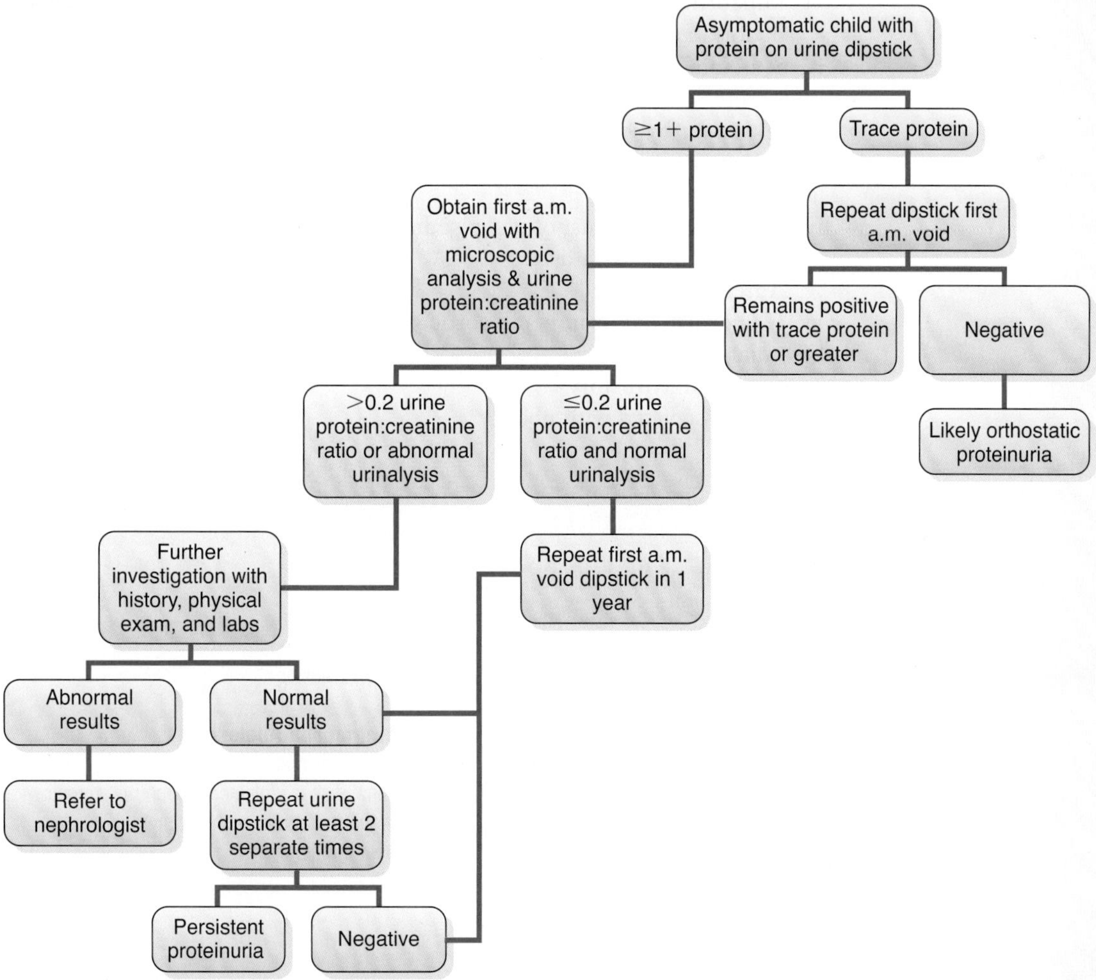

b. C3 and C4 levels: low complement levels are consistent with postinfectious GN, MPGN, or lupus nephritis
c. Labs including ANA, HIV, and ASO titers may be warranted
2. Radiologic testing
a. Renal ultrasound is first line
b. VCUG indicated for abnormal ultrasound or recurrent febrile UTIs
3. Other testing
a. Referral to nephrologist once persistent proteinuria is diagnosed
b. Kidney biopsy for persistent or worsening proteinuria

III. Approach to Hypertension

A. Background information
1. HTN is defined as a BP >95th percentile based on normal values for child's age, gender, and height, verified on ≥3 occasions
2. Differential diagnosis (Box 7-1)
a. Intrinsic renal disease
i. Acute (i.e., postinfectious) or chronic GN (i.e., lupus)
ii. Congenital structural abnormalities (i.e., ureteropelvic junction [UPJ] obstruction)
iii. Acute kidney injury (AKI), including during injury resolution
iv. PKD
v. Acute or chronic pyelonephritis, with renal scarring
vi. Renal dysplasia
vii. Wilms tumor
viii. Hemolytic-uremic syndrome (HUS)
b. Cardiovascular
i. Small- or large-vessel renal artery thrombosis
ii. Coarctation of aorta
iii. Midaortic syndrome (multiple vessel narrowing anywhere along course of aorta and its branches)
iv. Systemic vasculitides
c. Endocrine
i. Hyper- or hypothyroidism
ii. Hyperparathyroidism
iii. Pituitary tumors
iv. Pheochromocytoma, often episodic in nature, may be seen in patients with neurofibromatosis
v. Adrenal tumors
vi. Glucocorticoid or mineralocorticoid (aldosterone) excess syndromes
d. Essential HTN
i. Strong family history
ii. Often associated with obesity

BOX 7-1

Differential Diagnosis of Childhood Hypertension

Neonatal Period
Renal artery thrombosis (large-vessel or small distal branch stenosis)
Coarctation of the aorta
Inherited tubulopathy
Endocrine cause (thyroid, adrenal)
Central nervous system cause

Younger Children
Intrinsic renal disease (glomerulonephritis, chronic pyelonephritis)
Coarctation of the aorta
Renal vessel thrombosis
Essential hypertension

Older Children and Adolescents
Essential hypertension
Intrinsic renal disease (glomerulonephritis, chronic pyelonephritis, reflux nephropathy)
Renal vessel thrombosis

e. Central nervous system (CNS) disorders (e.g., tumors, bleeding, increased intracranial pressure [ICP])
f. Medications and ingestions: sympathomimetics (common cold medications), illicit drug use, stimulants used to treat attention-deficit hyperactivity disorder (ADHD), anabolic steroids, oral contraceptives
g. Tumors (Wilms, neuroblastoma, pheochromocytoma)
h. Others (hypercalcemia, anxiety, pain)

B. Historical questions
1. Symptoms of headaches, blurry vision, or dizziness?
2. Abdominal pain is often a presenting symptom in younger children
3. Swelling of eyes and legs in addition to dark-colored urine suggests GN
4. Flushing, sweating, palpitations, and episodic symptoms are concerning for an endocrine cause (e.g., thyroid disease or pheochromocytoma)
5. Rash, joint symptoms, and weight loss are symptoms associated with vasculitis
6. Urinary symptoms including polyuria, polydipsia, and nocturia are seen with renal concentrating defect in association with chronic intrinsic renal disease
7. In younger children, ask about neonatal course including umbilical lines, which predispose to renal vascular disease via microthrombi
8. Family history of childhood-onset HTN associated with tubulopathies, whereas adult onset is more consistent with essential HTN
9. Careful social history to assess for exposures, medications, drug use, diet (high salt intake), and exercise as risk factors for essential HTN

C. Physical examination findings
1. Vital signs
a. Ideally, BP should be recorded in upper extremity (UE) with proper-sized cuff, with patient sitting, calm, and comfortable
b. Assess heart rate to consider endocrine or medication causes
c. Check height: short stature may occur with chronic kidney disease (CKD)
2. Overall appearance and skin
a. Assess for flushing, acanthosis nigricans, obesity
b. Skin exam looking for café-au-lait spots indicating neurofibromatosis
3. Head and neck exam
a. Fundoscopic exam looking for retinal changes or papilledema
b. Thyroid examination
c. Tonsillar hypertrophy may be seen as cause of sleep apnea
4. Cardiovascular exam
a. Assess for murmurs and abdominal bruits
b. Femoral pulses to rule out coarctation (also consider if leg BP is lower than arm BP by $\geq$10 mm Hg)
5. Abdominal exam: flank masses or abdominal masses are concerning for tumors (Wilms and neuroblastoma), multicystic dysplastic kidneys, or PKD
6. GU exam: ambiguous genitalia to assess for adrenal etiology

D. Laboratory testing and radiologic imaging
1. Laboratory data
a. Urinalysis
i. Urine dipstick to assess for hematuria, proteinuria, infection, and urine-concentrating ability (specific gravity)
ii. If hematuria, perform urine microscopy on spun urine sample to look for casts or crystals
b. Serum electrolytes
i. Low potassium occurs with Liddle syndrome and renin excess
ii. High potassium in Gordon syndrome
iii. Albumin if concerned for GN, edema
c. Essential HTN: fasting glucose, lipids, and HbA1c if patient has metabolic syndrome
d. Plasma renin/aldosterone, thyroid hormones, and pheochromocytoma evaluation (catecholamine testing) if secondary HTN is suspected or if HTN remains severe

QUICK HIT

The younger the age and the higher the BP, the less likely the etiology is essential HTN.

QUICK HIT

Essential HTN is often associated with obesity, the metabolic syndrome, sleep apnea, and a positive family history of HTN.

QUICK HIT

An appropriate-sized BP cuff should cover 80% of the circumference of the upper arm and 2/3 the distance of the upper arm from the shoulder to elbow.

QUICK HIT

All new patients, regardless of age, need a 4-extremity BP to rule out coarctation of the aorta.

QUICK HIT

Signs of Cushing syndrome include ↑ BP, upper body obesity, thin and fragile skin, increased fat around the neck, and stretch marks.

QUICK HIT

BUN and creatinine to assess renal function.

QUICK HIT

Doppler ultrasound examination can often miss renal artery stenosis, especially smaller vessel disease.

e. Endocrine studies: adrenocorticotropic hormone (ACTH), parathyroid hormone (PTH), and cortisol
2. Radiologic imaging
   a. Renal ultrasound: highly informative test in children with HTN to assess kidney size and for presence of cysts, signs of CKD, and evidence of large-vessel disease
   b. Magnetic resonance angiography (MRA) or CT angiography can also be used to assess renal and thoracic/abdominal vessels if concerned for stenosis; however, gold standard remains angiography, requiring vascular access in femoral vein
   c. Echocardiogram (Echo) is useful to assess for left ventricular hypertrophy and end-organ damage from long-standing HTN
   d. Sensitive and specific abdominal imaging is often required if pheochromocytoma or an abdominal mass is suspected
   e. Consider sleep study if history concerning for sleep apnea

DISEASE SPECIFIC

IV. Acute Kidney Injury

A. General characteristics
1. Abrupt decline in renal function resulting in a decrease in glomerular filtration rate (GFR) usually characterized by 1 or all of the following
   a. Increased BUN
   b. Increased serum creatinine levels
   c. Decreased urine output (although can have nonoliguric AKI)
2. Dysfunction attributed to insult and consequent structural or functional changes
3. Results in disturbance of normal renal function including impaired nitrogenous waste excretion, water and electrolyte homeostasis, and acid–base regulation
4. Cause
   a. Etiology of derangements is related to where insult occurs in kidney, including in vasculature, glomerulus, renal tubules, and urinary tract
   b. Classified into 3 broad categories
      i. **Prerenal** (most common): severe volume depletion leads to decreased renal blood flow (RBF); nephrons remain structurally intact
      ii. **Intrinsic**: cytotoxic, ischemic, or inflammatory renal insults result in structural/functional damage to glomerulus/tubules with release of renal afferent vasoconstrictors
      iii. **Postrenal**: obstruction of urine
         (a) Initially causes increase in tubular pressure proximal to obstruction, thereby decreasing filtration driving force
         (b) This increase in pressure, in turn, causes renal damage, resulting in decreased renal function (Table 7-3)

TABLE 7-3 Etiologies of Acute Renal Failure

Prerenal	Intrinsic	Postrenal
Volume depletion	**Vascular**	**Urinary tract obstruction**
Gastrointestinal losses (vomiting, diarrhea)	Renal artery or vein obstruction	Posterior urethral valves
Renal losses (diuretics, polyuria)	Hemolytic-uremic syndrome	Renal stones
Cutaneous losses (burns, Stevens-Johnson syndrome)	Vasculitis	Tumors
Hemorrhage	**Glomerular**	Strictures
Decreased effective circulating volume	Acute glomerulonephritis	Obstructed Foley catheter
Congestive heart failure	**Tubular**	
Liver disease	Acute tubular necrosis	
Nephrotic syndrome	**Interstitial**	
Shock	Acute interstitial nephritis	
	Infection	
	Systemic disease (sarcoid, lupus, lymphoma, leukemia)	

TABLE 7-4 **Nephrotoxic Agents**

Drug Class	Specific Drugs
Antimicrobials	Aminoglycosides, amphotericin, acyclovir, penicillins, cephalosporins, sulfonamides, rifampin
Nonsteroidal anti-inflammatory drugs (NSAIDs)	Ibuprofen, naproxen
Immunosuppressive agents	Calcineurin inhibitors, indinavir, methotrexate, pentamidine, cisplatin, ifosfamide
Psychiatric	Lithium
Antihypertensives	ACE inhibitors, ARB
Other	Radiocontrast agents

ACE, angiotensin-converting enzyme; ARB, angiotensin receptor blocker.

5. Risk factors for increased severity: during periods of depressed RBF, kidneys are particularly vulnerable to further insults
   a. Pre-existing renal disease
   b. Chronic medical problems
   c. Hospitalization
   d. Exposure to nephrotoxic agents (Table 7-4)
6. Pathophysiology
   a. Driving force for glomerular filtration is pressure gradient from glomerulus to Bowman space
   b. Glomerular pressure is primarily dependent on RBF and is controlled by combined resistances of renal afferent and efferent arterioles
   c. Regardless of cause of AKI, reductions in RBF represent common pathologic pathway for decreasing GFR

B. Clinical features
1. Historical question to establish the underlying diagnosis
   a. Has the child had decreased drinking, decreased urine output, vomiting, or diarrhea? *Severe dehydration can cause AKI*
   b. Is the child taking medications? *Nephrotoxic medications cause AKI*
2. Physical exam findings: pay careful attention to volume status (i.e., do they appear fluid depleted or overloaded) and for findings from systemic diseases that can cause renal dysfunction (e.g., rashes, arthritis, abdominal masses)

C. Diagnosis
1. Differential diagnosis: depends on classification
2. Laboratory findings (Table 7-5)
3. Radiology and pathology findings
   a. Renal ultrasound
      i. Depending on etiology of AKI, renal ultrasound may reveal kidney enlargement and dilation of collecting system
      ii. Doppler studies of renal vasculature can also show decreased flow in diseases that obstruct RBF
   b. Renal radioisotope scan: delineates areas of normal or low perfusion associated with poor renal function and areas of parenchymal damage by showing delay in accumulation of radioisotope
   c. CT scan of abdomen and pelvis: may reveal masses or other structural abnormalities that could be contributing to AKI
4. Other findings
   a. Renal biopsy: pathologic findings depend on underlying etiology

D. Treatment: medical management
1. Maintaining renal perfusion and fluid and electrolyte balance
2. Controlling BP
3. Treating anemia
4. Providing adequate nutrition

QUICK HIT

Nonsteroidal anti-inflammatory drugs, antibiotics like gentamicin and vancomycin, and antihypertensives like angiotensin-converting enzyme inhibitors, diuretics, and β-blockers are among the drugs that can cause AKI.

QUICK HIT

Normal serum concentrations of creatinine vary by age: infant = 0.2–0.5 mg/dL, child = 0.3–0.7 mg/dL, and adolescent = 0.5–1.0 mg/dL.

QUICK HIT

Fractional excretion of sodium (FENa) differentiates prerenal AKI from intrinsic injury. To calculate: FENa = [(urine sodium × serum creatinine)/(serum sodium × urine creatinine)] × 100.

QUICK HIT

In patients with mild reversible AKI, or in whom the cause is understood, further imaging may not be warranted.

TABLE 7-5 Laboratory Abnormalities in Acute Kidney Injury

Serum Electrolyte Derangements	Urine Electrolyte and Sediment Derangements	Other Laboratory Studies
Hyponatremia	Low urine sodium (prerenal)	CBC • Anemia, may be seen with hemolytic-uremic syndrome • Severe hemolysis may result in AKI • Eosinophilia may be seen in interstitial nephritis
Hyperkalemia (occurs due to decreased renal excretion)	Fractional excretion of sodium • <1%: prerenal etiology • >2%: intrinsic etiology	Streptococcal antibodies (ASO, anti-DNAse B) to rule out poststreptococcal GN
Metabolic acidosis (occurs due to decreased urinary excretion of hydrogen ions)	Urine osmolality • High in prerenal • Low in intrinsic renal causes	Complement studies (C3 and C4) • Low C3: poststreptococcal GN, membranoproliferative GN • Low C3 and C4: systemic lupus erythematosus
Hyperphosphatemia (occurs due to decreased renal excretion)	Red blood cell casts are diagnostic for GN	Hepatitis B and C panels as a possible cause for postinfectious GN
Elevated BUN and creatinine	Hematuria • GN • Renal vein thrombosis • Renal calculi	Serologic studies • Antineutrophil cytoplasmic antibodies (ANCAs) • Antinuclear antibodies (ANAs) • Anti–glomerular basement membrane (GBM) antibodies
Elevated uric acid levels in tumor lysis syndrome	Proteinuria may be seen with glomerular disease White blood cells with granular or waxy casts with mild to moderate proteinuria suggest tubular or interstitial disease Urine eosinophils may suggest interstitial nephritis	

AKI, acute kidney injury; ASO, antistreptolysin O; BUN, blood urea nitrogen; CBC, complete blood count; GN, glomerulonephritis.

QUICK HIT

Mortality rates are variable and depend on underlying cause rather than AKI itself.

QUICK HIT

Medical management may be necessary for a prolonged period to treat the sequelae of AKI, including CKD, HTN, renal tubular acidosis, and urinary concentrating defects.

QUICK HIT

GFR is an index of functioning renal mass and is often estimated from creatinine-based formulas.

5. Adjusting medications for degree of renal impairment
6. Initiating renal replacement therapy (dialysis) when indicated
7. Whether a patient with AKI should be cared for on the wards or in an intensive care unit (ICU) depends on his or her clinical severity

E. Duration/prognosis
1. Prognosis for recovery of renal function depends on underlying cause of AKI
   a. Recovery is likely if AKI is secondary to prerenal causes, HUS, acute tubular necrosis (ATN), acute interstitial nephritis, or tumor lysis
   b. Recovery is unusual when AKI is due to rapidly progressive GN, bilateral renal vein thrombosis, or bilateral cortical necrosis

V. Chronic Kidney Disease

A. Characteristics
1. Definition
   a. GFR <60 mL/min/1.73 m^2, abnormal renal pathology, or kidney damage lasting ≥ 3 months
   b. 5 stages
2. Epidemiology
   a. Incidence of 6–12 per million children
   b. Prevalence of 20–75 per million children
3. Cause
   a. Glomerular disease
   b. Renal dysplasia/obstructive uropathy
   c. Vascular disease
4. Genetics: several inherited diseases are associated with developing CKD
   a. Congenital nephrotic syndrome
   b. Early-onset focal segmental glomerulosclerosis (FSGS)
   c. *WT1* mutations (Frasier and Denys-Drash syndromes)

d. PKD (autosomal recessive or dominant)
e. Nephronophthisis/medullary cystic kidney disease
f. Alport syndrome (hematuria and deafness)
g. Others (e.g., Dent disease, cystinosis)
5. Risk factors for progression include HTN and proteinuria
6. Pathophysiology
a. Usually develops as a consequence of a primary renal insult
b. Rate of kidney disease progression is variable, being fast in glomerular disease and slower in renal dysplasia/obstructive uropathy
c. Kidney damage is often associated with proteinuria, which causes inflammation and further renal damage.

B. Clinical features
1. Historical findings
a. Is there a history of recurrent UTIs?
b. Is there a family history of deafness (Alport syndrome: progressive hereditary nephritis and deafness)
c. Is there a history of polyuria, polydipsia, or nocturia, suggesting a renal concentrating defect, as seen in renal dysplasia?
d. Is there a history of chronic nonsteroidal anti-inflammatory drug (NSAID) use?
e. Is there a history of growth delay?
f. Are there rashes or joint symptoms as may occur with SLE?
g. Are there constitutional symptoms (fatigue, weight loss, nausea) suggesting severe renal dysfunction?
2. Physical exam findings
a. General appearance and vital signs
i. Assess for signs of dehydration including tachycardia, dry mucous membranes, sunken fontanelle, and weight loss
ii. Assess for poor growth or inadequate weight gain
b. Abdominal exam: careful abdominal exam for palpable kidneys, which may indicate PKD or bruit as seen in renal vascular disease
c. Musculoskeletal examination
i. Observe for edema associated with nephrotic syndrome
ii. Signs of rickets due to metabolic bone disease
iii. Joint inflammation suggesting SLE or other systemic disorders
iv. Sacral dimple or midline defects over lumbosacral region that may be sign of tethered cord and possible neurogenic bladder
d. GU exam: assess genitalia for appropriate development
e. Skin exam: pallor if significant anemia
f. Respiratory and cardiovascular exam: rales (e.g., fluid overload) or pericardial friction rub (e.g., severe uremia)
g. Eyes: fundoscopic exam should be performed to look for signs of HTN

C. Diagnosis
1. Differential diagnosis
a. Very broad, representing final common pathway of many renal diseases
b. Divide into general categories
i. Glomerular/inflammatory
ii. Dysplasia/obstructive
iii. Vascular (i.e., HUS)
2. Laboratory findings (Table 7-6)
3. Radiology findings
a. Renal ultrasound
i. Can assess renal size and identify structural anomalies
ii. Also evaluate for renal cysts, presence of nephrocalcinosis or renal calculi, and any evidence of obstruction and hydronephrosis
iii. Determine degree of corticomedullary differentiation
b. Bladder ultrasound
i. Look for thickened bladder wall (e.g., posterior urethral valves [PUVs])
ii. High postvoid residual may signify bladder dysfunction

QUICK HIT
The U.S. has one of the highest prevalence rates of kidney disease, including the need for dialysis, in the world.

QUICK HIT
The most common cause of CKD in children is congenital anomalies of the kidney, including obstructive uropathy, renal dysplasia, reflux nephropathy, and PKD.

QUICK HIT
Proteinuria both serves as a marker of kidney damage and causes further renal scarring through inflammatory pathways.

QUICK HIT
Recurrent UTI is an extremely rare cause of CKD. However, it is associated with reflux nephropathy.

QUICK HIT
Kidneys may be palpable in a relaxed normal newborn, but it is difficult to do. Outside of the newborn period, palpable kidneys warrant a renal ultrasound.

QUICK HIT
Ear pits and tags are often associated with renal abnormalities.

TABLE 7-6 Laboratory Assessment in Chronic Kidney Disease

Assessment	Laboratory Test Components	Typical Findings in Chronic Kidney Disease
Simple urinalysis (dipstick analysis)	Blood Protein Specific gravity Leukocyte esterase Glucose	Hematuria Proteinuria Dilute urine: concentrating defects Pyuria Glucosuria: tubular dysfunction
Urine microscopy	Casts Crystals	Red cell casts: glomerulonephritis White cell casts: glomerulonephritis, pyelonephritis Calcium, uric acid
Urine protein assessment	First-morning-void urine protein:creatinine ratio 24-hour urine collection (more difficult to perform in children)	>0.2 is abnormal >2 is nephrotic Quantify proteinuria
Basic metabolic panel	Creatinine Blood urea nitrogen Bicarbonate Potassium	Assess kidney function in context of muscle mass Elevated due to renal dysfunction, gastrointestinal bleeding, steroids, catabolic states Acidosis Hyperkalemia
Complete blood count	Hemoglobin Platelet count	Anemia Thrombocytopenia in hemolytic-uremic syndrome
Nutrition	Serum albumin	Low in poor nutrition and nephrotic syndrome
Iron studies	Ferritin Iron Transferrin	Acute phase reactant, so may be elevated in iron deficiency Iron deficiency anemia Low transferrin saturation
Bone disease	Parathyroid hormone Vitamin D Calcium Phosphate	Hyperparathyroidism 25-OH deficiency Hypocalcemia Hyperphosphatemia
Cardiovascular	Fasting lipid panel	Hypercholesterolemia from chronic kidney disease or nephrotic syndrome

QUICK HIT

Sensorineural hearing loss in Alport syndrome is very rare in infancy, but commonly presents before age 30 years.

QUICK HIT

Calcitriol is 1,25-OH vitamin D. In chronic kidney disease, the kidney is less efficient at metabolizing 25-OH vitamin D to 1,25-OH vitamin D. Therefore, these patients may not respond to simple vitamin D supplementation and need calcitriol.

QUICK HIT

In severe kidney disease, a PTH too high leads to renal osteodystrophy; a PTH too low leads to adynamic bone disease.

c. Nuclear medicine scanning
   i. Dimercaptosuccinic acid (DMSA) scan to identify cortical scarring
   ii. Technetium-99m mercaptoacetyltriglycine (MAG-3) study will look for obstruction
   iii. Diethylene triamine pentaacetic acid (DTPA) to calculate GFR
d. Hearing screen: Alport syndrome is cause of hereditary nephritis associated with sensorineural hearing loss
e. Echo: Identifies left ventricular hypertrophy due to long-standing HTN

D. Treatment
1. Therapy
   a. Anemia: recombinant erythropoietin and iron supplementation
   b. Bone disease
      i. Calcium supplementation to prevent renal osteodystrophy
      ii. Restrict dietary phosphate and use phosphate binders (e.g., calcium carbonate)
      iii. Vitamin D analogs (calcitriol) may be added if PTH is too high
   c. Cardiovascular disease: aggressive treatment of HTN to prevent cardiovascular damage and to slow the progression of renal disease
      i. Low-salt diet and daily exercise are encouraged
      ii. Lipid-lowering therapy may be added as needed

d. Electrolyte abnormalities
   i. Hyperkalemia is treated with Lasix, Kayexalate, and dialysis
   ii. Patients with CKD who are not getting dialysis often receive sodium citrate or sodium bicarbonate to protect against bicarbonate loss from the kidney and metabolic acidosis
e. Nutrition: maximize nutrition, which may require caloric supplements and tube feeding; growth hormone (GH) is approved for use in CKD
f. Psychosocial: provide counseling for children and families, monitor school performance, and provide physical and occupational therapy
g. Renal replacement therapy may included hemodialysis, peritoneal dialysis, and kidney transplant

2. Complications
   a. Cardiovascular disease remains primary cause of morbidity and mortality for both children and adults with CKD
   b. Poor growth is common due to anemia, acidosis, chronic inflammation, metabolic bone derangements, poor nutrition, and uremia
   c. Although kidney transplant is goal if end-stage renal disease (ESRD) develops, transplant patients still live with many risks, including rejection, infection, malignancy, and a high rate of cardiovascular disease
3. Prognosis
   a. Depends on underlying renal disease and individual patient factors
      i. Glomerular disease typically progresses faster
      ii. Dysplasia typically progresses slower
   b. Renal progression often accelerates during periods of rapid growth (infancy and adolescence), as diminished renal mass must try to keep up with increased metabolic waste products from growing child
4. Prevention
   a. *Aggressive treatment of HTN* includes keeping BP <90th percentile; some advocate <50th percentile to maximize renal protection
   b. *Aggressive treatment of proteinuria*: angiotensin-converting enzyme (ACE) inhibitors and angiotensin receptor blockers (ARBs) are preferred

> **QUICK HIT**
> Children on dialysis have a worse quality of life than do children with cancer.

> **QUICK HIT**
> Transplantation should be the goal for every child on dialysis.

> **QUICK HIT**
> During the 2 periods of rapid growth, infancy and puberty, the rate of CKD progression will increase.

> **QUICK HIT**
> ACE inhibitors are preferred for CKD.

VI. Nephrotic Syndrome

A. Characteristics
1. Definition
   a. Characterized by following clinical and laboratory findings
      i. Proteinuria
      ii. Hypoalbuminemia
      iii. Edema
      iv. Hyperlipidemia
   b. Group of renal diseases that are result of **injury to glomerular filtration barrier**, thus leading to increased permeability of membrane to large and small proteins
   c. Diffuse foot process effacement on electron microscopy; minimal changes (minimal change disease [MCD]), FSGS, or mesangial proliferation on light microscopy
2. Epidemiology
   a. **Primary nephrotic syndrome**: nephrotic syndrome without systemic disease
      i. More common in children age <6 years
      ii. **Idiopathic nephrotic syndrome** is most common form of nephrotic syndrome in children
         (a) >90% of children present between ages 1–10 years
         (b) Includes MCD, primary FSGS, and mesangial proliferation
   b. **Secondary nephrotic syndrome**
      i. Associated with systemic disease or secondary to another process that causes glomerular injury
      ii. Includes membranous nephropathy (SLE or medication induced; i.e., NSAIDs), secondary FSGS from nephron loss secondary to renal scarring or hypoplasia, postinfectious GN, and vasculitis (HSP, Wegener granulomatosis, SLE)

> **QUICK HIT**
> The typical presentation of minimal change disease is nephrotic syndrome in a child age <6 years, absence of HTN and absence of gross hematuria, normal complement levels, and normal renal function.

> **QUICK HIT**
> The lack of findings on microscopy are why we call it "minimal change disease." In reality, this disease often relapses, can be very frustrating, and often requires prolonged courses of steroids.

3. Genetics: steroid-resistant nephrotic syndrome
   a. Some patients with familial and sporadic cases have *NPHS2* mutation, which encodes for podocin, a membrane protein in glomerular podocytes; these patients frequently progress to ESRD
   b. *WT1* mutation: Wilms tumor suppressor gene in sporadic cases (Frasier or Denys-Drash syndrome)
   c. *NPHS1* mutation: encodes nephrin, associated with Finnish-type congenital nephrotic syndrome, a severe form that presents within first 3 months of life
4. Pathophysiology of nephrotic syndrome

B. Clinical features
1. Symptoms and signs
   a. Present with edema often after minor illness/event (URI, insect bite)
      i. Dependent edema, often periorbital or sacral in morning with LE (including scrotal edema) developing by evening
      ii. Generalized edema and anasarca are possible
   b. Abdominal pain and/or peritonitis
   c. Dyspnea due to pleural effusions or ascites
   d. Headache, irritability, malaise, and fatigue
   e. HTN and gross hematuria are infrequent
   f. Tachycardia, peripheral vasoconstriction, orthostatic BP, and oliguria are possible due to decreased effective circulating volume (Figure 7-3)

C. Diagnosis
1. Differential diagnosis: all are causes of generalized edema
   a. Heart failure
   b. Hypoalbuminemia (e.g., protein-losing enteropathy, kwashiorkor)
   c. Acute GN, renal failure
   d. Cirrhosis
   e. Sepsis or severe burns
   f. Eye swelling often mistaken for seasonal allergies
2. Laboratory findings: establish nephrotic range proteinuria and hypoalbuminemia, and hyperlipidemia
   a. Urinalysis: screening test; quantitative protein excretion studies if **3+/4+**
   b. Urinary protein excretion of >50 mg/kg/day or 40 mg/m²/hr or total protein:creatinine ratio >2 mg protein/mg creatinine on a spot urine
   c. Serum albumin <3 g/dL; may be <1 g/dL
   d. Hyperlipidemia: especially elevated serum total cholesterol, but triglycerides and total lipids may be elevated as well
   e. CBC: increased hemoglobin and hematocrit due to hemoconcentration and thrombocytosis, which may contribute to hypercoagulability
   f. Electrolytes: hyponatremia secondary to decreased water excretion
   g. BUN, creatinine

QUICK HIT

Edema is more common in gravity-dependent areas of the body.

QUICK HIT

When a patient presents with periorbital edema, do not assume it is due to seasonal allergies; *always* check a urinalysis to evaluate for nephrotic syndrome.

QUICK HIT

A trace of 1+ for protein on a urine dipstick is very unlikely to be nephrotic syndrome.

QUICK HIT

Start with a protein: creatinine ratio. A 24-hour urine is challenging to obtain in children.

QUICK HIT

Hyperlipidemia in nephrotic syndrome occurs because
1. ↓ protein stimulates protein production in the liver, resulting in ↑ production of lipoproteins.
2. Lower levels of lipoprotein lipase result in decreased lipid catabolism.

FIGURE 7-3 Five-year-old girl with nephrotic syndrome.

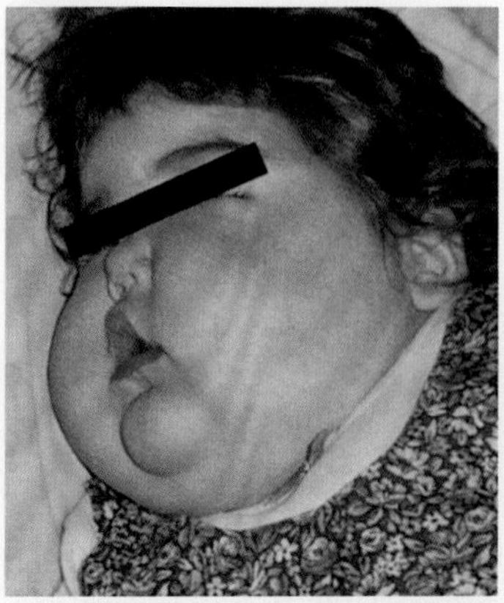

(From Fleisher GR, Ludwig W, Baskin MN. *Atlas of Pediatric Emergency Medicine*. Philadelphia: Lippincott Williams & Wilkins; 2004.)

h. ANA for children age >10 years or with signs of SLE
i. Hepatitis B and C and HIV as infectious causes of nephrotic syndrome
j. Complement studies: helpful in diagnosis of specific entity or systemic disease presenting with nephrotic syndrome
   i. Low C3: MPGN and postinfectious GN
   ii. Low C3 and C4: lupus nephritis

3. Renal biopsy is indicated for children with characteristics inconsistent with MCD, which include
   a. Age <1 year and >10 years old
   b. HTN, gross hematuria, or elevation of serum creatinine
   c. Abnormal complement levels
   d. Extrarenal symptoms (malar rash, purpura, recurrent fever, arthritis)
   e. Renal failure
   f. Steroid-resistant nephrotic syndrome

D. Treatment
1. Therapy
   a. Steroid-sensitive nephrotic syndrome occurs in >90% with MCD
   b. Steroid-resistant nephrotic syndrome: patients should have renal biopsy to determine underlying cause and guide future therapy; these patients have an increased risk of developing ESRD
   c. Immunosuppressive therapy is generally *not* effective in treating children with genetic causes (*NPHS2*, *NPHS1*, or *WT1* mutations)
   d. Management
      i. Initial therapy: prednisone 2 mg/kg/day for 6 weeks, followed by 1.5 mg/kg every other day for an additional 6 weeks
      ii. First relapse: prednisone 2 mg/kg/day until negative urine protein × 3 days, followed by a taper over 1 month
      iii. Frequent relapses: prednisone 2 mg/kg/day until urine protein negative for 3 consecutive days, a taper over 2–3 months; immunosuppressive agents (e.g., cyclophosphamide) may be used to sustain remission
      iv. **Steroid-dependent disease**: prednisone unless toxicity develops; immunosuppressive agents (e.g., cyclophosphamide, cyclosporine) may be used to reduce steroid dependence
      v. **Steroid-resistant disease**: based on renal biopsy's histologic findings; steroids stopped, but no optimal approach exists
         (a) **Second-line agents**: tacrolimus, cyclosporine, mycophenolate, rituximab
2. Complications
   a. 4%–5% of children with MCD eventually develop **ESRD** or die from complications, likely from progressing to FSGS
   b. Complications due to long-term steroid use include growth impairment, cataracts, excessive weight gain, osteoporosis (not proven in children), and suppression of the hypothalamic–pituitary axis (HPA)
   c. Side effects are also possible from use of steroid-sparing medications
   d. Impaired immunity and increased risk of infection
      i. Increased risk of infection due to encapsulated organisms (i.e., *Streptococcus pneumoniae*) in addition to gram-negative organisms and some viruses, including varicella and measles
      ii. Patients may present with spontaneous bacterial peritonitis, pneumonia, or overwhelming sepsis
   e. Thrombosis secondary to hypercoagulability
3. Duration/prognosis
   a. Steroid-responsive nephrotic syndrome
      i. 30% will never relapse; cured with 1st course of steroids
      ii. 30%–40% have frequent relapses (>4/year)
      iii. 90% respond within 4 weeks of starting steroids
      iv. Factors associated with better prognosis
         (a) Shorter response time to steroids
         (b) No relapse within first 6 months of treatment

QUICK HIT

Majority of children with idiopathic nephrotic syndrome are responsive to **glucocorticoids**; most of these patients have MCD.

QUICK HIT

There is some support to identify genetic mutations before starting therapy to avoid unnecessary exposure and side effects from immunosuppressive therapy.

QUICK HIT

Angiotensin antagonism: ACE inhibitors and angiotensin II receptor blockers slow progression of proteinuric renal failure in adults; there are no data in children, but these are used for children with persistent proteinuria.

QUICK HIT

Response to steroids, rather than histologic features on renal biopsy, is better at predicting long-term prognosis.

VII. Glomerulonephritis

A. Characteristics

1. Definition: variety of renal disorders characterized by inflammation of glomeruli or small blood vessels of kidneys, which manifests as hematuria, proteinuria, and RBC casts; various degrees of HTN and renal insufficiency
   a. Injury is typically immunologically mediated; can be due to primary renal disease, systemic diseases, infection, or other inciting event
   b. Categorized into several different pathologic patterns
2. Epidemiology
   a. In U.S., GN represents 10%–15% of glomerular diseases and comprises 25%–30% of all cases of ESRD
   b. Worldwide, IgA nephropathy is most common cause of GN
   c. Incidence of PSGN has decreased in most Western countries but is more common in developing countries
3. Etiology (Figure 7-4)
   a. Primary GN
      i. MPGN: idiopathic form exists although more commonly secondary to SLE, hepatitis B, and hepatitis C
      ii. **Rapidly progressive GN (RPGN)**: clinical syndrome with progressive loss of renal function over short days to months
      iii. **Berger disease (IgA nephropathy)**: most common cause of primary GN; most common in Caucasians and Asians; 40%–50% of patients present with hematuria following URI
   b. Secondary GN
      i. **Acute postinfectious GN (PIGN)**: symptoms usually develop 1–3 weeks after an acute infection
         (a) Most common cause is **group A β-hemolytic strep (PSGN)**
         (b) Less commonly, staphylococci, mycobacteria, Epstein-Barr virus (EBV), cytomegalovirus (CMV), hepatitis B, coxsackievirus, rubella, and rickettsial infections
      ii. **Systemic disease**: including **HSP**, granulomatosis with polyangiitis (formerly Wegener granulomatosis), hypersensitivity vasculitis, polyarteritis nodosa, **collagen vascular diseases**, and cryoglobulinemia

QUICK HIT

Antibiotic treatment of group A β-hemolytic strep infections *does not* reduce the risk of acute PSGN.

FIGURE 7-4 **Categorization of glomerulonephritis.**

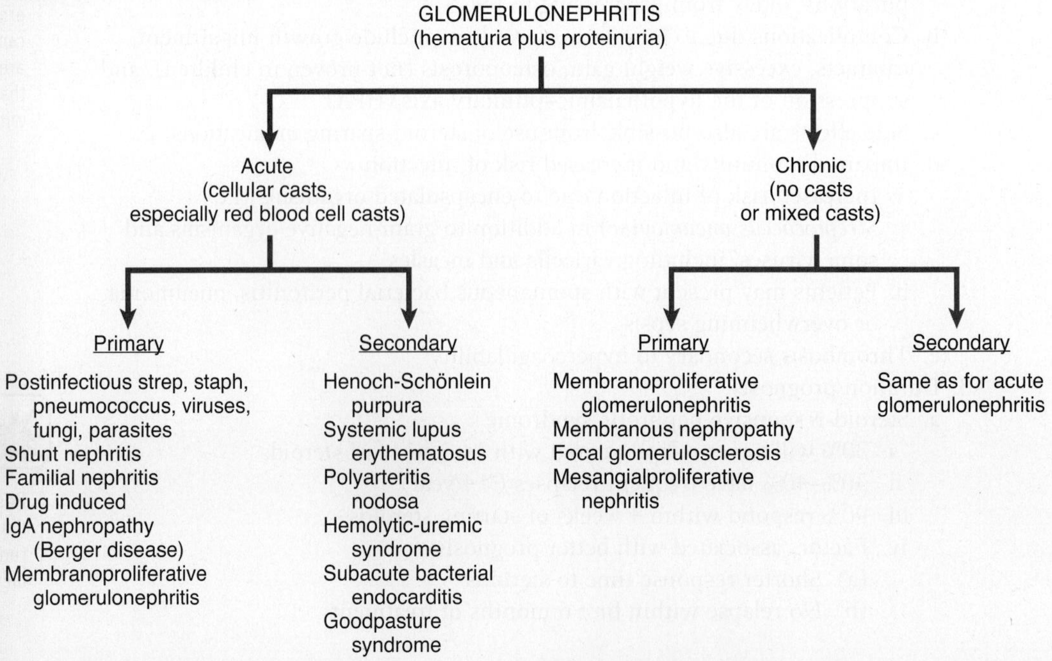

TABLE 7-7 History and Physical Exam Findings in Glomerulonephritis

History	Physical Exam Findings
Dark-colored urine	Signs offluid overload • Periorbital and/or lower extremity edema • Hypertension, rates or dyspnea, ascites, weight gain
Underlying systemic disease • History of sinusitis, rash, hemoptysis, arthralgias	Rash
Recent infection • Usually 1–4 weeks prior to admission	Pallor
Nonspecific symptoms • Fever, fatigue, sore throat, abdominal or flank pain	Joint edema or erythema
Facial, eyelid, lower extremity edema	Altered mental status
Shortness of breath	Pharyngitis, impetigo, or other indications of upper respiratory tract infection
Poor appetite, changes in weight	Heart murmur

iii. Miscellaneous causes, including Guillain-Barré syndrome, irradiation of Wilms tumor, diptheria, tetanus, and pertussis (DTaP) vaccine, and serum sickness

4. Risk factors
   a. Individuals with various medical disorders are at greater risk for developing GN: group A streptococcal (GAS) infections, collagen vascular diseases, vasculitis
   b. Some medications predispose to GN (e.g., NSAIDs)
5. Pathophysiology
   a. May be caused by primary renal disease or systemic disease
   b. Glomerular lesions can be result of immune complex deposition
   c. Structural changes in glomerulus
      i. Can be **focal**, **diffuse**, **segmental**, or **global**
      ii. Can be result of **proliferation** of **endothelial**, **mesangial**, and **epithelial cells**, leading to increased number of cells in glomerular tuft
      iii. May cause glomerular basement membrane thickening
      iv. May lead to irreversible injury indicated by sclerosis
   d. Functional changes
      i. Proteinuria, hematuria, reduction in GFR, and RBCs and RBC casts in urine
      ii. Decreased GFR and sodium and water retention lead to **expansion of intravascular volume**; edema; and, consequently, **systemic HTN**

QUICK HIT

PSGN and HUS are examples of glomerulonephritis where renal biopsy is rarely indicated.

B. Clinical features: history and physical exam findings consistent with GN are shown in Table 7-7

C. Diagnosis
1. Differential diagnosis: important to consider underlying cause of GN
   a. Renal (acute renal failure, nephrotic syndrome, interstitial nephritis)
   b. Systemic (HUS, rheumatic fever, endocarditis, rhabdomyolysis)
2. Laboratory findings of GN (Table 7-8)
3. Other findings
   a. Renal biopsy
      i. Confirms diagnosis, evaluates extent of injury, and has prognostic implications
      ii. Not necessary for diagnosis of PSGN
   b. Renal ultrasound to evaluate kidney size
   c. Other studies can be considered based on clinical presentation and concern for underlying causes

QUICK HIT

Acute PSGN will initially present with a low complement (C3) level; this should normalize within 6 weeks.

D. Treatment
1. Therapy: *target therapy to underlying etiology of GN*
   a. Sodium and fluid restriction
   b. Monitoring of renal function, BP, and urinalysis
   c. Consultation with nephrologist may be indicated

TABLE 7-8 Laboratory Evaluation in Patients with Glomerulonephritis

Urine Studies	Serum Studies	Other Studies

• Urinalysis and sediment
  • Gross or microscopic hematuria
  • Red blood cell casts
  • Urine protein > 100 mg/m^2 per day
  • Sterile pyuria and/or WBC casts
• Urine electrolytes, fractional excretion of sodium (FENa)
	• Serum electrolytes
	  • Na, K, CO_2, Ca, Mg, Phos
	• Blood urea nitrogen
	• Serum creatinine
	• CBC
	• Blood culture
	• Erythrocyte sedimentation rate
	• Viral serologies
		• Complement levels
		  • Low C3: PSGN
		  • Low C3 and C4: SLE, shunt nephritis, nephritis due to subacute bacterial endocarditis
		• ANA, anti-DNA antibodies
		• ASO, anti-DNAse B antibodies
		• ANCA, IgA, GBM antibodies

ANA, antinuclear antibody; ANCA, antineutrophil cytoplasmic antibody; ASO, antistreptolysin O; CBC, complete blood count; PSGN, poststreptococcal glomerulonephritis; SLE, systemic lupus erythematosus; WBC, white blood cell.

2. Complications: may require close monitoring in inpatient or ICU setting
   a. Hypertensive encephalopathy
   b. Pulmonary edema
   c. Significant renal failure or uremia requiring dialysis
3. Duration/prognosis
   a. Most patients completely recover
   b. Mortality of acute GN in pediatric patients reported at 0%–7%
   c. Sporadic cases of acute nephritis can progress to chronic form
   d. Favorable long-term prognosis in acute PSGN
      i. *>98% of patients asymptomatic after 5 years*
      ii. CKD reported in 1%–3% of cases
   e. Prognosis for nonstreptococcal PIGN depends on underlying pathogen; worse in patients with significant proteinuria, HTN, and significant elevations of creatinine
   f. Other causes of GN have outcomes varying from complete recovery to complete renal failure

QUICK HIT

Histologic hallmark is **interstitial inflammatory cell infiltration**, including neutrophils, lymphocytes, and eosinophils.

QUICK HIT

The list of drugs that can cause interstitial nephritis is long. NSAIDs, a variety of antibiotics, diuretics, and antivirals are the most common.

MNEMONIC

Causes of Eosinophilia on CBC
N = neoplasm, nephritis
A = allergy/asthma
A = Addison disease
C = collagen vascular disease, chlamydia
P = parasites

VIII. Interstitial Nephritis

A. Definitions
   1. Renal injury resulting in acute or chronic decline in renal function
   2. Involves inflammation of renal interstitium
B. Cause/pathophysiology
   1. Multiple causes involving 3 main categories
      a. Drugs
      b. Infection
      c. Autoimmune disease
C. Clinical presentation
   1. Patients may present with range of features, from asymptomatic elevation of BUN and creatinine, to AKI with generalized symptoms
   2. Generalized symptoms include fever, rash, arthralgia, as well as malaise, anorexia, nausea, vomiting, flank pain, polyuria, and polydipsia
D. Testing
   1. Diagnosis includes obtaining a thorough history
      a. Recent medications or drug use
      b. Recent illness
   2. Laboratory evaluation
      a. CBC may reveal eosinophilia
      b. **Urine eosinophils** may be seen
      c. Basic metabolic panel to assess elevation in BUN and creatinine
      d. Urinalysis may reveal proteinuria, WBCs, RBCs, and WBC casts; RBC casts are *not* seen
      e. Dilute urine (low specific gravity) is often a clue

3. May require renal biopsy for pathologic evaluation
4. May need ophthalmology exam (tubulointerstitial nephritis/uveitis syndrome)

E. Therapy
1. Disease self-limited when cause determined and eliminated
2. Supportive care indicated: hydration with fluid and electrolyte management, symptomatic treatment of fevers and other systemic symptoms; rarely, dialysis
3. Expect improvement within several weeks
4. Steroid and immunosuppressive use controversial and usually reserved for complex, biopsy-confirmed cases

QUICK HIT

It is critical to stop any medications that might be causing interstitial nephritis, but in some cases, such as mild nephritis from acyclovir, the drug may be continued if therapy is important and other options do not exist.

IX. Renal Tubular Acidosis (RTA)

A. Characteristics
1. Definition: group of transport defects in nephron characterized by inability to either reabsorb bicarbonate or excrete hydrogen
2. Pathophysiology
   a. Type 1 (distal RTA): impairment in hydrogen ion secretion in distal tubule leads to inability to acidify urine, resulting in a urine pH >5.5
      i. Plasma HCO_3^- is usually <15 mEq/L
      ii. Potassium reabsorption is impaired, leading to **hypokalemia**
      iii. Hypercalciuria and decreased citrate excretion often present
      iv. May be primary or secondary
      v. Secondary type 1 RTA may result from various disorders (cirrhosis, autoimmune disease, sickle cell disease) or drug exposures (lithium, amphotericin B)
   b. Type 2 (proximal RTA): impairment in HCO_3^- reabsorption in proximal tubules leading to urinary bicarbonate wasting and acidosis
      i. Normal bicarbonate reabsorption threshold reset leading to bicarbonate wasting
      ii. Urine pH <5.5 if plasma HCO_3^- concentration depleted from ongoing losses; urine pH >7 if HCO_3^- concentration is normal
      iii. Usually associated with increased urinary excretion of glucose, uric acid, phosphate, amino acids, citrate, Ca, K, and protein (generalized proximal tubular dysfunction = Fanconi syndrome)
      iv. Various inherited and acquired etiologies including Fanconi syndrome, drugs (sulfa, acetazolamide, tetracycline), vitamin D deficiency, renal transplantation, and heavy metal exposure
   c. Type 4 (generalized RTA): occurs secondary to aldosterone deficiency or impairment of distal tubule's response to aldosterone
      i. Urine pH is usually appropriate for serum pH (usually <5.5 when there is serum acidosis)
      ii. Plasma HCO_3^- is usually >17 mEq/L
      iii. Aldosterone deficiency (reduced K secretion and hyperkalemia)
      iv. Most common type of RTA; typically occurs sporadically
      v. Factors that can lead to type 4 RTA include ACE inhibitor or ARB use, CKD (diabetic nephropathy), congenital adrenal hyperplasia, critical illness, HIV nephropathy, obstruction, and medications (cyclosporine, potassium-sparing diuretics, NSAIDs)

QUICK HIT

RTA is associated with a normal serum anion gap metabolic acidosis.

QUICK HIT

Type 2 RTA can lead to rickets secondary to losses of calcium and phosphate in the urine and alterations in vitamin D metabolism.

QUICK HIT

Aldosterone "resorbs Na and spits out K." For type 4 RTA, acidosis is usually mild, and high K is the bigger concern.

B. Clinical features
1. History: important to inquire about the following during a history
   a. Polyuria, inadequate weight gain, constipation, or generalized weakness
   b. History of renal stones or bone disease
   c. Thorough family and medication history
2. Physical exam: following may be seen in patient with RTA
   a. Signs of growth retardation, muscle weakness, abnormal reflexes, dehydration (tachycardia, delayed capillary refill, dry mucous membranes)
   b. Growth retardation develops secondary to metabolic acidosis, which interferes with major aspects of insulin–growth hormone (insulin-like growth factor) axis

QUICK HIT

RTA is a rare and often unrecognized cause of failure to thrive (FTT) in an infant.

C. Diagnosis
1. Differential diagnosis: consider the following in child with normal anion gap metabolic acidosis
   a. Distal RTA
   b. Congenital hypothyroidism
   c. Obstructive uropathy
   d. Renal dysfunction
   e. Bicarbonate loss: proximal RTA, diarrhea, other gastrointestinal (GI) causes, medications (magnesium sulfate, calcium chloride)
   f. Acid loading: ammonium chloride, arginine hydrochloride
2. Laboratory findings
   a. Fresh spot urine pH
   b. Serum electrolytes and blood gas
      i. Metabolic acidosis with serum total CO_2 <17.5 mEq/L for all types of RTA
      ii. May see compensatory respiratory alkalosis
      iii. Hyperchloremia and normal anion gap
      iv. Normal BUN and creatinine (Table 7-9)
      v. ↑ K is expected in type 4 RTA
   c. Urine electrolytes
      i. Hypercalciuria, hypocitraturia, and potassium wasting are associated with type 1 RTA
      ii. Urinary excretion of glucose, uric acid, phosphate, amino acids, citrate, Ca^{2+}, K, and protein in type 2 RTA
   d. Plasma renin and aldosterone levels
3. Radiology findings: renal ultrasound or abdominal CT: nephrocalcinosis in undiagnosed or untreated/inadequately treated RTA

D. Treatment
1. Therapy: consists of correction of pH and electrolyte abnormalities
   a. Type 1 RTA: administration of an alkali is mainstay
      i. Typically treat with sodium bicarbonate, Bicitra (citric acid + sodium citrate), or potassium citrate
      ii. Correction of acidosis usually corrects hypokalemia
   b. Type 2 RTA: requires larger and more frequent dosing of alkalizing agents such as Bicitra
      i. Large doses of alkali are required due to substantial losses of HCO_3^- that occur in urine

QUICK HIT

Type 1 RTA, urine pH consistently >5.5
Type 2 RTA, urine pH <5.5

QUICK HIT

Type 1 RTA is associated with a positive urine anion gap: $Na^+ + K - Cl^-$.

TABLE 7-9 **Renal Tubular Acidosis Types and Characteristics**

	Type 1 RTA	Type 2 RTA	Type 4 RTA
Derangement	Impairment in hydrogen ion secretion in the distal tubule	Impairment in HCO_3^- reabsorption in the proximal tubules	Aldosterone deficiency or poor response to aldosterone by distal tubule
Urine pH	>5.5	<5.5	<5.5
Plasma HCO_3	<15 mEq/L	<17 mEq/L	<17 mEq/L
Potassium	Low	Normal or low	High
Urine electrolytes	Elevated Ca, and K, low citrate	Elevated glucose, uric acid, phosphate, amino acids, citrate, Ca, K	
Aldosterone	Normal	Normal	Normal or low
Causes	Primary, autoimmune diseases, sickle cell, exposure to lithium, amphotericin B	Inherited, Fanconi syndrome, drug exposures, vitamin D deficiency, renal transplantation, heavy metal exposure	Obstructive uropathy, ACE inhibitor or ARB use, CKD, CAH, exposure to cyclosporine, heparin, K-sparing diuretics, NSAIDs

ACE, angiotensin-converting enzyme; ARB, angiotensin receptor blocker; Ca, calcium; CAH, congenital adrenal hyperplasia; CKD, chronic kidney disease; K, potassium; NSAIDs, nonsteroidal anti-inflammatory drugs; RTA, renal tubular acidosis.

ii. Potassium supplementation
iii. Thiazide diuretics to induce diuresis and raise proximal tubule threshold for HCO_3^- wasting

c. Type 4 RTA
   i. Major treatment goal is to lower serum potassium level via low-potassium diet and drugs to promote potassium loss (loop diuretics, fludrocortisone)
   ii. Alkali therapy usually not required; mild acidosis is usually corrected by correcting serum potassium levels

d. Treatment of concomitant abnormalities (K, Ca^{2+}, phosphate)

2. Complications: include growth failure, weakness, dehydration, and complications from other electrolyte abnormalities (hyperkalemia, hypocalcemia)
3. Prognosis
   a. Type 1 RTA: response to therapy varies with accelerated growth in some after a few months of therapy and others requiring 1 or more years of therapy before achieving documented improvement of linear growth
   b. Type 2 RTA: compliance may be issue given amount of medication needed to correct acidosis
   c. Threshold for bicarbonate reabsorption can mature with age in type 2, proximal RTA, and in some patients can return to normal
   d. Type 4 RTA: no data available on long-term outcome; prognosis entirely dependent on underlying cause
   e. Hyperkalemia and acidosis can worsen as renal function declines, leading to eventual development of an anion gap metabolic acidosis
   f. Renal replacement therapy should be considered if conservative measures fail to control hyperkalemia or acidosis
4. Surveillance/prevention: close monitoring of serum bicarbonate concentration, urinary calcium:creatinine ratio, and linear growth; goal is to maintain serum bicarbonate >22 mEq

QUICK HIT

Severe hyperkalemia with peaked T waves on electrocardiogram is a rare emergency.

X. Rickets

A. Characteristics
1. Definition
   a. Failure or delay in mineralization of growing skeleton caused by calcium, vitamin D, or phosphorus deficiency in children
   b. **Osteomalacia** describes similar condition in adolescents whose growth plates have already closed
2. Epidemiology: 5 per million children between ages 6 months and 5 years have rickets, and peak prevalence is between ages 6–18 months
3. Cause: poor mineralization of epiphyseal cartilage and consequent growth retardation from conditions that lead to hypocalcemia and hypophosphatemia (decreased intake; malabsorption; and/or increased excretion of calcium, phosphorus, or vitamin D)
4. Genetics: genetic abnormalities include following disorders
   a. Vitamin D dependency type I and II (defective synthesis of hormone or hormone-receptor function)
   b. X-linked hypophosphatemic rickets
   c. Renal tubule disorders (Fanconi syndrome)
5. Risk factors
   a. Infants who are breastfed, especially those who receive little to no formula or vitamin supplementation
   b. Darkly pigmented skin
   c. Cities in northern latitudes, due to less sunlight exposure
   d. Vegan diets without adequate attention to nutrition
6. Pathophysiology
   a. Appropriate levels of both calcium and phosphorous are essential for optimal bone mineralization
      i. Calcium homeostasis is controlled in intestines
      ii. Phosphate homeostasis is regulated in kidneys

QUICK HIT

Incidence of vitamin D deficiency is increasing in the United States, and rickets is 1 of the most frequent childhood diseases in developing countries.

QUICK HIT

Breast milk contains little vitamin D. Vitamin D supplementation is important in breastfeeding infants.

QUICK HIT

Infants who breastfeed from mothers with risk factors are also at risk.

FIGURE 7-5 Characteristic bowing of the legs associated with rickets.

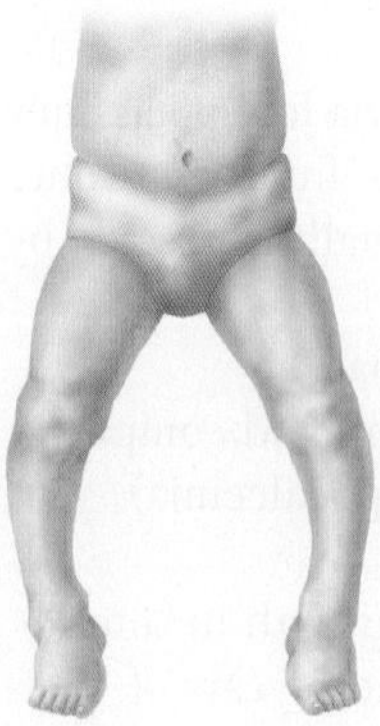

(From Bickley LS, Szilagyi P. *Bates' Guide to Physical Examination and History Taking.* 8th ed. Philadelphia: Lippincott Williams & Wilkins; 2003.)

QUICK HIT

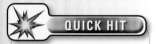

Rickets is typically characterized by a low calcium, low phosphorus, or both.

QUICK HIT

While rickets may be noted incidentally on x-ray, radiography is not needed to make the diagnosis of rickets.

QUICK HIT

Early treatment of rickets is essential to minimize bony deformities and growth retardation.

b. Vitamin D plays an important role in bone mineralization
c. Derangement at any level of calcium, phosphorous, or vitamin D homeostasis can result in rickets

B. Clinical features
1. Historical findings
a. Obtain thorough dietary history
b. Elicit any history of frequent fractures, delayed dentition, weakness, poor weight gain, seizures, and developmental delay
c. Obtain family and medication history (e.g., sibling with rickets)
2. Physical exam findings (Figure 7-5)

C. Diagnosis
1. Differential diagnosis
a. Nutritional deficiency (vitamin D deficiency, hypocalcemia, or hypophosphatemia)
b. Metabolic bone disease (vitamin D–resistant rickets, vitamin D–dependent rickets, congenital rickets, and osteogenesis imperfecta [OI])
c. Renal disease and RTA
d. Other causes including nonaccidental trauma, accidental trauma, prematurity, hyperphosphatasia, and primary chondrodystrophy
2. Laboratory findings
a. Patient with rickets should have calcium, phosphorus, PTH, and alkaline phosphatase concentrations measured
b. Renal function tests (RFTs) and 25-OH vitamin D and 1,25-OH vitamin D levels should also be obtained
3. Radiographic findings: osteopenia, spinal abnormalities (scoliosis, kyphosis, lordosis), coxa vara, pelvic deformities, and cupping/widening of distal ends of radius and ulna (Figure 7-6)

D. Treatment
1. Therapy: should be tailored to particular condition
a. Vitamin D–deficient rickets
i. Vitamin D supplementation, although sunlight and ultraviolet irradiation are therapeutic
ii. Response to therapy can be demonstrated radiographically within 2–4 weeks of onset of treatment
b. Vitamin D–resistant (X-linked hypophosphatemia) rickets requires therapy with oral phosphate and vitamin D to prevent secondary hyperparathyroidism
c. Renal failure patients should receive 1,25-OH vitamin D
d. Symptomatic hypocalcemia (tetany) requires oral administration of calcium chloride, calcium lactate, or calcium gluconate
e. Orthopedic correction of skeletal deformities may be required

FIGURE 7-6 Rachitic rosary on chest x-ray (*arrows*).

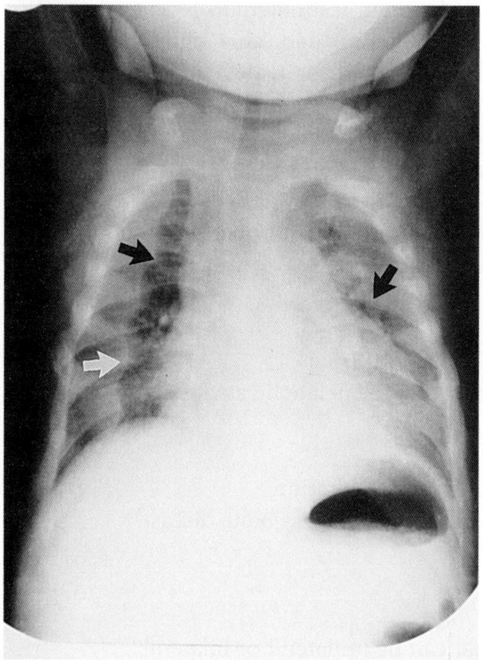

(From Yochum TR, Rowe LJ. *Yochum and Rowe's Essentials of Skeletal Radiology.* 3rd ed. Philadelphia: Lippincott Williams & Wilkins; 2004.)

2. Complications: hypocalcemia, seizures, skeletal deformities, and growth delay
3. Duration/prognosis
    a. Early diagnosis prevents sequelae such as motor developmental delay
    b. Bony deficiencies may persist for months to years despite treatment if severe deformities have occurred
4. Prevention
    a. Stress need for dietary supplementation with vitamin D in breastfeeding infants
    b. Target high-risk groups
        i. African American breastfeeding infants
        ii. Breastfeeding infants whose mothers avoid skin exposure (e.g., mother wearing burqas)
        iii. Children who have low intakes of milk and dairy products
        iv. Infants who live in northern areas where colder winter weather limits outdoor activities
    c. Dietary supplementation helps to speed healing process

> **QUICK HIT**
> Supplementation with sufficient amounts of vitamin D begins healing process within a few days, and healing progresses slowly over several months.

XI. Proximal Tubular Dysfunction (Fanconi Syndrome)

A. Definition
1. Disturbance of proximal renal tubule leading to inappropriate excretion of glucose, amino acids, phosphate, bicarbonate, and uric acid into urine
2. One cause of **Type 2** RTA

B. Epidemiology: can occur at any age; inherited causes manifest within first 12 months of life

C. Cause/pathophysiology
1. Inherited
    a. Primary (idiopathic): due to sporadic mutation (most cases) or familial
    b. Secondary: cystinosis, tyrosinemia, Wilson disease, Lowe syndrome (X linked), galactosemia, fructose intolerance, glycogen storage disorders, vitamin D–dependent rickets
2. Acquired
    a. Intrinsic renal disease, nephrotic syndrome, shock, nutritional abnormalities, hyperparathyroidism

> **QUICK HIT**
> Cystinosis occurs almost exclusively in Caucasians and is most common cause of Fanconi syndrome in children.

b. Drugs: salicylates, cisplatin, ifosfamide, gentamicin, outdated tetracyclines, valproate, deferasirox, amphotericin
c. Toxins: glue sniffing, heavy metals (copper, lead, mercury)

D. Clinical presentation: polyuria, polydipsia, vomiting and other signs and symptoms indicative of dehydration, bone deformities, inadequate weight gain

E. Testing
1. Differential diagnosis: consider other causes of polyuria, polydipsia (DM or diabetes insipidus [DI]), rickets, and FTT
2. Laboratory findings
a. Excessive loss in urine of amino acids, glucose, phosphate, bicarbonate
b. Further investigations required to identify the cause (liver function tests [LFTs], copper, lead levels)

F. Therapy
1. Mainstay is replacement of substances lost in urine
a. Repletion of sodium bicarbonate to correct metabolic acidosis due to excessive loss of bicarbonate
b. Repletion of potassium
2. Oral or intravenous (IV) fluids to address dehydration
3. Phosphate and vitamin D supplementation to address bone disease
4. Cysteamine therapy for cystinosis

QUICK HIT

Physical exam findings in Fanconi syndrome: children can often present with severe rickets and growth retardation.

QUICK HIT

Common laboratory abnormalities in Fanconi syndrome include hypokalemia, hypophosphatemia, and hyperchloremic metabolic acidosis.

XII. Renal Vein Thrombosis

A. Definition: thrombosis of renal vein that can be unilateral or bilateral

B. Cause/pathophysiology: often unknown, but risk factors are those associated with Virchow triad (endothelial injury, hypercoagulability, venous stasis)

C. Testing
1. Laboratory findings
a. CBC to assess platelet count and hemoglobin
b. Basic metabolic panel to assess for renal dysfunction
c. Urinalysis to assess for hematuria and proteinuria (nephrotic syndrome)
d. Serum albumin to assess for nephrotic syndrome
2. Radiology findings
a. Direct venography is gold standard but invasive
b. Ultrasonography: evaluate for decreased renal vein flow, increased vascular resistive indices, loss of corticomedullary differentiation, and enlarged kidney
c. MRA or CT angiography: can offer increased sensitivity but takes longer to perform (MRA) or exposes child to radiation (CT)

D. Therapy: depends on presentation and extent of disease as well as assessment of risks and benefits of anticoagulation; always treat underlying disease
1. Unfractionated/low-molecular-weight heparin therapy
2. Local thrombolysis or surgery (especially if thrombosis is bilateral)

QUICK HIT

Renal vein thrombosis is the most common location for non–catheter-associated thrombosis in the neonatal period.

QUICK HIT

Doppler ultrasound is often useful screening tool if index of suspicion is high.

QUICK HIT

Clinical presentation: classic triad of renal vein thrombosis *in neonates* is palpable abdominal mass, gross hematuria, and thrombocytopenia.

XIII. Hemolytic-Uremic Syndrome

A. Characteristics
1. Defined as triad of *microangiopathic hemolytic anemia, AKI, and thrombocytopenia*
2. Epidemiology
a. Mainly affects children age <5 years
b. Most common cause of AKI in children
c. Incidence is 1–2 cases/100,000
d. Mortality is low (3%–5%) with D+ (plus diarrhea) HUS but nears 25% with D− (minus diarrhea) HUS
3. Causes
a. D+HUS
i. *Escherichia coli* serotype O157:H7 is most common cause in children; acquired by eating undercooked meats, nonpasteurized milk, and fruits or vegetables, or contact with farm animals (petting zoos)
ii. *Shigella dysenteriae* type 1 is another cause and may result in more severe disease

QUICK HIT

Avoid use of antibiotics and antimotility agents during the diarrheal illness; they increase the chance of developing HUS by keeping the toxins in the gut for longer!

b. D–HUS (atypical HUS)
   i. Includes group of various etiologies
   ii. *S. pneumoniae* is a leading cause
   iii. Drugs and toxins (e.g.., cyclosporine, tacrolimus, clopidogrel)
   iv. Other infections including HIV
   v. Genetic causes have been
      (a) Inherited deficiencies of von Willebrand factor–cleaving protease or complement factors
      (b) Inherited deficiency of vitamin B_{12} metabolism
      (c) Other familial inherited disorders
c. Secondary HUS: diseases associated with microvascular injury including SLE, antiphospholipid-antibody syndrome, and malignant HTN

4. Risk factors: eating undercooked hamburgers and age <5 years
5. Pathophysiology
   a. Microvascular injury with endothelial cell damage is characteristic
      i. In classic D+ forms of HUS, toxin causes direct damage to endothelial cells → intravascular thrombogenesis → decreased GFR
      ii. Platelet aggregation → consumptive thrombocytopenia
      iii. Microvascular injury and partial vascular occlusion → mechanical damage to RBCs → microangiopathic hemolytic anemia
   b. Genetic causes may be triggered by inciting event like infection

B. Clinical features
1. Historical findings
   a. Typically present with abdominal pain, preceded by bloody diarrhea (in 90%), vomiting, and fever
   b. Acute onset of pallor, irritability, and lethargy follows initial illness
   c. Oliguria can be seen early
   d. Neurologic symptoms like seizures, irritability, or altered mental status
2. Physical exam depends on organ systems involved
   a. Abdominal pain is prominent and exam may demonstrate acute abdomen with signs of peritonitis with potential for pancreatitis
   b. GI bleeding is often noted; bowel perforation is possibility
   c. Cardiac involvement occurs in about 10% of cases
      i. Symptoms may include congestive heart failure (CHF) mainly due to volume overload and arrhythmias
      ii. Acute respiratory failure (acute respiratory distress syndrome) may also rarely occur
3. Vital signs may demonstrate fever, HTN, or tachycardia (related to fever or dehydration)

C. Diagnosis
1. Differential diagnosis
   a. Other causes of microvascular injury and bleeding including **TTP** and **disseminated intravascular coagulation (DIC)** can present similarly
   b. **Gastroenteritis** in general can present similarly to HUS but does not typically have associated laboratory findings
   c. Autoimmune processes like **SLE** and **antiphospholipid syndrome** can have findings similar to HUS
2. Laboratory findings
   a. CBC will demonstrate **thrombocytopenia** (usually 20,000–100,000/mm^3), **anemia** (may be mild initially but quickly progresses), and **leukocytosis**
      i. Reticulocyte count typically high
   b. Prothrombin time (PT) and partial thromboplastin time (PTT) are normal
   c. Coombs test for autoimmune hemolysis is typically negative; **haptoglobin** will be *low*, supporting hemolytic process
   d. Urinalysis with microscopic hematuria and proteinuria
   e. Stool cultures for ***E. coli* O157:H7** are positive >90% of time if obtained during 1st week of illness

QUICK HIT

Thrombotic thrombocytopenic purpura (TTP) has similar presenting clinical symptoms but often has greater CNS involvement, fever, and a more gradual onset.

QUICK HIT

D+HUS causes 95% of HUS in children.

QUICK HIT

Outbreaks of HUS have been associated with petting zoos.

QUICK HIT

HUS is preceded by diarrhea (often bloody) in 90% of cases.

QUICK HIT

Patients may present with dehydration or fluid overload depending on whether the gastroenteritis or renal insufficiency dominates and what overall fluid intake is.

QUICK HIT

Peripheral blood smear with schistocytes, Burr cells, and helmet cells, demonstrating hemolysis.

QUICK HIT

Haptoglobin binds to free hemoglobin. If the level is low, this implies RBCs are hemolyzing.

QUICK HIT

Despite the low platelet counts, platelet transfusions are not indicated because they are almost immediately consumed and can worsen the course; despite the low counts, serious bleeding is rare. Platelets should only be given for invasive procedures or acute bleeding.

f. **Renal panel** will demonstrate **elevated BUN and creatinine**
g. Hemolysis (**elevated lactate dehydrogenase** and **indirect bilirubin**)
3. Imaging studies are not indicated

D. Treatment
1. Therapy is primarily supportive
a. Fluid and electrolyte management; dialysis is indicated for refractory acidosis, hyperkalemia, fluid overload, and/or uremia
b. HTN control
c. Seizure control
d. RBC transfusion to keep hemoglobin >7 g/dL
e. Consultation with nephrologist or hematologist
2. Most common complications are proteinuria, renal insufficiency, and HTN
3. Prognosis for patients with D+HUS is generally good with complete recovery, *but* if residual HTN or renal insufficiency persists beyond 1 year, they require close follow-up due to risk of CKD
a. Mortality <5%
b. Adult prognosis worse than kids
4. Prevention of D+HUS is best achieved with good handwashing to prevent spread of infection

XIV. Urolithiasis

A. Characteristics
1. Defined as **calculi** or **stones** present anywhere along urinary tract
2. Relatively uncommon in children and adolescents
a. Account for 1/1,000–1/7,600 hospital admissions for children
b. Children typically have higher concentrations of inhibitors of crystal formation, contributing to low incidence
c. Commonly incidental finding due to use of improved radiography
d. Slight male preponderance compared to females
3. Causes are often multifactorial
a. Urine of patients with calcium and uric acid stones contains high levels of cholesterol, cholesterol ester, and triglycerides
b. Metabolic factors are most common cause, followed by urinary tract abnormalities and infection as next most common
i. Common metabolic factors: high urinary concentrations of calcium, oxalate, uric acid, or cysteine
ii. Structural abnormalities (e.g., UPJ obstruction, ureteroceles, PUVs) lead to urinary stasis and increased risk of urolithiasis
iii. With infection, many bacteria produce **urease**, which increases urine pH, predisposing to stone formation
4. Risk factors: anything that causes urinary stasis, obstruction, infection, or abnormalities in concentration and/or the formation of calcium, oxalate, cysteine, or uric acid (Box 7-2)

QUICK HIT

Calcium oxalate and calcium phosphate crystals are the most common cause of urolithiasis in children.

BOX 7-2

Risk Factors for the Development of Urolithiasis

Distal renal tubular acidosis
Medullary sponge kidney
Autosomal dominant polycystic kidney disease
Cystinosis
Wilson disease
Inflammatory bowel disease or other gastrointestinal diseases
Cystic fibrosis
Premature infant
Use of certain pharmacologic agents (i.e., loop diuretics predispose to calcium oxalate crystals)
Certain diets may predispose to urinary stones (i.e., high-calcium diet, ketogenic diets)

5. Pathophysiology
   a. Balance between factors that promote and factors that inhibit crystallization determines development of stones
   b. Multiple steps are involved in stone formation including crystallization, crystal growth, aggregation, and adherence of crystals to epithelium

B. Clinical features
1. Historical findings
   a. Obtain thorough personal (recurrent UTIs, previous stones, chronic medical problems, anatomic kidney abnormalities), family, diet, and medication (including herbal supplements and over-the-counter [OTC] medications) history
   b. Screen for signs of infection
2. Physical exam findings: vital sign abnormalities include HTN related to underlying kidney disease or pain, tachycardia related to pain or fever, or fever with infection

C. Diagnosis
1. Differential diagnosis: other processes that can cause hematuria and pain including HUS, GN, IgA nephropathy, PKD, urethral foreign body, trauma, UTI, or pyelonephritis
2. Laboratory workup recommended for urinary stones includes
   a. Spot urinalysis to assess pH and presence of RBCs or WBCs, leukocyte esterase, or nitrite (often present with infection)
   b. Urine measurement of calcium and creatinine
      i. Subsequent calculation of urine calcium:urine creatinine ratio
      ii. Calcium crystals are most common cause of urolithiasis, although can also consider other substances (i.e., uric acid, oxalate, and cysteine and compare to urine creatinine)
   c. Consider sending serum electrolytes, BUN, creatinine, calcium, phosphorus, total protein, albumin, PTH, and vitamin D studies
   d. Consider sending CBC if suspicious for infection
3. Radiology findings
   a. **Ultrasound** should be first line and is effective for identifying urinary tract stones
   b. If ultrasound is negative but suspicion for stones and symptoms persists, can consider noncontrast spiral abdominal CT
   c. Abdominal x-ray may identify some radiopaque urinary stones
4. Determining composition of stones is important element in diagnosis and requires collection of stone either by straining urine, examining diapers for stones, or obtaining via procedure
5. Nephrologist consultation is often indicated for metabolic workup

D. Treatment
1. Medical therapy options
   a. Enteral or parenteral hydration is key in management of stones with goal of *increasing urine output* (goal mL/day varies depending on age)
   b. **Analgesics** for pain management
   c. If stone is small (<5 mm), may consider allowing time for it to pass
   d. Dietary modification is sometimes indicated depending on stone type
   e. Urine alkalinization with sodium bicarbonate or potassium citrate may be necessary with some stones, specifically uric acid stones
   f. Low-salt diet can help reduce stone risk
   g. In patients with chronic interstitial disease (inflammatory bowel disease), decreased fat absorption causes calcium to saponify. Now, oxalate may be free to be absorbed, resulting in oxalate stones. These patients may ironically benefit from calcium supplementation.
2. Surgical therapy
   a. Indicated for large stones (>5 mm) that are causing or have potential to cause obstruction; urologist should be involved in these cases
   b. Include **extracorporeal shock wave lithotripsy (ESWL)**, **ureteroscopic lithotripsy** or **removal**, or **percutaneous ultrasonic lithotripsy**

> **QUICK HIT**
> Classic presentation is *intense pain that starts in back and radiates down to groin or lower abdomen*; check for presence of back pain on physical exam by checking for costovertebral angle tenderness.

> **QUICK HIT**
> Older children typically present with flank pain and hematuria, whereas younger children typically present with more nonspecific symptoms like irritability and vomiting.

> **QUICK HIT**
> While uncommon, absence of RBCs in urinalysis does not rule out nephrolithiasis.

> **QUICK HIT**
> In older children and in adults, a urine calcium:urine creatinine ratio >0.2 may indicate hypercalciuria.

> **QUICK HIT**
> Gout is extraordinarily rare in children, and urate stones are unlikely outside of rare metabolic diseases (Lesch-Nyhan syndrome).

FIGURE 7-7 Kidney and ureter showing hydronephrosis and kidney stone obstructing ureter.

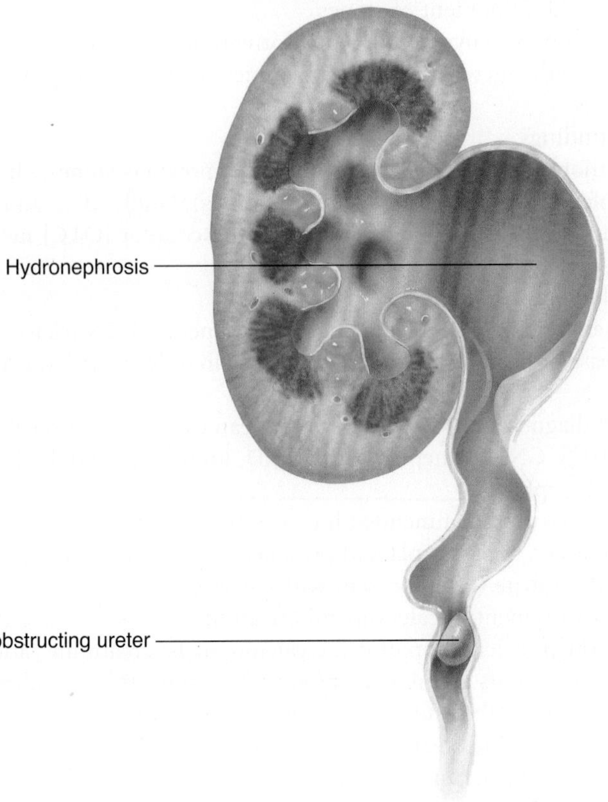

(Asset provided by Anatomical Chart Co.)

3. Complications are uncommon but can be related to untreated renal outflow tract obstruction, causing renal failure, or infected stones, causing sepsis (Figure 7-7)
4. Prognosis is generally very good if recommendations are followed, but recurrence rates are high, especially in children with metabolic abnormalities
5. Prevention of urolithiasis hinges on adequate hydration

> **QUICK HIT**
> Adenovirus is a common cause of transient hemorrhagic cystitis.

XV. Hemorrhagic Cystitis

A. Defined as acute or chronic bleeding of bladder
B. Caused by *damage to bladder transitional epithelium and blood vessels* by
   1. Viruses (i.e., adenovirus, BK virus, influenza) have been implicated and are more often seen in children receiving immunosuppression
   2. Medication/chemical toxin exposure (i.e., cyclophosphamide, penicillins, dyes, insecticides)
   3. Radiation (although uncommon in pediatric population)
   4. Trauma

> **QUICK HIT**
> Clots almost always imply a nonrenal source of blood.

C. Clinical presentation
   1. Typically presents as sudden onset of gross hematuria, dysuria, frequency, and urgency, often associated with clots
   2. May present with new-onset incontinence
D. Testing
   1. Urinalysis and urine culture should be obtained
      a. Urinalysis will have WBCs (termed sterile pyuria) and RBCs
      b. Bacterial urine culture will typically be negative
      c. Send viral urine studies if suspicious for viral etiology
   2. Renal and bladder ultrasound should be obtained to rule out other potential causes for hematuria

3. Consider sending CBC to evaluate hemoglobin and platelet count and/or coagulation studies to evaluate PT, PTT, and international normalized ratio (INR)
4. Cystoscopy if there is clot retention or persistent unexplained bleeding

E. Therapy
1. If viral etiology in immunocompetent patient, process is usually self-resolving
2. If viral etiology in immunocompromised patient, consider antiviral therapy
3. If secondary to cyclophosphamide, mesna disulfide, which inactivates cyclophosphamide metabolites, and adequate hydration can protect bladder
4. Bladder irrigation may be warranted in more severe forms

XVI. Rhabdomyolysis

A. Definitions
1. Injury and breakdown of muscle tissue
2. Release of muscle cellular components into circulation

B. Cause/pathophysiology
1. Causes
   a. Inherited
   b. Acquired (may be exertional)
2. Pathophysiology
   a. Destruction of muscle fiber cells leads to displacement of cellular contents and alteration in electrolyte balance (K, Ca, phosphorus)
   b. Resultant kidney injury due to ischemia from dehydration coupled with tubule damage from myoglobin breakdown products

C. Clinical presentation
1. Myalgias
2. Urine color change (red or brown)
3. May have range of associated systemic symptoms: fever, chills, malaise, vomiting, or rare mental status changes, such as delirium or confusion

D. Testing
1. Diagnosis includes obtaining thorough history to review past medical history and recent history of exposure, injury, or exertion
2. Laboratory evaluation
   a. **Creatine kinase (CK)** markedly elevated
   b. Basic metabolic panel
      i. Electrolyte disturbance: hyperkalemia, hypocalcemia, hyperphosphatemia common
      ii. Metabolic acidosis possible
      iii. AKI: elevated BUN and creatinine
   c. Urinalysis positive for blood but without RBCs on microscopy: indicative of **myoglobinuria**

E. Therapy
1. Aggressive fluid hydration
2. Electrolyte management
3. Alkalinization of urine controversial; has been shown effective in preventing AKI in some animal studies

QUICK HIT

Patients with sickle strait may be at increased risk for rhabdomyolysis after strenuous exercise.

QUICK HIT

Urine may often be the color of cola in rhabdomyolysis.

QUICK HIT

Renal damage from rhabdomyolysis is rare if the CK <10,000.

XVII. Urinary Retention

A. Definition: inability to fully empty bladder with voiding

B. Causes/pathophysiology
1. Behavioral: voluntary holding often associated with potty training or dysfunctional voiding and stool patterns
2. Infection
3. GU tract obstruction: anatomic abnormality, trauma
4. Medication: pseudoephedrine, antihistamines, antidepressants
5. Neuromuscular disease
6. Recent surgery

C. Clinical presentation
1. History of inability to void or decreased volume of urine
2. Lower abdominal pain in pelvic area

QUICK HIT

Constipation is likely the most common cause of urinary retention.

QUICK HIT

If treating constipation relieves urinary retention, imaging is not indicated.

D. Testing
   1. Ultrasound
      a. Evaluate for hydronephrosis or hydroureter
      b. Document postvoid residual volume
   2. VCUG may be indicated to evaluate anatomy
   3. Urodynamic testing in consultation with urologist
E. Therapy
   1. Acute treatment
      a. **Catheterization** to relieve pressure and empty bladder
      b. If infection is cause, antibiotic treatment indicated
   2. Chronic treatment depends on cause and may include intermittent catheterization, surgery, or behavioral modification
   3. Stool softeners or behavioral therapy for constipation-induced urinary retention

QUICK HIT

VUR is most common urologic abnormality in children.

XVIII. Vesicoureteral Reflux (VUR)

A. Characteristics
   1. Definition: retrograde flow of urine from bladder into the upper urinary tract
   2. Epidemiology
      a. Present in approximately 1% of newborns
      b. Higher incidence (20%) in children with febrile UTI
      c. Incidence same in girls and boys
      d. Diagnosed more frequently in young infants and toddlers
   3. Cause
      a. Primary VUR
         i. Inadequate closure of ureterovesical junction during bladder contraction
         ii. Usually result of a genetically short ureter segment where it inserts through bladder wall
      b. Secondary VUR
         i. Abnormally high bladder pressure does not allow closure of ureterovesical junction during contraction
         ii. Associated with anatomic (e.g., PUVs) or functional (e.g., neurogenic bladder) obstruction
         iii. Postkidney transplant after surgical implantation of ureter

QUICK HIT

VUR must be ruled out in young children presenting with recurrent UTI.

   4. Genetics
      a. Unknown mode of inheritance
      b. Increased prevalence in patients with sibling or parent with VUR
   5. Risk factors
      a. Febrile UTI
      b. Genetic predisposition
      c. Anatomic abnormality, such as PUVs
   6. Pathophysiology
      a. Abnormally short or malfunctioning ureterovesical junction is unable to block flow of urine into ureter
      b. Urine flows retrograde into upper urinary tract
      c. Infected urine refluxing into kidney can cause renal scarring and inhibition of normal kidney growth
B. Clinical features
   1. Historical findings
      a. Generally asymptomatic
      b. May be associated with symptoms indicative of UTI, including fever, fussiness in an infant, urinary frequency, dysuria, and vomiting
   2. Physical exam findings
      a. Generally normal exam
      b. May have signs of UTI, such as suprapubic tenderness
C. Diagnosis
   1. Laboratory findings
      a. Urinalysis may show signs of infection, such as positive leukocyte esterase, nitrite, or elevated WBC count on microscopy

b. Urine culture may be positive for infection
c. May have abnormal electrolytes or elevated creatinine
2. Radiology findings
a. Renal ultrasound may show hydronephrosis and/or hydroureter (prenatal ultrasound may be suggestive of diagnosis)
b. Contrast VCUG or radionuclide cystogram (RNC) used to evaluate for presence and severity of VUR
i. Graded using International Reflux Study Group (IRSG) classification system (Figure 7-8)
(a) Grade I: reflux into ureter without dilation
(b) Grade II: reflux into ureter and collecting system without dilation
(c) Grade III: reflux into ureter and collecting system with mild dilation of ureter and blunting of calyces
(d) Grade IV: reflux into ureter and collecting system with more significant dilation of ureter and blunting of calyces
(e) Grade V: massive reflux with dilation and tortuosity of ureter and dilation of collecting system
ii. Severity grading: grades I–II (mild); grade III (moderate); grades IV–V (severe)
D. Treatment
1. Therapy
a. Medical
i. Promptly treat UTI with antibiotics
b. Surgical
i. Urology consultation recommended for severe VUR
ii. Ureteral reimplantation is surgical procedure of choice
2. Complications
a. Recurrent pyelonephritis
b. Renal scarring
i. Associated with reflux of infected urine
ii. Higher rate with increasing severity of VUR
iii. May lead to CKD or kidney failure if bilateral
3. Duration/prognosis
a. Most VUR resolves spontaneously within several years
b. Severe VUR less likely to spontaneously resolve
4. Prevention
a. No means of prevention of VUR but may be able to prevent some complications by promptly diagnosing and treating UTIs
b. Prophylactic antibiotics are controversial as they do not prevent renal scarring

QUICK HIT

Ultrasound is gaining acceptance as the primary screening method for VUR. VCUG should be performed on children with abnormal ultrasound.

QUICK HIT

Generally, surveillance of VUR over time is indicated, due to high rate of spontaneous resolution.

QUICK HIT

VUR results in renal scarring. Patients with frequent UTI without reflux very rarely proceed to CKD.

FIGURE 7-8 **Vesicoureteral reflux grading system.**

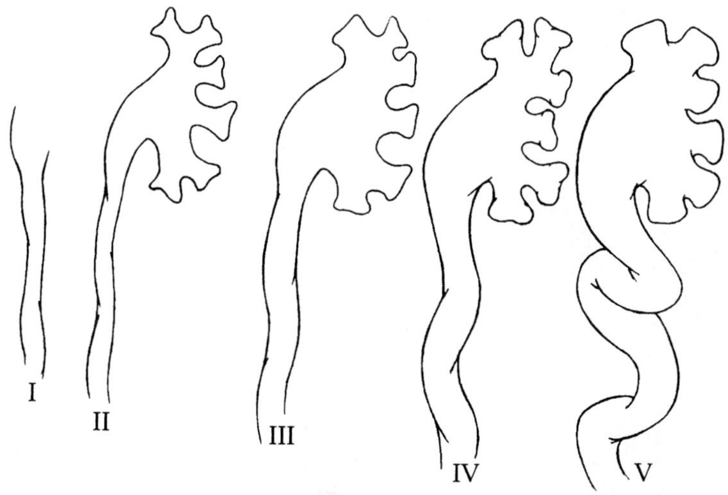

(From Blackbourne LH. *Advanced Surgical Recall.* 2nd ed. Baltimore: Lippincott Williams & Wilkins; 2004.)

Diseases of the Renal and Genitourinary System

XIX. Posterior Urethral Valves

A. Definition: anatomic abnormality involving membranous folds of posterior urethra, found in *males*

B. Cause/pathophysiology
   1. Persistence of urogenital membrane during embryologic development
   2. Valve obstructs urinary flow
      a. Leads to distention of GU tract upstream including bladder hypertrophy, hydroureter, hydronephrosis, and ultimately CKD if not repaired
      b. Potter sequence may result if severe enough to cause oligohydramnios and impaired lung development in utero

QUICK HIT

Infants with PUV may be extremely sick and require emergent relief from obstruction.

C. Clinical presentation
   1. Often diagnosed on routine prenatal ultrasound
   2. Presentation is variable depending on degree of urethral obstruction
   3. Infants and children may present with UTI, abdominal distention, straining with urination, or poor urinary stream/dribbling

D. Testing
   1. Laboratory evaluation includes basic metabolic panel to evaluate electrolytes and kidney function (BUN, creatinine)
   2. Radiology studies
      a. Ultrasound may reveal urinary tract dilation and hydronephrosis, renal dysplasia, and thickened, trabeculated bladder
      b. VCUG shows dilated urethra during voiding phase (Figure 7-9)
      c. Radionuclide scans assess degree of obstruction and kidney parenchyma

QUICK HIT

Any infant boy who doesn't make a strong urinary stream should raise concern for PUV. If a parent has not been "hit" during a diaper change, it is worth considering.

E. Therapy
   1. Correct electrolyte abnormalities
   2. Acutely remove obstruction with Foley catheter
   3. Cystoscopy with ablation of valves; after treatment, children may develop postobstructive diuresis and need to be monitored closely
   4. CKD and bladder dysfunction may result, requiring dialysis and transplant care

QUICK HIT

UPJ obstruction occurs in 1/500 live births and is more common in boys.

XX. Ureteropelvic Junction Obstruction

A. Definition
   1. Partial or total blockage of urinary flow at any level along urinary tract
   2. Most common anatomic cause of antenatally detected hydronephrosis

B. Pathophysiology
   1. Congenital UPJ obstruction usually caused by intrinsic stenosis of upper segment of ureter causing obstruction of urinary flow, resulting in hydronephrosis

FIGURE 7-9 **Voiding cystourethrogram revealing a posterior urethral valve (*white arrow*).**

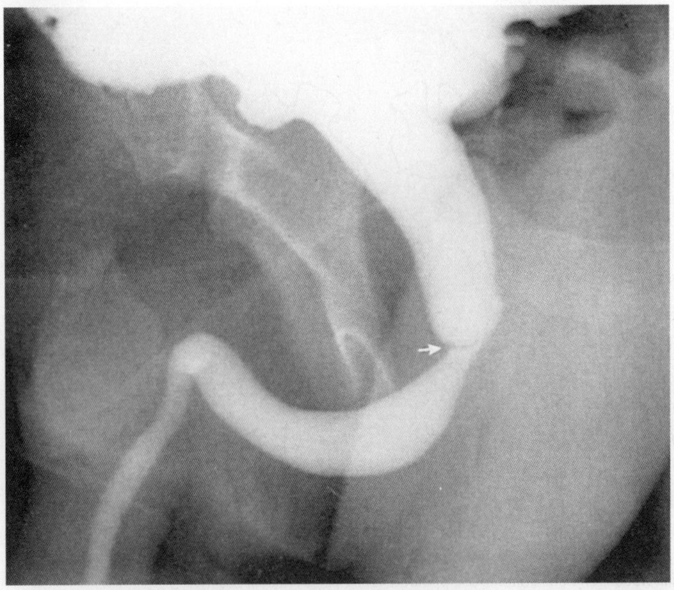

(From Eisenberg RL. *An Atlas of Differential Diagnosis.* 4th ed. Philadelphia: Lippincott Williams & Wilkins; 2003.)

2. Extrinsic compression from aberrant or accessory renal artery is less common
C. Clinical presentation
1. Most are identified during antenatal period with routine ultrasound screening
2. Newborns may present with abdominal mass, UTI, hematuria, and FTT
3. Older children can present with intermittent flank or abdominal pain, +/− nausea and vomiting
D. Diagnosis and evaluation
1. Diagnosis is suspected when ultrasound reveals hydronephrosis
2. Diuretic renography and CT scan are not routinely needed
3. VCUG is used to evaluate for VUR and PUVs in boys; 10% of patients with UPJ obstruction have VUR
E. Therapy: goal is to preserve renal function while avoiding unnecessary surgery
1. No randomized controlled studies to determine optimal management, so it is currently based on best expert opinion
2. Many asymptomatic patients with unilateral obstruction can be followed with serial ultrasounds and diuretic renography

QUICK HIT

UPJ obstruction can be an incidental finding of hydronephrosis while being evaluated for mild renal injury, hematuria, renal calculi, or HTN.

QUICK HIT

In symptomatic patients, surgical intervention with pyeloplasty of atretic or stenotic section is used to relieve obstruction.

XXI. Polycystic Kidney Diseases

A. Characteristics
1. Definition
a. Autosomal recessive PKD: **congenital** inherited disorder that involves dilation of **collecting ducts** and hepatic fibrosis
b. Autosomal dominant PKD: inherited disorder *often diagnosed in adulthood* that involves cyst formation in multiple organs, including kidney (*all parts of nephron*), liver, pancreas, and cardiovascular system (Figure 7-10)

QUICK HIT

When autosomal dominant PKD is diagnosed *in children*, it is often an incidental finding on imaging.

FIGURE 7-10 **Polycystic kidney.**

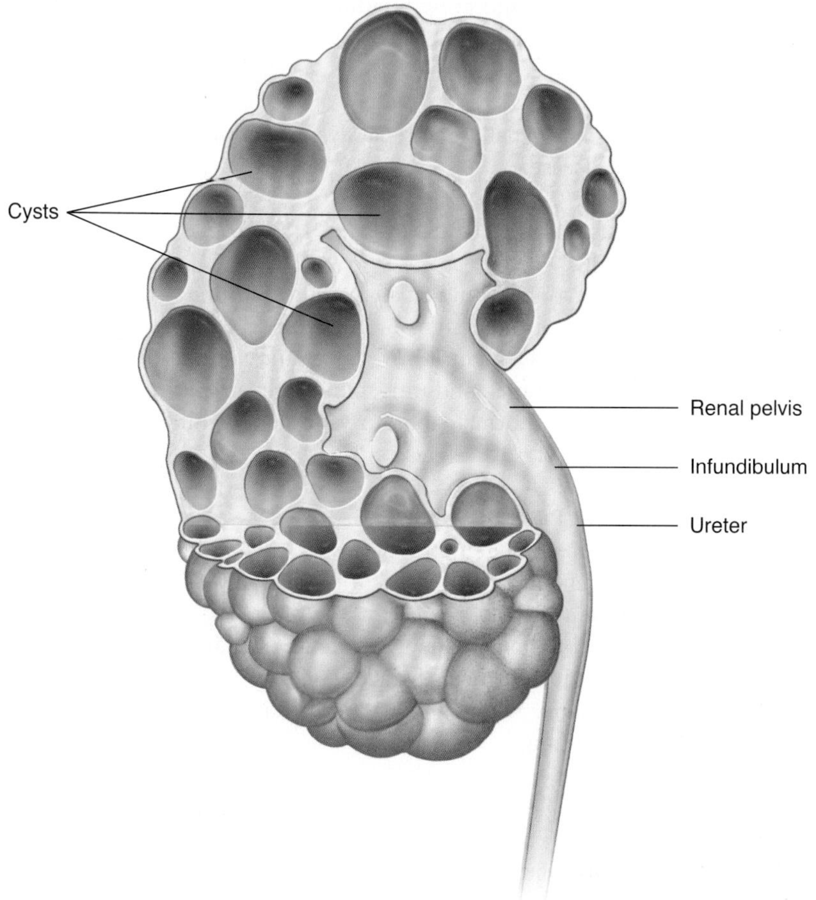

(Asset provided by Anatomical Chart Co.)

2. Epidemiology
   a. Autosomal recessive PKD: rare disease (1:20,000)
   b. Autosomal dominant PKD: frequent genetic cause of ESRD in adults
      i. May be diagnosed in children
      ii. Symptoms generally increase with age
   c. Both autosomal recessive PKD and autosomal dominant PKD equally affect all ethnicities and both sexes
3. Cause: abnormal structural proteins in the formation of renal cilia lead to structural abnormalities and cyst formation
4. Risk factors
   a. Autosomal recessive PKD: family members but not parents affected
   b. Patients with autosomal dominant PKD have at least 1 affected parent
5. Pathophysiology
   a. Both fibrocystin (abnormal in autosomal recessive PKD) and polycystin (abnormal in autosomal dominant PKD) can lead to abnormal renal cilia
   b. Disruption of renal cilia leads to cyst formation
      i. Autosomal recessive PKD: cysts originate in *collecting ducts of kidney*
      ii. Autosomal dominant PKD: cysts originate *anywhere in nephron*

B. Clinical features
1. Historical findings
   a. Autosomal recessive PKD
      i. May be found incidentally, including on prenatal ultrasounds prior to onset of symptoms
      ii. Abdominal distention most common symptom
      iii. May also present with HTN, oliguria, respiratory distress
   b. Autosomal dominant PKD often found incidentally in childhood with development of symptoms generally not occurring until 4th decade of life
2. Physical exam findings
   a. Autosomal recessive PKD: elevated BP, palpable abdominal mass or enlarged liver, poor feeding, and growth failure
   b. Autosomal dominant PKD: elevated BP, costovertebral angle tenderness, hematuria

C. Diagnosis
1. Differential diagnosis: simple renal cysts, renal dysplasia, tuberous sclerosis, glomerulocystic kidney disease
2. Laboratory findings
   a. Genetic testing available for mutations in *PHKD1*, *PKD1/2*
   b. Autosomal recessive PKD
      i. Renal profile with hyponatremia or increased creatinine
      ii. Urinalysis with proteinuria or signs of infection
      iii. Evaluation of liver involvement: LFTs, coagulation studies, CBC (focusing on platelet count), and ultrasound of liver/spleen
   c. Autosomal dominant PKD: normal laboratory studies in childhood
3. Radiology findings
   a. Ultrasound
      i. Autosomal recessive PKD
         (a) Enlarged echogenic bilateral kidneys with ductal dilation
         (b) Hepatic enlargement with fibrosis or portal HTN
      ii. Autosomal dominant PKD
         (a) Cysts occur throughout kidney, unilateral or bilateral
         (b) Specific criteria for diagnosis by age
   b. CT and magnetic resonance imaging (MRI) are alternative options for equivocal ultrasound findings

D. Treatment
1. Therapy
   a. Autosomal recessive PKD
      i. Respiratory support, dialysis, eventual renal transplantation, and antihypertensives

QUICK HIT

In childhood, autosomal recessive PKD is usually severe and autosomal dominant PKD is usually asymptomatic.

QUICK HIT

A solitary cyst is usually a benign finding and not consistent with PKD.

QUICK HIT

Autosomal recessive PKD is often diagnosed on prenatal ultrasound and can be associated with pulmonary hypoplasia due to oligohydramnios.

QUICK HIT

There is no specific therapy for PKD. Treatment is supportive.

ii. Nephrectomy generally *not* indicated unless severe pulmonary restriction due to enlarged kidneys
b. Autosomal dominant PKD: also treat supportively, with close monitoring for cyst progression and extrarenal complications
2. Complications
a. Autosomal recessive PKD: respiratory failure, recurrent UTIs, progressive hepatic fibrosis with portal HTN, bacterial cholangitis
b. Autosomal dominant PKD: progressive HTN, cardiovascular disease
3. Duration/prognosis
a. Autosomal recessive PKD
i. Survival higher for children diagnosed after age 1 year
ii. Prognosis depends on severity of renal and hepatic dysfunction at time of diagnosis
iii. Can live into adulthood
b. Autosomal dominant PKD: patients diagnosed earlier in life more likely to progress to ESRD
4. Prevention: genetic counseling available to families with history of PKD

XXII. Phimosis and Paraphimosis

A. Definitions
1. Phimosis: tight foreskin that cannot be retracted to expose glans penis
2. Paraphimosis: retracted foreskin in an uncircumcised (or partially circumcised) male that is not able to return to its normal position, often caused by foreskin retraction for cleaning, infections, sexual activity, or instrumentation
B. Pathophysiology: paraphimosis occurs when foreskin becomes entrapped behind coronal sulcus and impedes lymphatic and venous flow from constricting ring, leading to venous engorgement
C. Clinical presentation
1. History findings include swelling of penis, pain, irritability in infant, dysuria, and decreased urinary stream
2. Physical exam includes edema and tenderness of glans penis, painful swelling of distal retracted foreskin, and color change if penis is ischemic
D. Diagnostic testing: none as diagnosis is clinical
E. Therapy: timely reduction of foreskin over glans penis via manual retraction; may ice before to decrease swelling and induce vasoconstriction
1. Pain control and topical anesthetics are critical
2. If arterial compromise is present, immediate reduction and urologic consultation; requires dorsal slit procedure to relieve congestion
3. Prevention: teach parents of young, uncircumcised boys not to forcefully retract phimotic foreskin, and teach adolescents to return foreskin to normal position after cleaning and sexual intercourse

XXIII. Priapism

A. Definition: persistent erection of penis, usually lasting >4 hours, not associated with sexual stimulation
1. Relatively rare, occurs in 1.5:100,000 men; common in sickle cell disease
B. Pathophysiology
1. Ischemic (most common): prolonged erection results in compartment syndrome
2. Nonischemic: less common
a. Result of fistula between cavernosal artery and corpus cavernosum
b. Often result of penile trauma from needle injury or blunt injury (biking), which occurs up to 72 hours after injury
c. Not an emergency because cavernous blood is well oxygenated
d. 2/3 of cases will resolve spontaneously if untreated
C. Clinical presentation
1. Clinical diagnosis
2. History should include duration of erection, recurrence of symptoms, history of sickle cell disease, perineal trauma

QUICK HIT

Phimosis is normal in young uncircumcised males when foreskin is still fused to glans; infection can cause this in older children.

QUICK HIT

Young infants may display similar symptoms with **hair tourniquet syndrome**, in which a constricting hair becomes wrapped around the penis, causing pain and vascular compromise.

QUICK HIT

The most common associated diagnosis in children who experience priapism is sickle cell disease.

QUICK HIT

Long-term sequelae and subsequent erectile dysfunction are associated with duration of priapism; tissue damage can occur in 4–6 hours and significant damage by 12 hours.

QUICK HIT

Ischemic priapism often presents with a painful and rigid erection, whereas nonischemic priapism is often associated with a history of trauma and is less painful and rigid.

D. Diagnostic testing
  1. Doppler ultrasound: minimal or absent flow is seen in ischemic priapism; normal-to-high flow in nonischemic priapism
  2. Hemoglobin electrophoresis for blood dyscrasias and sickle cell disease

E. Therapy
  1. Current treatment is based on case reports/series and expert opinion as no definitive randomized controlled treatment studies exist
  2. Pain control
  3. Ischemic priapism is an emergency and requires urologic intervention

QUICK HIT

Nonischemic priapism is not urgent; conservative management until it spontaneously resolves (days) is acceptable.

XXIV. Testicular Torsion

A. Definition: painful twisting of spermatic cord leading to testicular ischemia and potential loss
  1. Peak incidence of testicular torsion is in neonates and teenagers, with 65% occurring in boys between ages 12 and 18 years
  2. Incidence of testicular torsion is 1:4,000 in males age <25 years

B. Pathophysiology
  1. Inadequate fixation of testes to tunica vaginalis allows increased mobility and twisting, which causes venous compression and subsequent edema of testicle, ultimately leading to ischemia and necrosis
  2. Bell clapper deformity: lack of attachment to tunica vaginalis leads to transverse lie of testicle within scrotum (often bilateral) (Figure 7-11)

C. Clinical presentation
  1. History: patients will complain of abrupt onset of constant scrotal pain, lower abdominal and inguinal pain, nausea, and vomiting (90%)
  2. Physical exam: edematous, indurated, and erythematous scrotum
  3. Intermittent torsion: presents as acute, intermittent, and sharp testicular pain and swelling with rapid resolution and long intervals without pain

D. Diagnostic testing
  1. Clinical diagnosis; further testing is recommended to clarify diagnosis if it does not delay treatment
  2. Doppler ultrasound will provide information on testicular size as well as arterial flow to testes and epididymis
  3. Nuclear scan is available to measure testicular perfusion, although it is used less frequently and may delay therapy
  4. Urinalysis and CBC may be considered

QUICK HIT

Testicular torsion is a common and serious cause of acute scrotal pain in children and adolescents.

QUICK HIT

Affected testicle is tender, swollen, and slightly elevated (shortening of cord from twisting), and cremasteric reflex is absent.

QUICK HIT

Prehn sign: elevation of the testicle relieves the pain in epididymitis but has no effect on or aggravates the pain in testicular torsion.

QUICK HIT

Testicle viability depends on the duration and degree of torsion (after 12 hours, there is only a 20% chance of viability).

QUICK HIT

Torsion of the appendix of the testicle occurs in boys age 7–12 years. There is a nontender testicle with a palpable tender mass and a "blue dot sign" when the appendix appears gangrenous through the scrotum. Treatment is usually only supportive care.

FIGURE 7-11 **Testicular torsion.**

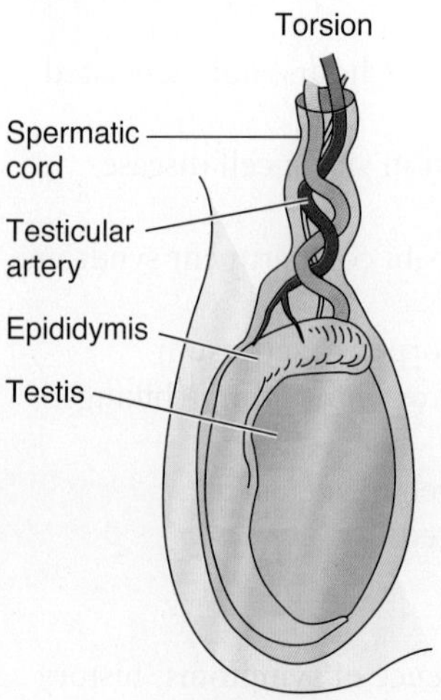

(From Porth CM. *Pathophysiology Concepts of Altered Health States.* 7th ed. Philadelphia: Lippincott Williams & Wilkins; 2005.)

E. Therapy
  1. Immediate consultation with urologist
  2. Pain management as needed
  3. Viable testicle: surgical detorsion and fixation (orchiopexy) of both testes; contralateral testicle at risk for bell clapper deformity
  4. Nonviable testicle: orchiectomy to remove the testicle
  5. Fertility controversial, with some studies reporting decreased and others with no change in fertility after unilateral torsion

XXV. Undescended Testicle (Cryptorchidism)

A. Definition: testicle that is not within scrotal sac and cannot be manipulated down; 10% are bilateral

B. Cause/pathophysiology
  1. Occurs when testicle stopped along its normal descent into scrotum; may be in abdomen, inguinal canal, or outside external ring
  2. Pathophysiology: not well understood; thought to be related to interaction of mechanical and hormonal effects

C. Clinical presentation
  1. Most descend spontaneously; prevalence is 1% by age 1 year, and most will descend in first 6 months of life
  2. Noted on routine physical exam; absence of testicle in scrotal area
  3. Careful examination for features of genetic syndrome or hypospadias

D. Diagnostic testing: when undescended testicles are present bilaterally or hypospadias is found, there may be disorder of sexual development
  1. Ultrasound to look for gonads and to exclude uterus in phenotypic males
  2. Lab evaluation varies with age and may include electrolytes, luteinizing hormone, follicle-stimulating hormone, Müllerian-inhibiting substance, karyotyping, and 17-OH progesterone

E. Therapy
  1. Orchiopexy: viable undescended testicle is manipulated into scrotum and sutured in place; nonviable testes are removed; refer to urology at age 6 months
  2. Hormonal therapy: administration of human chorionic gonadotropin intramuscularly is approved in the United States; most likely to work in distal located undescended testicle

QUICK HIT

Undescended testes should not be confused with **retractile testes**, which are in suprascrotal location and can be manipulated down into scrotal sac.

QUICK HIT

2%–5% of full-term and 30% of premature infants are born with an undescended testicle.

QUICK HIT

Changes in fertility occur in undescended testicles early, as young as age 1 year.

QUICK HIT

Routine exam of the newborn male includes palpation of the testes.

QUICK HIT

Testis is untorsed by lateral rotation: "open like a book."

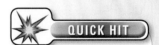

QUICK HIT

If undescended testes are not corrected, there is a risk for testicular neoplasm, decreased fertility, torsion, hernia, and trauma.

8 Fluids and Electrolytes

SYMPTOM SPECIFIC

I. Approach to Dehydration

A. Definition: water deficit due to decreased intake and/or excessive losses (Box 8-1)

B. Historical questions

1. Questions should focus on intake and losses of fluids and minerals
   a. Has your child been hot, overdressed, or overbundled?
   b. Has your child suffered vomiting or diarrhea?
   c. How many wet diapers in the last day? How many times did your child urinate today? *Looking for inadequate urine output or excessive urination as in the case of diuretic use or diabetes mellitus (DM) and diabetes insipidus (DI)*
   d. Has your child had decreased intake or retention of fluids? *Children do not always have unlimited access to water or may not be able to verbalize or act on their thirst; they are dependent on caregivers to appreciate needs and to supply fluids*
   e. Has your child had fever? *Children will sweat excessively when the fever breaks*

C. Physical examination findings (Table 8-1)

D. Lab work needed to begin therapy

1. Chemistry panel: in many cases of dehydration, no laboratory data are necessary
   a. Bicarbonate is most reliable single lab in determining degree of dehydration (lower in more severe dehydration)
   b. Serum sodium will further classify type of dehydration
      i. Hyponatremic: Na^+ <130 mmol/L
      ii. Isonatremic: Na^+ 130–150 mmol/L
      iii. Hypernatremic: Na^+ >150 mmol/L

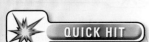

QUICK HIT
Hypovolemia may be more appropriate term because it is rarely only water content that is deficient but also electrolytes.

QUICK HIT
Higher surface area relative to volume ratio in children, especially young infants, and thus more insensible losses.

QUICK HIT
Insensible losses are through the skin and respiratory system. They are called "insensible" because they are difficult to measure routinely.

QUICK HIT
The treatment of dehydration should occur simultaneously with the diagnostic workup. In many cases, the treatment of dehydration may begin prior to establishing definitive diagnosis.

BOX 8-1

Common Causes of Dehydration in Children

- The most common etiology is from gastroenteritis, with losses due to vomiting and diarrhea
- Fever increases insensible fluid losses from skin and respiratory system
- Diabetic ketoacidosis, which causes vomiting due to ketosis and excessive urine output due to hyperglycemia
- Diabetes insipidus, which causes excessive urinary water losses due to deficient antidiuretic hormone
- Absence of intact thirst mechanism
- Environmental exposure to heat and excessive sweating
- Restriction of fluid intake
  - Voluntary from painful oral lesions or pharyngitis
  - Involuntary (because infants and young children are dependent on caregivers for oral intake)
  - Severe food restriction in cases of anorexia
- Diuretic use
- Burns: increase insensible losses from skin
- Increased respiratory rate such as in respiratory distress

TABLE 8-1 **Physical Examination Findings that Characterize the Severity of Dehydration**

Symptom*	Minimal or No Dehydration	Mild to Moderate Dehydration**	Moderate to Severe Dehydration**
% Dehydration	Infant: 1%–5% Child: 1%–3%	Infant: 6%–9% Child: 3%–6%	Infant: >10% Child: >6%
Mental status	Well, alert	Normal, fatigued or restless, irritable	Apathetic, lethargic, unconscious
Thirst	Drinks normally	Thirsty	Drinks poorly
Heart rate	Normal	Normal to increased	Tachycardic
Pulse	Normal	Normal to increased	Weak, thready
Fontanelle	Normal	**Sunken**	**Deeply sunken**
Eyes	Normal	Slightly sunken	Deeply sunken
Tears	Present	**Decreased**	**Absent**
Mucous membranes	Moist	Dry	Parched
Skin/skin turgor	Normal/instant recoil	Dry/recoil	Clammy, tenting present
Capillary refill	<2 seconds	**2–3 seconds**	**>3 seconds**
Extremities	Warm	Cool	Cold, mottled, cyanotic
Urine output	Normal to decreased	Decreased	Minimal

*The presence of any three symptoms of dehydration is sensitive and specific for a deficit of at least 5%. Only one finding is specific but not sensitive.

**Finding a bicarbonate level of <17 improves the sensitivity for moderate and severe categories of this clinical scale even further.

c. Blood urea nitrogen (BUN) and creatinine usually both elevated but less *specific* than bicarbonate
d. Glucose may be necessary to evaluate for hypo- or hyperglycemia
2. Serum lactate may be helpful in severe dehydration, especially when hypovolemic shock is possible/likely; suggests anaerobic metabolism secondary to cardiovascular compromise

E. Treatment
1. Estimate the degree of dehydration (mild/moderate/severe dehydration) by physical exam (see Table 8-1)
2. Best way to determine degree of dehydration is to compare *well weight* with *current weight* (although well weight often is not available)
3. In some conditions such as DM, patient has lost fluid and electrolytes *in addition* to fat and muscle; *well weight* may not be reliable in these cases and may *overestimate* dehydration
4. **Oral rehydration therapy (ORT)**
   a. First line in **uncomplicated mild and moderate dehydration**
   b. Contraindications for ORT include shock or concerns for an acute abdomen
   c. Goal: 50–100 cc/kg oral rehydration solution (ORS) over 4 hours
   d. Examples of ORS: Infalyte, Pedialyte, and World Health Organization rehydration fluids
   e. Fruit juices or sport drinks contain more glucose and negligible amounts of sodium and chloride and are not suitable alternatives for ORT; may also promote diarrhea
5. Intravenous (IV) rehydration
   a. *Standard therapy for severe dehydration/hypovolemic shock and for those patients who cannot tolerate ORT*

QUICK HIT

When a patient is dehydrated, an increase in heart rate will initially maintain blood pressure in the normal range. Hypotension indicates severe dehydration/volume depletion and requires immediate isotonic fluid therapy.

QUICK HIT

Young children with gastroenteritis are at risk for hypoglycemia due to smaller glycogen stores.

QUICK HIT

The degree of dehydration = (well weight − current weight)/well weight × 100%. For example, if a patient weighed 10 kg at a well-child visit last week and now weighs 9 kg, he or she is 10% dehydrated.

QUICK HIT

Often an antiemetic, in particular, **ondansetron**, can be given to improve tolerance of ORS in cases of gastroenteritis (contraindicated in prolonged QTc syndrome).

QUICK HIT

Give small frequent amounts of appropriate ORS if vomiting. Often, child will do well when fed 5–10 mL at a time by syringe.

QUICK HIT

ORSs maximize the gut's absorption of water and electrolytes by avoiding hyperosmolarity and making the sodium-to-carbohydrate ratio ideal for the gut's sodium/glucose cotransporter channels.

QUICK HIT

Give a 20-cc/kg bolus of normal saline or lactated ringer (LR) up to 3× with re-evaluation of patient between each bolus.

QUICK HIT

Initial bolus should always be normal saline or LR, as these quickly replenish the intravascular space.

QUICK HIT

Development of rales on lung exam or hepatomegaly may indicate patient is not tolerating rapid fluid therapy.

QUICK HIT

The cause of hyponatremia is determined by examining the patient's osmolality, volume status, and urine sodium.

QUICK HIT

Most cases of hyponatremia are hypotonic.

FIGURE 8-1 **This picture depicts the placement of an intraosseous (IO) needle in a patient's tibia. Fluid infused into the marrow cavity enters the circulation by way of venous sinusoids. Intravenous medications may be administered via an IO needle.**

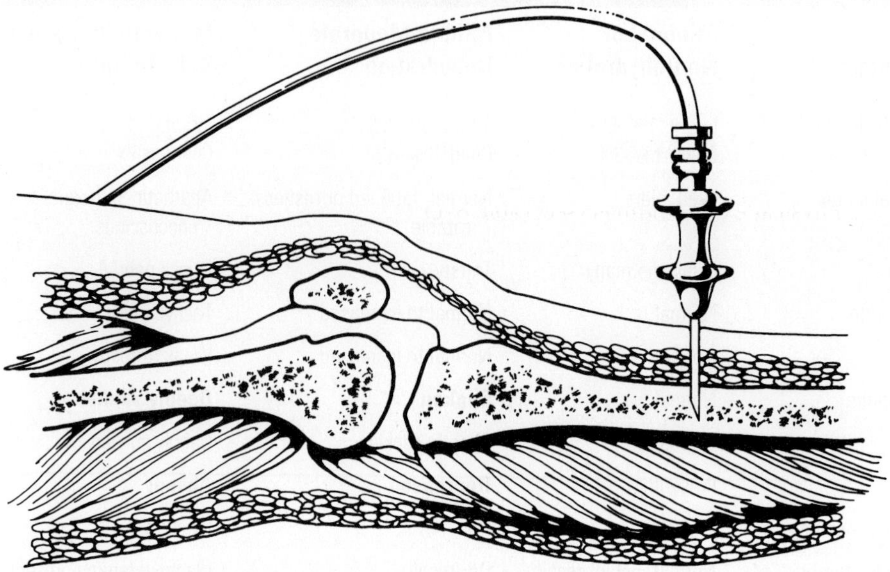

(From *Nursing Procedures*. 4th ed. Ambler, PA: Lippincott Williams & Wilkins; 2004.)

b. Rate of delivery depends on degree of dehydration and size of vessel cannulated
   i. Boluses are given over 5–10 minutes in urgent/emergent situations
   ii. Given over 20–30 minutes if less urgent
c. IV placement can be problematic in small patients; may require central venous access by experienced practitioners

6. **Intraosseous (IO) fluid administration**
   a. Used in severe dehydration or hypovolemic shock when IV access cannot be obtained
   b. American Heart Association (Pediatric Advanced Life Support) Guidelines recommend IO route in shock if IV access cannot be obtained in 5 minutes (Figure 8-1)
   c. Can administer any fluid or medicine via IO that can be given IV
7. **Subcutaneous rehydration therapy** (SCRT): also known as "**clysis**"; old technique finding renewed interest
   a. Alternative route of fluid administration for infants and children with mild to moderate dehydration, especially those unable to tolerate enteral fluids
   b. Administered with butterfly needle or angiocatheter, typically in interscapular region, often augmented with recombinant hyaluronidase
   c. Ease of use, safety, and reduced cost support use of this modality in many emergent settings
   d. Contraindicated in severe dehydration and hypovolemic shock, cardiac and renal disease, and hypocoagulable states

DISEASE SPECIFIC

II. Hyponatremia

A. Characteristics
   1. Definition
      a. Serum sodium <135 mEq/L
      b. Hyponatremia is usually synonymous with hypo-osmolality (serum osmolality <280 mEq/kg) because sodium is predominant osmole in extracellular volume
   2. Epidemiology: hyponatremia may be present in as many as 20% of infants and children hospitalized for gastroenteritis and volume depletion

B. Clinical features
  1. Historical findings
    a. How long has your child been ill? *Questions should focus on disease duration and severity, in addition to past history, medications, and family history when appropriate (see Approach to Dehydration)*
    b. Has your child had vomiting and diarrhea? Altered mental status? *Severity of hyponatremia and acuity in rate of fall will determine symptoms, which may include nausea and vomiting, anorexia, lethargy, muscle cramps, headaches, disorientation or agitation, and acute respiratory failure*
  2. Physical exam findings (see Table 8-1)
    a. Focus on assessing volume/hydration status and severity of illness (see Approach to Dehydration)
    b. Findings will also vary depending on severity and may include altered mental status, decreased tendon reflexes, hypothermia, and seizures
C. Diagnosis (Box 8-2)
D. Treatment
  1. Therapy for syndrome of inappropriate antidiuretic hormone (SIADH) secretion
    a. Water restriction
      i. Due to obligatory loss of water from skin and respiratory tract (insensible losses) and, even in setting of maximal antidiuretic hormone (ADH) secretion, obligatory excretion of water in urine (usually 10 mL/kg/day or greater), serum sodium has to increase if amount of water ingested is less than amount of water excreted

QUICK HIT

Mild hyponatremia (Na = 130–135 mEq/L) is common in dehydrated patients with conditions that cause SIADH (e.g., pneumonia). Do *not* withhold fluids in these patients.

BOX 8-2

Causes of Hyponatremia

Hypovolemic Hyponatremia (total body water ↓, total body Na^+ ↓↓)

Hypovolemic due to renal sodium loss > free water loss
- Osmotic diuresis (e.g., mannitol)
- Diuretic excess
- Salt-wasting dieresis
- Adrenal insufficiency
- Pseudohypoaldosteronism
- Hypovolemic due to extrarenal loss of sodium in excess of free water loss
- Vomiting/diarrhea
- Cerebral salt-wasting syndrome
- Third spacing conditions
  - Pancreatitis
  - Burns
  - Muscle trauma
  - Peritonitis
  - Large pleural effusions
  - Ascites

Euvolemic Hyponatremia (total body water ↑, total body Na^+ unchanged)

SIADH
- Tumors
- Pulmonary disease
- CNS disorders (especially meningitis) (rare)
- Drugs (rare)
- Gastroenteritis
- Postoperative surgical patients

Water intoxication (psychogenic polydipsia)

Hypervolemic Hyponatremia (total body water ↑↑, total body Na^+ ↑)
- Congestive heart failure
- Cirrhosis
- Renal failure

QUICK HIT

Recheck Na^+ at least every 2 hours to make sure you are not correcting too fast.

QUICK HIT

If a 50-kg adolescent admitted with meningitis develops seizures and is found to have a serum sodium level of 115 mEq/L, rapid correction is necessary. Correcting the Na^+ by increasing by 5 mEq/L should stop the seizures; 1 mL/kg of 3% saline will raise the serum Na^+ 1 mEq/L. Usually 2–6 mL/kg of 3% saline is used.

QUICK HIT

Because ADH has a short half-life of <10–15 minutes, the sodium level is typically rapidly corrected by isotonic fluid in this setting, and water restriction is not necessary.

QUICK HIT

You should check Na^+ *at least* every 2 hours. Goal is no more than 12 mEq/L/day.

QUICK HIT

Too rapid correction of hyponatremia can cause central pontine myelinolysis.

QUICK HIT

Increase in ECF tonicity from hypernatremia causes water to move out of cells, leading them to shrink; brain can be most vulnerable, which, in acute severe hypernatremia, can lead to serious neurologic complications.

ii. 15 mL/kg/day (e.g., 300 mL/day in 20-kg child) is reasonable starting point, and it can be increased or decreased depending on clinical response

b. Loop diuretics (furosemide, bumetanide, torsemide): increase urinary free water excretion
   i. Used along with water restriction, because they indirectly increase ADH release and increase thirst, and if patients are allowed free access to water, sodium level will not improve
   ii. Thiazide agents impair urinary dilution and typically will worsen hyponatremia
   iii. Should not be administered to patients with volume depletion

c. IV 3% sodium chloride (NaCl)
   i. Will rapidly increase serum sodium and is indicated in acute, severe symptomatic hyponatremia
   ii. In patients who are comatose, who have acute decline in neurologic function, and who are having seizures, IV 3% NaCl (which contains 513 mEq/L, called *hypertonic saline*) is particularly indicated

d. ADH receptor antagonists
   i. Demeclocycline, lithium carbonate
   ii. Tolvaptan and conivaptan are expensive and do not improve mortality in adults with hyponatremia, and pediatric drug safety data are limited

2. Treatment based on selected causes of hyponatremia
   a. Increased ADH due to decrease in intravascular volume
      i. Always treat with correction of underlying condition (diarrhea, vomiting, osmotic dieresis) and administration of isotonic fluid until intravascular volume is normalized
      ii. Then, calculate extracellular fluid (ECF) sodium deficit and correction for sodium derangement to determine sodium needs for next 24 hours
   b. Increased ADH due to an effective decrease in circulating volume (e.g., congestive heart failure)
      i. Correct of underlying condition (i.e., inotropic agents, diuretics)
      ii. Water restriction is also helpful
   c. SIADH: most challenging cause of hyponatremia to treat effectively
      i. In short term (transient ADH increases due to postoperative state, pain, nausea, or temporary pulmonary or central nervous system [CNS] diseases), water restriction and treatment of underlying condition are typically all that is necessary, and condition will spontaneously resolve
      ii. In chronic cases (e.g., CNS tumors causing persistent hyponatremia), water restriction will be effective, but may be poorly tolerated by patient; use of demeclocycline or vasopressin V_2 receptor antagonist on chronic basis may be indicated

III. Hypernatremia

A. Characteristics
   1. Definition: serum $[Na^+]$ >150 mEq/L
   2. Epidemiology (incidence varies widely): generally low (1%–2%) but much higher in intensive care unit (ICU) setting
   3. Pathophysiology and accompanying causes (Box 8-3 and Table 8-2)
      a. Generally reflects water loss in excess of sodium or sodium gain in excess of water
      b. Cerebral adaption: beginning almost immediately; however, there is increased generation and uptake of "osmolytes" by brain cells, causing water to move back into cells and restoring cell volume

B. Clinical features
   1. How long has your child been sick? Has your child had altered mental status? Has your child had fewer wet diapers? Less drinking? *Historical findings: questions should delineate disease duration and severity, in addition to past history, medications, and family history when appropriate (see Approach to Dehydration)*

BOX 8-3

Causes of Hypernatremia

Hypovolemic hypernatremia (total body water ↓↓, total body Na^+ ↓), most common

Renal losses
- Intrinsic renal disease
- After relief of urinary obstruction
- Loop diuretics
- Osmotic diuresis (mannitol, glucose in DKA, urea from high-protein feedings, or in recovering obstructive nephropathy or recovering acute tubular necrosis)

Extrarenal losses
- Diarrhea
- Excessive insensitive losses
- Burns

Euvolemic hypernatremia (total body water ↓, total body Na^+ unchanged)

Renal losses
- Diabetes insipidus (central or nephrogenic)

Extrarenal losses
- Moderate insensitive losses
- Hypodipsia
- Essential hypernatremia (= reset osmostat, all reported idiopathic cases <13 years old)

Hypervolemic hypernatremia (total body water ↑, total body Na^+ ↑↑)

Hypertonic solutions, improperly prepared formula, salt tablets
Hypertonic dialysate
Mineralocorticoid excess (mild hypernatremia)
Apparent mineralocorticoid excess (mild hypernatremia)

TABLE 8-2 Common Causes of Pediatric Diabetes Insipidus

Central Diabetes Insipidus (CDI)	Nephrogenic Diabetes Insipidus (NDI)
Congenital	Congenital (more common)
Septo-optic dysplasia (sporadic or familial)	X-linked (♂ >> symptoms than ♀)
	Autosomal dominant
	Autosomal recessive
Acquired (more common)	Acquired
Idiopathic (≈50% of cases)	Lithium toxicity
Encephalitis	**After relief of obstructive nephropathy**
Meningitis	Chronic kidney disease
Cerebral hemorrhage or infarction	After acute tubular necrosis
Granulomas (tuberculosis, sarcoidosis, Wegener)	Polycystic kidney disease
Tumors	Cystinosis
Histiocytosis	Amyloidosis
Trauma	Drugs (demeclocycline, cidofovir, foscarnet, didanosine, amphotericin B, ifosfamide)
Iatrogenic (neurosurgical, brain radiation therapy)	Protein malnutrition

2. Physical exam aims at assessing volume/hydration status and severity of illness (see Approach to Dehydration)
   a. Skin may feel "doughy"
   b. Severity of signs is due to degree of hypernatremia and its chronicity
   c. May present with high-pitched cry, irritability, lethargy, muscle weakness, and coma

C. Diagnosis
1. Laboratory findings (if unable to determine etiology from the history)
   a. Urine osmolality (Uosm): Uosm usually >600–800

QUICK HIT

Newborns of first-time breastfeeding mothers are at risk for hypernatremic dehydration.

QUICK HIT

Infants and young children are particularly susceptible to hypernatremia due to an inability to communicate thirst or access water, higher surface area–to–volume ratio with consequent larger insensitive losses, and higher incidence of diarrhea/vomiting.

QUICK HIT

Isolated findings on physical exam can be nonspecific. When assessing volume/hydration status, it is important to correlate a constellation of findings with the patient's history.

QUICK HIT

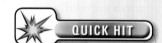

Due to water shifts from the intracellular to the extracellular space, the circulating blood volume is preserved. In hypernatremic dehydration, the physical exam may underestimate the degree of dehydration/volume depletion.

QUICK HIT

A serum Na >150 mEq/L indicates hypernatremia. An Na >170 mEq/L is an emergency but can be dangerous if you lower it too quickly.

QUICK HIT

Hyperosmolality stimulates ADH release.

QUICK HIT

Rapid resuscitation with hypotonic or hypertonic solutions is contraindicated due to potential cerebral edema or demyelination, respectively.

QUICK HIT

Calculations are only estimates. Check Na^+ level *at least* every 2 hours to make sure you are not correcting too fast.

QUICK HIT

Rate of correction should generally *not exceed 0.5 mmol/L/hr or 12 mmol/L/24 hr.*

QUICK HIT

Too rapid correction of hypernatremia can result in brain edema and brain herniation.

QUICK HIT

Another way to guide therapy: predicted change in $[Na^+]$ = (infusion fluid $[Na^+]$ – serum $[Na^+]$)/(total body water + 1) per 1,000 mL infused.

b. Uosm <300 → either lack of ADH (central diabetes insipidus [CDI]) or resistance to ADH (nephrogenic diabetes insipidus [NDI])
c. Water deprivation followed by DDAVP (desmopressin = synthetic vasopressin analog) administration will distinguish between CDI and NDI
   i. Uosm will more than double in complete CDI
   ii. Uosm will increase by >10% in partial CDI
   iii. Uosm will not significantly increase in complete NDI
d. Other labs
   i. BUN, creatinine to assess renal function
   ii. Other electrolytes can be abnormal (K^+, HCO_3, Ca^{++})
   iii. Urine Na^+ usually <20 mmol/L in volume depletion (some exceptions: loop diuretics, osmotic diuresis, intrinsic renal disease)

D. Treatment
1. Emergently restore moderate to severe volume deficit (if present); solution of choice is isotonic (0.9%) saline (crystalloid)
2. Restore serum tonicity and maintain volume repletion (see Appendix)
   a. Oral (or nasogastric tube [NGT]) water is preferred
3. Treat underlying cause
   a. Hypervolemic hypernatremia
      i. Remove sodium
      ii. Stop offending agent
      iii. Loop diuretic (e.g., furosemide)
      iv. Hemodialysis or peritoneal dialysis if needed in renal failure
   b. Chronic therapy for CDI
      i. Complete CDI: DDAVP, oral or nasal
      ii. Partial CDI: DDAVP, chlorpropamide, clofibrate, or carbamazepine (potentiate release of vasopressin)
   c. Chronic therapy for NDI (not as effective as for CDI)
      i. Remove offending drug
      ii. Correct hypokalemia or hypercalcemia
      iii. Thiazides
         (a) Possibly by causing volume contraction →
         (b) ↑ proximal tubule sodium and water reabsorption →
         (c) ↓ water delivery to collecting duct
         (d) Also inhibits diluting segment of nephron
      iv. Nonsteroidal anti-inflammatory drugs can be well tolerated and are used in combination with thiazides
      v. Amiloride may be helpful in lithium-induced NDI (blocks Na^+ channel in renal collecting duct, site of lithium reabsorption)
4. Complications
   a. Hypernatremia
      i. Symptoms can progress to seizures, coma, and death
      ii. Rare cases of osmotic demyelination (pontine and extrapontine) have been reported in severe cases
   b. Rapid correction of hypernatremia (usually >0.7 mmol/L/hr), especially after brain adaptation is established
      i. Rapid ↓ ECF tonicity → rapid shift of water back into cells → brain cell edema → brain volume ↑
      ii. But, cranium cannot expand → brain herniation
5. Prognosis: very good in developed countries with rapid access to health care, with low risk for neurodevelopmental compromise
6. Prevention
   a. Close clinical monitoring of breastfeeding newborns, including lab work if excessive weight loss
   b. Monitor $[Na^+]$ if risk factors for hypernatremia exist (see Box 8-3)

IV. Hyperkalemia

A. Definition: serum K^+ levels **>5 mEq/L**

B. Causes and pathophysiology
  1. Red cells may lyse during the blood draw or on the way to the lab.
    a. Red blood cell (RBC) hemolysis
    b. Metabolic acidosis causes H^+ to enter cells and potassium to exit cells in order to maintain electroneutrality
    c. In diabetic ketoacidosis (DKA), insulin deficiency and hyperosmolality from hyperglycemia promote exit of potassium from cells
    d. Hyperosmolality from mannitol therapy or hypernatremia results in **solvent drag** (i.e., phenomenon in which rapid exit of water from cells causes intracellular potassium to be "dragged" out of cells)
    e. Increased tissue breakdown results in release of intracellular potassium in these conditions
      i. Rhabdomyolysis
      ii. Tumor lysis syndrome
      iii. Crush injuries
      iv. Hypothermia leading to tissue necrosis
    f. β-Blockers decrease Na^+/K^+ ATPase activity, thereby causing potassium to leave cells
    g. Exercise causes potassium to be released from muscle cells
    h. Digitalis overdose results in inhibition of Na^+/K^+ ATPase activity
  2. Decreased urinary potassium excretion
    a. Decreased urinary flow rate and impaired Na^+/K^+ ATPase activity
      i. Prerenal intravascular volume depletion
      ii. Acute kidney injury
      iii. Chronic kidney disease
    b. Hypoaldosteronism
      i. Decreases Na^+/K^+ ATPase activity, resulting in decreased movement of serum potassium into cells
      ii. Decreases number of potassium channels in luminal membrane of principal cells, resulting in decreased potassium secretion
      iii. Decreases number of sodium channels in luminal membrane of principal cells, leading to decreased reabsorption of sodium and decreased potassium secretion
      iv. Type 4 renal tubular acidosis (RTA) (see Chapter 7)
    c. Medications that inhibit **renin–angiotensin–aldosterone system**, resulting in hypoaldosterone state
      i. Angiotensin-converting enzyme (ACE) inhibitors
      ii. Angiotensin receptor blockers (ARBs)
      iii. Calcineurin inhibitors (cyclosporine, tacrolimus)
  3. Ureterojejunostomy: attachment of ureters to jejunum results in absorption of urinary potassium in jejunum
  4. Increased dietary intake of potassium salts
  5. Pseudohyperkalemia
    a. Venipuncture trauma causes RBC hemolysis
    b. Hereditary spherocytosis
    c. Familial pseudohyperkalemia causes leakage of potassium from RBCs due to increased temperature during specimen collection
    d. Leukocytosis (white blood cells [WBCs] $>100{,}000/mm^3$) results in movement of intracellular potassium out of WBCs after clotting
    e. Thrombocytosis (platelets $>400{,}000/mm^3$) results in movement of intracellular potassium out of platelets after clotting
  6. Hyperkalemic periodic paralysis: autosomal dominant disorder that develops after cold exposure, fasting, ingestion of potassium, or rest after exercise

C. Clinical features
  1. Historical and physical exam findings
    a. *Irregular heart rates, arrhythmias*
    b. Weakness of extremities, ascending muscle weakness: begins with legs and progresses to trunk and arms

QUICK HIT

A "false-positive" high K^+ from serum is extremely common in children. Consider if the child truly has a reason for hyperkalemia.

QUICK HIT

Insulin promotes movement of potassium into cells.

QUICK HIT

Catecholamines and β-agonists, such as albuterol, cause potassium to shift into cells by stimulating Na^+/K^+ ATPase activity.

QUICK HIT

Decreased urinary flow rate results in impaired urinary potassium secretion.

QUICK HIT

Serum potassium levels increase by 0.15 mEq/L for every $100{,}000/mm^3$ increase in platelet count.

FIGURE 8-2 Diagnostic evaluation of hyperkalemia.

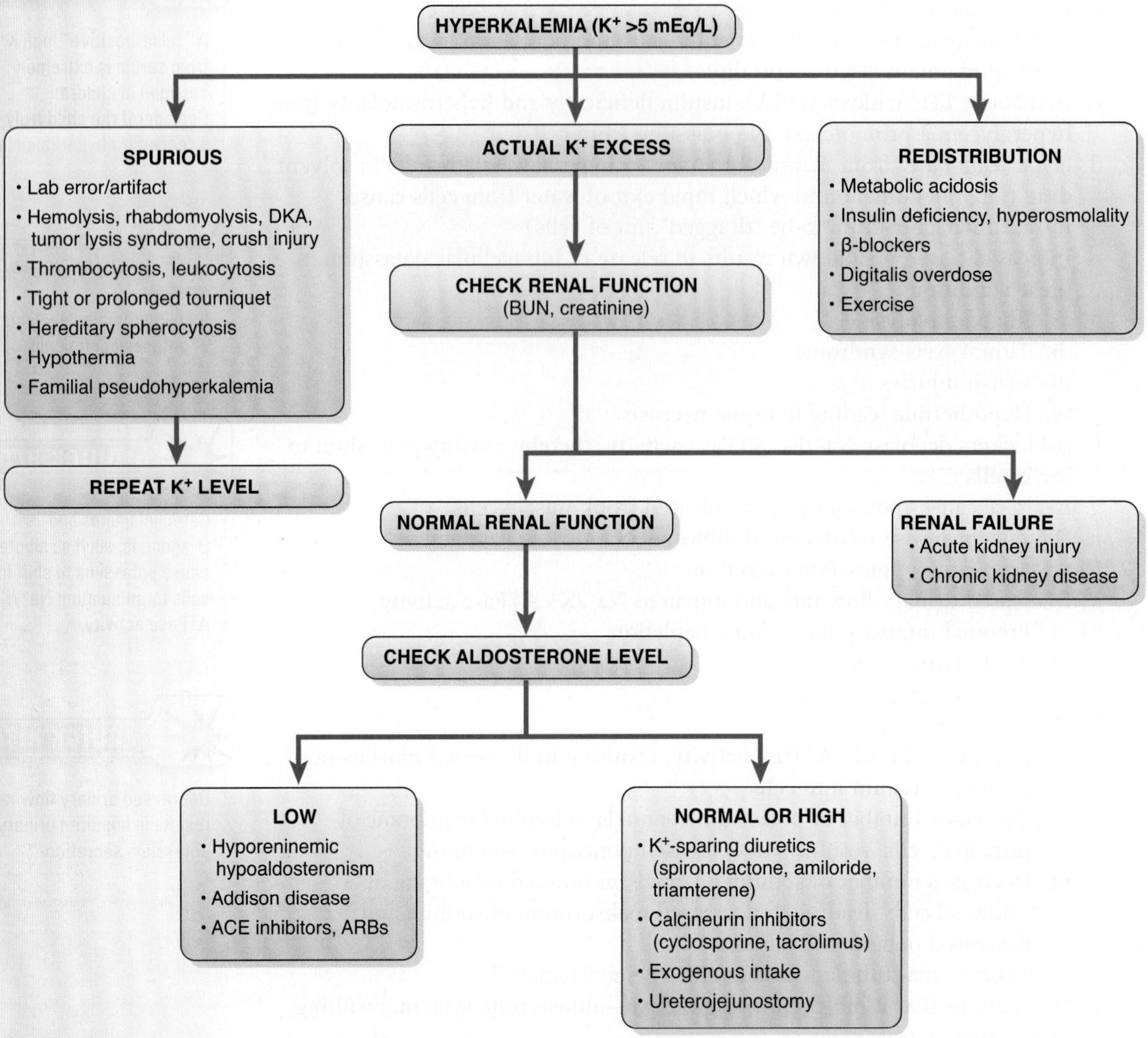

ACE, angiotensin-converting enzyme; ARBs, angiotensin receptor blockers; DKA, diabetic ketoacidosis

QUICK HIT

Signs and symptoms usually occur when serum K^+ concentration is **≥7.0 mEq/L.**

c. Oliguria, edema, hypertension in renal dysfunction
d. Symptoms are reversible with correction of hyperkalemia

D. Diagnosis
1. Workup (Figure 8-2)
2. Electrocardiogram (ECG) findings: low P wave, prolongation of PR interval, widening of QRS complex, and peaked T waves (Figure 8-3)

E. Treatment (Box 8-4)

QUICK HIT

K^+ >6.0 can cause life-threatening arrhythmias, due to disruptions in the electrical conduction system of the heart, resulting in ventricular fibrillation and arrest.

BOX 8-4

Treatment of Hyperkalemia

1. Shift potassium intracellularly
   a. Insulin *and* glucose
   b. Sodium bicarbonate (increases pH)
   c. β_2-Agonists, such as albuterol and epinephrine
2. Remove potassium
   a. Kayexalate (absorbs potassium in colon)
   b. Diuresis if renal function intact; give normal saline and furosemide
   c. Dialysis if severe renal impairment
3. Cardiopulmonary monitoring during therapy is essential

FIGURE 8-3 **Electrocardiogram changes for hyperkalemia and hypokalemia.**

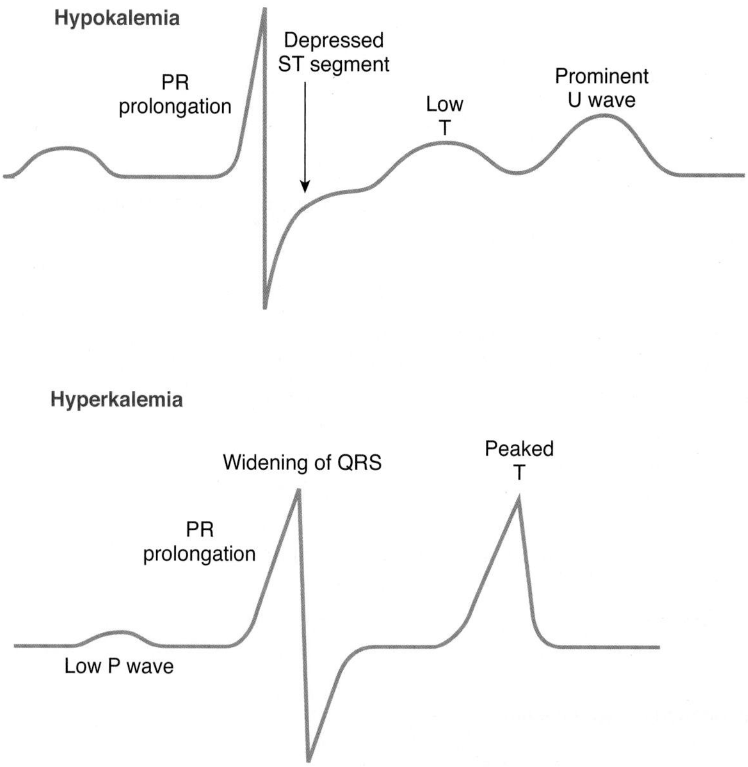

QUICK HIT

For any $K^+ > 6.0$, first give calcium chloride or calcium gluconate to stabilize cardiac muscle membrane potentials.

QUICK HIT

Calcium chloride and calcium gluconate can be caustic to veins and cause tissue necrosis if extravasation occurs, so a central line is preferred particularly during rapid infusion rate.

V. Hypokalemia (serum K^+ levels <3.5 mEq/L)

A. Causes and pathophysiology
  1. Movement of extracellular K^+ into cells
    a. Metabolic alkalosis causes H^+ to leave cells, resulting in potassium entering cells to maintain electroneutrality
    b. β_2-Adrenergic agonists increase Na^+/K^+ ATPase activity, resulting in potassium entering cells
    c. Hyperinsulinemia
    d. Acute increase in RBC or WBC production
    e. Hypothermia
    f. Hypokalemic periodic paralysis: autosomal dominant disorder that develops after high-carbohydrate diet or heavy exercise
  2. Increased urinary K^+ excretion
    a. Hyperaldosteronism
      i. Increases Na^+/K^+ ATPase activity, resulting in movement of potassium into cells and then into urinary lumen
      ii. Increases number of potassium channels in luminal membrane of principal cells, resulting in increased potassium secretion
      iii. Increases number of sodium channels in luminal membrane of principal cells, leading to increased reabsorption of sodium and increased potassium secretion
    b. Polyuria washes away urinary potassium, thereby creating concentration gradient allowing for additional secretion of potassium into urinary lumen
    c. Increased sodium delivery to cortical collecting duct (CCD) results in reabsorption of sodium and development of electrochemical gradient (negative charge from chloride in urinary lumen) that promotes potassium secretion
    d. RTA
      i. Type 1: distal RTA
      ii. Type 2: proximal RTA
    e. Bartter syndrome: congenital renal defect in $Na/K/Cl^-$ cotransporter in thick ascending loop of Henle, presents with growth failure, metabolic alkalosis, hypokalemia, and hypercalciuria defect

QUICK HIT

The most common causes of hypokalemia in pediatric patients are vomiting, the use of diuretics in patients with heart disease and chronic lung disease, and DKA.

QUICK HIT

Bartter syndrome manifests symptoms similar to furosemide poisoning.

QUICK HIT

Gitelman syndrome manifests symptoms like thiazide poisoning.

QUICK HIT

Signs and symptoms usually occur when serum potassium concentration is **≤2.5 mEq/L**.

QUICK HIT

↓ K^+ in combination with ↓ Mg^{2+} can cause torsades de pointes.

QUICK HIT

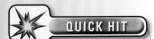

Oral potassium replacement is safer, but efficacy is slower compared to IV.

QUICK HIT

Give IV K^+ if $K^+ < 2$, if there are ECG changes, or if you cannot use the GI tract.

QUICK HIT

IV K^+ repletion should be given with caution because it can be caustic to veins and result in tissue necrosis if extravasation occurs; therefore, a central line is preferred.

f. Gitelman syndrome: defect in Na/Cl^- cotransporter in distal tubule
g. Medications
i. Loop diuretics
ii. Thiazides
iii. Acetazolamide
iv. Amphotericin B
3. Increased gastrointestinal (GI) losses
a. Increased stool losses from diarrhea, laxative abuse
b. Increased gastric losses from vomiting, NGT suction, pyloric stenosis
4. Decreased dietary intake of potassium

B. Clinical features
1. Historical and physical exam findings
a. Bradycardia, irregular heart rate, arrhythmias
b. Muscle cramps and weakness of extremities due to skeletal muscle and neuromuscular dysfunction; rhabdomyolysis may occur.
c. Respiratory depression
d. Ileus: abdominal distension
e. Polyuria, hypokalemia impairs ability to reabsorb hydrogen ions in kidney, causing concentration defect
f. Symptoms are reversible with correction of hypokalemia

C. Diagnosis
1. Workup (Figure 8-4)

FIGURE 8-4 **Diagnostic evaluation of hypokalemia.**

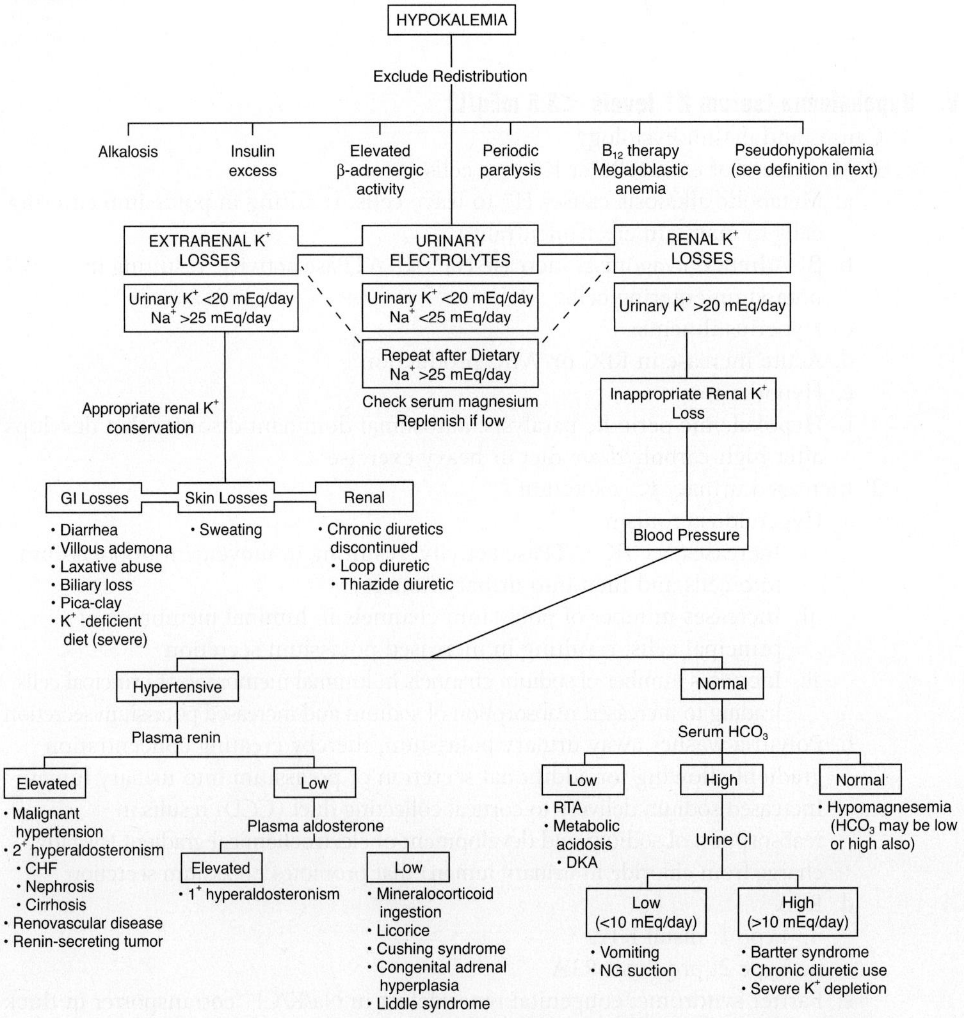

CHF, congestive heart failure; DKA, diabetic ketoacidosis; GI, gastrointestinal; NG, nasogastric; RTA, renal tubular acidosis.

2. ECG findings: flattened or inverted T waves, ST depression, presence of U wave (see Figure 8-3)
   a. Life-threatening arrhythmias can occur (less often than in hyperkalemia)
   b. When patient is on digitalis and has hypokalemia, cardiac arrhythmias are more likely

D. Treatment
1. Potassium replacement
   a. Potassium chloride; preferred if there is alkalosis present
   b. Potassium bicarbonate; preferred if there is acidosis present
   c. Potassium phosphate
   d. Potassium acetate (IV only)
2. Potassium-sparing diuretics
   a. Spironolactone
   b. Amiloride
   c. Eplerenone
3. Cardiopulmonary monitoring during therapy is essential

VI. Anion Gap Metabolic Acidosis

A. Characteristics
1. Definition: decreased blood pH and decreased plasma bicarbonate concentration, resulting in increased plasma acidity
2. Results from increased acid generation from either endogenous or exogenous source
3. Causes
   a. Ketoacidosis
   b. Lactic acidosis
4. Pathophysiology: plasma acid accumulation overwhelms physiologic compensatory mechanisms
   a. Bicarbonate buffer system maintains acid–base homeostasis as described by Henderson-Hasselbalch equation: $H^+ + HCO_3^- = H_2CO_3 = H_2O + CO_2$
   b. As more acid moves into system, CO_2 forms and is removed by lungs
   c. As more acid accumulates, kidney absorbs more HCO_3^-
   d. When these mechanisms are overwhelmed, buffer system shifts to left, with acid accumulation

B. Clinical features
1. Some nonspecific physical findings associated with metabolic acidosis
   a. Generalized weakness and pain
   b. Nausea, vomiting, and diarrhea
   c. Confusion
   d. Impaired myocardial function
   e. Hyperkalemia
   f. Decreased pulmonary blood flow
   g. Right shift in oxygen–hemoglobin dissociation curve, diminishing affinity of hemoglobin for oxygen and increasing oxygen delivery to tissue

C. Diagnosis (Box 8-5)
1. Often 1st clue of metabolic acidosis is low serum HCO_3^- on venous sample
2. Arterial blood gas (ABG) is necessary to determine overall acid–base status
3. Measurement of pH and partial pressure of carbon dioxide (PCO_2) through ABG makes it possible to differentiate between metabolic compensation of respiratory alkalosis and primary metabolic acidosis
4. To assess respiratory compensation to metabolic acidosis, use the Winter formula: expected partial pressure of carbon dioxide in arterial blood ($PaCO_2$) (mm Hg) = (1.5 × measured HCO_3^- [mEq/L]) + 8 ± 2
   a. Predicts expected respiratory compensation ($PaCO_2$ level) to metabolic acidosis: if $PaCO_2$ does not fall within acceptable range, then patient has another primary acid–base disorder
   b. If $PaCO_2$ is as predicted, then patient has simple metabolic acidosis with appropriate secondary hypocapnia

QUICK HIT

Metabolic acidosis can be divided on basis of serum anion gap into **increased anion gap metabolic acidosis ("gap" acidosis)** and **nonanion gap metabolic acidosis.**

QUICK HIT

Serum anion gap is a useful test in determining the etiology of metabolic acidosis. **Serum anion gap** = (Na^+) − [(Cl^-) + (HCO_3^-)]. The normal value is ~12 ± 2.

QUICK HIT

The MUDPILES mnemonic is a ubiquitous, although by no means comprehensive, memory aid for some of the causes of metabolic acidosis:
- M: Methanol
- U: Uremia (chronic kidney disease)
- D: Diabetic ketoacidosis
- P: Propylene glycol, Paraldehyde
- I: Infection, Iron, Isoniazid, Inborn errors of metabolism
- L: Lactic acidosis
- E: Ethylene glycol, Ethanol
- S: Salicylates

QUICK HIT

For *every* patient with acidosis, calculate anion gap to know whether it is gap or nongap acidosis.

QUICK HIT

NOTE: Metabolic acidosis can, and often does, coexist with other acid–base disturbances.

QUICK HIT

A large anion gap (>20 mmol/L) always indicates primary metabolic acidosis; the body does not generate large anion gaps as a compensatory mechanism.

Fluids and Electrolytes

BOX 8-5

Approach to Blood Gas Interpretations

Look at the pH:
The abnormality that is causing a shift on either side of 7.4 is the primary abnormality. So a pH of 7.2 indicates that the primary abnormality is an acidosis, and a pH of 7.5 indicates alkalosis as the primary abnormality. The body does not "overcompensate."

Look at the $PaCO_2$ and the serum bicarbonate for the respiratory and metabolic components:
- If the pH is alkalotic, or >7.4, then either a lowered $PaCO_2$ (<35) indicates a primary respiratory alkalosis or a raised bicarbonate (>26) indicates a metabolic alkalosis.
- If the pH is acidotic, or <7.4, then either a high $PaCO_2$ (>45) indicates a primary respiratory acidosis or a low bicarbonate (<22) indicates a primary metabolic acidosis is the primary disorder.

Calculate the anion gap for any acidosis.
The body does not generate a large anion gap to compensate for a primary disorder. If there is a large gap (>20 mmol/L), there is a primary metabolic acidosis.

Calculate the delta-delta.
First, calculate the excess anion gap (total anion gap – normal anion gap [12 mmol/L]) and add this to the measured bicarbonate concentration for the delta-delta, which estimates the baseline bicarbonate. If the sum is greater than a normal serum bicarbonate (30 mmol/L), there is an underlying metabolic alkalosis. If the sum is less than a normal serum bicarbonate (23 mmol/L), there may be an underlying nonanion gap metabolic acidosis.

Calculate the expected respiratory compensation for acute metabolic acidosis.
Use Winter's formula once you identify a metabolic acidosis to assess respiratory compensation. Expected $PaCO_2$ (mm Hg) = (1.5 × measured HCO_3^- [mEq/L]) + 8 ± 2

QUICK HIT

Failure to compensate for metabolic acidosis can be a sign of impending respiratory failure.

c. If actual $PaCO_2$ is higher than calculated $PaCO_2$, then patient has metabolic acidosis with respiratory acidosis
d. If actual $PaCO_2$ is lower than calculated $PaCO_2$, then patient has metabolic acidosis with respiratory alkalosis

D. Therapy
1. Correction of underlying conditions, whether ingestions, inborn errors of metabolism, shock
2. Provision of supportive care while underlying conditions are being treated (e.g., mechanical ventilation may be necessary if patient is fatigued from prolonged hyperventilation such as in DKA)
3. Sodium bicarbonate is sometimes used to treat severe refractory acidosis; contraindicated with hyperammonemia because bicarbonate may increase cellular influx of ammonia in brain

VII. Nonanion Gap Metabolic Acidosis

A. Characteristics
1. Definition: nonanion gap or "hyperchloremic" metabolic acidosis occurs whenever there is failure to excrete acid in urine, or from loss of bicarbonate ions from GI tract or renal tubules
2. Pathophysiology
a. Anion gap reflects unmeasured anions in body
i. Total number of cations = total number of anions in body
ii. Therefore, fall in serum HCO_3^- concentration must be offset by concurrent rise in concentration of other anions
b. If anion accompanying excess acid is chloride, then *fall in serum bicarbonate value must be matched by rise in serum chloride concentration* (anion gap will remain normal as can be seen from equation above)
c. Normal kidney excretes H^+ ions in urine coupled with ammonia (NH_3); therefore, estimation of urinary ammonium (NH_4^+) concentration

MNEMONIC

H = Hyperalimentation
A = Acetazolamide*
R = RTA
D = Diarrhea
U = Ureteroenteric fistula
P = Pancreaticoduodenal fistula
*More common in adults

(unmeasured cation) by calculating urinary anion gap can help distinguish *renal* from *extrarenal* causes ($U_{AG} = [U_{NA} + U_K] - U_{Cl}$)
   i. A positive gap implies lots of NH_4^+, hence decreased urine excretion of ammonium, and thus an intrarenal problem
   ii. A negative gap implies increased NH_4^+ excretion and an extrarenal problem

B. Clinical features
   1. History
      a. Has your child had growth failure, dehydration, or weight loss? Has your child had sore muscles? *Children with RTA clinically present with* ***nonspecific symptoms*** *such as growth failure, dehydration, anorexia, muscle cramps, myalgias, polyuria, polydipsia, constipation, and recurrent vomiting*
      b. Has your child had diarrhea? *Children with* ***GI losses*** *of bicarbonate will present with history of* ***diarrhea*** *or surgical history of* ***ureteral anastomosis*** *or* ***enterostomies***
   2. Physical exam
      a. Flank tenderness and hematuria related to **nephrocalcinosis** and **renal stones** may be seen with distal (type 1) RTA
      b. Patients with proximal (type 2) RTA in association with Fanconi syndrome may also present with **rickets** from **renal calcium** and **phosphate wasting** and glucosuria in the setting of normoglycemia

C. Diagnosis
   1. **Renal origin** (see Chapter 7, Renal Tubular Acidosis)
   2. **Extrarenal origin**
      a. Diarrhea
         i. Intestinal secretions beyond stomach are **rich in bicarbonate**, and **accelerated loss** of these secretions as diarrhea will lead to metabolic acidosis; because bicarbonate absorption within colon occurs in electroneutral exchange for Cl^-, loss of bicarbonate from diarrhea also results in rise in serum chloride
         ii. Volume loss also leads to **increased absorption of NaCl** from kidney, resulting in hyperchloremic nonanion gap acidosis
      b. GI–ureteral connections
         i. Surgical diversion of ureter into ileum or colon may be seen in patients with abdominal or bladder tumors or for treatment of neurologic bladder dysfunction; **urinary chloride** entering GI tract causes **activation of GI anion-exchange pump**, leading to chloride absorption and bicarbonate loss in stool
         ii. Hyperchloremic nonanion gap metabolic acidosis develops in up to **80%** of these patients
   3. Laboratory and radiology findings
      a. Laboratory values will reflect **low serum pH**, a low pCO_2 secondary to respiratory compensation, and serum electrolyte concentrations consistent with nonanion gap hyperchloremic metabolic acidosis
      b. Serum potassium level is typically low in most cases, except for patients who present with type 4 RTA
      c. Urinary electrolytes are needed to calculate urinary anion gap
      d. Radiology findings: **renal ultrasound** may be considered if you suspect **nephrocalcinosis**, which suggests diagnosis of distal RTA

D. Treatment
   1. Children with RTA usually require **lifelong oral alkali therapy** to maintain their pH in normal range and normalize growth (see Chapter 7, Renal Tubular Acidosis for further discussion)
   2. Children with diarrhea will require treatment of their primary condition and **correction** of their **volume and bicarbonate deficiency**; in most cases, acidosis resolves with improvement of diarrhea

QUICK HIT

Urinary anion gap = (urine Na^+ + urine K^+) urine Cl^-. A negative urinary anion gap indicates an extrarenal cause for the nonanion gap metabolic acidosis. A positive urinary anion gap indicates a renal cause.

QUICK HIT

Failure to thrive associated with metabolic acidosis in an infant should alert the clinician to the possibility of RTA.

QUICK HIT

A similar clinical picture (hyperchloremic nonanion gap acidosis) may be seen in patients suspected of occult laxative abuse.

QUICK HIT

Serum anion gap must be determined 1st in all cases of metabolic acidosis.

QUICK HIT

Determination of the serum and urinary anion gaps are necessary to determine the etiology of metabolic acidosis.

> **QUICK HIT**
> In a hospitalized patient with long-standing nasogastric suctioning, consider metabolic alkalosis as a potential problem.

> **QUICK HIT**
> If etiology of metabolic alkalosis is not apparent based on history/physical exam, urinary chloride (Cl^-) can help guide the differential.

> **QUICK HIT**
> Remember K^+ and H^+ are "swapped" across the cell wall. If the body has low K^+, it will pull K^+ out of cells by swapping for $H^+ \rightarrow$ alkalosis.

> **QUICK HIT**
> Alkalosis leads to poor tissue oxygen delivery (hypoxemia) as oxygen–hemoglobin dissociation curve shifts to left.

> **QUICK HIT**
> Alkalosis can cause hypocalcemia because as albumin binds more free calcium during alkalosis.

> **QUICK HIT**
> Erosion of tooth enamel, from repeated exposure of the teeth to acidic gastric secretions, should prompt consideration of bulimia nervosa in the differential.

VIII. Metabolic Alkalosis

A. Characteristics
1. Definition: metabolic disturbance associated with tissue pH >7.45, resulting from loss of hydrogen ions or gain in serum bicarbonate (HCO_3^-)
2. Epidemiology: in hospitalized patients, this is common acid–base disorder, often associated with gastric fluid losses or diuretic administration
3. Pathophysiology: generation of metabolic alkalosis mainly involves kidneys and GI tract
   a. Loss of gastric secretions rich in hydrochloric acid (HCl)
      i. Normally, pancreatic HCO_3^- release neutralizes gastric secretions
      ii. In absence of HCl delivery to duodenum, pancreatic HCO_3^- release is attenuated, leading to net systemic HCO_3^- gain
   b. Chronic diuretic therapy
      i. Leads to enhanced NaCl delivery to CCD
      ii. Principal cells of CCD reclaim this sodium, setting up net lumen negative charge
      iii. Lumen negativity enhances both urinary H^+ and K^+ losses
      iv. Total body Cl^- depletion also stimulates electroneutral uptake of filtered HCO_3^- by nephron
      v. Vascular depletion concentrates serum HCO_3^- (termed **contraction alkalosis**)
   c. Mineralocorticoid excess
      i. Na^+ reabsorption by principal cells is stimulated, leading to increased H^+ and K^+ urinary losses
      ii. Congenital upregulation of principal cell sodium uptake provides similar effects
      iii. Aldosterone also directly increases H^+/ATPase pump activity on α-intercalated cells of CCD
      iv. Cortisol has greater affinity and activation of mineralocorticoid receptor, stimulating H^+ and K^+ secretion
4. Risk factors
   a. Vomiting or continuous nasogastric (NG) suctioning
   b. Loop or thiazide diuretic usage
   c. Hypokalemia
      i. Shifts H^+ from extracellular to intracellular space
      ii. Promotes urinary retention of K^+ at expense of H^+
   d. Renal failure patients taking alkali compounds
   e. Antacid or calcium carbonate ingestion
   f. Cushing syndrome (excess mineralocorticoid)

B. Clinical features
1. Symptoms and signs will vary depending on etiology
2. Dehydration may present with tachycardia, postural hypotension, dry mucous membranes, poor skin turgor, and weight loss
3. If hypokalemia is present, patient may have myalgias, generalized weakness, and/or life-threatening cardiac arrhythmias
4. Hypocalcemia can present as jitteriness, irritability, muscle spasms, tetany, tingling, change in mental status, convulsions, or coma
5. Chemoreceptor inhibition within medullary respiratory center leads to hypoventilation with potential bouts of apnea
6. In congenital adrenal hyperplasia (CAH), infants may show hypertension and growth retardation; female newborns may develop virilization
7. Patients with Cushing syndrome may have cushingoid facies, buffalo hump, hirsutism, obesity, acne, and abdominal striae
8. Increased mineralocorticoid levels typically present with hypertension and weight gain

C. Diagnosis
1. Differential diagnosis: can be divided into low urinary chloride excretion (<10 mEq/L) and normal urinary chloride (>20 mEq/L) excretion

a. Low urinary chloride excretion (or, chloride-responsive individuals)
   i. Loss of gastric secretions rich in HCl due to excessive vomiting, GI obstruction, or continuous NG suction
   ii. Thiazide or loop diuretics enhance urinary H^+ and K^+ excretion; also promote urinary chloride loss and total body chloride depletion
   iii. Bartter and Gitelman syndromes (see Hypokalemia)
   iv. Antacids, in combination with sodium polystyrene administration, enhance bicarbonate uptake in large intestine
   v. Cystic fibrosis commonly leads to volume depletion during infancy and high chloride losses in their sweat
   vi. Rare, autosomal recessive form of severe secretory diarrhea (**congenital chloridorrhea**) has significant intestinal Cl^- losses and HCO_3^- reclamation
b. Normal urinary chloride excretion (chloride-resistant individuals)
   i. Hyperreninemic state from renal artery stenosis or renin-secreting tumors leads to activation of angiotensin–aldosterone system
   ii. Primary hyperaldosteronism
   iii. Constitutively active mineralocorticoid receptor defect
   iv. 11α-hydroxysteroid dehydrogenase type 2 enzymatic deficiency
   v. Liddle syndrome
   vi. CAH
   vii. Excess licorice ingestion (containing glycyrrhizic acid)

2. Laboratory findings
   a. Elevated serum bicarbonate: although serum HCO_3^- rises during respiratory acidosis compensation, consider when plasma HCO_3^- exceeds 35 mEq/L
   b. ABG with high pH and high HCO_3^-
   c. Check urinary chloride (see Diagnosis)
   d. Hypokalemia and hypocalcemia

D. Treatment
1. Therapy
   a. Fluid resuscitation for hypovolemic shock
   b. Blood pressure and arrhythmia medications may be required
   c. KCl supplements to replenish both low potassium and chloride concentrations
   d. Acetazolamide, a carbonic anhydrase inhibitor, can decrease proximal tubular HCO_3^- reabsorption in patients with fluid excess or in postcardiac surgery
   e. Patients with renal failure may require dialysis to correct alkalosis
   f. Discontinuation of diuretic therapy or switching to K^+-sparing diuretics may be helpful when continuous diuretic administration is warranted
   g. If HCl administration becomes imperative, placement of central line is critical because severe tissue necrosis can occur following extravasation
2. Prognosis
   a. If treated promptly and hypoxia is avoided, there is low likelihood of long-term complications
   b. Untreated severe metabolic alkalosis can lead to heart failure, seizures, or coma

IX. Hypomagnesemia

A. Characteristics
1. Definition: serum magnesium (Mg) level **<1.5 mg/dL** (normal 1.8–2.5 mg/dL)
2. Pathophysiology
   a. Mg, second most abundant intracellular cation
   b. **Essential ion in fundamental metabolic processes**
      i. DNA and protein synthesis
      ii. Adenosine triphosphate (ATP) metabolism
   c. Levels **maintained within narrow range**
3. Causes (Table 8-3)

B. Clinical features
1. **Most often asymptomatic**
2. Symptoms: Mg <1.2 mg/dL, often **associated hypocalcemia, hypokalemia**

QUICK HIT

In a 4- to 12-week-old infant with protracted emesis, consider pyloric stenosis and obtain electrolytes. A hypochloremic, hypokalemic metabolic alkalosis will be seen. Fluid status and metabolic derangements should be corrected with normal saline before a pylorotomy is performed.

QUICK HIT

If a patient has metabolic alkalosis and hypercalcemia, consider milk–alkali syndrome from excessive calcium carbonate intake for peptic ulcer therapy.

QUICK HIT

Liddle syndrome is a rare, gain-of-function mutation in the apical Na channel of the CCD principal cells, leading to volume expansion, hypertension, alkalosis, and hypokalemia.

QUICK HIT

Alkalosis requires close monitoring in ICU when pH >7.55.

QUICK HIT

Infants with pyloric stenosis require surgical correction after normalization of their metabolic alkalosis and electrolyte deficit.

QUICK HIT

In infants with pyloric stenosis, nothing by mouth (NPO) status and IV fluids usually reverse the alkalosis.

QUICK HIT

Administration of glucocorticoids, to suppress pituitary adrenocorticotropic hormone release, is beneficial in the treatment of patients with primary hyperaldosteronism.

QUICK HIT

Patients with hypokalemia often don't respond to replacement therapy if hypomagnesemia is not corrected as well!

QUICK HIT

In the parathyroid gland, Mg is needed as a cofactor for the release of parathyroid hormone.

QUICK HIT

Only 1% of total body magnesium is extracellular (95% in bone), making serum magnesium an insensitive test. However, it is still the most practical test in the clinical setting.

QUICK HIT

Magnesium supplements can be confusing. Magnesium citrate is for constipation, not Mg supplementation.

QUICK HIT

↓ PTH causes ↑ PO_4 from kidney, and ↓ Ca from bone vitamin D causes ↑ PO_4 *and* ↑ Ca absorption.

TABLE 8-3 **Causes of Hypomagnesemia**

Decreased Intake	Decreased Intestinal Absorption	Increased Renal Excretion	Endocrine/ Metabolic Causes
Starvation/ malnutrition Alcoholism Parenteral nutrition	Chronic diarrhea Malabsorptive states Enteric fistula Bowel resection Nasogastric tube suction Laxatives	Diuretics Acute tubular necrosis Renal failure Polyuria Glycosuria Genetic wasting syndromes (e.g., Bartter/Gitelman) Aminoglycosides Amphotericin B Chemotherapeutics	Diabetes mellitus Phosphate depletion Parathyroid hormone abnormalities

C. Diagnosis/lab findings
   1. Low serum Mg
   2. Serum calcium and potassium: low levels often seen concurrently
      a. Hypocalcemia secondary to decreased parathyroid hormone (PTH) release
      b. Hypokalemia: Mg is responsible for maintaining K^+ transmembrane gradient
   3. Urinary fractional excretion of magnesium (FEMg)
      a. FEMg <2%, increased resorption and likely not renal
      b. FEMg >3% (normal renal function) indicates renal Mg wasting

D. Treatment
   1. Mild hypomagnesemia/ongoing losses
      a. Oral replacement with Mg salts
      b. Consider parenteral replacement if underlying seizure or cardiac disorder, hypokalemia, hypocalcemia
   2. Severe hypomagnesemia/symptomatic: parenteral magnesium sulfate

X. Hyperphosphatemia

A. Characteristics
   1. Definition/background
      a. Serum phosphorus (generally defined as **>4.5 mg/dL**)
      b. Most phosphorus (99%) found in bones and **intracellular space**
      c. Main functions: cellular metabolism (ATP), skeletal mineralization, maintains cell structure (phospholipid membrane), performs intracellular signaling, forms backbone of RNA and DNA, acts as pH buffer in serum and urine
   2. Causes
      a. Decreased renal excretion
         i. Most common cause
         ii. 90% of filtered load is reabsorbed in **proximal tubule**
      b. Hypoparathyroidism increases phosphorus resorption (↓ PTH = ↑ PO_4)
      c. Thyroid hormone (thyrotoxicosis) and growth hormone (acromegaly) increase phosphorous resorption
      d. Vitamin D intoxication increases intestinal absorption of phosphorus and calcium
      e. Cell lysis releases high levels of intracellular phosphorus and potassium (e.g., tumor lysis syndrome, rhabdomyolysis, acute hemolysis) (Table 8-4)
   3. Pathophysiology
      a. Phosphorus homeostasis balanced by 3 organs: intestines, kidneys, bones
         i. Vitamin D controls GI tract's phosphorus absorption
         ii. PTH inhibits kidney's reabsorption of phosphorus (increasing renal excretion) and increases release of phosphorus from bones into blood

TABLE 8-4 Causes of Hyperphosphatemia

↑ Absorption/Intake	↓ Excretion/Elimination	↔ Transcellular Shifts
Enema and laxatives Cow's milk in infants Vitamin D intoxication Treatment of hypophosphatemia Other meds high in phosphorus: liposomal amphotericin B, fosphenytoin	Renal failure Hypoparathyroidism or pseudohypoparathyroidism Hyperthyroidism Acromegaly Familial tumoral calcinosis	Tumor lysis syndrome Rhabdomyolysis Acute hemolysis Malignant hyperthermia (with anesthesia) Crush injury Diabetic ketoacidosis and lactic acidosis

QUICK HIT

Hyperuricemia and hypocalcemia occur with both tumor lysis syndrome and rhabdomyolysis. An elevated creatine phosphokinase suggests rhabdomyolysis, whereas an indirect hyperbilirubinemia with elevated lactate dehydrogenase distinguishes hemolysis.

b. Hyperphosphatemia can precipitate with calcium (calcification) in the blood vessels, especially if serum [phos] × serum [Ca] >70
c. Calcification causes hypocalcemia, causing **renal dysfunction**, mitral and aortic stenosis, hypertension from vascular deposits, heart block, and other organ dysfunction

B. Clinical features (physical exam findings of symptomatic hypocalcemia from hyperphosphatemia): tetany, seizures, hyperreflexia, paresthesias, bradycardia, hypotension, left ventricular dysfunction, arrhythmias

C. Diagnosis
1. Serum phosphorus is <1%; therefore, lab value not always accurate reflection of total body phosphorus
2. Pseudohyperphosphatemia can result from hyperglobulinemia (e.g., multiple myeloma), hyperlipidemia, or hyperbilirubinemia (free serum phosphorus concentration, unbound by protein, remains normal in this case)

D. Treatment
1. Acute hyperphosphatemia in asymptomatic individual with normal renal function resolves spontaneously
2. Phosphate binders (e.g., aluminum hydroxide, calcium carbonate, resins)
3. Dietary restriction
4. IV fluids (especially helpful with tumor lysis syndrome and rhabdomyolysis)
5. Rarely, dialysis is required

9 Hematologic Diseases

Hematologic Diseases

QUICK HIT

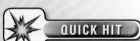

Normal Hgb values vary by age. Newborn infants have higher baseline normal values, which then drop by age 2 months (called the **physiologic nadir**) and rise back to adult baseline normal levels by adolescence.

QUICK HIT

Children fed purely goat's milk diets are at risk for folate deficiency with associated megaloblastic anemia.

QUICK HIT

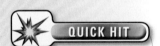

Exposures to toxins should be inquired about because certain substances can cause anemia, especially lead, in young children.

QUICK HIT

Risk factors for lead exposure in children include living in a house with old pipes and/or peeling paint chips and children with pica who live in contaminated areas.

SYMPTOM SPECIFIC

I. Approach to Anemia

A. Definition: reduction in hemoglobin (Hgb) or hematocrit (Hct) below 2 standard deviations from mean for age and gender

B. Differential diagnosis can be divided into 3 main categories
   1. Impaired red blood cell (RBC) production
   2. ↑ RBC destruction
   3. Blood loss

C. Historical findings
   1. General symptoms associated with anemia including fatigue, listlessness, ↓ energy, headaches, poor appetite, and shortness of breath/exercise intolerance
   2. Detailed nutritional history should be performed
   3. History of pica, the ingestion of nonnutritional substances (e.g., dirt, clay, paint chips, etc.), is associated with anemia
   4. Recent history of infection
   5. Medication history of certain agents associated with anemia
   6. Detailed and specific evaluation for sources of blood loss
   7. Ask about exposures associated with hemolytic anemia
   8. Detailed family history for presence of hereditary anemias

D. Physical signs
   1. General
      a. Pallor, fatigue and lethargy, dizziness, palpitations, dyspnea
      b. Tachycardia or hypotension if anemia is acute
   2. Failure to thrive (FTT) with growth failure can be a sign of chronic anemia

E. Diagnosis
   1. Mean corpuscular volume (MCV) varies by age
      a. Anemias are generally classified as
         i. Microcytic (MCV < 70 fL)
         ii. Normocytic (MCV 70–85 fL)
         iii. Macrocytic (MCV > 90 fL)
      b. Reticulocyte count measures number and percentage of immature RBCs
         i. Elevation suggests that marrow response to level of anemia is appropriate. An elevated reticulocyte count suggests the anemia is related to peripheral red cell destruction or blood loss.
         ii. If patient is anemic and reticulocytes are low or normal, it suggests primary RBC production defect in marrow
      c. Peripheral blood smear should be evaluated in newly diagnosed patient (Figure 9-1A–C)
         i. RBCs can have specific inclusions with specific diagnoses
         ii. Shape of RBCs can point toward diagnosis
            (a) Hemolytic anemias will often have **schistocytes**, helmet-shaped cells, and RBC fragments

FIGURE 9-1 **A. Basophilic stippling (ribosomal aggregates within RBC that stain purple; seen in iron deficiency anemia, lead poisoning, thalassemias, and certain enzyme deficiencies. B. Heinz bodies (made up of denatured Hgb seen in thalassemia, asplenic patients, and disorders of unstable Hgb). C. Howell-Jolly bodies (round small nuclear remnants seen in asplenic patients, megaloblastic anemias, and severe iron deficiency anemia).**

A B C

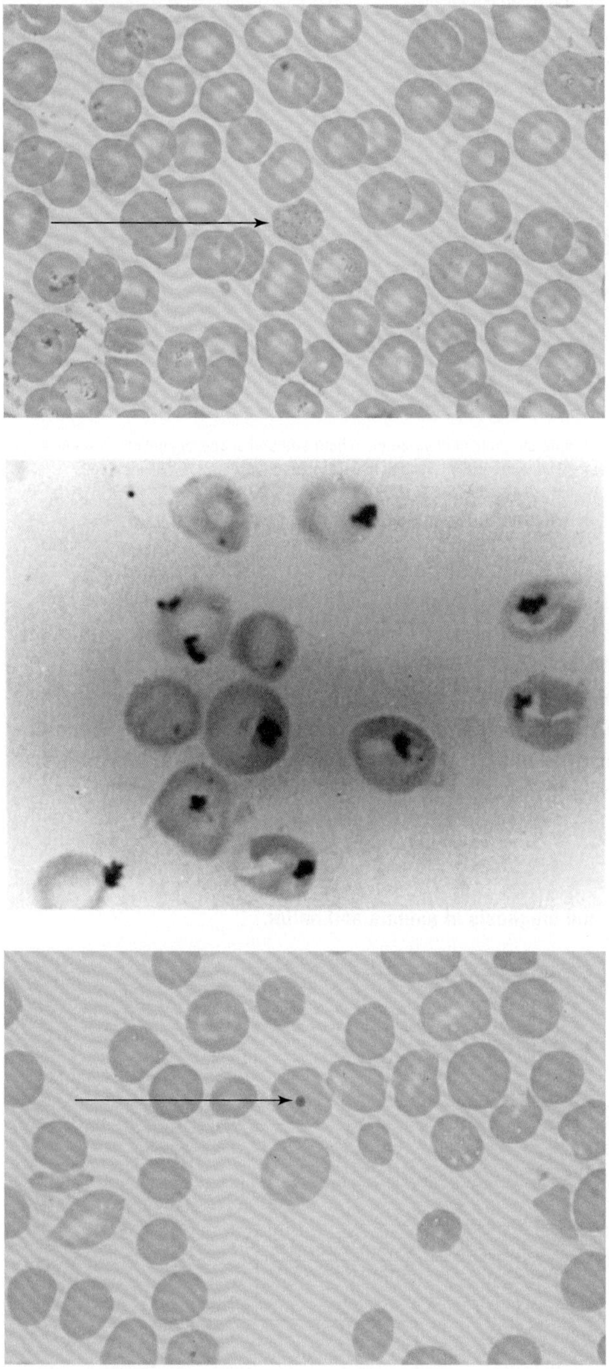

(**B:** From MacDonald MG, Mullett MD, Seshia MMK. *Avery's Neonatology Pathophysiology & Management of the Newborn.* 6th ed. Philadelphia: Lippincott Williams & Wilkins; 2005. **C:** From Anderson SC, Poulsen KB. *Anderson's Atlas of Hematology.* Philadelphia: Wolters Kluwer Health/Lippincott Williams & Wilkins; 2003.)

QUICK HIT

Infants and children with severe anemia usually have a hyperdynamic precordium and a systolic flow murmur heard best in the upper anterior chest.

QUICK HIT

Diffuse abdominal tenderness is associated with inflammatory colitis, Crohn disease, and ulcerative colitis, all of which can cause anemia from chronic GI blood loss.

QUICK HIT

When evaluating an anemic patient, the first place to turn when approaching diagnosis is the MCV, which refers to the size of the RBCs, the reticulocyte count, and the peripheral blood smear.

QUICK HIT

Account for severe anemia by calculating the "corrected reticulocyte count" = reticulocyte count × (actual Hct/normal Hct). A normal corrected reticulocyte count is generally 1%–2%.

(b) **Spherocytes** or **elliptocytes** can signify specific RBC membrane abnormalities

(c) Sickle-shaped cells suggest sickle cell anemia

iii. Normal RBCs have area of central pallor

(a) RBCs that have ↑ central pallor are hypochromic (Figure 9-2)

(i) Seen most commonly in iron-deficiency anemia

(ii) Thalassemia can also have hypochromic RBCs

FIGURE 9-2 **The peripheral blood smear in fully developed iron-deficiency anemia exhibits erythrocytes rich in central pallor.**

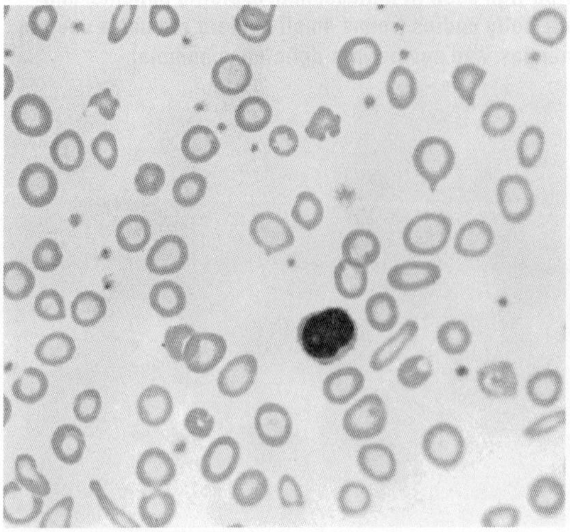

Although virtually all erythrocytes are microcytic, note the prominent variation in both size and shape, typical of iron-deficiency anemia. (From McClatchey KD. *Clinical Laboratory Medicine*. 2nd ed. Philadelphia: Lippincott Williams & Wilkins; 2002.)

(b) Hyperchromic RBCs can be seen in certain RBC membrane abnormalities or megaloblastic anemia

2. Evaluate remainder of complete blood count (CBC) to determine if platelet count and white blood cell (WBC) count are normal (Figure 9-3)
   a. If other hematopoietic cell lines are affected, this implies bone marrow production or infiltration defect, such as malignancy or aplastic anemia
   b. Suppression of multiple hematopoietic cell lines can also be secondary to global bone marrow suppression by infection or autoimmune disease

FIGURE 9-3 **Approach to the workup and diagnosis of anemia and pallor.**

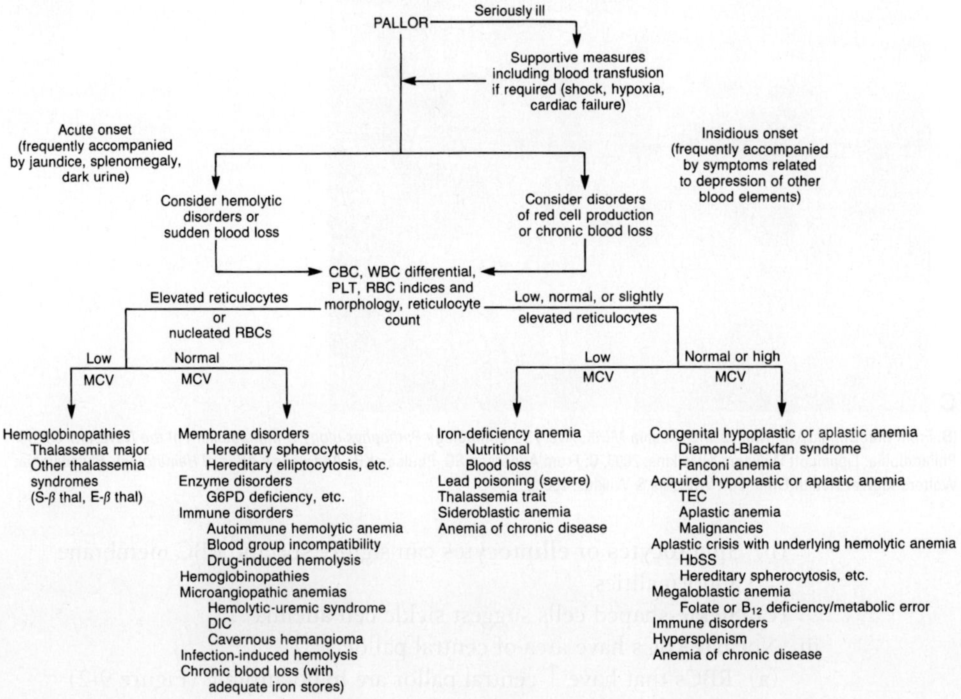

CBC, complete blood count; DIC, disseminated intravascular coagulation; G6PD, glucose-6-phosphate dehydrogenase; MCV, mean corpuscular volume; PLT, platelet count; RBC, red blood cell; TEC, transient erythroblastopenia of childhood; WBC, white blood cell.

3. **Mentzer index** = MCV ÷ RBC count: helps distinguish iron deficiency from β-thalassemia
   a. <13: thalassemia
   b. >13: iron deficiency

II. Approach to Bleeding Disorders

A. Differential diagnosis
   1. Hemophilia (factor 8 or 9 deficiency)
   2. von Willebrand disease
   3. Acquired clotting factor deficiency: disseminated intravascular coagulation (DIC), vitamin K deficiency, and liver failure
   4. Acquired thrombocytopenia: DIC, idiopathic thrombocytopenic purpura (ITP), thrombotic thrombocytopenic purpura (TTP), hemolytic-uremic syndrome (HUS)
   5. Congenital thrombocytopenia, bone marrow suppression or failure
   6. Platelet dysfunction due to rare platelet function disorders or medication effect
   7. Fibrinogen disorders
   8. Other coagulation factor deficiency

B. Historical findings
   1. Establish sites of bleeding
      a. Distinguish between mucosal bleeding and deep tissue or joint bleeds
      b. Bleeding limited to single site suggests local phenomenon as opposed to systemic or inherited bleeding disorder
   2. Document bleeding duration and severity
   3. Severe inherited bleeding disorders typically present in infancy
   4. Bleeding complications associated with injury or procedures (e.g., circumcision), if extensive, can imply inherited bleeding tendency
   5. History of recent infection can be associated with autoimmune-mediated thrombocytopenia
   6. Family history of bleeding symptoms is helpful (Table 9-1)

C. Physical examination findings
   1. Petechiae (Figure 9-4)
   2. Purpura
   3. Ecchymoses
      a. Bruising overlying bony structures (e.g., anterior tibial surfaces) can be acquired through normal childhood play and does not indicate bleeding disorder
      b. Patients with bleeding disorders often present with large ecchymoses without history of trauma

QUICK HIT

A rough rule of thumb is that in iron deficiency, the marrow cannot produce RBCs, so RBC count is low, whereas in thalassemia, RBC production is preserved, but the cells are small and fragile.

QUICK HIT

Mucosal bleeding is more likely to represent a platelet disorder or von Willebrand disease, whereas deep tissue bleeds are more common in hereditary factor deficiencies such as hemophilia.

QUICK HIT

When interviewing a patient with menorrhagia, ask how often she must change her pad or tampon.

QUICK HIT

Normal patients may develop scattered petechiae above the nipple line with ↑ thoracic pressure due to vomiting, coughing, or straining.

Hematologic Diseases

TABLE 9-1 Laboratory Abnormalities in Bleeding Disorders

Condition	PT	PTT	Platelet Count
ITP	Unaffected	Unaffected	Decreased
von Willebrand disease	Unaffected	Can be prolonged	Unaffected or decreased
Vitamin K deficiency	Prolonged	Unaffected or mildly prolonged	Unaffected
Hemophilia (types A and B)	Unaffected	Prolonged	Unaffected
Factor VII deficiency	Prolonged	Unaffected	Unaffected
Factor XIII deficiency	Unaffected	Unaffected	Unaffected
DIC	Prolonged	Prolonged	Decreased

DIC, disseminated intravascular coagulation; ITP, immune-mediated thrombocytopenia; PT, prothrombin time; PTT, partial thromboplastin time.

FIGURE 9-4 Petechiae.

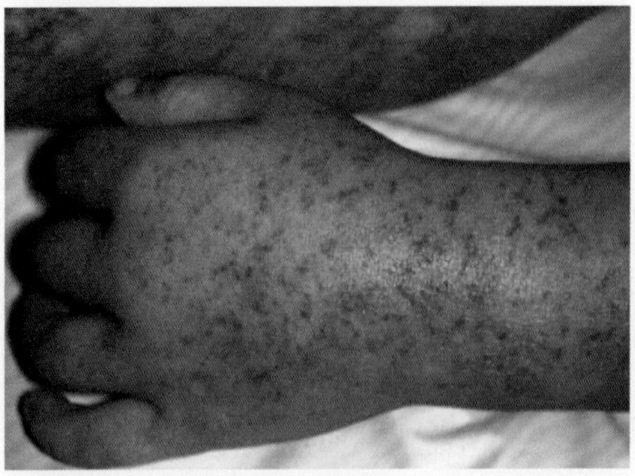

These tiny skin hemorrhages occurred in a child with low platelet count (thrombocytopenia). (From McConnell TH. *The Nature of Disease Pathology for the Health Professions.* Philadelphia: Lippincott Williams & Wilkins; 2007.)

QUICK HIT

The only coagulopathy that presents with an isolated prolonged PT is factor VII deficiency.

4. Hepatosplenomegaly
   a. Hematologic malignancies can present with bleeding and are often associated with enlarged liver and/or spleen
   b. Splenomegaly can also result in consumptive thrombocytopenia that can lead to bleeding
5. Hematomas
6. Hemarthrosis

D. Diagnosis (Table 9-2)
1. Prothrombin time (PT)/international normalized ratio (INR)
   a. Assesses extrinsic coagulation pathway: factors I, II, V, VII, and X
   b. INR standardizes result of PT from institution to institution
2. Partial thromboplastin time (PTT)
   a. Assesses intrinsic and common coagulation pathway: factors I, II, V, VIII, IX, X, XI, and XII

TABLE 9-2 **Blood Components Used for Transfusion**

Product	Content	Comments
Whole blood	Blood plus anticoagulant/preservative (citrate, phosphate, dextrose, and adenine)	1 unit = 500 mL (423 mL blood + 77 mL anticoagulant/preservative)
Packed RBCs (pRBCs)	Whole blood – plasma and platelets	Hematocrit is usually 70%–80%; can be stored for ~5 weeks; 1 unit pRBCs ranges from 220 mL to 260 mL
Washed RBCs	pRBCs with residual plasma removed and replaced with saline	Must be transfused within 24 hours; used in patients requiring multiple transfusions and in those with history of allergic transfusion reactions
Leukoreduced RBCs	Removal of residual WBCs from pRBCs by centrifugation, washing, freezing, deglycerolization, or filtration	Used to minimize febrile, nonhemolytic transfusion reactions
Fresh frozen plasma	Liquid portion of whole blood that is separated from RBCs	Contains coagulation factors (II, V, VII, VIII, IX, X, XI), protein C, protein S, and antithrombin III + electrolytes, albumin, immunoglobulin, and complement in physiologic amounts; used to replace clotting factors
Cryoprecipitate	Cold, insoluble remnant of 1 unit of fresh frozen plasma	Contains factor I (fibrinogen), factor VIII, vWF, and factor XIII; typically used for patients with hypofibrinogenemia
Platelets	1 unit of platelets is derived from 1 unit of whole blood; volume is ~40 mL	Platelets can be transfused singly (single donor) as for small infants or pooled to meet transfusion requirements of older children and adults

RBCs, red blood cells; vWF, von Willebrand factor; WBCs, white blood cells.

b. Prolonged PTT can be due to inherited factor deficiency or inhibitor to specific factor (e.g., antiphospholipid antibody or heparin)
3. Platelet function analyzer (PFA-100): a screening tool for platelet dysfunction
4. History, presentation, and screening laboratory results can determine whether other testing is required

> **QUICK HIT**
> Estrogen-containing oral contraceptives are associated with clot formation.

III. Approach to Clotting Disorder

A. Differential diagnosis
1. Acquired thrombophilia due to sepsis, dehydration, malignancy, vascular injury, drug induced, or lupus anticoagulant
2. Inherited disorders that predispose to the development of thrombosis, including antithrombin deficiency, protein C or S deficiency, factor V Leiden mutation, prothrombin gene mutation, hyperhomocysteinemia, dysfibrinogenemias

B. Historical findings
1. History must identify symptoms of thrombosis that require immediate intervention
   a. Signs of a neurovascular event: altered mental status, weakness, numbness, visual changes, altered speech
   b. Signs of pulmonary embolism (PE): dyspnea, chest pain
2. Timing of symptoms can help determine clot acuity
3. Establish whether patient recently started new medications
4. Family history is essential

> **QUICK HIT**
> Families may not recognize symptoms of hypercoagulability, so be sure to ask about miscarriages, strokes, and heart attacks in addition to PE and DVT.

C. Physical examination findings vary by site of thrombus
1. Deep venous thrombosis (DVT) of extremities presents with limb swelling, pitting edema, and tenderness to palpation
2. If arterial blood flow is compromised, cyanotic changes in skin distal to thrombotic insult can be seen
3. Patients with PE have tachycardia, hypoxia, diaphoresis, and ↓ pulses
4. Patients with neurovascular events often have focal neurologic findings, including altered mental status, seizure, dysarthria, paresthesia, weakness, and altered tone and reflexes

> **QUICK HIT**
> Imaging studies are the gold standard, but certain laboratory studies can be helpful to diagnose a clot. An elevated D-dimer supports the diagnosis of a thrombus but has a high false-positive rate (↑ sensitivity but ↓ specificity).

D. Diagnosis
1. If stroke is in differential, emergent head imaging
2. Spiral computed tomography (CT) used to diagnose PE
3. Doppler ultrasound is diagnostic test of choice for DVT
4. Hypercoagulable workup should include testing for inherited disorders of thrombophilia

> **QUICK HIT**
> Lab testing should not hold up treatment of clotting emergencies, but anticoagulation alters diagnostic testing results. Whenever possible, the labs should be drawn before starting medications.

DISEASE SPECIFIC

IV. Iron-Deficiency Anemia

A. Characteristics
1. Anemia due to iron deficiency or chronic blood loss with insufficient iron stores to respond to ↓ in RBCs
2. Iron is an essential component of Hg molecule; when the body is deficient in iron, fewer RBCs can be made, and those present are ineffective in oxygen transport
3. Most common form of anemia and most common nutritional deficiency worldwide
4. Multiple causes
   a. Nutritional
      i. Most commonly associated with inadequate intake during periods of rapid growth (infancy and adolescence)
      ii. Strict vegetarians are at risk
      iii. Infants who ingest large amounts of whole milk are at risk
   b. Blood loss
      i. Gastrointestinal (GI)
         (a) Patients with inflammatory bowel disease at high risk
         (b) Patients with ulcers, gastritis/colitis, varices, polyps, Meckel diverticulum, hemorrhoids, or parasitic infections
         (c) Celiac disease
         (d) History of small bowel resection

> **QUICK HIT**
> A hypercoagulable workup is indicated in any patient with an unexplained thrombus, an individual who has a history of more than 1 thrombosis, or a highly suspicious family history.

QUICK HIT

A thrombophilia workup will be altered by recent transfusion of blood products. In this case, the workup can be postponed until the patient is no longer requiring blood products or has completed anticoagulant therapy.

QUICK HIT

Gastric acidity helps with absorption of iron. Ascorbic acid and citrate will accentuate absorption of iron, whereas bran, tannins, plant phylates, and antacids will ↓ absorption.

QUICK HIT

Lead and iron have complex interactions, and anemia from lead poisoning is typically only at high levels. However, iron deficiency is common in patients with lead poisoning, and iron studies should be checked in these patients.

QUICK HIT

The reticulocyte count is usually normal unless there is active frank bleeding, in which case it can be elevated.

QUICK HIT

Anemia is a late finding in iron deficiency; the first abnormalities are low ferritin, low MCV, and elevated TIBC.

QUICK HIT

The serum iron is not a helpful test in the diagnosis of iron deficiency anemia because it is subject to wide variability based on several factors including age, gender, time of day, and recent iron ingestion.

ii. Menstrual
(a) Dysfunctional uterine bleeding
(b) Normal adolescent females with heavy or frequent menses and inadequate iron in diet
iii. Genitourinary

B. Clinical features
1. Historical findings
a. Symptoms of anemia
b. Pica (persistent ingestion of nonnutritive substances) common in infants and young children
c. History of excessive milk intake
d. Menorrhagia or other symptoms of blood loss
e. Children with long-standing iron-deficiency anemia may present with poor school performance and learning difficulty
2. Physical exam findings
a. Signs of anemia, including pallor, tachycardia, cardiac murmur
b. Long-standing anemia can result in growth delay, cardiac hypertrophy, splenomegaly, and koilonychia (spoon-shaped nails)

C. Diagnosis
1. CBC
a. MCV will be low in later stages
b. Hypochromic RBCs are seen on peripheral blood smear
c. RBC distribution width (RDW) is elevated
d. Platelet count can be elevated due to reactive thrombocytosis
2. Iron studies
a. Ferritin is body's storage protein for iron and will be low
b. Total iron-binding capacity (TIBC) reflects percentage of iron-binding sites present on transferrin (iron transport protein) and is elevated in iron deficiency anemia (Table 9-3)
c. Serum iron does not accurately reflect stores and is not helpful

D. Treatment
1. Therapy
a. Correction of any mechanisms underlying blood loss
b. Iron supplementation at dose of 4–6 mEq/kg/day of **elemental** iron
c. Restrict whole milk to 6–8 oz/day in young children

TABLE 9-3 **Evaluation of Microcytic Anemia**

	Iron Deficiency	Lead	Thalassemia Trait	Chronic Disease
Hemoglobin	↓	Normal or ↓	↓	↓
MCV	Normal or ↓	Normal or ↓	↓	Normal or ↓
RDW	Normal or ↑	Normal or ↑	Normal	Normal
Number of RBCs	↓	↓	Normal or ↓	↓
FEP	↑	↑	Normal	↑
Serum iron	↓	Normal	Normal	↓
TIBC	↑	Normal	Normal	Normal or ↓
% Transferrin saturation	↓	Normal	Normal or ↑	↓
Ferritin	↓	Normal	Normal	Normal or ↑

FEP, free erythrocyte protoporphyrin; MCV, mean corpuscular volume; RBC, red blood cell; RDW, RBC distribution width; TIBC, total iron-binding capacity.

From Ludwig S, Shah SS. *Pediatric Complaints and Diagnostic Dilemmas: A Case-Based Approach.* Philadelphia: Lippincott Williams & Wilkins; 2004.

d. ↑ high iron–containing foods
e. Give iron with vitamin C–containing foods to ↑ iron absorption
f. Avoid foods that inhibit absorption of iron
g. Blood transfusions if severely anemic and signs of cardiovascular compromise, although they are usually not necessary

2. Oral iron therapy is often implicated as cause of constipation, but this is unlikely at standard dosing
3. Duration/prognosis
    a. Most patients will respond to iron supplementation and dietary modification
    b. Response to iron supplementation
        i. Reticulocytosis is seen after 7–10 days of iron supplementation
        ii. ↑ in Hgb seen within 2 weeks
        iii. Resolution of anemia usually takes 4–6 weeks
    c. Treatment should continue for at least 3 months after resolution of anemia to replete body stores of iron
4. Prevention (based on American Academy of Pediatrics recommendations)
    a. Infants should be breastfed until at least age 5–6 months if possible
    b. Iron supplementation after age 5–6 months for breastfed infants
    c. Nonbreastfed infants should be given iron-fortified formula
    d. 1st foods introduced in infancy should be iron-fortified cereals
    e. No whole milk until after 1st birthday

V. Anemia of Chronic Disease

A. Definition
1. Normocytic, normochromic anemia secondary to chronic unrelated illness
2. Multiple chronic illnesses have been linked to anemia of chronic disease

B. Cause/pathophysiology
1. Due to impairment in delivery of iron from reticuloendothelial system to bone marrow precursors, which leads to impairment of RBC production
2. Inflammation should be present to make diagnosis

C. Diagnosis
1. Anemia is typically normocytic and normochromic, although it can be mildly microcytic in some cases
2. Normal reticulocyte count and RDW
3. Iron studies may be useful to rule out iron deficiency

QUICK HIT

Anemia of chronic disease is differentiated from iron deficiency anemia by ↓ or normal TIBC and normal or ↑ ferritin.

VI. Sickle Cell Disease (SCD)

A. Characteristics
1. Autosomal recessive disorder of Hgb caused by point mutation of codon 6 of β globin gene on chromosome 11, which results in substitution of amino acid valine with glutamate resulting in production of sickle hemoglobin (HbS)
2. HbS is less soluble than the normal adult hemoglobin (HbA) and, when deoxygenated, causes distortion in RBCs, which appear as sickle shapes
3. Sickle-shaped RBCs are prematurely destroyed, resulting in hemolytic anemia
4. Sickle-shaped RBCs also ↑ blood viscosity, impede blood flow, and generate microthrombi, which can lead to occlusion in microvasculature
5. Predominates in African populations because carrier state is protective against malaria

B. Clinical features
1. Historical findings
    a. History should be focused on complications of SCD
        i. Number of previous hospitalizations and complications
        ii. History of admission to intensive care unit (ICU) or intubation
        iii. Where patient's vaso-occlusive crises tend to occur and what pain medications are effective
        iv. How often patient has required RBC transfusions
        v. Complete infectious history due to high risk of severe infection
        vi. Respiratory symptoms can be sign of acute chest syndrome
        vii. History of neurologic symptoms may be sign of stroke
    b. Family history of any hemoglobinopathy, including carriers

QUICK HIT

A vaso-occlusive crisis is typically characterized by stabbing or throbbing pain.

BOX 9-1

Acute Complications of Patients with Sickle Cell Disease

- Vaso-occclusive pain crisis in long bones, back, chest, ribs, or other areas
- Stroke
- Splenic infarction and sequestration
- Occlusion of the pulmonary vasculature, which can lead to acute chest syndrome and pneumonia
- Cardiomegaly and myocardial dysfunction
- Priapism
- Dactylitis (inflammation of finger or toe)
- Aplastic crisis
  - Related to infection
  - Shut down of red blood cell production in the marrow

Hematologic Diseases

QUICK HIT

Patients who present with a severely painful erection that has lasted for 4 hours or more require urgent intervention; priapism is a medical emergency!

2. Physical exam findings
   a. Patients often have evidence of chronic, hemolytic anemia including baseline systolic ejection murmur and mild jaundice or scleral icterus
   b. Acute chest syndrome is associated with chest pain and respiratory distress
   c. Vaso-occlusive crisis presents with warmth, swelling, and tenderness to palpation in affected area
   d. Neurologic findings including hemiparesis, gait abnormalities, or speech deficits may be sign of ischemic event or stroke
   e. Splenomegaly at baseline, although rapidly enlarging spleen is sign of acute splenic sequestration
   f. Patients with aplastic crisis can present with acute onset of pallor
   g. Priapism (Box 9-1)

C. Diagnosis
1. Laboratory findings
   a. Can be diagnosed *in utero* by chorionic villus sampling (CVS) or testing of fetal fibroblasts with amniocentesis
   b. Most patients in U.S. are diagnosed via newborn screen Hgb electrophoresis, which will identify HbS variant
   c. Anemia
      i. Normocytic, normochromic anemia with baseline Hgb of 7–10 g/dL
      ii. Should have elevated reticulocyte counts unless experiencing aplastic crisis
      iii. Patients can have elevated neutrophil and platelet counts
      iv. Peripheral blood smear will reveal characteristic sickle-shaped cells with evidence of hemolysis and nucleated RBCs
   d. Patients with fever should have blood cultures to rule out bacteremia
2. Radiology findings
   a. Cardiomegaly on chest radiograph at baseline
   b. Chest x-ray (CXR) will reveal infiltrate in patients with acute chest syndrome
   c. In patients with fever and pain not improving with analgesia, magnetic resonance imaging (MRI) or bone scan to evaluate for osteomyelitis may be indicated
   d. Diffusion-weighted MRI with fluid-attenuated inversion recovery (FLAIR) sequences is better modality to evaluate for stroke in sickle cell patients than noncontrast head CT

QUICK HIT

Differentiating pneumonia from acute chest syndrome is challenging in sickle cell patients, but treat for both if new infiltrate is present on CXR.

D. Treatment
1. Therapy
   a. General health maintenance of sickle cell patients
      i. Lifelong folic acid supplementation: 1 mg/day
      ii. Transcranial Doppler ultrasounds every 6 months from ages 2 to 16 years to identify risk of stroke
      iii. Ophthalmology evaluation yearly to screen for retinopathy

BOX 9-2

Common Long-Term Complications of Sickle Cell Disease

Cholecystitis
Retinopathy
Avascular necrosis
Sensorineural hearing loss
Leg ulcerations
Nephrotic syndrome and renal failure
Hepatic necrosis and cirrhosis
Myocardial dysfunction and pulmonary hypertension

iv. Dental screening every 6 months
v. Vaccinations with polyvalent pneumococcal, hepatitis B, hemophilus influenza type B (Hib), and yearly influenza vaccines are especially important
vi. Penicillin prophylaxis from age 8 weeks to 5 years due to ↑ risk of sepsis because of baseline splenic dysfunction

b. Hydroxyurea is recommended for patients with severe phenotype and multiple episodes of vaso-occlusive complications by increasing production of fetal hemoglobin (HbF) and increasing solubility of HbS
c. Chronic RBC transfusions for patients with multiple vaso-occlusive complications
d. Emergent treatment of specific crises
   i. Vaso-occlusive/pain crisis should be treated immediately with adequate analgesia using nonsteroidal anti-inflammatory drugs (NSAIDs) and narcotics as needed
   ii. Acute chest syndrome is treated with hydration, pain relief, broad-spectrum antibiotics; packed RBC transfusion may be indicated if patient shows signs of respiratory decompensation
   iii. Splenic sequestration is treated with packed RBC until spleen returns to baseline
   iv. Stroke requires urgent intervention with immediate exchange transfusion
   v. Priapism should be managed with ↑ fluid intake, analgesics, and evaluation by pediatric urologist
   vi. Patients are at ↑ risk of infection with encapsulated organisms, and when fever above 101.5°F is present, broad-spectrum parenteral antibiotics are administered pending blood culture results

2. There are many long-term complications of SCD, and all organ systems are affected (Box 9-2)

VII. Thalassemias

A. Characteristics
1. Definition
   a. Inherited microcytic hemolytic anemia due to abnormal Hgb synthesis
   b. Normal predominant HbA is tetramer made up of 2 α globin chains and 2 β globin chains
   c. Human genome has 4 α globin genes and 2 β globin genes
   d. Thalassemia syndromes result when 1 or more of globin genes mutates; clinical phenotype determined by which and how many genes are mutated
2. Epidemiology
   a. α Globin mutations predominate in people of Southeast Asian and African descent, whereas β globin mutations predominate in people of Mediterranean and Southern and Southeast Asian descent
   b. Mutations are protective against malaria
3. Pathophysiology
   a. ↓ production of either β or α globin chains leads to relative excess of corresponding chains needed to form tetramer

QUICK HIT

Bone marrow transplant is the only curative treatment currently available but poses significant risks and is only indicated in certain cases.

QUICK HIT

Patients with sickle cell anemia are at ↑ risk for osteomyelitis. The most common pathogen that leads to osteomyelitis in SCD patients is from *Staphylococcus* species, although sickle cell patients do have greater frequency of osteomyelitis secondary to salmonella than does the general population.

b. Buildup of excess chains leads to precipitations and deposits in RBCs, which causes hemolysis
c. RBC life span is shortened, resulting in ↑ erythropoiesis, bone marrow expansion, and ↑ iron absorption and overload

B. Clinical features: range from asymptomatic to severe anemia depending on number of genes affected
1. Historical findings
a. Patients with thalassemia minor (1 β gene mutated), patients who are silent carriers of α globin mutations (1 α gene mutation), and patients with α thalassemia trait (2 α genes mutated) are generally asymptomatic
b. Patients with clinically significant thalassemia can present with symptoms of hemolytic anemia including FTT, lethargy, poor feeding, and periods of jaundice (especially with infection)
2. Physical findings
a. Signs of anemia: pallor, tachycardia, and systolic ejection murmur
b. Jaundice
c. Hepatosplenomegaly
d. Short stature and puberty delay
e. Patients with β-thalassemia major (mutations in both β globin genes) will have typical dysmorphic facies due to extramedullary hematopoiesis and bone marrow expansion (Figure 9-5)

FIGURE 9-5 **Thalassemia major. Characteristic facies of thalassemia major. Note prominent malar eminences, producing an apparent depression of the nose, and enlargement of the maxilla with upward protrusion of the lip, exposing the upper teeth.**

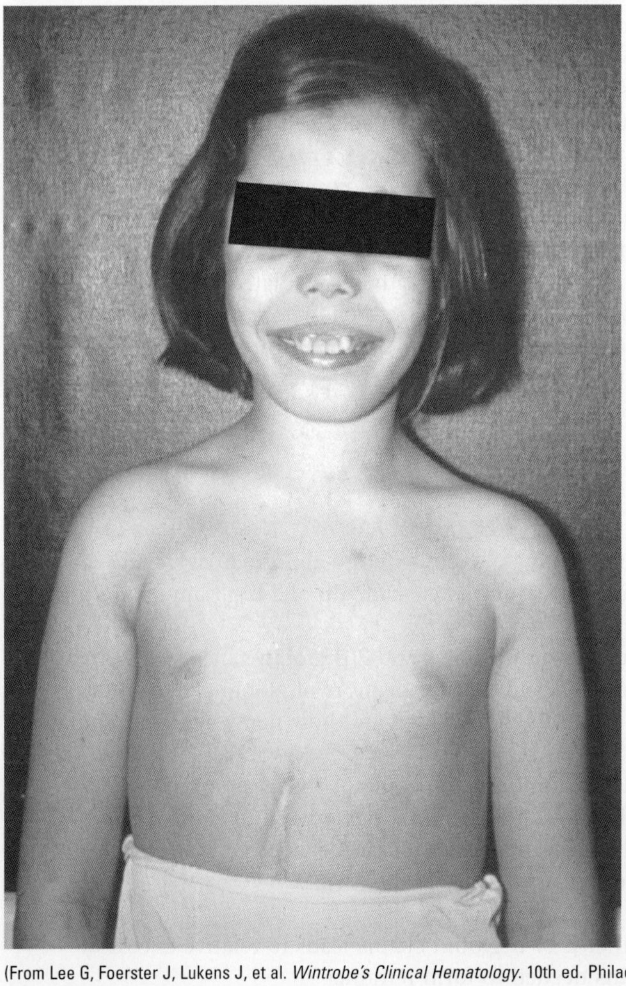

(From Lee G, Foerster J, Lukens J, et al. *Wintrobe's Clinical Hematology*. 10th ed. Philadelphia: Lippincott Williams & Wilkins; 1998:1422, with permission.)

C. Diagnosis
  1. Laboratory findings
    a. Diagnosis is made based on Hgb electrophoresis
      i. Typical HbA: 97% HbA, 1%–3% HbA2, and <1% HbF
      ii. β-Thalassemia patients will have elevated percentage of HbA2 and HbF depending on extent of mutations present
      iii. α-Thalassemia patients will have ↑ percentage of Hgb Barts and HbH depending on extent of mutations present
    b. Microcytic, hypochromic anemia; level of baseline Hgb is dependent on extent of mutations present
    c. Peripheral blood smear will reveal target cells, ↑ nucleated RBCs, ↑ reticulocytes, and basophilic stippling
    d. Ferritin is often elevated
  2. Radiology findings: Bones show general widening of medullary space with thinning of bone cortices

D. Treatment
  1. Therapy
    a. Folic acid supplementation
    b. Avoidance of oxidizing agents
    c. Transfusions only if necessary
    d. Splenectomy if patient has hypersplenism with ↑ transfusion requirements
    e. All patients should receive genetic counseling.
    f. Other care is directed by specific thalassemia syndrome
      i. Patients with thalassemia minor and patients who are silent carriers of α globin mutations or with α-thalassemia trait are asymptomatic
      ii. Hydrops fetalis (4 α gene mutations)
        (a) Intrauterine transfusions if diagnosed before fetus suffers demise from congestive heart failure (CHF)
        (b) Chronic transfusions
        (c) Bone marrow transplant
      iii. HbH disease (3 α gene mutations); patients do not usually require chronic transfusions
      iv. Thalassemia major (mutations in both β globin genes)
        (a) Patients require chronic transfusions approximately every 3–4 weeks
        (b) Chronic transfusions ↑ oxygen delivery to body to allow for normal growth and development
        (c) Transfusions should begin when Hgb falls below 7 g/dL and are used to maintain Hgb between 9 g/dL and 12 g/dL
  2. Most complications due to chronic anemia with excessive iron overload, extramedullary hematopoiesis, and bone marrow expansion

MNEMONIC

LUNATIcs are a cause of RBC basophilic stippling
Lead poisoning
Unstable hemoglobin
Nucleotide deficiency (pyrimidine 5′-nucleoidase deficiency)
Anemia caused by arsenic poisoning and megaloblastic anemia (e.g., vitamin B_{12} or folate deficiency)
Thalassemia
Iron deficiency

QUICK HIT

Patients on chronic transfusion protocols will suffer from severe iron overload, which results in severe morbidity and requires chelation therapy!

VIII. Hereditary Red Cell Membrane Defects

A. Definitions
  1. Large, heterogeneous group of inherited disorders with shortened RBC half-life and hemolytic anemia
  2. Most common RBC membrane defect is hereditary spherocytosis
  3. Other defects include hereditary elliptocytosis, hereditary pyropoikilocytosis, Southeast Asian ovalocytosis, and hereditary stomatocytosis

B. Cause/pathophysiology
  1. Caused by genetic abnormalities that result in abnormal membrane proteins
  2. Protein defects lead to abnormally shaped RBCs, which leads to hemolysis and premature clearance by reticuloendothelial system

C. Clinical presentation
  1. Anemia, jaundice, reticulocytosis, splenomegaly, or gallstones
  2. Many patients will present in neonatal period with prolonged jaundice

D. Diagnosis
  1. CBC and peripheral blood smear, with evidence of hemolysis and abnormally shaped RBCs
  2. Osmotic fragility testing and spectrin content to confirm diagnosis

E. Therapy
1. Primary treatment is splenectomy for severe cases; splenectomy ↑ RBC half-life and ↓ hemolysis
2. Patients may require chronic transfusions
3. Many patients are asymptomatic, although they will have Hgb levels slightly lower than that of general population
4. Most patients will be placed on folate supplementation
5. Patients with inherited RBC membrane defects have elevated risk of cholelithiasis and may require cholecystectomy at some point

QUICK HIT

Patients with RBC membrane disorders can suffer hemolytic crises in the setting of viral infection. These patients often present with abrupt onset of severe jaundice and anemia and worsening splenomegaly.

IX. Glucose-6-Phosphate Dehydrogenase (G6PD) Deficiency

A. Characteristics
1. G6PD is essential enzyme in production of nicotinamide adenine dinucleotide phosphate (NADPH) through pentose phosphate shunt
   a. NADPH maintains body's reserve of reduced glutathione, which cleans up free radicals from oxidative stress
   b. G6PD deficiency results in acute hemolytic anemia with oxidative stress
2. Prevalence estimated at 0.5%–2.9% in the United States
3. Caused by mutation in *Gd* gene on long arm of X chromosome and is inherited in X-linked pattern
4. Children with G6PD deficiency are clinically and hematologically normal at baseline, but, in presence of certain agents, they can develop life-threatening hemolytic anemia
   a. In absence of adequate G6PD, Hgb and other proteins within RBC precipitate at times of oxidative stress, leading to cell membrane damage
   b. Intravascular hemolysis ultimately results
5. Stresses associated with hemolytic crisis include
   a. Infection
   b. Ingestion of fava beans (**favism**)
   c. Exposure to certain oxidative agents including many medications (acetylsalicylic acid [ASA], sulfa-containing compounds, nitrofurantoin, and others)

QUICK HIT

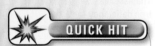

Trimethoprim-sulfamethoxazole, an antibiotic commonly used for mild urinary tract infections, is contraindicated in patients with G6PD deficiency.

QUICK HIT

G6PD-associated hemolytic crisis can be triggered by infection, certain foods, and medications, particularly antibiotics. Be sure to ask about medications and exposures in any patient presenting with unexplained hemolytic anemia.

B. Clinical features
1. Acute hemolytic crisis can present with irritability progressing to fatigue and lethargy, fever, nausea, abdominal pain, or diarrhea and tea- or cola-colored urine
2. Physical exam findings
   a. Signs of anemia: pallor, tachycardia, and systolic ejection murmur
   b. Signs of hemolysis: jaundice, tender splenomegaly, hepatomegaly
   c. In severe cases, signs of hypovolemic shock may be present
   d. Prolonged neonatal jaundice

QUICK HIT

Consider G6PD deficiency in any male infant with prolonged or refractory neonatal jaundice.

C. Diagnosis
1. Peripheral smear will show evidence of hemolysis and elevated reticulocyte count
2. Indirect hyperbilirubinemia and elevated lactate dehydrogenase (LDH)
3. Low haptoglobin (haptoglobin binds free Hgb released in serum)

D. Treatment
1. Focused on prevention of hemolytic crisis by teaching patients what foods, medications, and substances to avoid
2. With severe, symptomatic anemia, patients may benefit from blood transfusion
3. Splenectomy can be helpful in patients who develop chronic hemolytic anemia

QUICK HIT

Patients should be educated to recognize the signs and symptoms of hemolytic crisis so they can seek immediate medical attention!

X. Pyruvate Kinase Deficiency (PKD)

A. Definitions
1. Extremely rare autosomal recessive disorder in erythrocyte metabolism, which results in chronic hemolytic anemia
2. Pyruvate kinase is enzyme essential for production of adenosine triphosphate (ATP) in erythrocytes (through final step of glycolysis)
   a. Erythrocytes deficient in ATP cannot maintain normal electrolyte homeostasis and suffer intracellular buildup of Na^+ is the likely etiology
   b. Leads to rigid membrane and premature hemolysis

B. Clinical presentation
   1. Severity of hemolytic anemia varies widely among affected patients, although extent of anemia is typically stable throughout patient's life
   2. Patients usually exhibit unconjugated hyperbilirubinemia and splenomegaly
   3. Morbidities include kernicterus, FTT, iron overload, and gallstones

C. Diagnosis
   1. Lab abnormalities include macrocytic anemia, reticulocytosis, and indirect hyperbilirubinemia
   2. Diagnosis is made by pyruvate kinase function testing or DNA testing

XI. Transient Erythroblastopenia of Childhood (TEC)

A. Definition
   1. TEC is self-limited, pure RBC aplasia thought to be brought on by viral illness
   2. Exact mechanism is unknown but is thought to be result of autoantibodies directed against RBC precursors that develop following viral infection

B. Clinical presentation: affects otherwise healthy children between 6 months and 4 years
   1. Presents with pallor and fatigue and may report recent viral syndrome ~1–2 months prior to anemia onset
   2. Activity level is usually not reflective of anemia, which can be severe

C. Diagnosis
   1. Normocytic anemia with low or absent reticulocytes
   2. Patients have normal iron studies
   3. WBC and platelet counts are usually within normal limits
   4. Patients can be difficult to distinguish from patients with inherited RBC aplasia

D. Therapy
   1. Because TEC is self-limited, most patients recover without intervention
   2. In cases of severe or symptomatic anemia, blood transfusions may be beneficial

> **QUICK HIT**
>
> TEC, as a diagnosis, is rare in children younger than age 6 months and older than age 4 years.

> **QUICK HIT**
>
> TEC is easily confused with severe iron deficiency anemia because they both typically present in otherwise healthy toddlers. Remember: TEC is usually normocytic, whereas iron deficiency is microcytic.

XII. Diamond-Blackfan Anemia (DBA)

A. Definition: rare, autosomal dominantly inherited anemia characterized by erythroid aplasia, congenital anomalies, and predisposition to malignancy

B. Clinical presentation
   1. Most patients present in infancy with profound anemia and reticulocytopenia
   2. Associated with multiple congenital anomalies
   3. Patients have predisposition to malignancy
   4. Overall 40-year survival is 75%

C. Diagnosis
   1. DBA is a clinical diagnosis supported by macrocytic anemia and scant RBC precursors in bone marrow
   2. Genetic testing is available for 4 known genes associated with DBA, which account for ~45% of cases

D. Therapy
   1. ~30% of patients develop spontaneous hematologic remission in 1st decade of life
   2. Glucocorticoids and RBC transfusion are primary treatments
   3. Hematopoietic stem cell transplantation is curative and is considered in patients with a human leukocyte antigen–matched sibling or patients who develop acute myeloid leukemia (AML)/myelodysplastic syndrome or aplastic anemia

> **QUICK HIT**
>
> DBA is characterized by a congenital inability to make RBCs. As a result, patients present in infancy with macrocytic anemia, low or absent reticulocytes, and congenital abnormalities. It is very unlikely to be the diagnosis in a patient who presents with new onset anemia over the age of 1 year.

XIII. Autoimmune Hemolytic Anemia (AIHA)

A. Characteristics
   1. Characterized by immune-mediated destruction of RBCs
   2. Classified by etiology as either primary (idiopathic) or secondary
      a. Primary AIHA affects 1 in 80,000 people per year; can affect all age groups, including infants
      b. Secondary AIHA is associated with multiple disease states including other autoimmune diseases (e.g., systemic lupus erythematosus, Crohn disease, juvenile idiopathic arthritis), lymphoproliferative disorders, malignancies, and *Mycoplasma* infection

3. Autoantibodies responsible for development of primary AIHA are classified as *warm* or *cold agglutinins*, referring to temperature at which antibody has highest activity
   a. Warm reactive AIHA
      i. Most common form of primary AIHA
      ii. Antibodies most often immunoglobulin (Ig) G, which poorly activates complement
      iii. Results in extravascular hemolysis
   b. Cold reactive AIHA
      i. Antibodies typically IgM, which fixes complement well
      ii. Results in intravascular hemolysis

B. Clinical features
1. Patients present with symptoms of hemolytic anemia, including fatigue, dyspnea, and dark urine
   a. Many patients will report recent viral syndrome
   b. Adolescent patients may exhibit symptoms of other autoimmune disorders
2. Physical exam findings
   a. Symptoms of anemia: pallor, tachycardia, systolic ejection murmur
   b. Symptoms of hemolysis: scleral icterus, jaundice, and tender splenomegaly
   c. In severe cases, hypoxia and hepatomegaly can be seen as result of cardiac failure brought on by profound anemia

C. Diagnosis
1. Laboratory findings
   a. Most important laboratory finding is direct antiglobulin test (**Coombs test**)
   b. With hemolytic anemia, low haptoglobin or elevated LDH is seen
   c. Spherocytes and schistocytes are seen on peripheral blood smear
   d. Reticulocytes may be elevated or low; variance depends on autoantibody adherence to reticulocytes and RBC maturity

> **QUICK HIT**
>
> A "direct" Coombs test finds antibodies that are *directly* attached to the RBC membrane. An "indirect" Coombs test evaluates patient plasma against a standard panel of RBCs in the lab, indicating what proteins the patient's antibodies are binding to, thereby guiding choice for blood for transfusion.

D. Treatment
1. Therapy
   a. Need to treat patients with AIHA depends on severity and acuity of anemia
   b. Transfusion should be reserved for patients with severe, symptomatic anemia and hemodynamic instability, because autoantibodies present in patient's serum will destroy transfused RBCs and endogenous cells
   c. Corticosteroids are first-line treatment for AIHA; more effective for AIHA due to IgG than IgM
   d. For patients with hemodynamic instability and poor response to steroids, exchange transfusion or plasmapheresis can also be used
   e. For patients who are refractory to steroids or develop chronic AIHA, there are several alternative therapies
      i. Surgical intervention with splenectomy is effective in 60% of cases
      ii. Immunomodulation can be effective
2. Complications
   a. Most severe complication of AIHA is cardiovascular collapse and death from precipitous and uncompensated drop in Hgb
   b. Overall, there is 10% mortality associated with AIHA
3. Most children with AIHA do well and respond to therapy
4. Patients younger than age 2 years and older than age 12 years and patients with secondary AIHA are more likely to develop refractory disease and complications

XIV. Aplastic Anemia

A. Definition
1. Inherited or acquired disorder with ↓ production of normal hematopoietic precursors in bone marrow resulting in acute or chronic myelosuppression
2. Can either be idiopathic or caused by multiple exposures
   a. Viral infection: HIV, hepatitis, Epstein-Barr virus (EBV), cytomegalovirus, others

b. Medications: chemotherapy, chloramphenicol, NSAIDs, others
c. Toxins: benzene, ionizing radiation, pesticides
3. Exact pathophysiology is unknown, although related to autoimmune T cell–mediated destruction of hematopoietic precursors

B. Clinical presentation is related to the level of myelosuppression
1. Pallor and fatigue from anemia
2. ↑ bleeding and bruising secondary to thrombocytopenia
3. ↑ infections and fever due to neutropenia

C. Diagnosis
1. CBC with differential will reveal cytopenias
2. Bone marrow biopsy is diagnostic and shows marrow hypocellularity
3. Screen for viruses associated with aplastic anemia and for inherited bone marrow failure syndromes

D. Treatment: involves supportive care with transfusions as necessary
1. Many patients will respond to immunosuppressive therapy with steroids, antithymocyte globulin, and cyclosporine
2. Hematopoietic stem cell transplant can be curative for patients who recur despite immunosuppressive therapy

XV. Folic Acid and Vitamin B_{12} Deficiency

A. Characteristics: associated with development of megaloblastic macrocytic anemia

B. Cause/pathophysiology
1. Folate and vitamin B_{12} are essential cofactors for erythropoiesis
2. Vitamin B_{12} deficiency is more commonly related to malabsorption than it is to nutritional deficiency (e.g., may be seen in Crohn disease)
3. Deficiency leads to development of abnormal chromatin and enlarged nuclei, which leads to apoptosis
4. Bone marrow is hyperactive secondary to stimulation by erythropoietin

C. Clinical presentation
1. Symptoms and signs of anemia
2. Irritability
3. GI features including glossitis and anorexia, weight loss, and FTT

D. Diagnosis
1. Peripheral blood smear will reveal large RBCs with hypersegmented neutrophils
2. MCV is high for age and often above 100 fL; RDW is elevated
3. Platelet and WBC counts may be low
4. ↓ serum B_{12} level in patients with vitamin B_{12} deficiency

E. Treatment: involves replacement of cofactor and treatment of underlying disorder, if present

XVI. von Willebrand Disease (vWD)

A. General characteristics
1. Congenital bleeding disorder caused by quantitative or qualitative defect of von Willebrand factor (vWF)
2. Most common inherited bleeding disorder; most cases are autosomal dominant
3. vWF is large protein synthesized and stored in endothelial cells, platelets, and megakaryocytes
4. vWF has 2 important functions in hemostasis
   a. Binds to platelets and exposed subendothelial structures at sites of vascular injury, initiating platelet adhesion for primary hemostasis
   b. Acts as carrier protein for factor VIII, protecting it from destruction within circulation and releasing it to participate in fibrin clot production

B. Clinical features
1. Historical findings
   a. Inquire about typical bleeding symptoms (Box 9-3) seen in vWD
   b. Ask about bleeding related to surgical procedures
   c. Obtain detailed family history of bleeding

QUICK HIT

All 3 major cell lines in the CBC are usually affected by aplastic anemia.

QUICK HIT

Folate supplementation may mask the hematologic effects of vitamin B_{12} deficiency but will *not* prevent progression of neurologic abnormalities caused by the deficiency.

QUICK HIT

Goat's milk is notoriously low in folate, and individuals on pure goat's milk diets are at high risk for folate deficiency.

QUICK HIT

Folate is needed from preconception to 1 month of gestation to prevent neural tube defects.

QUICK HIT

In severe cases, vitamin B_{12} deficiency can cause neurologic symptoms, in particular subacute combined degeneration of the spinal cord and dementia.

QUICK HIT

Serum folate level is not as helpful as RBC folate level, which reflects the actual tissue level and will be low in patients with folate deficiency.

QUICK HIT

Easy bruising is a very common complaint in pediatrics. Questioning should focus on location of bruising, spontaneous bruising, and associated hematomas to determine if the patient is likely to have an inherited bleeding disorder.

BOX 9-3

Symptoms of von Willebrand Disease

- Easy bruising
  - Spontaneous bruising
  - Bruising in unusual locations: face, chest, abdomen, back
  - Bruises that expand significantly or become hematomas
- Skin bleeding
  - Lacerations or minor cuts in skin with prolonged bleeding
  - Excessive scarring
- Mucous membrane bleeding
  - Frequent episodes of epistaxis
  - Nosebleeds that last longer than 10 minutes
  - Bleeding from gums when brushing teeth
  - Dental bleeding when teeth erupt or are extracted
  - Bright red blood in stools or emesis
  - Melena
- Menorrhagia
  - Increased bleeding with menses and increased duration of menses

QUICK HIT

Symptoms that result from interference with normal platelet function, such as vWD, typically manifest as mucous membrane bleeding, whereas bleeding from clotting factor deficiencies, such as hemophilia, presents with severe joint, muscle, or other soft tissue bleeds.

QUICK HIT

Excessive water retention can lead to hyponatremia and seizures, which can be life threatening; therefore, water restriction should be advised when prescribing DDAVP.

2. Physical exam findings
   a. Detailed skin examination to document location, size, and color of bruising and presence of petechiae or hematomas
   b. Evidence of recent bleeding in mouth or nose

C. Diagnosis
   1. CBC and PT/INR/PTT should be done as screen; however, these are usually normal in vWD
   2. PFA-100 measures ability of vWF–platelet complex to form a platelet plug and is usually prolonged in vWD
   3 Testing for vWF includes sending vWF antigen, ristocetin cofactor, and vWF multimer analysis
   4. Desmopressin (DDAVP) challenge determines if patients respond to DDAVP

D. Treatment
   1. Appropriate therapy depends on type of vWD
      a. DDAVP is the treatment of choice for vWD type 1 but is generally only needed for times of extensive bleeding or before surgical or dental procedures. Most patients have very mild bleeding symptoms and do not require the medication on a routine basis.
         i. Synthetic analogue of vasopressin and stimulates endothelial cell release of vWF, increasing vWF and factor VIII levels by 2–4×
         ii. Has antidiuretic properties; temporary **syndrome of inappropriate antidiuretic hormone secretion** is noted side effect
         iii. Administered intravenously (IV) or intranasally, acts within 15 minutes with peak effect in 30–60 minutes, and dose can be repeated once in 8–12 hours
      b. vWF-containing replacement products for severe bleeding symptoms
         i. Types of replacement products
            (a) Factor VIII concentrate
            (b) vWF highly purified concentrate
            (c) Cryoprecipitate
      c. Antifibrinolytic therapy (aminocaproic and tranexamic acids) inhibits fibrinolysis and stabilizes clot that has formed
      d. Topical agents (thrombin or fibrin sealant)
   2. Complications include bleeding, which can be severe especially in patients with types 2 and 3 disease

XVII. Hemophilias

A. General characteristics
   1. Hemophilia A and B are bleeding disorders caused by inherited clotting factor deficiencies
      a. Hemophilia A results from deficiency of factor VIII
      b. Hemophilia B results from deficiency of factor IX
   2. 2nd most common bleeding disorder after vWD
   3. Both hemophilia A and B are inherited in an X-linked recessive fashion and, therefore, affect males nearly exclusively; females can be carriers
   4. Pathophysiology
      a. Both factors VIII and IX are key components of **intrinsic clotting cascade**, which is activated in the presence of endothelial damage (Figure 9-6)
      b. Without the activity of factor VIII or IX, body's ability to create stable clot after endothelial damage is severely limited

B. Clinical features
   1. Historical findings
      a. Clinical features of hemophilia A and B are indistinguishable
      b. Detailed family history for affected male relatives
      c. Recurrent hemorrhage (spontaneous or secondary to minor trauma) into joints and soft tissue

QUICK HIT

Factor IX Leyden is a rare type of hemophilia B in which severe bleeding as a child significantly improves following puberty.

QUICK HIT

If a female patient presents with symptoms typical of hemophilia (deep tissue bleeds or joint bleeds), the diagnosis of type 2N vWD (a mutation in the von Willebrand antigen that causes inability to bind to the factor VIII molecule) should be considered.

FIGURE 9-6 The clotting cascade.

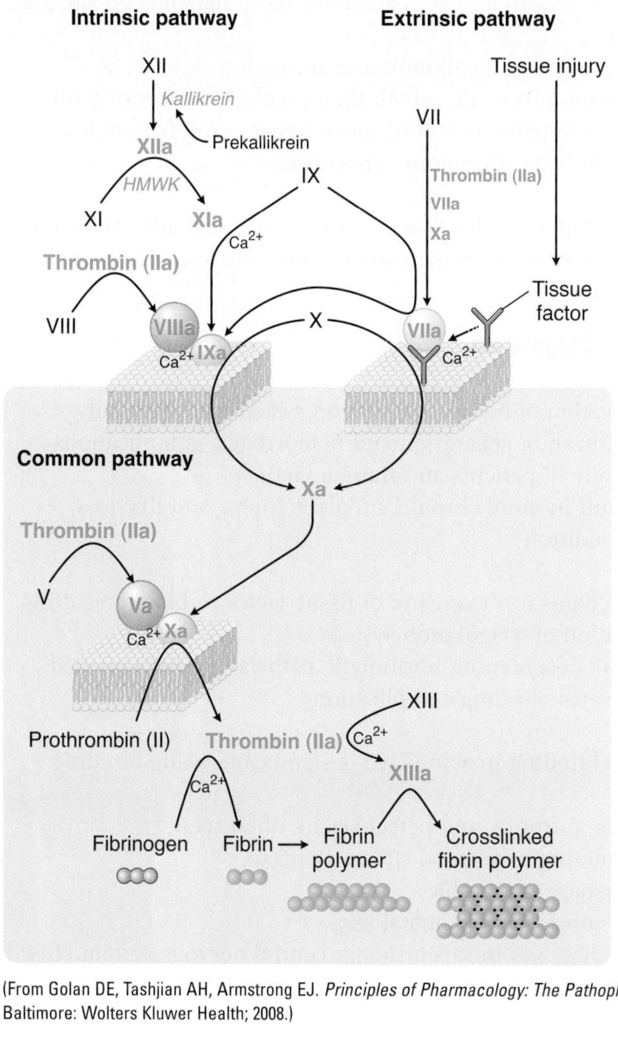

(From Golan DE, Tashjian AH, Armstrong EJ. *Principles of Pharmacology: The Pathophysiologic Basis of Drug Therapy.* 2nd ed. Baltimore: Wolters Kluwer Health; 2008.)

QUICK HIT

A normal prenatal history without bleeding complications does not rule out the diagnosis of hemophilia; most patients with mild hemophilia do not have excessive bleeding with circumcision and may go years without having symptoms or being diagnosed.

QUICK HIT

The average age for first presentation of hemarthrosis is 10 months.

QUICK HIT

The typical presentation for hemophilia is a male patient with joint bleeding in the setting of isolated mild trauma and a positive family history.

QUICK HIT

Newborns will have low factor IX levels at baseline because liver synthetic function has not matured. However, factor VIII levels should be normal or high because factor VIII is not produced by the liver.

QUICK HIT

DDAVP, which is used primarily for the treatment of vWD, may also be used to treat mild hemophilia A because it acts to release vWF and factor VIII from platelets and endothelial cells, thereby increasing factor VIII levels 2–5-fold.

d. Internal or external hemorrhage is possible; location and degree of hemorrhage depends on severity of hemophilia
e. Male infants with hemophilia may present with excessive bleeding in newborn period including intracranial hemorrhage or bleeding after circumcision and separation of umbilical stump

2. Physical exam
   a. Considered if severe acute blood loss with minor trauma in a male patient
   b. Exam should focus on identifying site of bleed
      i. Hemarthrosis will present with joint swelling and warmth, ↓ range of motion, pain with passive movement
      ii. Hematomas on skin may be seen, but usually not bruising and petechiae
      iii. Internal GI bleed may show peritoneal signs such as rebound and guarding
      iv. Intracranial bleeding may present with focal neurologic signs

C. Diagnosis
1. Abnormally prolonged activated partial thromboplastin time (aPTT) will be seen, whereas PT, INR, and bleeding time should all be normal
2. Confirmation of diagnosis can be made by obtaining specific factor assays: adults and children should have factor levels that approach or are above 100%

D. Treatment
1. Therapy
   a. Factor replacement is standard of care
      i. IV replacement of factor VIII or IX to therapeutic plasma levels allows for effective hemostasis with bleeding
      ii. Fresh frozen plasma (FFP) and cryoprecipitate have scant available _factor VIII or IX and are usually unhelpful
      iii. Plasma factor level required to stop an active bleed depends on site and severity of bleed
   b. Patients are at risk of developing alloimmune antibodies (known as *inhibitors*) against factor VIII or IX, which then preclude treatment with factor replacement; these patients will be given bypass products such as recombinant factor VII or prothrombin concentrate
2. Complications
   a. Severe recurrent bleeding episodes that can lead to hemorrhage and death
   b. Risk of chronic arthropathy and degenerative joint disease secondary to multiple recurrent joint bleeds

XVIII. Disseminated Intravascular Coagulation

A. General characteristics
1. DIC is widespread activation of body's coagulation system, paradoxically resulting in both microthrombi generation and hemorrhagic complications
2. Usually seen with severely ill patients and trauma victims
3. Low-grade DIC can result in more chronic, indolent course and due to a variety of pathologic conditions
4. Pathophysiology
   a. Major triggering mechanism is exposure of tissue factor to blood, resulting in widespread activation of coagulation system
   b. Following widespread coagulation, fibrinolytic pathway is also activated, which further aggravates bleeding complications

B. Clinical features
1. Most common historical finding in acute DIC is significant, acute bleeding
2. Physical findings
   a. Bruising, ecchymoses, purpura, and petechiae are often seen
   b. Oozing from venipuncture or surgical sites may occur
   c. Postoperative hemorrhage is possible
   d. GI bleeding is more common in neonatal DIC
   e. Intrapulmonary bleeding and intraventricular central nervous system (CNS) hemorrhage may also be seen in neonate
   f. Microvascular thrombosis resulting in end-organ damage

TABLE 9-4 **Distinguishing Other Coagulation Disorders from DIC**

Lab Test	Vitamin K Deficiency	Liver Disease	DIC
PT	Prolonged	Prolonged	Prolonged
aPTT	Prolonged	Prolonged	Prolonged
Platelets	Normal	Normal	Decreased
Fibrinogen	Normal	Variable	Very low
FSP	Normal	Normal or high	Very high
Factors	Low II, VII, IX, X	Low I, II, V, VII, IX, X	Variable
Blood Smear	Normal RBCs	Target cells possible	Schistocytes

aPTT, activated partial thromboplastin time; DIC, disseminated intravascular coagulation; FSP, fibrin-split products; PT, prothrombin time.

C. Diagnosis (Table 9-4)
  1. Laboratory findings
    a. Prolonged PT and aPTT
    b. ↓ fibrinogen
    c. ↑ fibrin-split products (FSP) and ↑ D-dimer
    d. CBC will reveal thrombocytopenia and possibly signs of hemolytic anemia
D. Treatment
  1. Therapy
    a. Treatment of the underlying cause is the most important aspect
    b. Replacement of consumed products: platelets, FFP and cryoprecipitate
  2. Complications of DIC can be severe and include hemorrhage, thrombosis, and death

XIX. Vitamin K Deficiency

A. Definitions
  1. Vitamin K is lipid-soluble vitamin supplied by leafy, green vegetables necessary for production of factors II, VII, IX, and X
  2. Impaired production of these coagulation factors results in bleeding
B. Cause/pathophysiology
  1. Vitamin K initiates carboxylation of amino acid glutamate on certain clotting factors, which is necessary for appropriate function
  2. Vitamin K–dependent clotting factors that are not carboxylated have short half-lives and are removed from the circulation quickly, resulting in low serum values
  3. Newborns are at ↑ risk as vitamin K is not readily transported across the placenta
C. Clinical presentation
  1. Symptoms can include GI bleeding, bruising, or intracranial hemorrhage
  2. After delivery, newborns can present with cephalohematomas or internal bleeding
  3. After day 1 of life, infants can present with GI bleeding, umbilical stump bleeding, or internal bleeding
  4. Vitamin K deficiency can occur due to malabsorption or liver disease
D. Diagnosis
  1. Prolonged PT (due to low factor VII) and prolonged PTT (due to low factor IX)
  2. Specific deficiency of vitamin K–dependent factors (factors II, VII, IX, and X)
  3. If other factor levels are ↓, consider primary liver dysfunction as diagnosis
E. Treatment
  1. All newborns receive vitamin K prophylaxis at birth
  2. Human daily dietary requirement of vitamin K is 1 mcg/kg
  3. Vitamin K replacement may be given orally, intramuscularly, or IV

QUICK HIT

The risk of viral transmission with factor replacement is now extremely low due to viral screening improvements. HIV and hepatitis C were commonly transmitted in the past, but this has become extremely rare with the current products available.

QUICK HIT

In low-grade DIC, symptoms are not overt: platelet counts, fibrinogen levels, and clotting factor levels may be normal or only mildly ↓.

QUICK HIT

The clinical signs and symptoms of DIC are often difficult to recognize in a severely ill patient with multiple other comorbidities; therefore, a high index of suspicion should be maintained for at-risk children and sick neonates.

QUICK HIT

Lab abnormalities in DIC can vary.

QUICK HIT

The underlying cause for DIC should be determined as soon as possible, and treatment should be instituted rapidly!

QUICK HIT

Warfarin acts by interfering with vitamin K regeneration, thereby decreasing factor levels and allowing for anticoagulation.

> **QUICK HIT**
> Breast milk is low in vitamin K, which further aggravates the risk of deficiency in breast-feeding infants.

> **QUICK HIT**
> Factor VIII is unique in that its level remains normal in the setting of liver dysfunction.

> **QUICK HIT**
> Acute ITP can occur at any age in both sexes, but it has a bimodal distribution with peaks among boys age 1–6 years and women age 30–40 years.

> **QUICK HIT**
> Patients with acute ITP have a normal physical exam aside from bleeding symptoms.

XX. Immune-Mediated Thrombocytopenia (ITP)

A. Characteristics
1. Autoimmune-mediated clearance of circulating platelets by antibodies that develop against platelet glycoproteins
2. Antibody-coated platelets are prematurely cleared by reticuloendothelial macrophages in spleen, resulting in macrothrombocytopenia with platelet counts possibly dropping to numbers well below 20,000/mm^3
3. Acute ITP (80% of all cases of ITP)
   - i. Platelet count returns to normal within 6 months of diagnosis and does not recur
   - ii. Spontaneously resolves without therapy in some cases
   - iii. Commonly associated with antecedent viral illness or vaccinations
4. Chronic ITP
   - i. Platelet count persists at low levels beyond 6 months
   - ii. More likely to be associated with baseline autoimmune dysfunction or other chronic illness
   - iii. More common in adolescents and not associated with antecedent viral illness

B. Clinical features
1. Historical findings
   - a. Acute onset of hemorrhagic symptoms in otherwise well child
   - b. Ask about preceding viral illness
   - c. Extensive history needed to rule out inherited bleeding disorder
   - d. In acute disease, parents will report ↑ bruising, prolonged epistaxis, and new-onset petechial rash over days leading into presentation
2. Physical exam findings
   - a. Should be completely normal aside from hemorrhagic manifestations
   - b. Intracranial hemorrhage extremely rare (<0.5% of cases)
   - c. Hepatosplenomegaly and lymphadenopathy are NOT present and warrant more aggressive and cautious workup

C. Diagnosis
1. Differential diagnosis
   - a. Malignancy: main illness to rule out is childhood leukemia
     - i. Patients with acute lymphoblastic leukemia (ALL) can have thrombocytopenia at diagnosis, but this will usually be in conjunction with drop in other hematopoietic cell lines
     - ii. Patients who present with leukemia often have hepatosplenomegaly, lymphadenopathy, and/or fever
   - b. Other non–immune-mediated causes of thrombocytopenia
     - i. Infection
     - ii. Drug-mediated thrombocytopenia
     - iii. Splenomegaly can lead to ↑ platelet consumption but usually also with anemia and neutropenia
     - iv. Congenital thrombocytopenia due to marrow production defects
     - v. Platelet function disorders
     - vi. Wiskott-Aldrich syndrome
       - (a) X-linked recessive disorder associated with thrombocytopenia and immunodeficiency
       - (b) Platelets are small, unlike in ITP, which is associated with large platelets
2. Laboratory findings
   - a. CBC with differential
     - i. Platelet count should be <20,000/mm^3; mean platelet volume is commonly elevated
     - ii. Hgb is only low if there has been severe bleeding
     - iii. WBC should be normal
   - b. Bone marrow biopsy can show ↑ numbers of megakaryocytes but is absolutely unnecessary if diagnosis is clear

c. In chronic cases in which thrombocytopenia has not resolved for >1 year, more thorough workup with bone marrow biopsy or evaluation for autoimmune disease may be indicated

D. Treatment
  1. Therapy
    a. Treatment of acute ITP is directed at temporarily alleviating thrombocytopenia until autoantibodies are cleared from plasma
    b. Observation without treatment if platelet count is >10,000/mm^3; serial CBC evaluations and strict precautions against head injury
    c. Platelet transfusion is usually contraindicated unless emergent bleeding is present because transfused platelets will be coated by autoantibodies and cleared as easily as endogenous platelets
    d. Avoid platelet-inhibiting medications (e.g., ASA, ibuprofen)
    e. Treatment options
      i. IV immunoglobulin (IVIG)
        (a) Competitive inhibition of Fc receptors on splenic macrophages ↓ clearance of platelets
        (b) Platelets remain coated with antibody but continue to function
      ii. Anti-D immunoglobulin
        (a) Patients must be Rh+
        (b) Competitive inhibition of Fc receptors on macrophages by RBCs coated with Rh antibody
        (c) Patients can become anemic from hemolysis, so Hgb should be checked 1 week following administration
      iii. Steroids
        (a) Downregulation of immune system ↓ antibody production and ↓ uptake by splenic macrophages
        (b) Patients receiving steroids prior to treatment for leukemia can have worse outcome; therefore, before using steroids, treating physician should be absolutely confident of ITP diagnosis

XXI. Hypercoagulability

A. Characteristics
  1. Thrombosis develops from excessive generation of or ineffective breakdown of thrombin
  2. Multiple secondary risk factors that predispose patients to thrombosis have been identified (Box 9-4)
  3. Inherited mutations that predispose to thrombophilia usually do not present until adulthood
  4. Hereditary causes of thrombophilia include
    a. Antithrombin III (ATIII) deficiency
      i. ATIII functions to form complex with activated thrombin, Xa, IXa, and XIa, which neutralizes these activated clotting factors
      ii. Homozygous mutations are incompatible with life, whereas heterozygous patients have higher risk of venous thrombosis in 2nd decade of life

QUICK HIT

Bone marrow biopsy is not routinely indicated in acute ITP. It should be done if the diagnosis is unclear or the patient has other clinical findings of concern such as fever, hepatosplenomegaly, or lymphadenopathy. It is also indicated if thrombocytopenia has not resolved for several months.

QUICK HIT

Platelet transfusion is contraindicated in ITP unless there is life-threatening hemorrhage. Transfused platelets are coated easily by autoantibodies and cleared by the spleen effectively.

QUICK HIT

Therapy does not actually cure acute ITP; it leads to a temporary prevention of platelet clearance and resolution of symptoms until autoantibodies naturally are cleared over time from plasma.

QUICK HIT

A complete workup requires a large volume of blood and cannot be easily obtained until the patient is several months old; in this circumstance, testing parental blood may lead to a diagnosis.

BOX 9-4

Secondary Risk Factors that Predispose to a Hypercoagulable State

Malignancy	Liver disease
Smoking	Nephrotic syndrome
Estrogen-containing oral contraception	Asparaginase
Surgery/immobility	Steroids
Antiphospholipid antibody syndrome	Systemic lupus erythematosus
Indwelling catheters	Other autoimmune disease
Infection	Sickle cell disease
Burns	Vasculitides

b. Protein C and protein S deficiency
   i. Function to break down clotting factors Va and VIIIa
   ii. Heterozygosity poses slight ↑ in risk of venous thrombosis in 2nd decade of life, whereas homozygosity is associated with multiple thromboses in neonates (syndrome known as *neonatal purpura fulminans*)
c. Factor V Leiden mutation
   i. Leads to resistance in breakdown by protein C
   ii. Most common inheritable mutation with ↑ incidence in people of Northern European descent
   iii. ↑ risk for arterial and venous thrombosis in adulthood, but childhood thrombosis is rare
d. Prothrombin mutation
   i. Results in excess thrombin
   ii. ↑ risk of thrombosis in adulthood
e. *MTHFR* mutation
   i. Mutation in *5,10-methylenetetrahydrofolate reductase* gene (*MTHFR*), enzyme normally responsible for conversion of homocysteine to methionine
   ii. Patients with this mutation develop elevated levels of homocysteine, which damages blood vessel wall and predisposes to thrombosis in adulthood

QUICK HIT

Most children with thrombosis will have multiple risk factors that are responsible for excessive thrombin generation and/or ineffective breakdown of fibrin and thrombin. A single risk factor is usually not enough to cause thrombosis in a child.

B. Treatment
1. Therapy
   a. For newly diagnosed thrombosis, anticoagulation will be instituted for 3 months, assuming clot resolves
   b. Certain clinical situations, such as presence of multiple risk factors or multiply recurrent thromboses, require long-term anticoagulation
   c. Heparin
      i. Naturally occurring substance that accentuates ATIII activity
      ii. Given as infusion with frequent monitoring of PTT, which will become prolonged; infusion escalated or held based on desired PTT
      iii. Effect can be cleared by discontinuing infusion or by administration of protamine sulfate, which is neutralizing antidote

QUICK HIT

Heparin does not participate in acute clot degradation; rather, it prevents further clot formation and propagation, allowing for natural breakdown of a thrombotic lesion by the fibrinolytic system.

   d. Low-molecular-weight heparin
      i. Results in more efficient breakdown of factor Xa
      ii. Administered daily via subcutaneous injection
      iii. In children, monitor anti-Xa levels for therapeutic effect and adjust dose to maintain levels between 0.5–1 units/mL
      iv. Effect can be rapidly cleared by administration of protamine sulfate, which is neutralizing antidote
   e. Warfarin
      i. Oral anticoagulant that inhibits vitamin K
      ii. Therapeutic effect is monitored by following INR
      iii. Can take several days to achieve desired INR therapeutic target
      iv. Protein C and S production is also vitamin K dependent
         (a) Because warfarin also inhibits protein C and S, patients can be paradoxically hypercoagulable early in therapy
         (b) Patients will also be started on heparin until warfarin achieves desired therapeutic INR
      v. Antidote to warfarin is vitamin K
   f. Thrombolytic therapy
      i. Indicated for patients with life-threatening and recent arterial thrombosis
      ii. These agents actively break down an existing thrombus
      iii. Poses significant risk of bleeding and hemorrhage
2. Treatment should be instituted immediately to avoid neurovascular compromise and further ischemia
3. Preventive measures, such as avoiding immobility, tobacco use, and estrogen-containing medications, are essential

XXII. Neutropenia

A. Characteristics
   1. Absolute neutrophil count (ANC) below normal for age
   2. Neutropenia in children is usually secondary and can be due to variety of exogenous causes including infection, drug induced, or autoimmune disease
      a. Infection-mediated neutropenia
         i. Extremely common and usually due to ↑ neutrophil margination
         ii. Some infectious agents inhibit neutrophil production and maturation
         iii. This is usually benign and self-limited
      b. Drug-induced neutropenia
      c. Benign neutropenia of childhood is most common cause of neutropenia in pediatrics with no other identifiable risk factors
         i. Occurs most commonly in children younger than age 3 years with median age at diagnosis of 8 months
         ii. Caused by autoantibodies to neutrophils produced in response to medication or infection
         iii. Clinical picture is not in line with ANC; can be as low as 0
         iv. Some evidence that neutrophils are present and effective but are cleared or marginated into periphery before they can be measured, which accounts for relatively low incidence of serious infections in such patients
   3. Inherited disorders associated with impaired neutrophil production
      a. Cyclic neutropenia: autosomal dominant stem cell defect that leads to temporary neutropenia with associated infectious symptoms every 3 weeks
      b. Kostmann syndrome (congenital neutropenia): rare autosomal recessive disorder of neutrophil maturation that presents in infancy with multiple, severe infections with extremely low ANC ($<200/mm^3$)
      c. Shwachman-Diamond syndrome: extremely rare autosomal recessive disorder that causes multifactorial immunodeficiency, pancreatic insufficiency, neutropenia, orthopedic anomalies, and FTT

B. Clinical features
   1. Historical and physical exam findings are related to the ↑ risk of infection
   2. Oral ulcers and gingivitis, peritonitis, and stomatitis are common in patients with severe neutropenia

C. Diagnosis
   1. To be classified as neutropenic, patient's ANC should be
         i. Newborn: $<3{,}000/mm^3$
         ii. Infancy–age 2 years: $<1{,}000/mm^3$
         iii. Age >2 years: $<1{,}500/mm^3$
   2. Remainder of CBC and differential should be normal
   3. If suspected secondary (usually viral) neutropenia, repeat CBC with resolution of symptoms and, if neutropenia resolves, likely no further workup is needed
   4. Congenital disorders of neutropenia listed can be confirmed via genetic testing
   5. Patients suspected of having cyclic neutropenia should have CBC with differential performed twice weekly for 6 weeks to document cycle
   6. Antineutrophilic antibodies can be sent and will be positive in some cases of benign neutropenia of childhood. A negative test, however, does not rule out this disorder.

D. Treatment
   1. Therapy
      a. Benign neutropenia of childhood or other secondary causes of neutropenia
         i. Cautious observation until neutropenia resolves
         ii. If neutropenia is drug induced, stop medication
         iii. Granulocyte colony-stimulating factor (GCSF), IVIG, or prednisone can be given with severe, life-threatening infection
         iv. If patient is febrile, systemic antibiotics should be given for fever pending blood culture results

QUICK HIT

ANC = total WBC count (in thousands) × percentage of neutrophils and band forms within the CBC differential.

QUICK HIT

The most common cause of neutropenia in childhood is viral infection, whereas inherited neutrophil disorders are extremely rare.

QUICK HIT

Benign neutropenia of childhood is usually asymptomatic, despite extreme neutropenia.

b. Cyclic neutropenia
   i. GCSF during times of nadir if patient develops ANC $<200/mm^3$ and recurrent serious infections
   ii. Routine oral hygiene with rinses to prevent stomatitis
   iii. Antibiotics for infections
c. Kostmann syndrome
   i. Bone marrow transplant is curative
   ii. GCSF can raise neutrophil count
   iii. These patients should be on prophylactic antibiotics
d. Shwachman-Diamond syndrome
   i. GCSF and prophylactic antibiotics
   ii. Pancreatic enzyme supplementation
   iii. Bone marrow transplant

2. Complications
   a. Major complication of neutropenia is severe, life-threatening infection
   b. Patients with prolonged neutropenia are at risk for recurrent infections, chronic mouth sores, stomatitis, and gingivitis
   c. Kostmann and Shwachman-Diamond syndromes are both associated with ↑ risk of AML and/or myelodysplastic syndrome

Infectious Diseases

10

SYMPTOM SPECIFIC

I. Approach to Fever of Unknown Origin

A. Definition: pediatric fever of unknown origin (FUO) can be defined as fever >38.3°C (>100.4°F) for at least 8 days with no apparent diagnosis after initial outpatient or hospital evaluation
   1. Major diagnostic categories for FUO in children are infection, collagen vascular disease/inflammatory disorders, and neoplasm
      a. Infection: Epstein-Barr virus (EBV), cytomegalovirus (CMV), adenovirus, osteomyelitis, *Bartonella henselae* (cat-scratch disease), sinusitis, pneumonia, dental abscess, tuberculosis (TB), HIV, endocarditis, rickettsiae (e.g., Rocky Mountain spotted fever [RMSF])
      b. Inflammation: incomplete Kawasaki disease, systemic juvenile idiopathic arthritis (JIA), sarcoid, vasculitis (e.g., systemic lupus erythematosus [SLE])
      c. Malignancy: leukemia, lymphoma, neuroblastoma
   2. FUO is more likely due to an atypical presentation of a common condition than a typical presentation of an uncommon condition
   3. Cause of FUO commonly remains undetermined in >50%, but most of those without a specific cause identified recover uneventfully, suggesting a likely viral cause

B. Historical questions
   1. Most important key to diagnosing FUO is careful, thorough history and review of systems (ROS)
   2. Comprehensive exposure history is critical, including animal exposure, travel, sources of food and water, sick contacts, and medications (Table 10-1)

C. Physical exam and findings
   1. May hold clues to diagnosis but may be completely normal
   2. May be evolving; important to note historical exam findings even if not currently present

D. Laboratory testing and radiologic imaging
   1. Initially, should focus on differential diagnoses suggested by history and exam
      a. In children, early workup should focus on infectious etiologies as well as incomplete Kawasaki disease
      b. Typical initial labs are shown in Box 10-1

II. Approach to Fever in Newborn Infant

A. Background information
   1. Defined as rectal temperature >38°C in a neonate (age <28 days)
   2. Most cases of fever in neonate are secondary to self-limited viral infection (e.g., respiratory syncytial virus [RSV], enteroviruses)

> **QUICK HIT**
> FUOs are usually common disorders presenting atypically.

> **QUICK HIT**
> Cat-scratch disease (*B. henselae*) causes 5% of all cases of FUO.

> **QUICK HIT**
> In children, infection is by far the most common identified cause of FUO.

> **QUICK HIT**
> If fever lasts >3 weeks, likelihood of infectious etiology falls, and neoplasms and inflammatory disorders become more likely.

> **QUICK HIT**
> It is important to document fever reported by parent or patient, including how it was measured, how often it occurs, when it occurs, and if antipyretics are effective.

> **QUICK HIT**
> C-reactive protein (CRP) is normal with drug fever.

Table 10-1 Infectious Causes of Fever of Unknown Origin and Associated Exposures

Infection	Possible Associated Exposures
Bartonella henselae	Exposure to cats, especially kittens
Osteomyelitis	Exposure to methicillin-resistant *Staphylococcus aureus* or household members with history of abscesses/skin infections
Rocky Mountain spotted fever *Ehrlichia*	Tick exposure (this is not always well recalled and should be considered possible in any area where these diseases are endemic)
Tularemia	Tick exposure, rabbits, undercooked hunted meat
Salmonella	Undercooked poultry or eggs, cross-contamination of foods, reptile exposure/pets
Yersinia	Pork intestines (chitterlings), contaminated milk or water
Leptospirosis	Freshwater exposure (lakes, streams), urine of infected animals (dogs, rats, other wild mammals)
Tuberculosis	Travel to an endemic area, exposure to high-risk groups, exposure to symptomatic individual with chronic cough of unknown etiology
Brucella	Unpasteurized dairy products
Q fever	Unpasteurized milk, inhalation of dust contaminated by cat or sheep afterbirth
Histoplasmosis	Endemic to Ohio River Valley, lower Mississippi River, cave exploration, bird/bat droppings, construction with earth turnover
Blastomycosis	Endemic to Mississippi River and Ohio River basins and around the Great Lakes, recently flooded areas, rotting wood
Coccidioidomycosis	Endemic to the southwestern U.S. and central California (San Joaquin Valley)
Rat bite fever	Rat bite (also mouse, squirrels, cats, and weasels) or scratch, handling dead rats with open skin
Malaria	Travel to endemic areas especially without appropriate prophylaxis
Toxocara	Exposure to dog or cat feces (roundworm is shed in their stools)
Toxoplasmosis	Exposure to cat feces, raw/undercooked beef

Infectious Diseases

QUICK HIT

Medications commonly implicated in drug fever include antibiotics (especially β-lactam agents), ranitidine, antiepileptic drugs, opioids, and furosemide.

3. Goal is to identify newborns with serious bacterial infection such as urinary tract infection (UTI), bacteremia, meningitis, pneumonia, and bone and soft tissue infection
   a. 7%–13% of all newborns with fever will have a serious bacterial infection
   b. Virtually impossible to distinguish newborns with benign viral infections from those with serious bacterial infections by history and physical alone

BOX 10-1

Initial Laboratory and Radiologic Workup for Fever of Unknown Origin in Children

Laboratory tests

- Complete blood count with differential
- Erythrocyte sedimentation rate, C-reactive protein
- Liver enzymes and function tests (aspartate aminotransferase, alanine aminotransferase, albumin)
- Renal function tests
- Urinalysis and urine culture
- Epstein-Barr virus and cytomegalovirus serologies if compatible illness
- Specific testing for other diagnoses suggested by history and exam

Radiology tests

- Chest x-ray—given high percentage of FUO that are caused by lower respiratory tract infection
- Abdominal ultrasound—can be useful in assessing for systemic bartonellosis to look for microabscesses in liver and spleen as well as evaluating the genitourinary system
- Additional imaging should be guided by history, physical examination, and labs

FUO, fever of unknown origin.

B. Historical findings
  1. Antenatal/birth history risk factors for infection
    a. Maternal group B *Streptococcus* (GBS) colonization or infection and timing of peripartum antibiotic prophylaxis
    b. Maternal fever in perinatal period
    c. Maternal herpes simplex virus (HSV) infection
    d. Prolonged rupture of membranes
    e. Prematurity
  2. History of present illness
    a. Degree and duration of fever
    b. Method of measuring temperature
    c. Symptoms of upper respiratory infection (URI), such as cough
    d. Sick contacts
    e. History of bloody diarrhea or vomiting
    f. Feeding history
    g. History of lethargy
  3. Physical exam
    a. Vital signs: rectal temperature is most accurate, and pulse oximetry should be included
    b. Febrile or hypothermic infant
    c. Irritability or lethargy
    d. Full fontanelle is late finding for meningitis
    e. Tachypnea, respiratory distress, and hypoxia (pneumonia)
    f. Bone or joint tenderness (osteomyelitis or septic arthritis)
    g. Examine scalp at fetal scalp electrode site (HSV)
    h. Vesicular lesions (HSV)
    i. Pustular lesions (*Staphylococcus aureus*)

C. Evaluation
  1. Complete blood count (CBC) with differential
  2. Blood culture
  3. Urine analysis
  4. Catheterized urine culture
  5. Lumbar puncture (LP) with cerebrospinal fluid (CSF) sent for Gram stain, culture, protein, glucose, cell count with differential
  6. Chest x-ray (CXR) if respiratory symptoms are present
  7. Aspartate aminotransferase (AST), alanine aminotransferase (ALT), blood and CSF HSV polymerase chain reaction (PCR) if HSV infection is suspected
  8. Maintain low threshold for testing for HSV in febrile neonates age <21 days
  9. Appropriate viral studies based on epidemiology
  10. Stool culture if bacterial gastroenteritis is suspected

D. Treatment
  1. Start empiric antibiotics with ampicillin and gentamicin or ampicillin and cefotaxime to cover most common organisms
  2. Add clindamycin or vancomycin if bone or soft tissue infection is present to cover for *S. aureus*
  3. Delays in starting acyclovir in neonates with HSV are associated with higher mortality, so infants tested for HSV should receive acyclovir while awaiting CSF HSV PCR results

QUICK HIT

Two thirds of infants with serious bacterial infection will have a normal exam at presentation.

QUICK HIT

Neonates with meningitis or septic arthritis may have **paradoxical irritability** (i.e., crying when held, quiet when not disturbed).

QUICK HIT

Peripartum antibiotic prophylaxis prevents early-onset but not late-onset GBS infection. Infant mucosal GBS colonization, which predisposes to late-onset disease, is not eradicated by peripartum antibiotics.

QUICK HIT

Cerebrospinal fluid (CSF) pleocytosis (elevated white blood cell [WBC] count) is absent in >1/3 of neonates with central nervous system (CNS) infection caused by enteroviruses.

QUICK HIT

Neonates at high risk of bacterial infection have at least 1 of following:
- CSF WBC >8/mm^3
- Bacteria on CSF Gram stain
- Peripheral WBC >15,000/mm^3
- >10 WBC/high-power field (HPF) on urinalysis
- Band: neutrophil ratio >0.2

QUICK HIT

All febrile neonates should be admitted to hospital!

DISEASE SPECIFIC

III. Bacterial Meningitis

A. Definition: bacterial infection causes inflammation of **leptomeninges** (membranes that surround brain and spinal cord)
B. Epidemiology
  1. Incidence in U.S. has decreased in recent decades due to
    a. *Haemophilus influenzae* type b (Hib) vaccine
    b. *Streptococcus pneumoniae* (pneumococcal) conjugate vaccine

Table 10-2 Bacterial Pathogens Responsible for Bacterial Meningitis

Birth to 3 months
Group B *Streptococcus*
Escherichia coli
Listeria monocytogenes
Streptococcus pneumoniae (rare, but incidence increases after 1 month of age)
Neisseria meningitidis (rare)
3 months to 18 years
S. pneumoniae
N. meningitidis
Haemophilus influenzae type b
Gram-negative organisms (e.g., *E. coli, Klebsiella* spp.)
Mycobacterium tuberculosis (rare in U.S.)
Underlying conditions associated with specific organisms
Immunocompromised children – *S. pneumoniae, N. meningitidis*
Terminal complement deficiency – *N. meningitidis*
Congenital antibody deficiencies – *S. pneumoniae, H. influenzae* type b
T-lymphocyte deficiency – *L. monocytogenes*
Asplenia – *S. pneumoniae, N. meningitidis, Salmonella* spp.
Surgery – skin organisms, nosocomial pathogens

c. *Neisseria meningitidis* conjugate vaccine
d. Efforts to identify and treat GBS in pregnant women

2. Cause (Table 10-2) for common bacterial organisms that cause meningitis

C. Genetics
1. Children with certain immunodeficiency syndromes are at greater risk of meningitis (e.g., complement deficiency predisposes to meningitis caused by *N. meningitidis*)
2. Other risk factors
   a. CSF leak
   b. Asplenia (anatomic or functional)
   c. Immunodeficiency (HIV, malignancy, immunosuppressive drugs)
   d. Ventriculoperitoneal shunt or recent neurosurgery
   e. Penetrating head trauma

D. Pathophysiology
1. **Bacteria normally colonize the nasopharynx** (NP)
2. These bacteria then invade mucosa and enter bloodstream, leading to intravascular multiplication
3. Organisms then penetrate blood–brain barrier, causing inflammation in subarachnoid space, leading to damage of neuronal and auditory cells

E. Clinical features
1. Historical findings (symptoms)
   a. Infants typically have history of **inconsolable crying, hyper-** or **hypothermia, lethargy,** grunting, and poor feeding
   b. Older children typically have history of **fever, vomiting, headache,** photophobia, confusion, seizures, and **sore/stiff neck**
2. Exam findings (signs)
   a. In infants, bacterial meningitis may present with fever, hypothermia, irritability, respiratory distress, seizures, and bulging fontanelle
   b. Older patients present with fever and evidence of meningeal inflammation, such as vomiting, headache, or altered mental status

c. More specific signs of meningeal inflammation are **nuchal rigidity** and positive **Kernig** and **Brudzinski signs**
d. **Petechial** or **purpuric rash** is classically seen in *N. meningitidis* but can be seen in other causes of bacterial meningitis

F. Diagnosis
1. Differential diagnosis in children with fever and alteration of CNS function
a. Viral meningitis (e.g., enterovirus, arboviruses)
b. Encephalitis (e.g., HSV)
c. Postinfectious encephalitis (e.g., acute disseminated encephalomyelitis [ADEM])
d. Brain abscess
e. Rickettsial disease
f. Vasculitis
2. Laboratory
a. CBC, blood culture, and electrolyte panel should be obtained
b. **LP** is essential to make diagnosis
c. CSF analysis, including **Gram stain**, **aerobic culture**, **cell count with differential**, **glucose and protein concentrations**, and **various viral studies** are necessary to differentiate from other infectious and noninfectious etiologies
d. See Table 10-3 for interpretation of CSF findings
3. Radiology
a. Head computed tomography (CT) should be performed prior to LP if child has any focal neurologic deficits on exam or other signs of increased intracranial pressure (ICP) to exclude brain abscess, mass lesion, or other cause of increased ICP
b. Brain magnetic resonance imaging (MRI) should be performed in children who do not respond to therapy as expected to detect **brain abscess** or **subdural empyema**

G. Management
1. Therapy
a. **Antibiotic therapy**, **supportive care**, and **monitoring for complications** are management mainstays
b. Ideally, LP and blood culture should be performed before starting empiric antibiotic therapy
c. If patient is in respiratory distress, hypotensive, or otherwise critically ill, blood culture should be obtained and antibiotics should be immediately started and LP deferred
d. Antibiotic management
i. Antibiotics (especially β-lactam antibiotics) often require larger mg/kg dose when being used to treat bacterial meningitis to maximize concentration of antibiotics in CSF
ii. **Empiric antibiotic treatment** includes vancomycin and cefotaxime

QUICK HIT

Kernig sign is performed by bending hip and knee at 90° angles and is said to be positive if extension of knee causes back pain and resistance to straightening before an angle of 135°.

QUICK HIT

Brudzinski sign is performed by lifting patient's head while he or she is lying supine and is said to be positive if lifting of head causes involuntary lifting of legs.

QUICK HIT

Children with bacterial meningitis may develop hyponatremia due to syndrome of inappropriate antidiuretic hormone (SIADH) secretion.

QUICK HIT

Do not delay antibiotics while waiting for head CT. Administer antibiotics prior to head imaging because delay in antibiotic therapy is associated with worse outcomes.

TABLE 10-3 Typical Cerebrospinal Fluid Findings in Various Types of Meningitis

	WBC (per mm³)	% PMNs	CSF Glucose (mg/dL)	Protein (mg/dL)
Bacterial	>1,000	>85%–90%	<40	>100–150
Viral	20–500	20%–40%	Normal	Normal or <100
Fungal	<500	<10%–20%	<40	>100–200
Tuberculosis	<300	<10%–20%	<40	>200–300

CSF, cerebrospinal fluid; PMN, polymorphonuclear cells; WBC, white blood cell.

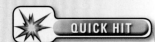

> **QUICK HIT**
> Ampicillin, vancomycin, and 3rd-generation cephalosporins have relatively good penetration into CSF, whereas aminoglycosides have poor CSF penetration.

> **QUICK HIT**
> Vancomycin is added to a 3rd-generation cephalosporin (e.g., ceftriaxone) for empiric treatment of bacterial meningitis in children over age 1 month to maximize coverage for possibility of highly resistant *S. pneumoniae*.

e. Corticosteroids
   i. Dexamethasone therapy decreases risk of neurologic and audiologic deficits in Hib meningitis
   ii. For *S. pneumoniae* meningitis, dexamethasone use is controversial, but recent data show no reduction in mortality
   iii. Corticosteroids, if used, must be given before or concurrently with 1st dose of antibiotics

H. Complications
1. Sensorineural hearing loss
2. Acute hydrocephalus
3. Vascular infarcts
4. Hemiparesis

I. Duration: in children with uncomplicated courses, duration of antibiotic therapy depends on causative organism
1. *S. pneumoniae* = 10–14 days
2. *N. meningitidis* = 5–7 days
3. Hib = 10 days
4. Gram-negative organisms = 21 days or longer
5. GBS or *Listeria* = 14 days or longer

J. Prognosis
1. Overall mortality rate in children = 5%–10%
2. Sensorineural hearing loss is important morbidity (seen in 20%–30% of patients with *S. pneumoniae* meningitis)

IV. Encephalitis

A. Definition
1. Inflammation of brain parenchyma caused by current or recent infections
2. Associated terms
   a. **Myelitis**: inflammation of spinal cord
   b. **Radiculitis**: inflammation of spinal roots
   c. **Meningoencephalitis** (or **encephalomyelitis**): inflammation at combination of locations
3. Acute process typically including **fever** and neurologic symptoms
4. Postinfectious encephalitis (i.e., **ADEM**) reflects an autoimmune response to previous viral infection
5. Encephalitis must be differentiated from **encephalopathy**, which has similar clinical symptoms but is not associated with inflammation
   a. Encephalopathy is typically not associated with fever
   b. Encephalopathy is caused by metabolic disorders, drugs, and toxins

B. Epidemiology
1. Viral encephalitis causes 19,000 hospital admissions and 1,400 deaths per year
2. Occurs primarily in children, older adults, and those exposed to arthropod vectors
3. Certain causes have seasonal increases due to increased exposure to mosquito or tick vectors

C. Cause
1. Viruses known to cause encephalitis
   a. Common: HSV, enteroviruses, arboviruses (e.g., West Nile virus)
   b. Less common: EBV, rabies, HIV, Japanese encephalitis
2. Bacteria known to cause encephalitis: *Bartonella henselae, Borrelia burgdorferi, Mycoplasma pneumoniae, Rickettsia rickettsii*
3. Encephalitis should be considered in a child who has fever, altered mental status, lethargy, or seizure

D. Risk factors
1. Exposure to infectious secretions via delivery → neonatal HSV encephalitis
2. Exposure to vectors (e.g., **mosquitoes**, **ticks**) → **arboviral** or **rickettsial** encephalitis
3. Exposure to **bats** or rabid animals → **rabies** encephalitis
4. Exposure to cats or **kittens** → ***B. henselae*** encephalitis

> **QUICK HIT**
> CSF WBC count is normal in encephalopathy but elevated in encephalitis.

> **QUICK HIT**
> HSV is leading cause of severe encephalitis in all age groups.

> **QUICK HIT**
> Animals at high risk of rabies include bats, skunks, foxes, and raccoons.

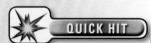

Infectious Diseases

E. Pathophysiology
 1. Mechanisms vary by tropism of virus or bacteria
  a. Virus can enter brain via hematogenous route, resulting in diffuse encephalitis (e.g., neonatal HSV)
  b. Virus and certain bacteria can enter via neuronal tracts causing focal encephalitis
  c. HSV outside newborn period can travel to frontal or temporal lobes from trigeminal ganglion via retrograde spread
 2. Viral invasion of brain parenchyma is thought to cause damage via cellular dysfunction, cytolysis, and inflammation
 3. Exaggerated autoimmune inflammatory response to viral or bacterial pathogen is thought to be responsible for ADEM

F. Clinical features
 1. Historical findings can range from subtle to severe
  a. Typically presents with some combination of fever, headache, nausea, vomiting, irritability, and personality changes
  b. Symptoms may progress to ataxia, hemiparesis, seizures, altered level of consciousness, coma
  c. Neonates and infants
   i. Fever, irritability, poor feeding, lethargy, and seizures
   ii. Neonates with HSV encephalitis may present with nonspecific findings such as irritability without fever
 2. Exam findings
  a. Neurologic exam can range from altered mental status to focal neurologic findings, including abnormalities of cranial nerves, strength, cerebellar function, and/or reflexes
  b. Decreased level of consciousness can be severe and include impaired respiratory drive and cardiorespiratory failure

> **QUICK HIT**
> In older children and adolescents, encephalitis can present initially with emotional lability.

> **QUICK HIT**
> Any patient with fever, focal neurologic findings, or seizures should raise suspicion for HSV encephalitis.

G. Diagnosis
 1. Signs of neurologic irritation: depressed level of consciousness, seizures, focal neurologic findings
 2. Signs of inflammation: fever, CSF pleocytosis, consistent neuroimaging or electroencephalogram (EEG)
 3. Differential diagnosis: patients with altered mental status require initial broad differential
 4. Laboratory
  a. CBC, blood culture, serum electrolytes
  b. CSF analysis for Gram stain, bacterial culture, glucose, protein, antibody/PCR studies for HSV, enterovirus, and arbovirus
  c. CSF findings vary with etiology
   i. CSF pleocytosis occurs in 60%; typically <200 cells/mm^3
   ii. CSF usually has lymphocyte predominance
   iii. Can have neutrophilic predominance in 1st 24–48 hours
   iv. Red blood cells (RBCs) in CSF ("a bloody tap")
    (a) Can occur from trauma during LP, intracranial hemorrhage, or hemorrhagic encephalitis from HSV
    (b) RBCs that decrease with each successive tube of CSF collected suggest traumatic LP
  d. Culture/antigen studies/PCR of NP specimens for respiratory viruses
  e. Consider other specific blood/CSF studies for other pathogens and diagnoses based on history, exam findings, and epidemiologic risk factors
 5. Radiology
  a. Brain MRI may reveal cerebral edema or inflammation of cerebral cortex, gray–white matter junction, or basal ganglia
  b. MRI may suggest specific causes: temporal lobe localization (HSV), white matter demyelination (ADEM), intracranial calcifications (CMV, toxoplasmosis)
 6. EEG helps distinguish encephalitis from subclinical status epilepticus

H. Management/therapy
  1. Some cases require aggressive supportive care
    a. Airway protection
    b. ICP monitoring
    c. Control of seizures
  2. Empiric antibiotics and antivirals are usually required while awaiting lab results
    a. Acyclovir should be used to empirically treat for HSV
    b. 3rd-generation cephalosporin ($\pm$ vancomycin) should be used to empirically treat for bacterial meningitis (see Bacterial Meningitis)
    c. Doxycycline if rickettsial infection is a consideration
I. Complications
  1. Status epilepticus
  2. Cerebral edema
  3. Syndrome of inappropriate antidiuretic hormone (SIADH) secretion
  4. Respiratory failure
  5. Disseminated intravascular coagulation (DIC)
J. Duration/prognosis
  1. Both depend on underlying cause
  2. Many cases resolve with few permanent sequelae over days to weeks
  3. Overall mortality from encephalitis is 3%–4%; overall morbidity is 7%–10%
  4. HSV encephalitis has higher risk of long-term complications
    a. Treated HSV encephalitis in neonates is associated with ~14% fatality rate; >50% of survivors have major neurologic sequelae
    b. Older children with treated HSV encephalitis have 28% mortality rate
K. Prevention
  1. Most causes are not preventable
  2. Vector-borne illness may be prevented by actions to decrease exposure to mosquitoes and ticks
  3. Risk of Japanese encephalitis can be decreased through vaccination

V. Preseptal Cellulitis

A. General characteristics
  1. Infection of anterior portion of eyelid sparing components of orbit such as ocular muscles (infection restricted to tissue anterior to orbital septum)
  2. Breakdown of skin or local trauma provides portal for bacterial entry
  3. Important to distinguish *preseptal cellulitis* from *orbital cellulitis* because orbital cellulitis is sight threatening if not treated promptly (Table 10-4)
B. Clinical features and diagnosis
  1. Eyelid erythema, edema, warmth, and tenderness
  2. Fever may be present

TABLE 10-4 Differences between Preseptal and Orbital Cellulitis

	Preseptal Cellulitis	Orbital Cellulitis
Pain with extraocular muscle movements	No	Yes
Proptosis	No	Yes
Chemosis	Generally no	Yes
Diplopia	No	Possible
Ophthalmoplegia	No	Possible
Eyelid swelling and erythema	Yes	Yes
Normal pupil reactivity	Yes	Possibly no

Infectious Diseases

3. Diagnosis is made clinically by history and physical
   a. If concern for orbital cellulitis, obtain CT scan of orbits and sinuses
   b. Blood culture rarely positive
4. Differential diagnosis includes orbital cellulitis, allergic reaction, insect bite, conjunctivitis, chalazia, and hordeolum

C. Treatment
1. Can be treated as an outpatient with oral antibiotics and close follow-up
2. Organism is rarely identified; most often, antibiotics are chosen empirically
3. Common organisms include skin flora (*Staphylococcus aureus, Streptococcus pyogenes*)
4. Community-acquired methicillin-resistant *Staphylococcus aureus* (CA-MRSA) is increasingly common; coverage for CA-MRSA should be included in empiric antibiotic regimen (e.g., clindamycin, trimethoprim-sulfamethoxazole plus amoxicillin)
5. Patients without improvement within 48 hours of antibiotic initiation should be admitted for intravenous (IV) antibiotics; also consider orbit CT to diagnose orbital cellulitis as well as otolaryngology or ophthalmology consultation
6. Complications and treatment failure are rare

> **QUICK HIT**
>
> Sinusitis can cause periorbital swelling by compression of superior or inferior ophthalmic veins. This can be distinguished from periorbital cellulitis by lack of tenderness of swollen areas.

VI. Orbital Cellulitis

A. Characteristics
1. Bacterial infection of orbit, posterior to orbital septum
2. Usually occurs as complication of acute or chronic sinusitis
3. Can present in all age groups but seen more often in young children
   a. Typically unilateral
   b. More common in winter due to higher incidence of sinusitis
4. Pathophysiology
   a. Anatomic characteristics of orbital structures allow extension of external ocular infections into deeper tissues
      i. Infection can spread from paranasal sinuses surrounding orbital cavity
      ii. Thin orbital septum divides soft tissues of eyelid (preseptal space) from soft tissues of orbit (postseptal space) and may be incomplete, allowing spread of infection
      iii. Orbital veins allow for hematogenous spread of infections
   b. Bacterial etiology (*Staphylococcus aureus, Streptococcus pyogenes,* anaerobes, *Streptococcus milleri* group bacteria)

> **QUICK HIT**
>
> Ethmoid sinus is separated from orbit by a thin lamina, a characteristic that makes ethmoid sinusitis most common cause of orbital cellulitis in all age groups.

B. Clinical features
1. Historical findings
   a. Both periorbital (preseptal) and orbital infections may be associated with fever, eye pain, swollen eyelids, and red eye
   b. Recent URI, trauma to eye, or sinus infection
   c. History of dental disease, previous eye surgery
2. Physical exam findings
   a. Fever, toxic appearance with eyelid edema, erythema
   b. Signs of increased orbital pressure including decreased eye movement, proptosis, decreased vision and papilledema, or other signs of optic nerve involvement

C. Diagnosis
1. Differential diagnosis
   a. Periorbital cellulitis
   b. Other causes of eyelid swelling such as allergic reactions, severe conjunctivitis, and edema due to hypoproteinemia must be considered
   c. Proptosis can be caused by inflammation or noninfectious masses (e.g., histiocytosis, leukemia, rhabdomyosarcoma)
2. Laboratory findings
   a. White blood cell (WBC) count, C-reactive protein (CRP), and erythrocyte sedimentation rate (ESR) elevated; none of these tests are routinely necessary
   b. Blood cultures may be reserved for ill-appearing patients
   c. Orbital, epidural abscess, and sinus fluid cultures obtained surgically are often positive

> **QUICK HIT**
>
> Pain with eye movement distinguishes orbital from periorbital cellulitis.

3. Radiology findings help guide management
   a. CT with contrast is preferred study for diagnosing orbital cellulitis
   b. MRI should be performed if there is concern for intracranial involvement or when clinical picture does not match CT findings
   c. Consider repeat CT if symptoms worsen or fail to improve after 48–72 hours of medical therapy

D. Treatment
1. Patients should be admitted for inpatient care by interdisciplinary team consisting of pediatrician or pediatric hospitalist and pediatric subspecialists (i.e., ophthalmologist, otorhinolaryngologist)
2. Medical management with empiric IV antibiotics
3. Coverage against staphylococcal and streptococcal species, including MRSA plus coverage for organisms typically associated with rhinosinusitis (ampicillin-sulbactam or clindamycin)
4. Antibiotic therapy for total of 10–14 days with switch to oral antibiotics once significantly clinically improved
5. Close observation for clinical improvement including careful daily eye exam
6. Surgical drainage of abscess to relieve increased pressure on orbit and to obtain cultures in the following situations:
   a. Complete ophthalmoplegia, significant visual impairment, or afferent pupillary defect
   b. Large subperiosteal abscess, well-defined orbital abscess, or large abscess with mass effect
   c. Poor response to initial medical management

E. Complications
1. Intracranial extension causing subdural empyema, intracranial abscess, or bacterial meningitis
2. Cavernous sinus thrombosis
3. Septic emboli of optic nerve may cause loss of vision
4. Prognosis is good with early and appropriate medical and surgical therapy

VII. Cervical Lymphadenitis

A. General characteristics
1. Enlargement and inflammation of neck lymph nodes
2. Distinguish lymphadenitis (inflammation; often bacterial) from lymphadenopathy (enlargement; rarely bacterial)
3. Common in childhood and peaks at ages 1–4 years
4. Usually caused by infections (Box 10-2)
5. Pathophysiology: microorganisms infiltrate mucosa in head and neck, follow lymphatic drainage, and eventually infect lymph node

B. Clinical features
1. Historical findings (symptoms)
   a. Duration of adenopathy: acute versus chronic
   b. Location of enlarged lymph node(s)
   c. Rate of enlargement
   d. Sick contacts with symptoms of respiratory infection (viral infections, mononucleosis, streptococcal pharyngitis, TB)
   e. Oral pain or lesions (HSV gingivostomatitis, herpangina, dental caries)
   f. Painful versus painless: malignant nodes tend to be firm and nontender
   g. Systemic symptoms, such as fever, weight loss, and fatigue
   h. Animal exposures (cat-scratch, tularemia, toxoplasmosis)
   i. Medications (phenytoin, isoniazid)
   j. Travel (higher risk of TB)
2. Physical exam findings (signs)
   a. Assess for signs of malignancy (i.e., other enlarged lymph nodes, hepatosplenomegaly)
   b. Identify potential causes of enlarged lymph nodes (e.g., pharyngitis, impetigo, dental caries or abscesses)

QUICK HIT

Enlarged lymph nodes due to malignancy tend to be located in posterior neck or supraclavicular region.

QUICK HIT

Kittens rather than older cats are most likely to transmit cat-scratch disease.

BOX 10-2

Causes of Lymphadenitis

Acute bilateral cervical lymphadenitis
- Rhinovirus
- Influenza
- Epstein-Barr virus (EBV)
- Cytomegalovirus (CMV)
- Enterovirus
- Adenovirus
- Parainfluenza
- Streptococcal pharyngitis

Acute unilateral cervical lymphadenitis
- *Staphylococcus aureus*
- Group A *Streptococcus* (GAS)
- Anaerobic bacteria
- Tularemia

Chronic lymphadenitis
- EBV
- CMV
- HIV
- Tuberculosis
- Nontuberculous mycobacterium
- Cat-scratch disease (*Bartonella*)
- Toxoplasmosis

Noninfectious causes of cervical lymphadenitis
- Kawasaki disease
- Leukemia
- Lymphoma
- Neuroblastoma
- Connective tissue disorders
- Juvenile idiopathic arthritis
- Medications
- Periodic fever, aphthous stomatitis, pharyngitis, and cervical adenitis (PFAPA)

c. Conjunctivitis as seen with adenovirus, Kawasaki disease, and Parinaud oculoglandular syndrome (caused by *B. henselae*)

C. Diagnosis
1. Acute bacterial infection of single cervical lymph node can be diagnosed clinically; if no response to antibiotics in 48–72 hours, consider needle aspiration
2. For chronic cervical lymphadenitis, laboratory evaluation is recommended
   a. CBC with differential, blood culture, ESR, CRP, complete metabolic panel serologies for **EBV**, CMV, *B. henselae*, and HIV
   b. Also consider tuberculin skin testing (TST) (i.e., purified protein derivative [PPD])
3. Surgical consult for excisional biopsy should be considered for persistent lymphadenopathy or with suspicion for malignancy or mycobacterial infection
4. Differential diagnosis: other structures in neck, such as brachial cleft cyst, cystic hygroma, or thyroid nodule may mimic enlarged lymph node

D. Treatment
1. For most viral URIs, only supportive care is needed
2. For unilateral lymphadenitis with signs and symptoms of bacterial infection, 10-day course of antibiotics (e.g., clindamycin) with coverage for group A β-hemolytic *Streptococcus* (GABHS) and CA-MRSA should be prescribed
3. Parental antibiotics are indicated for severe bacterial adenitis or if patient fails outpatient treatment
4. For fluctuant lymph nodes, incision and drainage are necessary
5. Cat-scratch disease will resolve without antibiotics over 6 weeks; azithromycin will reduce lymph node size initially but does not alter time to complete resolution
6. Excisional biopsy is curative in most cases of atypical mycobacterial infection

E. Complications
1. Fistula can develop with atypical mycobacterial infection
2. Bacteremia or disseminated infection
3. Acute glomerulonephritis (GABHS)

F. Prognosis is excellent, with symptoms usually resolving over 1–2 weeks

G. Prevention: infection control

QUICK HIT

Cystic hygromas transilluminate.

QUICK HIT

Trimethoprim-sulfamethoxazole provides good coverage against *S. aureus* (including MRSA) but poor coverage against group A streptococcus (GAS).

VIII. Infective Endocarditis (IE)

A. General characteristics
1. Infection of endocardium, valves, and related structures
2. Bacterial IE is most common
3. Most cases of noninfectious endocarditis are immune mediated
   a. Libman-Sacks endocarditis is typically associated with SLE
   b. Rheumatic fever
4. Children often have preexisting condition such as an indwelling catheter or congenital heart disease
5. Formerly, most common risk factor was rheumatic heart disease
   a. With decreasing prevalence, incidence of IE has also decreased
   b. Recent increase in cases of IE due to increase in survival and life expectancy of children with congenital heart disease

B. Pathophysiology
1. Turbulent blood flow leads to endocardial surface injury
2. Thrombus develops at injury site
3. During transient bacteremia, thrombus becomes infected
4. Subsequent local tissue damage, embolic phenomena, and secondary autoimmune sequelae

C. Clinical features
1. Historical findings
   a. In subacute infection, symptoms include prolonged low-grade fever, weight loss, fatigue, myalgias, nausea, vomiting, and abdominal pain
   b. In acute infection, child may be ill-appearing with high fever or sepsis
2. Physical exam findings (signs)
   a. New or changing heart murmur
   b. **Janeway lesions**: nontender, small nodules or macules on palms/soles
   c. **Roth spots**: retinal hemorrhages with pale center that are caused by immune complex–mediated vasculitis
   d. **Osler nodes**: tender, erythematous nodules on hands and feet
   e. Splinter hemorrhages: tiny lines located under nail
   f. Signs of embolic phenomena: cerebral infarction or hemorrhage, pulmonary embolism, and renal infarction
   g. Splenomegaly
   h. Petechiae

D. Diagnosis
1. Duke criteria (Box 10-3)
   a. Definite diagnosis requires 2 major criteria or 5 minor criteria or 1 major criterion and 3 minor criteria

BOX 10-3

Duke Criteria

Major criteria
- Persistently positive blood cultures with an organism associated with endocarditis ("persistently positive" is defined as 2 blood cultures collected 12 hours apart or 3 different positive blood cultures)
- Echocardiogram findings of dehiscence of prosthetic valve, abscess, or vegetations
- New valvular regurgitation

Minor criteria
- Predisposing heart condition
- Fever
- Positive blood culture that does not meet major criteria
- Echocardiogram that is consistent with endocarditis but does not meet major criteria
- Immunologic response: glomerulonephritis, Osler nodes, Roth spots, rheumatoid factor
- Vascular phenomena: arterial emboli, pulmonary infarcts, aneurysm, intracranial hemorrhage, conjunctival hemorrhage, Janeway lesions

   b. Possible diagnosis requires 3 minor criteria or 1 major criterion and 1 minor criterion
2. Laboratory data
   a. Patients with endocarditis have persistent bacteremia; 3–5 blood cultures should be collected in a 24-hour period
   b. ESR and CRP are elevated
   c. Rheumatoid factor is positive in 25%–50% of cases
   d. Low complement, hematuria, and proteinuria suggest immune complex glomerulonephritis, which occurs with bacterial endocarditis
   e. Anemia of chronic disease is often present
3. Echocardiography (echo)
   a. Identifies vegetations, valvular regurgitation, and pericardial effusion; ventricular function can also be assessed
   b. Transesophageal echo has higher sensitivity and should be considered for those who have suboptimal images on transthoracic echo
   c. Any patient with bacteremia caused by HACEK bacteria (Box 10-4) should undergo evaluation for endocarditis

E. Treatment
1. Most cases are infections with gram-positive cocci (see Box 10-4)
2. Vancomycin for empiric therapy; because most cases have positive blood cultures, treatment can be tailored to specific organism
3. Bactericidal antibiotic should be used
4. Several blood cultures should be obtained prior to initiating treatment
5. 4–6-week course of IV antibiotics is required
6. Blood cultures are monitored to document response to treatment
7. Surgical intervention is reserved for cases complicated by fungal endocarditis, congestive heart failure (CHF), and need for valve replacement

F. Complications
1. CHF: caused by worsening valvular regurgitation
2. Stroke
3. Aneurysms
4. Metastatic abscesses can develop in spleen, kidney, and brain
5. Vertebral osteomyelitis associated with *S. aureus* IE

G. Prognosis depends on severity of underlying heart disease and duration of infection
1. Prior to antibiotics, mortality was >90%
2. Now, IE has 20% mortality rate

H. Prevention
1. High-risk patients (e.g., artificial heart valves, unrepaired cyanotic congenital heart disease) should receive antibiotic prophylaxis during dental procedures
2. Single dose of amoxicillin recommended; cephalexin and clindamycin are alternatives for penicillin-allergic patients
3. Good oral hygiene is important part of prevention for high-risk patients

QUICK HIT

Q fever caused by *Coxiella burnetii* is an important cause of culture-negative endocarditis. Cattle, sheep, and goats are main sources.

BOX 10-4

Organisms That Cause Pediatric Infective Endocarditis

Gram-positive
- *Staphylococcus aureus*
- Viridans streptococci
- Coagulase-negative staphylococci
- Other streptococcal species
- *Enterococcus*
- Pneumococcus

Gram-negative (HACEK)
- ***H****aemophilus parainfluenzae*
- ***A****ggregatibacter*
- ***C****ardiobacterium hominis*
- ***E****ikenella corrodens*
- ***K****ingella kingae*

IX. Acute Rheumatic Fever (ARF)

A. General characteristics
1. Complication of pharyngitis by GABHS
2. Symptoms begin several weeks after episode of acute pharyngitis
3. Typically affects school-aged children (ages 5–18 years)
4. Virtually eradicated in U.S. and Western Europe due to widespread screening and treatment of GABHS pharyngitis

B. Clinical features
1. Major criteria (also known as **Jones criteria**)
   a. **Carditis**: main cause of long-term morbidity; occurs in 80% of ARF
      i. Pancarditis can lead to valvular insufficiency and stenosis
      ii. Mitral and aortic valves are most commonly affected
   b. **Polyarthritis**: migratory and affecting large joint (knees, ankles, elbows)
      i. Joints are exquisitely tender, erythematous, and swollen
      ii. Symptoms respond well to anti-inflammatory medications
   c. **Erythema marginatum**: annular rash with clear center
   d. Subcutaneous nodules: painless, pea-sized nodules found on extensor surfaces; rare (<2%)
   e. **Sydenham chorea**: sole symptom to occur months after episode of pharyngitis
2. Minor criteria: fever, arthralgia, elevated acute-phase reactants, prolonged PR or atrioventricular (AV) block on electrocardiogram (ECG)

C. Diagnosis
1. Confirmation of prior GABHS infection AND either 2 major or 1 major and 2 minor criteria; exception is Sydenham chorea, a late finding, often occurs in isolation
2. Differential diagnosis: poststreptococcal reactive arthritis, IE, juvenile rheumatoid arthritis, Lyme disease
3. Laboratory findings: rapid-antigen test, throat culture, antistreptolysin O (ASO), ESR, CRP
4. Other findings: ECG may show pericarditis or arrhythmia

D. Treatment
1. Therapy: course of treatment for acute GABHS infection
2. Followed by prophylaxis to prevent future GABHS infection with benzathine penicillin B every 4 weeks until age 18 years

E. Complications: rheumatic heart disease, most commonly mitral stenosis

QUICK HIT

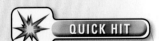

ARF is one of most common causes of acquired heart disease in children in developing nations.

MNEMONIC

Jones Criteria
Joints: migratory arthritis
♥: carditis
Nodules (subcutaneous)
Erythema marginatum
Sydenham chorea

X. Croup

A. General characteristics
1. Upper airway illness characterized by inflammation of larynx and trachea, especially subglottic area where trachea is "fixed" by firm cartilaginous ring
2. Also known as **laryngotracheitis**
3. Usually of viral etiology
   a. Common: parainfluenza, influenza
   b. Less common: RSV, human coronaviruses, enteroviruses, adenovirus
4. Most common in children ages 6 months to 3 years
5. Peak incidence in fall and winter
6. Risks for development of croup
   a. Family history
   b. Anatomic or acquired airway narrowing (e.g., history of intubation)

B. Clinical features
1. Symptoms: gradual onset of rhinorrhea, congestion, fever, hoarseness, barky cough, and, eventually, stridor
2. Signs on physical exam
   a. Mild disease: rhinorrhea, congestion, coryza, fever, hoarseness, barky cough, stridor with agitation
   b. More severe disease: tachypnea, stridor at rest, hypoxemia, respiratory distress with nasal flaring, grunting, and retractions

QUICK HIT

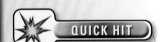

Stridor (inspiratory) indicates upper airway obstruction, whereas wheezing (expiratory) is more indicative of lower airway obstruction.

QUICK HIT

Improvement of symptoms of croup may follow change in temperature or humidity, such as going out in cool night air or being exposed to steam in a bathroom or a humidifier.

QUICK HIT

Stridor typically worsens with agitation and improves with calming. Stridor at rest is a key element in defining severity of disease.

BOX 10-5

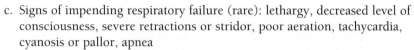

Differential Diagnosis of Stridor

- Epiglottitis
- Bacterial tracheitis
- Retropharyngeal or peritonsillar abscess
- Foreign body (ingested or aspirated)
- Allergic reaction/angioedema
- Upper airway anomaly or injury
- Diphtheria

c. Signs of impending respiratory failure (rare): lethargy, decreased level of consciousness, severe retractions or stridor, poor aeration, tachycardia, cyanosis or pallor, apnea

d. Always assess hydration status: tears, moist mucous membranes

C. Diagnosis

1. Clinical diagnosis most often appropriate

a. Differential diagnosis (Box 10-5): consider other diseases that present with upper airway obstruction and/or require specific therapies

2. Laboratory findings

a. Laboratory testing rarely indicated unless severe illness or need to evaluate for other etiologies

b. CBC may reveal elevated WBC count

c. Microbiologic testing not necessary but viruses likely detected on PCR of nasopharyngeal aspirate

3. Radiology findings

a. CXR not routinely required; obtain if recurrent or protracted course

b. Classic x-ray finding: "steeple sign" with subglottic narrowing (Figure 10-1)

D. Treatment

1. Mild croup

a. Supportive care: oral hydration, antipyretics

b. Dexamethasone: single oral dose of 0.6 mg/kg (max = 10 mg) prevents symptoms from worsening

2. Moderate/severe croup

a. Supportive care: humidified air (oxygen if hypoxemic)

b. IV fluids if not maintaining sufficient hydration orally (PO)

c. Dexamethasone as above: PO, IV, or intramuscular (IM)

d. Racemic epinephrine via nebulizer: requires observation for 3–4 hours after because some children relapse after drug wears off

E. Indications for hospitalization

1. Hypoxemia
2. Stridor at rest
3. Inability to maintain hydration PO
4. Barriers to return for care if worsening at home

F. Typical clinical course: 1–2 days of upper respiratory symptoms followed by worsening stridor and respiratory distress with gradual resolution over 3–5 days

G. Complications: secondary bacterial infection, hypoxemia; rarely respiratory failure, pulmonary edema, pneumothorax

H. Prevention: handwashing, limiting exposure to ill contacts

QUICK HIT

A "barky, seal-like cough" is a classic finding in mild croup; stridor is a classic finding in more severe cases requiring intervention.

QUICK HIT

A good "quick fix" for stridor at home is sitting with child in a steamy bathroom. Cold night air and cool humidifiers may also help. If stridor persists at rest, patients should be evaluated by a physician.

XI. Bronchiolitis

A. General characteristics

1. Primarily lower airway viral infection, most common in children age <2 years with peak incidence in winter months
2. Affects 20% of all infants; 2% require hospitalization (most common cause of hospitalization of U.S. children)
3. Rarely fatal; most commonly so in infants with underlying chronic conditions
4. Risk factors for increased severity

a. History of prematurity or underlying cardiac disease

b. Age <6 months during fall, winter, and early spring months

c. Daycare attendance or school-aged siblings

FIGURE 10-1 **Frontal radiograph of the neck shows a "steeple sign" (*arrows*) of the subglottic region.**

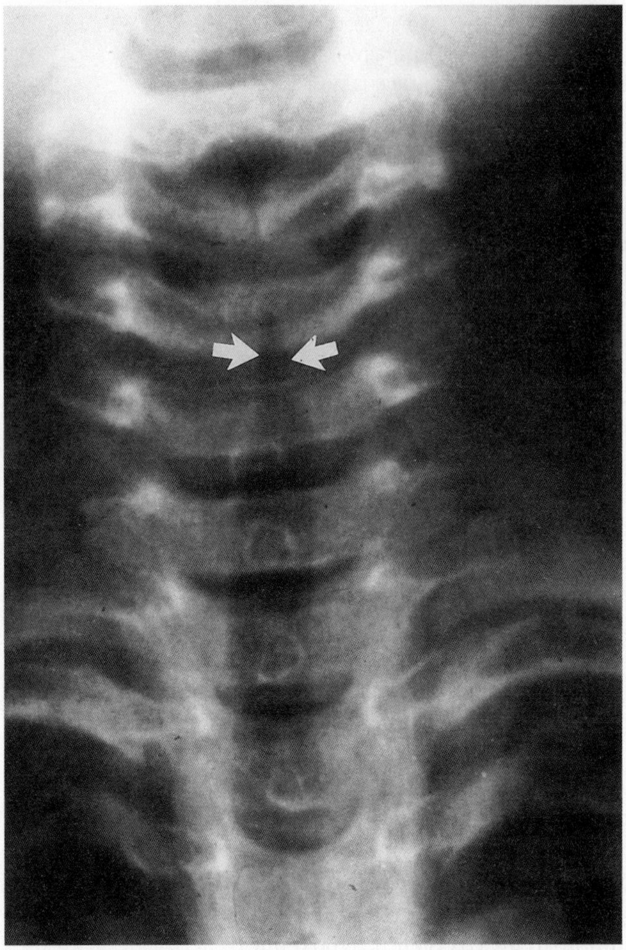

(From Daffner R. *Clinical Radiology: The Essentials*. 3rd ed. Philadelphia: Lippincott Williams & Wilkins; 2007.)

QUICK HIT

It is common for infants with bronchiolitis younger than age 2 months to present with apnea in absence of other symptoms.

QUICK HIT

During exam, listen with stethoscope at level of mouth and nose to distinguish between chest sounds and transmitted upper airway sounds. Sounds can radiate a long distance in a small child!

d. Lack of breastfeeding during early infancy
e. Smoking at home

5. Pathophysiology
   a. Predominantly viral (Box 10-6)
   b. Virus may infect upper airways and may cause purulent rhinorrhea
   c. Lower in airway, viral invasion results in inflammation and mucus that can obstruct infant's very small airway

B. Clinical features
   1. Historical findings (Box 10-7): questions should mostly focus on illness severity and duration
   2. Physical exam findings (Box 10-8)
      a. Normal vital signs vary based on patient age (see Appendix)
      b. Most critical signs for respiratory distress are mental status and severity of retractions on exam, which help distinguish "sick" versus "not sick"

BOX 10-6

Common Causes of Bronchiolitis

- Respiratory syncytial virus (RSV); most common
- Influenza virus (types A and B)
- Coronavirus
- Human metapneumovirus
- Rhinovirus
- Parainfluenza virus (types 1, 2, and 3)
- Adenovirus

BOX 10-7

Key Questions for History in Infants with Bronchiolitis

History of present illness

1. Description of upper and lower respiratory symptoms?
2. Presence of altered mental status, fever, cyanosis, apnea, fever, or vomiting or diarrhea?
3. Hydration status?
   a. How many ounces per feed? How often?
   b. If breastfed, does mom feel like the baby is eating well?
   c. Number of wet diapers in the last 24 hours?
4. Number of days of illness?

Past medical history

1. History of prematurity or underlying medical condition?
2. History of cigarette smoke exposure?
3. Diet history (breastfeeding versus formula fed)?

C. Diagnosis
   1. Differential diagnosis
      a. Children age >1 year may have asthma exacerbation triggered by viral illness; distinguishing these patients is difficult, and optimal management is controversial
      b. Pneumonia can be challenging to distinguish from bronchiolitis

QUICK HIT

Premature babies often have a "floppy" upper airway (tracheomalacia or laryngomalacia), which can contribute to increased illness severity and a prolonged disease course.

BOX 10-8

Key Physical Exam Findings in Infants with Bronchiolitis

Signs of dehydration

- Dry mucous membranes
- Decreased capillary refill (in very young infants, peripheral capillary refill may be delayed because of cold extremities; check capillary refill on the forehead or chest)
- Increased heart rate (inhaled therapies such as albuterol and racemic epinephrine also increase heart rate)
- Sunken fontanelle (moderate to severe dehydration)
- Decreased blood pressure (severe dehydration)
- Skin tenting (very rare, shows very severe dehydration)

Signs of respiratory distress

- Upper respiratory: cough, rhinorrhea, congestion (common; if not present, consider an alternative diagnosis)
- Retractions: suprasternal, intercostal, subcostal (indicates increased accessory muscle use and/or decreased lung compliance)
- Head bobbing and paradoxical breathing (belly distends while chest collapses on inhalation—more common in younger infants)
- Nasal flaring (indicates increased airway resistance)
- Grunting (body's method of creating positive end-expiratory pressure [PEEP] to reduce atelectasis)
- Wheezing (indicates lower airway obstruction; does not necessarily mean the child will respond to albuterol or has asthma)
- Rales (also known as crackles; high-pitched sound indicating alveolar involvement)
- Rhonchi (lower pitched sound indicating larger airway obstruction [nares, trachea, bronchi])
- Tachypnea
- Apnea (especially in young infants)
- Oxygen desaturation or cyanosis (<90% is typically considered "significant")
- Altered mental status, excessive drowsiness, or generally not interactive (may herald impending respiratory failure, especially in an infant with decreased or minimally increased respiratory effort)

Other

- Nonspecific viral exanthem or history of diarrhea indicating likely viral cause may limit need for testing

QUICK HIT

Bronchiolitis is generally a clinical diagnosis—labs and x-rays are not routinely required for diagnosis.

2. Laboratory findings: no testing routinely required
   a. Viral testing ("rapid viral panel")
   b. Blood culture
      i. Performed in infants age <2 months with fever; bacteremia is present in ~1%
      ii. Performed in children age >2 months with severe illness
   c. Urinalysis and urine culture should be performed in febrile infants age <2 months; UTI affects 2% of infants age >2 months with bronchiolitis
   d. LP not routinely required for infants age >1 month
   e. Also see page 257 for evaluation of febrile neonate
3. Radiology findings
   a. Chest radiography is not routinely required
      i. Peribronchial thickening (or "cuffing")
      ii. Hyperinflation
      iii. Atelectasis
      iv. Patchy, scattered infiltrates
      v. Pneumothorax (rare)
      vi. Atelectasis and infiltrate are difficult to distinguish
      vii. May lead to increased use of antibiotics, which do not help disease and may harm patient
      viii. Indicated in severely ill infants and those not following typical disease progression
4. Supplemental oxygen
   a. Assessment of oxygen saturation indicated in all patients
   b. Common transient desaturation not an indicator for oxygen therapy
   c. Patients admitted without oxygen requirement should have intermittent pulse oximetry with routine vitals rather than continuously, because transient dips are common in normal infants age <4 months

QUICK HIT

Hypoxia may be completely independent from respiratory distress, and an infant with a normal oxygen saturation may have impending respiratory failure. CO_2 and airway atelectasis are prime determinants of respiratory effort (i.e., work of breathing).

D. Treatment
1. Indications for hospitalization: poor hydration, increased respiratory distress, and impending respiratory failure
2. Primarily through respiratory support
   a. In child who persistently desaturates, continuous pulse oximetry and oxygen therapy are indicated to keep pulse oximeter value >90%
   b. For increased **work of breathing**, infants are often suctioned
      i. Suctioning should primarily be with saline and bulb
      ii. If severe, patients may require NP aspiration with wall suction
         (a) Relieves obstruction
         (b) Crying provides some **positive end-expiratory pressure (PEEP)**, which may relieve atelectasis
   c. If severely ill, infants may require continuous positive airway pressure (CPAP) to wash out carbon dioxide (CO_2) in airway dead space
      i. High-flow nasal cannula at rates >4 L/min may provide minimal positive pressure (less than CPAP) and also washes out CO_2 in airway dead space
      ii. Endotracheal intubation may be required

QUICK HIT

Grunting is body's method of creating PEEP to reduce atelectasis.

3. Most medicines found to be of limited or no benefit
   a. Steroids: not indicated in infants
      i. Do not benefit even subset of infants who respond to albuterol
      ii. Do not benefit infants with family history of asthma or eczema
   b. Albuterol (β-agonist causing bronchodilation)
      i. May lead to mild symptomatic improvement but does not affect course of illness in most patients
      ii. Trial may be warranted but discontinued if infant does not respond (most children do not)

c. Racemic epinephrine (combined α- and β-agonist)
   i. α-Agonist effect causes vasoconstriction, reducing airway edema and mucus production
   ii. May lead to mild symptomatic improvement but does not affect course of illness in most patients
   iii. Trial may be warranted; discontinue if infant does not respond
d. Hypertonic saline (nebulized)
   i. Reduces viscosity of mucus by osmotic pressure, allowing improved airway clearance
   ii. Several small studies have shown improvement of symptoms and reduced length of stay
   iii. No clear regimen established and variability of use among pediatric medical centers
e. Others: helium–oxygen inhaled mixture (heliox), ribavirin, and other expensive therapies may be of variable benefit and should be reserved for patients with severe illness in intensive care unit (ICU)

4. Close assessment of hydration status warranted in all patients
   a. Often have decreased oral intake; IV fluids may be warranted
   b. Dehydration common because of insensible losses through fever, vomiting, diarrhea, and tachypnea
   c. Inpatients should maintain adequate urine output (1 mL/kg/hr)
5. Duration
   a. Hospitalization typically lasts from 1 to 3 days but occasionally for weeks
   b. Symptoms peak on days 4 to 5; total duration of symptoms is 2 to 3 weeks
   c. Some may improve with respiratory function but be delayed in recovery of appetite, requiring longer hospital stays
6. Prevention
   a. Smoking cessation and handwashing lower risk of viral respiratory infections
   b. Selected infants may receive monthly doses of palivizumab (Synagis)
      i. Monoclonal antibody directed against RSV
      ii. Moderately effective (reduces likelihood of admission from ~8% to 4%) but extremely expensive
      iii. Indications for monthly administration during RSV season include infants younger than 2 years old who were born <32 weeks' gestation, cyanotic congenital heart disease, or severe pulmonary disease

XII. Pneumonia

A. Definition
   1. Inflammatory condition of lungs involving lung parenchyma
   2. Includes **fever, respiratory symptoms, and evidence of parenchymal lung involvement** on physical exam or chest radiography
   3. Community-acquired pneumonia (CAP) should be differentiated from hospital-acquired pneumonia because they are caused by different pathogens and require different empiric treatments
B. Epidemiology
   1. 3rd leading cause of death in children living in developing world
   2. In North America, annual incidence of pneumonia is 36–40 cases/1,000 population younger than age 5 years
C. Cause
   1. True prevalence of various causes of pneumonia is unknown because less invasive tests (e.g., blood cultures) are rarely positive and invasive tests (e.g., bronchoscopy) are not typically recommended or performed
   2. In 1st month of life, pneumonia is most often caused by GBS and gram-negative enteric bacilli
   3. In children younger than 5 years old, pneumonia is most often viral in etiology
      a. Common: RSV, influenza, parainfluenza, human metapneumovirus, adenovirus, human coronaviruses
      b. Rare: HSV, varicella-zoster virus, CMV, measles

4. Community-acquired bacterial pneumonia is seen in children of all ages
   a. Predominantly caused by ***Streptococcus pneumoniae***
   b. Other important bacterial pathogens
      i. ***Staphylococcus aureus***
      ii. *Moraxella catarrhalis*
      iii. Hib now rare cause of CAP due to introduction of conjugate vaccine in 1980s
   c. "**Atypical**" describes pneumonia that is not caused by typical bacterial pathogens mentioned above
      i. ***M. pneumoniae*** and ***Chlamydophila*** (formerly ***Chlamydia***) ***pneumoniae*** are 2 most common
      ii. Seen more often in school-aged children
      iii. Usually less severe clinical course than "typical" bacterial pathogens and often includes nonproductive cough, headache, pharyngitis
5. See Table 10-5 for pathogens that cause pneumonia

D. Genetics
1. No known genetic associations
2. Underlying cause of recurrent pneumonia includes genetic abnormalities such as **cystic fibrosis (CF)** and a number of **congenital immunodeficiencies**

E. Risk factors
1. Spread by droplet acquisition via respiratory passages
2. More common in lower socioeconomic classes and in winter due to crowding
3. Chronic diseases such as **congenital heart disease**, **CF**, **bronchopulmonary dysplasia**, **neuromuscular disease**, and **asthma** increase risk of severe disease

QUICK HIT

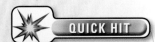

CA-MRSA has become an important pathogen in pediatric CAP. It often causes necrotizing pneumonia and empyema.

QUICK HIT

Because atypical pneumonia often has a mild to moderate clinical course not requiring hospital admission, it is sometimes referred to as "walking pneumonia."

Infectious Diseases

TABLE 10-5 Bacterial, Fungal, and Parasitic Pathogens Responsible for Pneumonia

Common Pathogens	Susceptible Host
Streptococcus pneumoniae	All ages outside of the immediate newborn period
Staphylococcus aureus	All
Streptococcus pyogenes	<5 years
Mycoplasma pneumoniae	>5 years
Chlamydia pneumoniae	>5 years
Chlamydia trachomatis	First 3 months of life
Group B *Streptococcus*	First 3 months of life
Gram-negative bacilli (e.g., *Escherichia coli*)	Newborns, immunocompromised hosts
Pseudomonas aeruginosa	Immunocompromised hosts, cystic fibrosis
Anaerobic organisms	Children at risk of aspiration
Uncommon Pathogens*	
Legionella pneumophila	Immunocompromised, inhalation of aerosol from infected water source
Coxiella burnetii	Exposure to farm animals (especially cattle, sheep, goats)
Chlamydia psittaci	Exposure to birds (especially parrots)
Mycobacterium tuberculosis	Travel to endemic areas, exposure to prison or homeless communities
Fungal infections: *Histoplasma capsulatum*, *Cryptococcus neoformans*	Immunocompromised, inhalation of soil contaminated with bird or bat guano
Pneumocystis jiroveci	HIV, severe immunodeficiency
Parasitic infections: *Toxoplasma gondii*, *Strongyloides stercoralis*	Exposure to undercooked meat, ingestion of contaminated feces (primarily cat) Exposure to endemic areas

*Some pathogens listed (e.g., *M. tuberculosis*) are widespread in developing countries.

F. Pathophysiology
   1. Results from invasion of virulent organism and failure of natural host defenses
   2. Often results from upper or lower respiratory tract viral infection that weakens host defenses and causes decreased respiratory compliance
      a. This environment increases risk of invasion of bacteria into lung parenchyma
      b. Infection causes local increase in WBCs, cellular debris, and respiratory fluid causing typical respiratory symptoms
   3. Bacterial and viral pneumonias cause different clinical and pathophysiologic manifestations
      a. **Typical bacterial** pathogens usually cause **lobar pneumonia** (inflammation and consolidation of lobe) or **bronchopneumonia** (infection of airways and surrounding interstitium)
      b. **Viral** and **atypical pneumonias** often cause bronchiolitis or interstitial pneumonitis (patterns can overlap)

G. Clinical features
   1. Historical findings (symptoms)
      a. **Neonates** and **infants**
         i. **Fever** and **lethargy** may be only symptoms
         ii. May have history of apnea
      b. Older children: history of fever, cough, and increased work of breathing provide more helpful clues to diagnosis
      c. History of fever found in most children with bacterial pneumonia
   2. Exam findings
      a. **Tachypnea**, **fever**, and **cough** are hallmarks
      b. Hypoxia and respiratory failure are seen in more severe cases
      c. Infants and young toddlers: focal lung findings may be absent
      d. Older children: **rales** (crackles), wheezing, rhonchi, or diminished breath sounds may be heard on auscultation
      e. In viral pneumonia, diffuse wheezes and **rhonchi** are common
      f. Atypical pneumonia often causes diffuse crackles and wheezing
      g. *Chlamydia trachomatis* pneumonia in infants
         i. Classically manifests as staccato cough and tachypnea
         ii. Infants usually have no history of fever
         iii. Often recent history of conjunctivitis

> **QUICK HIT**
>
> Abdominal pain can be primary presenting symptom of pneumonia in children due to referred pain from infection of lower lobe.

H. Diagnosis
   1. Can often be made clinically based on history and exam findings
   2. Laboratory and imaging studies are helpful in
      a. Moderate to severe cases to determine severity of illness and try to establish etiology
      b. Cases in which diagnosis is unclear
      c. Circumstances where complications are suspected (e.g., pleural effusion)
      d. Failure to improve on therapy
      e. Children with recurrent disease or chronic medical conditions (e.g., impaired immune function)
   3. Differential diagnosis
      a. Includes several infectious and noninfectious diagnoses, especially in younger children
         i. Anatomic abnormalities: bronchogenic cyst, pulmonary sequestration, congenital cystic malformation, vascular ring
         ii. Aspiration of gastric contents: predisposing factors include neurologic impairment, neuromuscular weakness, and tracheoesophageal fistula
      b. In infants: viral bronchiolitis can present similar to bacterial pneumonia with fever, tachypnea, and cough
      c. In toddlers: **foreign body aspiration** must always be considered, especially with asymmetric exam on auscultation
      d. Congenital lung malformations can appear as pneumonia on chest radiographs
      e. Segmental atelectasis seen in patients with asthma may mimic pneumonia on chest radiograph

4. Laboratory
   a. Laboratory studies are usually unnecessary in outpatients with uncomplicated pneumonia
   b. Blood cultures recommended for patients requiring hospitalization for CAP (3%–6% positive)
   c. CBCs are often obtained, but they are not reliable in distinguishing bacterial from viral causes of pneumonia
   d. Rapid viral testing (antigen, PCR) from NP swab is often helpful in children admitted to hospital
      i. Identifies **RSV**, **human metapneumovirus**, **adenovirus**, rhinovirus, human coronavirus, and **parainfluenza**, **influenza**
      ii. May help with cohorting of inpatients and predict illness course
      iii. Identification may also prompt clinician to discontinue unnecessary antibiotics
   e. *Mycoplasma* studies (either NP PCR or blood serologies) may be helpful because β-lactam antibiotics used against typical pneumonia organisms are ineffective against this organism, which lacks cell wall
   f. Various other laboratory studies are useful in specific circumstances or when looking for more unusual pathogens
      i. Sputum culture: helpful to identify typical bacterial pathogens in children who can produce sputum or when *Mycobacterium tuberculosis* is suspected
      ii. Serologies (e.g., *Coxiella burnetii*, *Toxoplasma gondii*)
      iii. Bronchoalveolar lavage (BAL)/lung biopsy: helpful to identify pathogens in children with serious illness who do not respond to empiric treatment or when diagnosis is unclear
5. Radiology
   a. Chest radiograph is helpful when diagnosis is unclear or there is suspicion of parapneumonic effusion
   b. CXR cannot always distinguish between viral and bacterial pneumonia
      i. Lobar consolidation or large pleural effusion is most likely caused by typical bacterial organism
      ii. Diffuse interstitial pattern suggests viral or atypical pneumonia

I. Management
1. General
   a. Many can be managed as outpatients with supportive care (e.g., antipyretics) and antimicrobials (when indicated)
   b. Decision to hospitalize depends on child's age, illness severity, and comorbidities; criteria include
      i. Significant tachypnea or hypoxia
      ii. Ill or toxic appearance
      iii. Signs of dehydration or inability to maintain hydration
      iv. Complicated pneumonia (e.g., effusion or empyema)
      v. Underlying medical disorder placing child at risk of severe illness
2. Outpatient management
   a. Supportive care
      i. Antipyretics
      ii. Encourage fluids and monitor for dehydration
      iii. Proper nutrition
   b. Empiric oral antimicrobials (Table 10-6)
      i. Amoxicillin
         (a) **1st-line agent for bacterial CAP** outside of newborn period
         (b) Effective against *Streptococcus pneumoniae* (most common etiologic agent for typical pneumonia)
         (c) "High-dose" amoxicillin (80–90 mg/kg/day divided into 2–3 daily doses) is recommended to overcome resistance seen in *Streptococcus pneumoniae*
         (d) Due to β-lactamase production, amoxicillin is ineffective against *Staphylococcus aureus* and many strains of *M. catarrhalis* and *H. influenzae*

Table 10-6 **Empiric Antibiotic Therapy for Community-Acquired Pneumonia**

Outpatient	**Oral Therapy**
Presumed bacterial pneumonia	Amoxicillin: 90 mg/kg/day divided in 2 doses **Alternatives:** Amoxicillin/clavulanate: 90 mg/kg/day divided in 2 doses 2nd- or 3rd-generation cephalosporin (cefdinir, cefuroxime, cefprozil)
Presumed atypical pneumonia	Azithromycin: 10 mg/kg/day on day 1 then 5 mg/kg/day for days 2–5 (max 500 mg on day 1; 250 mg on days 2–5)
Presumed influenza pneumonia	Oseltamivir (all ages) **OR** Zanamivir (>7 years of age)
Inpatient	**IV Therapy***
Presumed bacterial pneumonia (**fully immunized** against *Haemophilus influenzae* type b and *Streptococcus pneumoniae*)	Ampicillin: 150–200 mg/kg/day divided in 4 doses
Presumed bacterial pneumonia (**not fully immunized** against *H. influenzae* type b and *S. pneumoniae*)	Ceftriaxone: 50–100 mg/kg/day in 1–2 doses **OR** Cefotaxime: 150 mg/kg/day in 3 doses
Severe illness or suspicion of community-acquired methicillin-resistant *Staphylococcus aureus* (CA-MRSA) pneumonia	Either of the 3rd-generation cephalosporins mentioned directly above **PLUS** Clindamycin: 30–40 mg/kg/day divided in 3–4 doses (max 2 g/day) **OR** Vancomycin: 40–60 mg/kg/day divided in 3–4 doses (max 4 g/day)

*A macrolide should be added to the above regimens if it is unclear whether the patient has a bacterial community-acquired pneumonia (CAP) or atypical CAP.

ii. Amoxicillin-clavulanate: addition of clavulanate (β-lactamase inhibitor) expands coverage of amoxicillin to include *Staphylococcus aureus, M. catarrhalis,* and *H. influenzae* but does not alter coverage against pneumococcus

iii. Cephalosporins (e.g., cefuroxime axetil, cefdinir): 2nd and 3rd generations have activity against *Streptococcus pneumoniae, Staphylococcus aureus, M. catarrhalis*, and *H. influenzae*

iv. Macrolides (e.g., azithromycin)
   (a) Use in children suspected of having atypical pneumonia
   (b) Due to significant macrolide resistance in *Streptococcus pneumoniae*, macrolides should be added to β-lactam agents if *Streptococcus pneumoniae* and atypical bacteria are diagnostic considerations

v. Antiviral therapy
   (a) Should be started as soon as possible in children with moderate to severe CAP consistent with influenza
   (b) Oseltamivir and zanamivir are neuraminidase inhibitors with activity against most circulating strains of influenza A and B
   (c) Zanamivir is available as powder for inhalation; only approved for children age >7 years

3. Inpatient management
   a. Supportive care
      i. Antipyretics
      ii. IV fluids
      iii. Proper nutrition (PO, enteral feeding tube, parenteral nutrition)
      iv. Respiratory support: supplemental oxygen via nasal cannula to ventilatory support/intubation
   b. Empiric IV antibiotics (see Table 10-6)
      i. Typical regimens target ***Streptococcus pneumoniae*** with either **ampicillin** *or* **3rd-generation cephalosporin**

ii. Children who are not fully immunized against *Streptococcus pneumoniae* and Hib are at higher risk of pneumonia with these organisms; ampicillin monotherapy is not recommended for unimmunized children because many strains of *H. influenzae* are resistant due to β-lactamase production
iii. Empiric coverage for *Staphylococcus aureus* or CA-MRSA should be started in children who are ill appearing, have evidence of necrotizing pneumonia, or have pleural effusion/empyema
iv. Typical empiric coverage for suspected ***Staphylococcus aureus*** pneumonia includes **clindamycin** or **vancomycin** (based on local susceptibility patterns)
v. Macrolide antibiotic should be added to antibiotic regimen if diagnosis is unclear and atypical organisms are suspected

J. Complications (see XIII. Pneumonia Complicated by Pleural Effusion for discussion of pneumonia with pleural effusion or empyema)
   1. Empyema, pleural effusion, necrotizing pneumonia, lung abscess, and pneumatocele
   2. Patients with necrotizing pneumonia appear ill and may have evidence of significant respiratory distress or septic shock

K. Duration/prognosis
   1. No randomized controlled trials to determine exact length of treatment
   2. Uncomplicated pneumonia: 7–10 days of treatment are usually sufficient; route (IV or PO) depends on illness severity
      a. Most show clinical improvement in 24–48 hours
      b. Fever may persist after resolution of respiratory symptoms
   3. Prognosis is excellent; most patients recover without any long-term sequelae

L. Prevention
   1. Vaccination
      a. Hib and *S. pneumoniae* vaccination have been successful at reducing invasive infections due to these organisms (including pneumonia)
      b. Influenza vaccine reduces risk of influenza pneumonia
      c. Palivizumab (monoclonal antibody against RSV)
         i. Decreases risk of viral pneumonia caused by RSV
         ii. Expensive: only recommended for high-risk patients

XIII. Pneumonia Complicated by Pleural Effusion

A. Definitions
   1. **Parapneumonic effusion**: collection of fluid between parietal and visceral lung pleura associated with **underlying pneumonia**
   2. **Parapneumonic empyema**: collection of pus in pleural space associated with pneumonia
   3. Must be differentiated from pleural effusions caused by chyle (**chylothorax**), serous fluid (**hydrothorax**), or blood (**hemothorax**)
   4. Occur most often from typical bacterial pneumonia pathogens but can also occur from atypical bacteria and viruses
   5. "**Complicated pneumonia**" is used to describe serious complications from pneumonia, such as empyema, necrotizing pneumonia, lung abscess, or bronchopleural fistula

B. Epidemiology
   1. Pleural effusion is seen in **10%–15%** of children hospitalized with pneumonia
   2. ~20% of cases of pneumonia caused by *M. pneumoniae* are complicated by pleural effusions (usually small and bilateral)
   3. Most often seen in children <5 years old

C. Cause (see Box 10-9 for list of most common pathogens): bacterial etiology of parapneumonic effusions has shifted in last 30 years
   1. *S. pneumoniae* remains most common bacterial pathogen, but responsible serotypes have shifted away from those included in pneumococcal conjugate vaccine
   2. Hib is uncommon because of widespread use of Hib vaccine
   3. CA-MRSA has increased in recent years and is now important consideration when starting empiric antibiotics

BOX 10-9

Bacterial Pathogens Responsible for Pneumonia Complicated by Pleural Effusion

Streptococcus pneumoniae
Staphylococcus aureus (including MRSA)
Streptococcus pyogenes
Haemophilus influenzae
Mycoplasma pneumoniae
Mycobacterium tuberculosis
Mixed anaerobic organisms
Group B *Streptococcus* and gram-negative rods (neonates)

MRSA, methicillin-resistant *Staphylococcus aureus.*

D. Risk factors
  1. Chronic underlying medical conditions that impair normal lung function
    a. Neuromuscular disease (e.g., cerebral palsy, muscular dystrophy)
    b. Congenital or acquired lung structural abnormalities
    c. Heart or pulmonary vascular disorders
    d. CF
    e. Sickle cell disease
  2. Chronic underlying medical conditions that impair normal immune function
    a. Congenital or acquired immunodeficiencies
    b. Malignancy
E. Pathophysiology
  1. Pleural space is potential space between visceral and parietal pleura
  2. Normally, balance exists between **secretion** and **absorption** of pleural fluid by visceral and parietal pleura
  3. Pneumonia can cause fluid accumulation by altering this balance; occurs from
    a. Inflammation leading to increased capillary permeability with extravasation of pulmonary interstitial fluid into pleural space
    b. Direct extension of infection into pleural space
  4. Evolution of parapneumonic effusion can be differentiated into 3 phases
    a. **Exudative phase**: as effusion worsens, neutrophils and bacterial debris can accumulate, leading to pus in pleural space (**empyema**)
    b. **Fibrinopurulent phase**: as empyema progresses further, fibrinous pus coats pleurae, leading to decreased lung expansion; fibrinous bands can span pleural membrane, preventing fluid from flowing freely within pleural space (known as **loculations**)
    c. **Organizational phase**: further progression leads to fibroblast migration to pleurae, which causes nonelastic membrane to form (i.e., **pleural peel**)
F. Clinical features
  1. Historical findings
    a. Fever, cough, dyspnea, and malaise are common
    b. Other findings include chest pain, abdominal pain, and emesis
  2. Exam findings
    a. Tachypnea, retractions, grunting, and ill appearance
    b. Auscultation: decreased/absent breath sounds, **rales**, dullness to percussion, or pleural rub on affected side
    c. Splinting toward affected side
G. Diagnosis
  1. Typically made by combination of history, exam findings, and chest radiograph
  2. Differential (Box 10-10): any disease that alters normal hydrostatic/oncotic forces in pleural space can causes effusion
  3. Laboratory
    a. Blood culture
      i. Used along with pleural fluid culture to isolate organism
      ii. Positive in 10%–22% of patients

QUICK HIT

Anaerobic glycolysis causes pleural fluid from exudative phase to have a high lactate level and a low pH.

QUICK HIT

A child with parapneumonic effusion may sleep on affected side to splint it from pain.

BOX 10-10

Noninfectious Causes of Pleural Effusion

Increased capillary leak
Sepsis syndrome
Toxic shock syndrome
Vasculitis (e.g., juvenile idiopathic arthritis)
Malignancy (e.g., lymphoma)
Drugs (e.g., phenytoin, methotrexate)
Trauma

Increased hydrostatic pressure
Congestive heart failure
Sickle cell disease

Decreased oncotic pressure
Nephritic syndrome
Protein malnutrition

Lymphatic obstruction
Lymphangiectasia

Pleural inflammation
Pancreatitis
Mediastinitis

b. Pleural fluid analysis
   i. Gram stain
   ii. Bacterial culture: often negative due to prior antibiotic therapy
   iii. Cell count with differential
      (a) WBC >50,000/mm³ typical of empyema
      (b) WBC 10,000–50,000/mm³ typical in early parapneumonic effusion
      (c) WBC <10,000/mm³ typical of chronic effusion (i.e., malignancy)
      (d) Neutrophils predominate in bacterial infections
      (e) Lymphocytes predominate in *M. tuberculosis* infections
   iv. Biochemical analysis: pleural fluid pH, lactate dehydrogenase (LDH), protein, and glucose
      (a) Traditional tests of pleural fluid to differentiate **exudate** (i.e., inflammatory effusion, such as a parapneumonic effusion) from **transudate** (i.e., change in hydrostatic or oncotic pressure, such as nephritic syndrome)
      (b) In pediatrics, most pleural effusions are parapneumonic effusions (i.e., attributable to lung infection), making these tests less important
      (c) Can occasionally be helpful in differentiating routine parapneumonic effusion from empyema, which is more likely to have
         (i) pH <7.1
         (ii) Glucose <40 mg/dL
         (iii) LDH >1,000 International Units/mL
   v. Other tests
      (a) Cytology: when concern for malignancy
      (b) Acid-fast bacilli stains and culture: when concern for TB (along with TST or interferon-γ release assay [IGRA])
      (c) *M. pneumoniae* PCR

4. Radiology
   a. Although physical exam may be suggestive of pneumonia with pleural effusion, chest radiograph or chest ultrasound should be used to confirm fluid and determine size of effusion
   b. Lateral decubitus radiographs
      i. More sensitive for identification of pleural effusion than posteroanterior view
      ii. Can help differentiate loculated versus free-flowing fluid
   c. Ultrasonography: more accurately determines volume of pleural effusion and presence of loculations
   d. CT is often unnecessary but may be appropriate in severe cases to define disease extent

H. Management
   1. Depends on multiple clinical factors
      a. Clinical condition of patient
      b. Degree of respiratory compromise
      c. Size and character (e.g., loculated) of effusion

   d. Age of patient
   e. Presence of comorbid conditions
2. Antibiotic therapy with surgical drainage is typical treatment (in addition to supportive care)
3. Size of pleural effusion can be divided into small, moderate, and large and can often predict need for drainage or surgical intervention
   a. **Small**: <1 cm on lateral decubitus or <1/4 of hemithorax
      i. Usually respond well to antibiotic therapy alone
      ii. Drainage not typically needed
   b. **Moderate**: >1 cm on lateral decubitus but opacifies <1/2 of hemithorax
      i. Drainage often necessary for diagnostic and therapeutic purposes
      ii. Drainage likely needed with respiratory distress or empyema
   c. **Large**: opacifies >1/2 of hemithorax; drainage needed
4. Drainage/surgical intervention serves multiple purposes
   a. May relieve respiratory distress if effusion prevented lung expansion
   b. Allows fluid to be sent for Gram stain, bacterial culture, and other biochemical studies
   c. Allows for placement of chest tube for continued drainage
   d. Opportunity for loculations to be broken and purulent fibrinous material to be removed
5. Options for parapneumonic effusions
   a. **Thoracentesis** (i.e., needle aspiration): may be adequate for free-flowing pleural effusions but not typically recommended because of high failure rate with progression to complicated disease
   b. Chest tube with or without fibrinolytics
      i. Urokinase and tissue plasminogen activator are 2 commonly used fibrinolytics
      ii. Thought to be superior to chest tube alone
   c. **Video-assisted thoracoscopic surgery (VATS)**
      i. Camera enters pleural space through small chest wall incisions
      ii. Equivalent to chest tube with fibrinolytics in regard to
         (a) Length of hospital stay
         (b) Time required for resolution of infection
      iii. Should be used if chest tube therapy is not effective
   d. **Open chest debridement with decortication**
      i. May be necessary for advanced empyema
      ii. Increased morbidity when compared to VATS
      iii. Rarely necessary
6. Antimicrobial therapy
   a. Approach is similar to approach for CAP, because organisms are similar
   b. Key difference is that *S. aureus* (and MRSA) tends to be more common in CAP with effusion than CAP without effusion
   c. Antibiotics should be targeted toward bacteria identified by culture
   d. Empiric antibiotic treatment of pneumonia with pleural effusion includes ceftriaxone/cefotaxime + clindamycin or + vancomycin
   e. Optimal duration of antibiotic treatment may vary by pathogen, patient's age, response to treatment, extent of disease, and presence of comorbid conditions
   f. Children typically receive 2–4 weeks of antibiotic therapy; many experts recommend treating 7–10 days after fever resolution if drainage was done

I. Complications
   1. Bronchopleural fistula
   2. Pneumatocele
   3. Necrotizing pneumonia
   4. Pulmonary abscess

J. Duration/prognosis
   1. Mortality rate in otherwise healthy children is very low
   2. Clinical improvement usually seen in 2–3 days with pleural drainage and antibiotic treatment
   3. Most children recover completely without long-term pulmonary complications

QUICK HIT

Chest radiographs may take 6 months or more to normalize after pneumonia with pleural effusion.

> **QUICK HIT**
> 3 major endemic mycoses are most common cause of pulmonary fungal infection in immunocompetent individuals in U.S., with histoplasmosis causing largest number of cases.

XIV. Endemic Fungal Infections

A. General characteristics
1. Most common endemic fungal infections in U.S. are histoplasmosis, blastomycosis, and coccidioidomycosis
2. Occur in distinct geographic areas (Table 10-7)
   a. With endemic mycoses, most individuals are asymptomatic or have brief, self-limited illness; with histoplasmosis and coccidioidomycosis, only 5% of individuals develop significant symptomatic disease
   b. Extrapulmonary disease is even rarer but may involve skin or bone
3. Genetics and risk factors
   a. Infection
      i. Inhalation of dirt/dust (e.g., home renovation, outdoor landscaping, playing in barns)
      ii. Recreational activities (e.g., spelunking)
   b. Severe or disseminated disease
      i. Immunosuppression (especially cell-mediated immunity), inoculum size
      ii. Neonates/young infants, pregnant women, diabetics
4. Pathophysiology
   a. All 3 endemic mycoses cause pulmonary infection initiated by inhalation and are all dimorphic fungi that can shift from infective mold form at 25°C to yeast form at 37°C (body temperature), explaining why there is not person-to-person transmission
   b. After inhalation, fungus replicates in lower respiratory tract triggering host immune responses
   c. Immune response can lead to lymph node inflammation and mediastinal enlargement, causing airway compression and obstruction and symptoms
   d. In susceptible hosts, infection can also cause extrapulmonary disease

> **QUICK HIT**
> Pulmonary infections with endemic mycoses present similarly to CAP but will not respond to conventional antibiotic therapy.

> **QUICK HIT**
> Triad of fever, malaise, and mild cough is present in 90% of immunocompetent children with symptomatic histoplasmosis.

B. Clinical features
1. Complete history should include any possible predisposing conditions for severe/disseminated disease, complete ROS, and exposure history
   a. Key symptoms: fever, cough, chest pain
   b. Other symptoms: fatigue, headache, weight loss, night sweats
2. Complete physical examination should include careful pulmonary and chest exam and examination for evidence of extrapulmonary or disseminated disease
   a. Pulmonary infection: wheezing, asymmetry on auscultation due to airway compression from enlarged mediastinal lymph nodes
   b. Extrapulmonary: skin lesions (e.g., erythema nodosum), bone pain, hepatomegaly, splenomegaly

C. Diagnosis
1. Differential diagnosis
   a. CAP (bacterial)
   b. TB
   c. Noninfectious granulomatous diseases (such as sarcoidosis, Wegener granulomatosis)

TABLE 10-7 Geographic Distribution and Favorable Growth Conditions of Endemic Mycoses in the U.S.

Endemic Mycosis	Geographic Distribution
Histoplasmosis	Midwestern U.S. including states bordering the Ohio River and the Mississippi River valleys. Widest geographic distribution of all the endemic mycoses. Bird and bat excrement promote growth of *Histoplasma capsulatum* in soil.
Coccidioidomycosis	Southwestern U.S. including the San Joaquin Valley of central California, Arizona, New Mexico, and Texas. Hot summers, infrequent freezes, alkaline soil, and alternating periods of rain and drought (seen in the lower Sonoran life zone) best promote growth and aerosolization of *Coccidioides immitis*.
Blastomycosis	Midwestern and southeastern U.S. Acidic moist rich soil near waterways best supports the growth of *Blastomyces dermatitidis*.

d. Malignancy, primarily lymphoma
e. Disseminated/extrapulmonary disease can have broad differential diagnosis, including bacterial osteomyelitis and malignancy with bone involvement; disseminated disease can also present with septic picture in immunocompromised hosts

2. Laboratory diagnosis in 3 ways: sputum culture, antibody titers, and urine antigen testing (skin testing is also used, primarily in coccidioidomycosis)
3. Radiologic findings
   a. Diffuse or focal pulmonary infiltrates
   b. Mediastinal and/or hilar adenopathy suggests histoplasmosis
   c. Calcifications can be seen in histoplasmosis following resolution of illness
   d. Miliary pattern of disease can be seen in acute infection after exposure to heavy inoculum of organism

D. Treatment
1. Most immunocompetent individuals with endemic mycoses do not require treatment
2. Indications for treatment include prolonged disease, immunocompromise, disseminated or severe infection, and extrapulmonary infection
   a. For mild to moderate disease
      i. Itraconazole: levels should be monitored; many practitioners prefer liquid formulation due to superior bioavailability
      ii. Fluconazole can be used in coccidioidomycosis
   b. For severe disease and meningitis: amphotericin B
   c. Adjunctive therapy may include steroids, especially with severely enlarged mediastinal nodes with airway compression

E. Duration/prognosis
1. Duration dictated by clinical syndrome/disease severity and ranges from 6 to 12 weeks for mild to moderate disease to up to 1 year for meningitis, disseminated infection
2. With HIV+ patients and some other patients who are immunocompromised, lifelong itraconazole suppression after therapy is recommended

F. Prevention
1. Avoidance of high-risk activities and exposures, especially by immunocompromised individuals; if activities cannot be avoided, protective masks should be used
2. Antifungal prophylaxis may be appropriate in some cases

> **QUICK HIT**
>
> *Coccidioides* is an extremely hazardous organism in microbiology lab and can cause infection and death in lab personnel. Avoid culture if possible and notify lab in advance if culture must be sent.

XV. Tuberculosis

A. General characteristics
1. Infection with protean manifestations
2. Most commonly, disease is pulmonary, but extrapulmonary disease including meningitis, osteomyelitis, lymphadenitis, and genitourinary (GU) and peritoneal infection can occur, especially in immunocompromised individuals

B. Epidemiology
1. Transmitted person to person via mucus droplets that become airborne when person with active pulmonary infection coughs, sneezes, laughs, or sings; these droplets evolve into droplet nuclei that can remain suspended in air for hours, leading to effective transmission
2. Children age <10 years with pulmonary TB rarely infect others due to low bacterial numbers in their secretions and weaker force of cough
3. Risk of acquiring TB in childhood in U.S. is very low
4. TB in childhood has 2 peaks: age <5 years and age >14 years; infants and young children are at higher risk for disseminated disease and meningitis
5. Cause is *M. tuberculosis*, an aerobic, slow-growing, acid-fast bacillus

C. Genetics
1. Individuals with genetic immunodeficiencies affecting T cells or phagocytes are predisposed
2. Molecular basis of genetic control of TB infection is not fully understood

> **QUICK HIT**
>
> Between 30% and 50% of household contacts of a case of active TB develop reactive skin tests.

> **QUICK HIT**
>
> Because children acquire TB infection from adults, a TB infection in a child should trigger a public health investigation for TB-positive individuals in contact with that child.

D. Risk factors
  1. Exposure to high-risk groups: incarcerated or homeless individuals, IV drug users, nursing home residents and employees, health care workers, individuals born in high-prevalence countries or history of travel to such countries
  2. Immunocompromise: HIV, immunosuppressive medications, severe malnutrition
  3. Exposure to individual with known active pulmonary TB
  4. Birth in highly endemic country or travel to such countries

E. Pathophysiology
  1. TB droplet nuclei are inhaled and deposit in lung alveoli, where macrophages ingest bacteria and initiate cell-mediated T-cell response
     a. Immunocompetent patient
        i. Macrophages and T cells coordinate immune response, forming granuloma-containing TB infection, locally leading to latent infection (**Ghon focus**)
        ii. After 2–12 weeks, detection is possible with TST; often referred to as a PPD test
        iii. Successful immune response keeps infection in check without causing active disease, so called **latent TB infection (LTBI)**
     b. Immunocompromised patient
        i. Immune system fails to contain infection, and bacilli spread to other alveoli and disseminate via bloodstream to other sites (bone, joints, brain, lymph nodes, GU system)
        ii. These patients develop active TB infection and disease; TB meningitis may present acutely or subacutely in children
  2. Individuals who initially control TB infection and develop LTBI are at risk for developing active TB later, especially in context of immune suppression, which may be iatrogenic (tumor necrosis factor inhibitors)

F. Clinical features
  1. Historical findings
     a. Questions should focus on exposures, symptoms, duration of illness, and complicating clinical conditions
     b. Also do thorough ROS and take family history (Box 10-11)
  2. Physical exam findings
     a. Early pulmonary infection after exposure is often silent with no signs or symptoms; symptoms are more common in infants
     b. Focus on careful pulmonary exam and thorough examination for extrapulmonary manifestations of TB, including neurologic, lymph nodes, musculoskeletal, and abdominal exams

> **QUICK HIT**
>
> Fever for >14 days in a child should raise suspicion for possible TB.

G. Diagnosis
  1. Differential diagnosis
     a. Very broad, especially extrapulmonary disease
     b. For pulmonary TB, differential includes bacterial pneumonia, *Pneumocystis jiroveci* (formerly *Pneumocystis carinii*) pneumonia, fungal pneumonia, sarcoidosis, Wegener granulomatosis, and malignancy

BOX 10-11

Key Questions for History in Children at Risk for Tuberculosis

- Has the patient had fever? Night sweats? Cough? Shortness of breath? Chest pain? Hemoptysis? Decreased appetite/feeding? Weight loss? Fatigue? CNS symptoms such as headache, drowsiness, irritability, or loss of developmental milestones (in infants)?
- Duration of symptoms?
- Any chronic symptoms (>30 days) including joint pain/swelling, bone pain, or back pain?
- Has the patient been exposed to anyone with TB?
- Has the patient travelled or been exposed to high-risk groups?
- Any exposure to individuals with a chronic cough of unknown etiology?
- Family history: Is there any family history of TB even in family member the child has not met?
- Past medical history: Any predisposing conditions for TB such as immunocompromise or immune-suppressive medications, or any prior history of TB infection (latent TB infection or active disease)?

CNS, central nervous system; TB, tuberculosis.

2. Laboratory tests
   a. TST: 5 tuberculin units of PPD injected intradermally on volar surface of forearm
      i. Read at 48–72 hours postplacement; induration should be measured in millimeters
      ii. Interpretation depends on host factors and exposures (Box 10-12)
         (a) Positive TST reflects TB infection but does not distinguish between LTBI and active disease
         (b) Negative TST cannot rule out infection; false-negative tests may be caused by immunocompromise, malnutrition, steroids, recent TB infection (patient has not yet mounted immune response), overwhelming TB disease, and age <6 months
   b. Interferon-γ (IFN-γ) release assay (IGRA): measure adaptive T-cell response to TB infection by measuring specific IFN-γ responses to *M. tuberculosis*
      i. Advantages: results in 1 office visit
      ii. Disadvantages: Can have false-negatives for same reasons TST can; scant data exists for children, especially age <5 years of age, who are more likely to have indeterminate results
      iii. Best application is in distinguishing if positive TST is due to TB infection or recent BCG vaccination
   c. Culture: important diagnostic modality because allows recovery of organism for susceptibility testing, which is very important when source is unknown
      i. Only 40% of early morning gastric aspirates grow organism
      ii. Yield from gastric aspirate in children is superior to BAL
   d. Radiology findings: all patients with positive PPD should have CXR to look for active pulmonary disease
      i. CXR findings: mediastinal/hilar lymph node enlargement, calcification of parenchyma granuloma and associated lymph nodes (**Ghon complex**), evidence of bronchial obstruction with segmental hyperinflation (in endobronchial TB) sometimes evolving to emphysema with contiguous atelectasis, pulmonary infiltrates including lobar pneumonia pattern
      ii. Younger children may demonstrate military pattern
      iii. Upper lobe cavitary lesions and infiltrates are usually seen in adolescents with reactivated disease

QUICK HIT

As many as 10% of immunocompetent children with culture-documented TB infection have negative TST on initial testing.

QUICK HIT

False-positive TST can occur in setting of recent bacillus Calmette-Guérin (BCG) vaccination or nontuberculous mycobacterial infection.

QUICK HIT

M. tuberculosis from clinical specimens requires 4–6 weeks to grow with traditional methods; using newer automated systems can reduce time to 10–21 days.

BOX 10-12

Positive Tuberculin Skin Test Interpretations

A PPD of ≥5 mm induration is considered positive in
- HIV-infected persons
- A recent contact of a person with TB disease
- Persons with fibrotic changes on chest radiograph consistent with prior TB
- Patients with organ transplants
- Persons who are immunosuppressed for other reasons (e.g., taking the equivalent of >15 mg/day of prednisone for ≥1 month, tumor necrosis factor-α antagonists)

A PPD of ≥10 mm induration is considered positive in
- Recent immigrants (<5 years) from high-prevalence countries
- Injection drug users
- Residents of high-risk congregate settings
- Persons with clinical conditions that place them at high risk
- Children <4 years of age
- Infants, children, and adolescents exposed to adults in high-risk categories

A PPD of ≥15 mm induration is considered positive in
- Any person regardless of risk factors

PPD, purified protein derivative; TB, tuberculosis.

Infectious Diseases

QUICK HIT

LTBI prophylaxis is 70%–80% effective in preventing reactivation of TB infection.

MNEMONIC

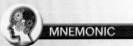

Empiric treatment for active TB infection is **RIPE**.
Rifampin
Isoniazid
Pyrazinamide
Ethambutol

MNEMONIC

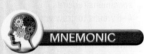

Remember isoniazid (**INH**) side effects.
Isoniazid
Neuropathy
Hepatitis

iv. Enlarged cardiac silhouette can be seen in TB pericarditis
v. Negative CXR with no evidence of extrapulmonary TB with +TST establishes diagnosis of LTBI

H. Treatment
1. Therapy
a. LTBI: isoniazid prophylaxis for 9 months; 3-month regimen with isoniazid + rifapentine is also effective
b. Active TB infection: treat empirically initially with 4-drug TB therapy
i. RIPE for 2 months and then isoniazid + rifampin for additional 4 months to complete 6 months of therapy
ii. Treatment for TB meningitis/CNS disease is 9–12 months
c. Therapy should be administered with directly observed therapy with health department support and supervision
d. In cases of multidrug-resistant TB, additional agents may be required
2. Complications of TB therapy
a. Isoniazid
i. Neuropathy, hepatitis (10% of child have ALT elevation; rarely severe); neuropathy can be prevented with pyridoxine (vitamin B_6) supplementation
ii. Some drug interactions
b. Rifampin: gastrointestinal (GI) upset; hepatitis; rash; orange staining of secretions, urine, and feces; thrombocytopenia; cholestatic jaundice
i. Many drug interactions
c. Pyrazinamide: GI upset, rash, hepatic dysfunction; well tolerated in children
d. Ethambutol: retrobulbar neuritis that presents with blurry vision and red/green color blindness; vision should be monitored on therapy

I. Prevention: prompt identification and effective complete treatment of active TB in communities by effective health department are critical to drive down TB incidence
1. BCG vaccine: used in many countries in young infants to decrease incidence of severe and disseminated TB in young children who are at greatest risk
a. Does not prevent primary pulmonary infection and establishment of LTBI and does not prevent reactivation
b. TST can be positive from BCG vaccination, but this effect wanes after time; TST results should be interpreted independent of BCG status
2. N-95 masks for health care workers caring for patients suspected of having TB
3. Negative-pressure isolation for patients admitted to hospital

QUICK HIT

Gastroenteritis often results in transient lactose intolerance due to disruption of normal villous anatomy and ability to absorb complex sugars.

XVI. Acute Gastroenteritis

A. General characteristics
1. Intestinal illness usually characterized by diarrhea, vomiting, and fever usually spread by fecal–oral route (spread also possible by asymptomatic hosts)
2. Mostly viral in etiology (Box 10-13) since improvements in public health have drastically reduced parasitic and bacterial causes in U.S.
3. Accounts for 7%–10% of childhood hospitalizations, mostly during winter
4. >95% hospitalizations are children age <5 years; 2% of children hospitalized at some point in childhood

BOX 10-13

Known Enteric Pathogens

- Viruses
  - Rotaviruses
  - Caliciviruses
  - Astroviruses
  - Adenoviruses (serotypes 40 and 41)
  - Picornaviruses
- Bacteria
  - *Campylobacter*
  - *Clostridium difficile*
  - *Escherichia coli*
  - *Salmonella*
  - *Shigella*
  - *Mycobacteria*
- Parasites
  - *Isospora belli*
  - *Cryptosporidium*
  - *Giardia*

5. Risk factors for severe disease: age <18 months, immunocompromise, malnutrition, underlying medical disease, decreased maternal antibodies (prematurity, nonbreastfed), large inoculum

B. Clinical features
  1. Symptoms: loose watery stools, vomiting, fever, anorexia, headache, abdominal cramps, myalgia, decreased ability to tolerate PO
  2. Signs on physical exam
    a. Evaluate hydration status: heart rate, blood pressure, moist mucous membranes, tears, mental status, skin turgor, capillary refill, weight change, fontanel in infants
    b. Look for signs of other diseases that may mimic gastroenteritis (e.g., appendicitis, inflammatory bowel disease, intussusception)

C. Diagnosis
  1. Clinical diagnosis usually sufficient, especially in mild cases in young children with no complicating factors
  2. Differential diagnosis: consider other diseases that may present with similar symptoms and/or require specific therapies
  3. Laboratory tests: often not indicated unless concern for other etiology or significant hypovolemia
    a. CBC: elevated WBC count or bandemia may indicate bacterial cause; anemia may indicate hemolysis
    b. Electrolytes: may be abnormal in hypovolemia
    c. Stool culture, leukocytes, ova and parasites: helpful if nonviral pathogen suspected
    d. Specific viral assays available but usually not necessary; may be helpful for cohorting hospitalized patients or in immunocompromised patients
  4. Radiology findings: usually not indicated unless concern for other etiology

D. Treatment
  1. Supportive care
    a. Oral rehydration ideal method if tolerated in mild to moderate dehydration
    b. IV rehydration indicated for PO intolerance or severe hypovolemia
  2. Medications
    a. Antimicrobials contraindicated unless treatable bacterial or parasitic pathogen identified
    b. Antidiarrheal agents not indicated in children due to limited efficacy and significant side effects
    c. Antiemetics
      i. Ondansetron shown in some studies to help decrease vomiting and need for IV fluids and hospitalization
      ii. Phenothiazines can help but have significant risks
      iii. Probiotic *Lactobacillus rhamnosus* (LGG) shortens duration of symptoms in immunocompetent children
      iv. Potentially helpful: zinc (in malnourished patients)

E. Typical clinical course: symptoms typically beginning 12 hours to 4 days after exposure and lasting 3–7 days

F. Complications: shock, hypoxemia, tissue acidosis, cerebral edema (from rapid drops in serum sodium with rehydration), severe disease in immunocompromised patients

G. Prevention
  1. Frequent handwashing by parent and child, especially after diaper changes and toilet use
  2. Diaper-changing areas separate from food preparation areas and cleaning of changing areas with alcohol or bleach solutions
  3. Water purification in areas without clean water supply
  4. Vaccination: oral live attenuated rotavirus vaccines very effective in preventing rotavirus infection and decreasing hospitalization rates from gastroenteritis

QUICK HIT

Blood/mucus in stool or a history of foreign travel/animal exposure is highly suggestive of bacterial or parasitic infection.

QUICK HIT

Frequent small amounts of an electrolyte-containing fluid are ideal for oral rehydration.

XVII. Intestinal Parasites

A. General characteristics
  1. Definition
    a. Inhabitants of GI tracts of humans and other animals and prefer intestinal wall, but many can survive and cause damage to other parts of body
    b. **Protozoa**: free-living, single-celled, eukaryotic cells that can exist in cyst or trophozoite form
    c. **Helminths**: worm-like organisms that consist of **nematodes** (roundworms), **trematodes** (flatworms), and **cestodes** (tapeworms)
  2. Epidemiology (Table 10-8)
    a. Enter body through ingestion of **infected water**, **contaminated food** (e.g., undercooked meat), ingestion of parasites via **contaminated hands** or **fingers** (e.g., finger sucking in toddlers) or **through skin absorption**
    b. Most often spread via stool of infected persons
    c. Secreted form of parasite may be immediately infectious if ingested by human host
    d. May be **endemic** to certain areas based on environmental or social factors; tend to be endemic in tropical or subtropical areas
    e. Occur sporadically or in **epidemics**
  3. Risk factors
    a. Untreated water
    b. Water supply contaminated by sewage
    c. Lack of handwashing
    d. Ingestion of raw or undercooked meat and fish
    e. Use of animal or human feces to fertilize crops
    f. Walking with bare feet in infected soil

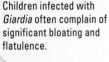

> **QUICK HIT**
> Children infected with *Giardia* often complain of significant bloating and flatulence.

B. Pathophysiology and life cycle
  1. Protozoa: cysts ingested with fecal–oral contamination
  2. Nematodes: eggs ingested after touching contaminated surfaces

C. Clinical features
  1. General
    a. Most intestinal parasite infections are **asymptomatic**
    b. Some are responsible for widespread morbidity within population (e.g., hookworm leading to chronic anemia and growth delay), although they may not have significant GI symptoms
  2. Historical findings (symptoms) and exam findings (signs): see Table 10-8

D. Diagnosis
  1. Differential
    a. Varies based on symptoms and geographical setting/travel history
    b. For children with diarrhea, vomiting, and abdominal pain, consider the following:
      i. Viral gastroenteritis (e.g., rotavirus, norovirus, adenovirus, astrovirus)
      ii. Bacterial gastroenteritis (e.g., *Salmonella* species, *Shigella* species, *Campylobacter jejuni*, *Escherichia coli*)
      iii. Other considerations (e.g., appendicitis, UTI, intussusception, pancreatitis)
  2. Laboratory
    a. Hemoccult stool test to look for presence of blood
    b. Stool **ova and parasites (O+P) test**
      i. 1 O+P has relatively low sensitivity (e.g., 50%–70% for *Giardia*)
      ii. 3 samples over 7–10-day period may be needed to identify parasite
      iii. Stool is examined microscopically for parasite cysts, helminth ova, and single-cell parasites (e.g., *Giardia* trophozoites)
    c. Rapid diagnostic tests (e.g., immunoassay, which requires only 1 specimen for *Cryptosporidium* species and *Giardia lamblia*)
    d. **Cellulose tape test** used to diagnose pinworm infection
      i. Parent can wrap cellulose tape around tongue depressor and apply to anus
      ii. Most sensitive if performed in early morning
      iii. Tape is examined microscopically for pinworm ova

TABLE 10-8 **Characteristics of Intestinal Parasites**

	Epidemiology	Transmission	Signs/Symptoms	Diagnosis	Treatment	Complications	Duration/Prognosis
Protozoa							
Entamoeba histolytica	10% of world population infected; majority asymptomatic	Fecal–oral	Abdominal pain, tenesmus, bloody diarrhea, fever, RUQ pain	O+P; look for trophozoites with ingested RBCs	Paromomycin for noninvasive infections (luminal agent) Metronidazole followed by paromomycin for invasive infections	Liver and pulmonary abscess; fulminant or necrotizing colitis (rare, 40% mortality); ameboma (granulation tissue mass around bowel)	Noninvasive infection has excellent prognosis if treated; invasive infection associated with significant morbidity and mortality
Giardia lamblia	~2.5 million cases a year in the U.S.	Drinking contaminated freshwater; day care centers	Nonbloody, foul-smelling diarrhea	O+P, enzyme immunoassay	Metronidazole	Chronic diarrhea with associated malnutrition	Excellent prognosis if treated; symptomatic giardiasis may occur in immunocompetent hosts
Cryptosporidium species	~750,000 infections in U.S. each year	Contaminated drinking water; can survive chlorine disinfection	Nonbloody diarrhea and abdominal pain	O+P, enzyme immunoassay	Nitazoxanide	Severe protracted diarrhea in immunocompromised hosts; biliary	Immunocompetent hosts usually have a self-limiting illness; immunocompromised patients can have a severe or prolonged illness
Cyclospora cayetanensis	Cause of travelers diarrhea; can cause severe disease in AIDS patients	Contaminated water or food (e.g., raspberries)	Watery diarrhea, vomiting, low-grade fever	O+P, PCR	TMP-SMX	Severe protracted diarrhea and biliary tract disease in immunocompromised hosts	Immunocompetent hosts usually have a decrease in severity over weeks; relapse can occur even if treated
Isospora belli	Seen in immunocompromised (especially AIDS) and outbreaks in institutionalized groups	Fecal–oral	Nonbloody diarrhea, abdominal pain	O+P, Entero-Test; may see eosinophilia	TMP-SMX	Severe protracted diarrhea in immunocompromised hosts	Usually self-limited in hosts with normal immune system; prolonged illness in those with HIV; relapse can occur even if treated

(continued)

TABLE 10-8 Characteristics of Intestinal Parasites *(Continued)*

	Epidemiology	Transmission	Signs/Symptoms	Diagnosis	Treatment	Complications	Duration/Prognosis
Nematodes							
Enterobius vermicularis (pinworm)	More than 30% of children around the world are infected	Fecal–oral; anal sex	Anal pruritus, vaginitis	O+P; scotch tape test	Pyrantel pamoate, mebendazole, albendazole	May increase risk of UTI, perianal cellulitis, rare cases of migration to appendix or fallopian tubes	Excellent prognosis if treated; rarely cause significant morbidity
Ancylostoma duodenale + *Necator americanus* (hookworm)	600 million infections worldwide	Enter the host through intact skin	Usually asymptomatic; vomiting, diarrhea; respiratory symptoms	O+P; 30%–60% develop eosinophilia	Mebendazole, albendazole	Anemia, protein deficiency, cognitive and growth retardation; pneumonitis	Excellent prognosis if treated prior to complications; significant morbidity if not treated
Ascaris lumbricoides (roundworm)	~25% of the world population infected	Fecal–oral	Often asymptomatic; abdominal pain, vomiting, cough, respiratory distress	O+P; eosinophilia may be present; visible worms may be in stool	Albendazole, mebendazole	Pneumonia, respiratory failure, bowel obstruction, migration of worms to appendix or biliary tree	Excellent prognosis if treated; 11%–67% of children in the developing world have a complication from the infection
Trichuris trichiura (whipworm)	600–800 million infections worldwide	Fecal–oral	Often asymptomatic; abdominal pain, bloody or mucous diarrhea	O+P	Albendazole or mebendazole PLUS ivermectin	Rectal prolapse, appendicitis, anemia, growth deficiency	Good prognosis if treated
Strongyloides stercoralis	Endemic in certain tropical/subtropical areas; seen in southeastern U.S.	Enter the host through intact skin when exposed to fecally contaminated soil	Dermatitis at site of infection; wheezing, cough; abdominal pain	O+P	Ivermectin	Abdominal obstruction; respiratory failure secondary to eosinophilic pneumonia (Löffler syndrome); autoinfection	Immunocompromised at high risk of autoinfection; high mortality if disseminated
Cestodes							
Diphyllobothrium latum	Most common in Scandinavia, former Soviet Union; seen in Northwestern U.S.	Ingestion of raw fish	Most asymptomatic; vomiting, diarrhea; abdominal pain	O+P	Praziquantel	Vitamin B_{12} deficiency leading to megaloblastic anemia (rare)	Excellent prognosis if treated

RBC, red blood cell; O+P, ova and parasites; PCR, polymerase chain reaction; RUQ, right upper quadrant; TMP-SMX, trimethoprim-sulfamethoxazole; UTI, urinary tract infection.

e. Entero-Test capsule ("string test")
  i. Gelatin capsule attached to string is swallowed by patient and pulled up 4 hours later
  ii. Duodenal mucus is then examined microscopically for parasites such as *Giardia* and *Strongyloides*
f. Peripheral eosinophilia
  i. Can represent invasive parasite infection (helminthic migration through tissues)
  ii. Parasites that stay within intestinal lumen rarely cause peripheral eosinophilia
g. Extreme eosinophilia (5,000 cells/mm^3 or >30%)
  i. Patients with invasive intestinal parasites
    (a) Hookworm
    (b) *Ascaris* infection
    (c) Whipworm
    (d) *Strongyloides stercoralis*
  ii. Nonintestinal parasitic infections
  iii. Nonparasitic causes of peripheral eosinophilia
    (a) Malignancy (e.g., eosinophilic leukemia)
    (b) *Coccidioides immitis*

E. Radiology
  1. CT or ultrasound of liver is often necessary if liver abscess is suspected
  2. Colonoscopy may be necessary to obtain tissue for pathology if diagnosis is uncertain
F. Management
  1. Therapy (see Table 10-8)
G. Prevention
  1. Wearing shoes to prevent parasites from entering skin
  2. Treating water and sewage to prevent fecal–oral transmission
  3. Handwashing to prevent fecal–oral transmission
  4. Cooking meat and fish thoroughly prior to eating
  5. Washing vegetables prior to eating
  6. Mass treatment of children in endemic areas reduces burden, but reinfection is likely

> **QUICK HIT**
> *Isospora belli* is unusual in that it is known to cause a peripheral eosinophilia even though it is a noninvasive intestinal parasite.

XVIII. Infectious Mononucleosis

A. Definition
  1. Clinical syndrome classically characterized by **fever**, **lymphadenopathy**, **tonsillar pharyngitis**, and **splenomegaly**
  2. Most often caused by **EBV**, member of herpesvirus family
B. Epidemiology
  1. EBV is ubiquitous in humans
  2. ~90%–95% of people develop seropositivity by early adulthood
  3. In U.S., 20%–50% of children will be seropositive by age 4 years in lower socioeconomic classes
  4. Spread in **oropharyngeal secretions** while person has acute infection or is still shedding virus after acute infection
  5. Common methods of spread include kissing, sharing drinks, and toddlers sharing toys
  6. Overall, <10% of children develop clinical signs of infection
C. Cause
  1. Infectious mononucleosis is predominantly caused by EBV
  2. **CMV**, another herpesvirus, causes identical syndrome but heterophile-antibody negative
  3. Other viral causes: HIV, adenovirus, human herpesvirus-6 (HHV-6), and toxoplasmosis
D. Risk factors
  1. Crowded conditions and low socioeconomic status increase risk for acquiring disease
  2. EBV may spread through sexual contact, but studies are inconclusive

> **QUICK HIT**
> Younger children usually have asymptomatic EBV infection.

> **QUICK HIT**
> Viral shedding of EBV can occur for up to 1 year after an acute episode.

E. Pathophysiology
  1. EBV contact with epithelial cells in oropharynx allows viral replication and spread through local lymph system via infected B cells
  2. Viral incubation lasts 4–8 weeks
  3. EBV-specific cytotoxic T cells help control acute infection (these cells represent "atypical lymphocytes" seen on manual differential or blood smear)
  4. After acute infection, EBV becomes lifelong infection, establishing latency with periodic reactivation
  5. Insufficient immune responses to initial infection may result in malignancy (e.g., Hodgkin lymphoma, Burkitt lymphoma)

QUICK HIT

The presence of antibodies to EBV nuclear antigen indicates past infection (>3 months ago).

F. Clinical features
  1. Historical findings
    a. **Malaise**, **fever**, and **pharyngitis**
    b. Headache and low-grade fever often precede more classic symptoms
    c. Fatigue can last up to 6 months in severe cases
    d. Many patients have mild disease: pharyngitis or tonsillitis without accompanying fever and malaise
    e. Young children can present with "**typhoidal form**": high fever, malaise, and lymphadenopathy

G. Exam findings
  1. Generalized or **cervical lymphadenopathy**: enlarged lymph nodes are usually firm and tender to palpation
  2. Pharyngeal inflammation and tonsillar exudates mimic streptococcal pharyngitis
  3. Splenomegaly
    a. ~50% of patients with infectious mononucleosis
    b. Rare risk of trauma-induced or spontaneous splenic rupture
  4. Hepatitis
    a. 25% have hyperbilirubinemia (usually conjugated)
    b. Mild to moderate hepatic transaminase elevation occurs in 80% of patients
  5. Rash
    a. 3%–19% of patients develop rash early in illness
    b. Most commonly, erythematous, macular, papular, or morbilliform
    c. Less commonly, urticaria or petechiae are seen

QUICK HIT

In patients with EBV, amoxicillin (and less commonly, other antibiotics) can cause an extensive, copper-colored, confluent rash that is maculopapular, pruritic, and occurs primarily on the chest but may include the palms and soles. This rash does *not* represent an amoxicillin hypersensitivity.

H. Diagnosis
  1. Differential diagnosis
    a. Infectious: HIV, HSV, *B. henselae*, toxoplasmosis
    b. Noninfectious: Kawasaki disease, lymphoma
  2. Laboratory tests
    a. EBV stimulates immune system to produce heterophile antibodies
    b. Detected using **spot agglutination assay** (often referred to as **monospot test**)
    c. Heterophile antibodies develop in majority of adolescents and adults with EBV infection but are less common in younger children
    d. Antibodies directed at viral capsid antigen (VCA) immunoglobulin (Ig) M and IgG are positive with acute infection; anti-early antigen appears at 1 month; and anti–Epstein-Barr nuclear antigen (EBNA) appears >6 weeks
      i. Presence of anti-EBNA always means past infection
    e. CBC classically shows lymphocytosis (>50% of leukocytes) and increased circulating atypical lymphocytes (>10%)
    f. Mild elevations in transaminases may be seen with both EBV and CMV
  3. Radiology: generally not necessary unless there is significant airway compromise or concern for splenic rupture

QUICK HIT

The "atypical lymphocytes" seen on peripheral smear in patients with EBV are the EBV-specific cytotoxic T cells.

I. Management
  1. Rarely requires more than supportive care with analgesia and antipyretics
  2. In severe cases of tonsillitis, short course of corticosteroids is often used to decrease swelling (although efficacy is unproven by available data)
  3. Antiviral medications (i.e., acyclovir, ganciclovir) do not alter clinical course

J. Complications
 1. Rare upper airway obstruction due to severe tonsillar enlargement; prompt consultation with otolaryngologist indicated
 2. Splenic rupture: rare but serious complication
 3. Hodgkin and Burkitt lymphomas associated with EBV infection

K. Duration/prognosis
 1. Most patients recover completely
 2. Fatigue may persist for weeks to months

L. Prevention
 1. Patients with confirmed mononucleosis: no full sports for at least 3 weeks after onset of illness (and spleen should no longer be palpable) to decrease risk of splenic rupture
 2. Some clinicians do not recommend return to sports until patient regains sense of well-being
 3. Imaging to determine splenic size not usually needed

XIX. Tickborne Infections

A. Characteristics
 1. Most common in U.S.: Lyme disease, RMSF, human monocytic ehrlichiosis (HME), human granulocytic ehrlichiosis (HGE), and tularemia
 2. Less common: tickborne relapsing fever, Colorado tick fever, southern tick-associated rash illness (STARI), tick paralysis, and babesiosis (Table 10-9)
 3. Epidemiology: seen across U.S. but have some geographic restrictions (see Table 10-9)
  a. Tick bites can occur year round, so clinician must have high index of suspicion in areas where disease is present
  b. History of known tick bite is often not consistent, especially when young nymph ticks cause infection because they are so small (1–2 mm)

QUICK HIT

A negative history for tick bites or removed ticks does not rule out tickborne infection.

TABLE 10-9 Vectors and Organisms of Tickborne Illness in the U.S.

Illness	Causative Organism	Vector	Geographic Distribution
Lyme disease	*Borrelia burgdorferi*	Black legged or deer tick (*Ixodes scapularis*)	Northeast U.S., Great Lakes region, small area northern California
Rocky Mountain spotted fever (RMSF)	*Rickettsia rickettsii*	Wood tick (*Dermacentor andersoni*) Dog tick (*Dermacentor variabilis*)	Limited to Western Hemisphere; all states except Maine, Hawaii, and Alaska Common to eastern and southern states
Human monocytic ehrlichiosis (HME)	*Ehrlichia chaffeensis*	Lone star tick (*Amblyomma americanum*)	South central U.S.
Human granulocytic ehrlichiosis (HGE)	*Anaplasma phagocytophilum*	Black legged or deer tick (*I. scapularis*)	Upper midwest and northeastern U.S.
Tularemia	*Francisella tularensis*	Lone star tick (*A. americanum*)	Rural areas, reported in all states but Hawaii; highest in south central and southeast U.S. Additional risk exposures include living or dead rabbits, squirrels, or other rodents
Babesiosis	*Babesia microti*	Black legged or deer tick (*I. scapularis*)	Northeast U.S.
Tickborne relapsing fever (TRF)	*Borrelia* spp.	Soft ticks (*Ornithodoros* spp.)	West of the Mississippi, primarily mountain states
Colorado tick fever	*Coltivirus* (RNA *Orbivirus*)	Wood tick (*D. andersoni*)	Rocky Mountain states
Southern tick-associated rash illness (STARI)	Unknown *Borrelia* species	Lone star tick (*A. americanum*)	South central U.S.

Infectious Diseases

4. Risk factors: outdoor exposures, dog exposures (ticks may transfer from dog to patient without outdoor exposures), prolonged tick attachment
   a. Severe illness may be seen in immunocompromised
   b. Risk factors for severe infection and increased mortality include prolonged symptoms prior to presentation (>5 days)
5. Pathophysiology
   a. Most tickborne illnesses: prolonged tick attachment (>24 hours) required to transmit infection
   b. RMSF: *R. rickettsii* enters skin and then spreads through bloodstream; most disease is due to infection and inflammation of endothelial cells of all major tissues and blood vessels, although many other cell types can also be infected
   c. Ehrlichiosis: WBCs are infected (granulocytes in HGE and monocytes in HME), which leads to perivascular inflammation and inflammation through mechanisms that are not fully understood
   d. Lyme disease: *B. burgdorferi* is inoculated into skin and starts to spread locally
      i. Days to weeks later, organism disseminated either hematogenously or lymphatically to multiple sites and can adhere to and infect many cell types
      ii. Organisms can persist in tissues for prolonged period, leading to symptoms sometimes several months after initial infection
   e. Tularemia: tick bite results in introduction of *Francisella tularensis* in skin and invasion of regional lymph nodes, which can then lead to hematogenous dissemination to other organs
      i. Organism can also be introduced by respiratory route, which results in fulminant pneumonia and sepsis
      ii. *F. tularensis* is intracellular parasite that can survive inside macrophages
   f. Babesiosis: parasite attaches to and infects RBCs (like in malaria) and can lead to hemolysis and acute renal failure
      i. Most cases are asymptomatic or mild and self-limited
      ii. Asplenia is a risk factor for severe disease

B. Clinical features
1. Historical findings: questions should focus on exposures/travel, severity, and duration; also do careful ROS
2. Physical exam findings
   a. Lyme disease: erythema migrans (classic rash) with 3 phases: early, localized; early, disseminated; and late disease (Table 10-10)
   b. Tularemia: regional tender adenopathy (ulceroglandular or glandular form)
   c. RMSF: classic petechial rash with peripheral distribution starting at ankles and wrists and moving centrally; palms and soles usually involved
   d. Ehrlichiosis: clinically presents almost identically to RMSF but only 1/3 of children have rash, which is usually maculopapular (usually in HME)
   e. *Ehrlichia* and RMSF can also cause CNS infection and may present with CNS symptoms and signs

QUICK HIT

In symptomatic patients with Lyme disease, 90% will have the classic erythema migrans rash.

QUICK HIT

As few as 10 organisms of *F. tularensis* can cause clinical disease, making *F. tularensis* a potential bioterrorism agent. Warn the lab if this organism is a possibility.

QUICK HIT

The triad of fever, headache, and rash is highly suggestive of tickborne infection.

QUICK HIT

In RMSF, rash begins 3–5 days after onset of symptoms; up to 15% have no rash or atypical rash.

QUICK HIT

Coinfection with *B. burgdorferi* (Lyme disease) and babesiosis is common in endemic areas. Doxycycline will treat both, but amoxicillin will only treat Lyme disease.

TABLE 10-10 **Stages of Lyme Disease**

Stage	Time of Onset/Presentation	Clinical Presentation
Early localized disease	8–14 days (range, 3–32 days)	Erythema migrans rash, fever, constitutional symptoms (myalgias, arthralgias, fatigue, headache), lymphadenopathy
Early disseminated disease	4–6 weeks (range, 3–10 weeks)	Erythema migrans rash (may be multiple), fever, constitutional symptoms, facial palsies (cranial nerve VII), meningitis, carditis (rare), radiculopathy
Late disease	2–12 months	Arthritis (usually recurrent, knee most common joint), peripheral neuropathy, CNS involvement

CNS, central nervous system.

f. STARI: erythema migrans, fever, and constitutional symptoms in an individual who has not been to an endemic Lyme area; most common in south central U.S.

C. Diagnosis
1. Differential diagnosis: extremely broad given nonspecific presentation of fever, constitutional symptoms
   a. Considerations include viruses (EBV, CMV, adenovirus, measles)
   b. More severe tickborne infections can mimic serious illnesses, such as meningococcemia (especially RMSF), toxic shock syndrome (TSS), sepsis, and Kawasaki syndrome
   c. Ulceroglandular tularemia may present similarly to *Bartonella* infection or lymphadenitis from bacterial or viral etiologies
   d. Babesia may mimic malaria in presentation
2. Laboratory findings
   a. CBC: leukopenia, thrombocytopenia, and, occasionally, anemia
   b. Liver function tests (LFTs): elevated AST, low albumin
   c. Most diagnostic studies have turnaround of days to weeks, so it is usually necessary to treat suspected tickborne illness empirically based on clinical suspicion because delayed time to treatment results in worse outcomes
   d. Multiple diagnostics exist (Table 10-11)
   e. CSF pleocytosis can be seen in RMSF, Lyme disease, HGE, and HME
3. Radiology studies: generally not part of initial evaluation of patient with tickborne infection (unless assessing for suppurative lymph nodes in tularemia)

D. Treatment
1. Therapy
   a. RMSF, ehrlichiosis (both HME and HGE), and tickborne relapsing: doxycycline in all ages, usually for 7–10 days with at least 3 days of therapy after defervescence
   b. Lyme disease and STARI
      i. Doxycycline for 14–21 days
      ii. Amoxicillin or cefuroxime for children age <8 years
      iii. IV ceftriaxone for 28 days in late disease meningitis and arthritis
   c. Tularemia: IV gentamicin for 7 days
   d. Babesiosis
      i. Quinine + clindamycin for at least 7 days
      ii. Most individuals with splenic function will not require treatment

> **QUICK HIT**
> RMSF and ehrlichiosis often present with hyponatremia, hypoalbuminemia, and thrombocytopenia.

> **QUICK HIT**
> Dental staining from a single 7–10-day course of doxycycline for treatment of rickettsial disease is likely not significant in children <8 years of age.

TABLE 10-11 Diagnostics for Tickborne Infections

Tickborne Infection	Available Diagnostics (Preferred Bolded)
Lyme disease	**Serology**—Enzyme-linked immunosorbent assay (ELISA) with confirmatory Western blot; many causes of false-positive ELISA, so Western blot must confirm all positive ELISA. Lyme titers must be interpreted in context of patient and likelihood of exposure. Serology persists for life and cannot distinguish active from resolved infection. Note in early localized disease, serology is negative and, if treated, patients may not develop a positive Lyme antibody. **PCR on joint fluid for Lyme arthritis**
Ehrlichiosis (HME, HGE)	**PCR**, serology, immunohistochemistry, morula on blood smear (insensitive)
RMSF	**Serology** (paired acute and convalescent ideal), current PCRs have suboptimal sensitivity, immunohistochemistry
Tularemia	**Serology**, culture (avoid culturing if possible and always notify lab if possible culture sent)
Babesiosis	**Demonstration of organism on thick/thin smears, serology**, PCR (not widely available)
STARI	Clinical diagnosis; no specific testing available; testing for Lyme disease is negative in STARI patients
Tick relapsing fever	**Dark-field examination of peripheral blood smear during febrile episode**; associated findings include elevated WBC, ESR, CSF pleocytosis
Colorado tick fever	**Viral isolation from blood, immunofluorescent exam of peripheral smear**, serology, PCR

CSF, cerebrospinal fluid; ESR, erythrocyte sedimentation rate; HGE, human granulocytic ehrlichiosis; HME, human monocytic ehrlichiosis; PCR, polymerase chain reaction; RMSF, Rocky Mountain spotted fever; STARI, southern tick-associated rash illness; WBC, white blood cell.

e. Colorado tick fever: supportive care
f. Tick paralysis: tick removal
2. Complications
a. RMSF: prolonged symptoms prior to starting therapy will result in slower response to therapy (in 1 study, therapy started after >5 days of symptoms increased mortality from 6.5% to 23%)
b. Lyme disease: patients may develop **Jarisch-Herxheimer reaction** (fever, rigors, malaise, diaphoresis) usually within 12 hours of treatment due to bacteriolysis; treat with nonsteroidal anti-inflammatory drugs
3. Duration/prognosis
a. If caught early and treated appropriately, most children with tickborne illnesses do well and recover with defervescence within 48–72 hours of starting therapy
b. Constitutional symptoms (myalgias, arthralgias, headaches) may persist for days to weeks in some patients

E. Prevention
1. Avoid tick-infested areas
2. Wear protective light-colored clothing (long pants, long sleeves)
3. DEET repellent
4. Spray clothing with permethrin
5. Promptly remove attached ticks and do regular tick checks after outdoor activity; transmission requires prolonged attachment

QUICK HIT

Pyelonephritis can lead to long-term complications, such as renal scarring, hypertension, and renal failure. Because it is difficult to differentiate pyelonephritis from cystitis in young children, they are generally considered and treated as indistinguishable in those age <2 years.

XX. Urinary Tract Infections

A. General characteristics
1. Infection of any part of urinary tract; generally caused by ascending infection beyond neonatal period
2. Prevalence ~7% in febrile young children but varies by subpopulation (see 4. Risk factors)
3. Usually caused by bacteria: *E. coli* (accounts for 85%), *Klebsiella*, *Proteus*, *Enterobacter*, *Citrobacter*, *Staphylococcus*, and *Enterococcus* species; rarely viral and fungal pathogens
4. Risk factors: personal or family history of childhood UTI, urinary tract or renal anatomic abnormality, vesicoureteral reflux (VUR), female sex, uncircumcised male, white race, age <1 year in boys and <4 years in girls, neurogenic bladder, catheterization, dysfunctional elimination, sexual activity in females, alteration of normal periurethral flora (recent antibiotic use, spermicide use in females)

QUICK HIT

Another potential source of fever does not rule out a UTI, so urine cultures may be helpful in young children with high fevers, even in the presence of a URI, otitis, or gastroenteritis.

B. Clinical features
1. Symptoms
a. Age <2 years: fever (especially >39°C) often only symptom; other symptoms include irritability, abdominal pain, poor feeding, elevated bilirubin, or poor growth in newborns
b. Age >2 years: fever, dysuria, frequency, urgency, incontinence, abdominal or back pain, hematuria; pyelonephritis suggested by fever, chills, flank pain, and vomiting
2. Signs

QUICK HIT

Nitrites are very specific but not very sensitive because urine must remain in the bladder >4 hours to form nitrites.

C. Diagnosis
1. Labs
a. Dipstick for macroscopic evaluation: blood, leukocyte esterase, and nitrites suggestive of UTI
b. Microscopic examination: presence of WBCs and bacteria highly suggestive of UTI
c. Urine culture: gold standard for diagnosis
i. Recommended for confirmation in any at-risk patient regardless of macroscopic and microscopic results
ii. Results with sensitivity help guide proper treatment; should be processed soon after collection

QUICK HIT

Catheterization or suprapubic specimens are necessary in non–toilet-trained patients; clean-catch specimens are adequate only in toilet-trained children.

d. Other labs: CBC, ESR, CRP can be helpful but not specific
   i. Serum creatinine (Cr) should be followed in patients with history of several UTIs to evaluate for renal damage
   ii. Blood culture and LP only for very ill children and neonates
2. Differential diagnosis: occult bacteremia (especially in young febrile infants), vulvovaginitis, urinary tract calculi, sexually transmitted disease, vaginal foreign body, appendicitis, Kawasaki disease, strep infection, dysfunctional elimination

D. Management
1. Antibiotic therapy: early empiric treatment in patients at high risk for UTI essential to preventing short- and long-term complications
2. Choice of antibiotic depends on likely organism (Gram stain may be helpful), history of prior sensitivities of cultured organisms, local resistance patterns, and recent antibiotic use
   a. 1st- or 3rd-generation cephalosporins are often used
   b. Culture and sensitivity results crucial for determining definitive therapy
   c. IV antibiotics and hospitalization indicated for age <2 months, ill appearance, failure to respond to or inability to tolerate PO medication (e.g., vomiting), dehydration, lack of adequate outpatient follow-up, immunocompromised patient
   d. Duration: 7–14 days for febrile children; 3–5 days for afebrile immunocompetent older children
3. Imaging workup
   a. Renal ultrasound to evaluate for renal abscess (during severe or nonresponding illness) and for obstruction or anatomic abnormalities (after acute illness) suggested in those age <2 years, poor response to antibiotics, recurrent febrile UTI, or family history of renal or urologic abnormality or hypertension
   b. Voiding cystourethrogram (VCUG) to detect VUR is warranted only in those with multiple UTIs, family history of renal or urologic abnormality, hypertension, poor growth, unusual pathogen, or abnormality on renal ultrasound

E. Complications: renal scarring leading to hypertension and decreased renal function (risks include recurrent UTIs, delay in treatment of UTIs, VUR, anatomic urinary obstruction, dysfunctional elimination), renal abscess, urosepsis

F. Prevention of complications from recurrent UTI
1. Controversial recommendations regarding prophylactic antibiotic use after febrile UTI; most advise it if VCUG is done and shows grades III–V VUR or potentially after recurrent UTI
2. Close follow-up after febrile UTI to ensure appropriate blood pressure and growth
3. After first febrile UTI, children should be evaluated promptly for any signs of recurrent infection

XXI. Skin and Soft Tissue Infections

A. **Cellulitis** and **erysipelas**
1. Infections of skin manifesting as skin erythema, edema, tenderness, and swelling; often with regional lymphadenitis and lymphangitis; may be complicated by abscess
2. Characteristics
   a. Cellulitis involves dermis and subcutaneous fat; often subacute in onset
      i. Commonly caused by β-hemolytic streptococci and *S. aureus*
      ii. Less commonly caused by gram-negative bacilli, *H. influenzae*, pneumococcus, meningococcus (Figure 10-2)
   b. Erysipelas involves upper dermis and superficial lymphatics and presents as raised area with clear demarcation from surrounding skin
      i. Generally acute in onset with fever and chills
      ii. Usually caused by β-hemolytic streptococci
      iii. Commonly complicated by bacteremia
   c. May involve vesicles, bullae, ecchymoses, petechiae, *peau d'orange*
3. Risk factors: compromise in skin barrier (wound, inflammation, current infections, eczema, edema), lymphatic obstruction

FIGURE 10-2 ***Haemophilus influenzae*** **type b periorbital cellulitis due to this invasive bacterial disease.**

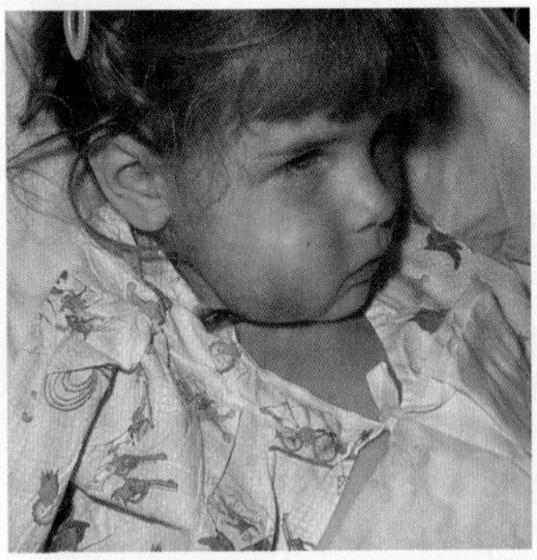

(Photo courtesy of American Academy of Pediatrics.)

4. Diagnosis
   a. Generally made clinically
   b. Cultures of blood, pus, or bullae useful in patients with large areas of involvement, systemic illness, immunodeficiency, animal bites
   c. Differential diagnosis: TSS, necrotizing fasciitis, osteomyelitis, erythema migrans, herpes zoster, contact dermatitis, allergic reaction, insect bite
5. Treatment
   a. Nonpurulent cellulitis
      i. Oral antibiotics if not systemically ill (e.g., cephalexin, clindamycin, doxycycline if age >8 years)
      ii. IV antibiotics if ill or for failed PO therapy
   b. Erysipelas
      i. Usually IV antibiotics to cover strep, with transition to PO when improved
      ii. Oral antibiotics for mild cases

B. **Impetigo** (superficial pyoderma)
1. Superficial bacterial infection manifesting as "honey-crusted" weeping lesions, mostly seen in children ages 2–5 years; usually caused by GABHS or *S. aureus* and very contagious
2. Risk factors: compromise in skin barrier (wound, eczema, minor trauma, scabies), warm and humid environment, crowding, poor hygiene, carriage of GABHS or *S. aureus*, immunocompromise
3. Variants
   a. Nonbullous (most common)
      i. Erythematous surrounding with papules progressing over 5–7 days to vesicles and then to pustules, which break down, forming classic thick golden-colored crust
      ii. Well-localized; usually without systemic symptoms
      iii. Often on face or extremities (Figure 10-3)

FIGURE 10-3 **Impetigo. Dried, stuck-on–appearing, "honey-crusted" lesions in a typical location.**

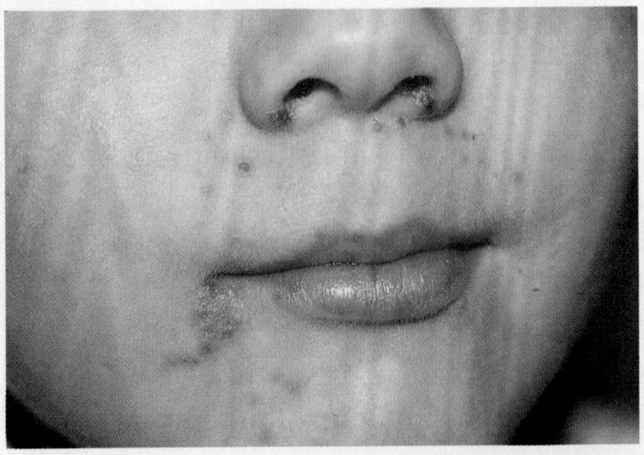

(From Goodheart HP. *Goodheart's Photoguide of Common Skin Disorders.* 2nd ed. Philadelphia: Lippincott Williams & Wilkins; 2003.)

Infectious Diseases

FIGURE 10-4 Bullous impetigo.

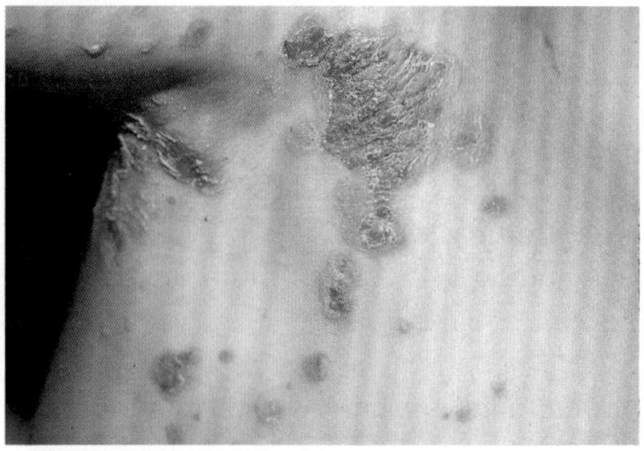

(From Goodheart HP. *Goodheart's Photoguide of Common Skin Disorders.* 2nd ed. Philadelphia: Lippincott Williams & Wilkins; 2003.)

b. Bullous
   i. Vesicles enlarge and form bullae, which break down forming darker brown and thinner crust
   ii. Usually fewer lesions than with bullous impetigo; more often on trunk (Figure 10-4)
c. **Ecthyma** (ulcerative impetigo): extends into dermis forming "punched-out" ulcers covered by yellow crust and surrounded by raised bluish purple coloring (Figure 10-5)

4. Diagnosis
   a. Generally made clinically
   b. Cultures of pus/bullous fluid may help if nonresponsive to empiric therapy
   c. Serologic testing not helpful for diagnosis
   d. Differential diagnosis: contact dermatitis, eczema, Stevens-Johnsons syndrome, herpes simplex, bullous pemphigoid
5. Treatment
   a. Topical antibiotics (such as mupirocin) or hydrogen peroxide cream if small area with no bullae
   b. Oral antibiotics for large areas or bullous lesions
   c. Choice based on local MRSA prevalence and susceptibility patterns; 7–10-day course
   d. Complications: **poststreptococcal glomerulonephritis** known complication even following appropriate treatment; usually occurs 1–3 weeks after
6. Prevention: handwashing

FIGURE 10-5 Ecthyma on the buttocks of a 13-year-old boy.

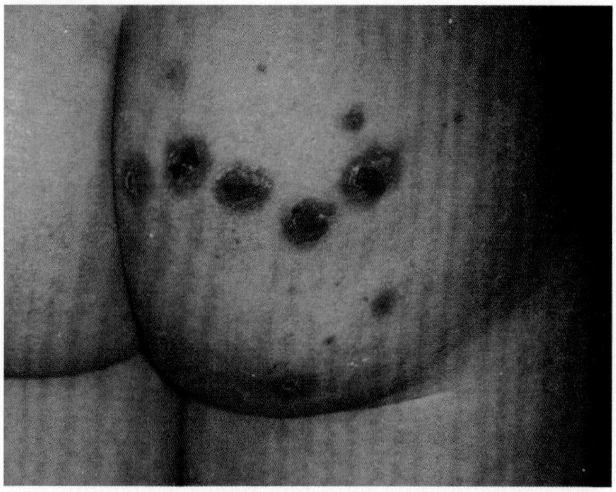

(From Sauer GC, Hall JC. *Manual of Skin Diseases.* 7th ed. Philadelphia: Lippincott-Raven; 1996.)

QUICK HIT

Doppler ultrasound is the best way to differentiate between an abscess near a major blood vessel and a vascular malformation, which is essential insofar as incising a vascular malformation can lead to life-threatening hemorrhage.

QUICK HIT

A specialist should be consulted for abscesses in the perirectal or pilonidal area, anterior or lateral neck, central face, breast, hand, or any area in close proximity to major nerves or vessels.

QUICK HIT

Studies have had conflicting conclusions about the benefit of antibiotics in short-term resolution and in decreasing recurrence rates.

C. Abscess
   1. Collection of pus within dermis and deeper skin tissue
      a. Presents with pain, tenderness, erythema, swelling, and fluctuance
      b. Often surrounded with cellulitis, with or without drainage and regional lymphadenopathy
      c. Fever and systemic symptoms less common
   2. Risk factors: *S. aureus* colonization, close contacts with abscesses, immunocompromise, breach in skin barrier (e.g., trauma, wound)
   3. Most commonly caused by *S. aureus* (including MRSA), but multiple other pathogens can be involved
   4. Diagnosis
      a. Generally made clinically, based on fluctuance or failure to respond to systemic antibiotic therapy
      b. Cultures of fluid indicated when abscess drained to help guide potential antibiotic therapy
      c. Ultrasound sometimes used to determine drainable fluid collections; predictive value uncertain in children
      d. Differential diagnosis: cellulitis with no drainable fluid collection, herpetic whitlow, kerion in tinea capitis, cyst, hidradenitis suppurativa, vascular malformation
   5. Treatment
      a. Incision and drainage: necessary element of treatment for majority of abscesses (although some small, spontaneously draining abscesses may be observed clinically for resolution first)
      b. IV or PO antibiotics (e.g., clindamycin, trimethoprim-sulfamethoxazole) indicated for large or multiple abscesses, systemic illness, immunocompromise, or poor response
      c. Recurrence in patients and close contacts is common problem; decolonization attempts with nasal mupirocin-chlorhexidine showers with or without antibiotics only transiently eradicate colonization
      d. Prevention: good handwashing, covering draining wounds to minimize contact and spread of contagious drainage, use of disinfectants on exposed surfaces, frequent washing, and not sharing linens/towels, etc.

XXII. Septic Arthritis

A. Characteristics: bacterial infection of synovium and joint space with subsequent inflammation (also called **pyogenic arthritis**)
B. Epidemiology
   1. 50% of cases occur in infants and children age <3 years
   2. Primarily occurs in lower extremities, typically in 1 joint
   3. Hip joint most commonly involved in infants; knee in older children
   4. *S. aureus* is predominant pathogen (Table 10-12)
C. Risk factors for infection
   1. Concomitant osteomyelitis
   2. Instrumentation of joint
   3. IV drug usage, sickle cell disease, and risky sexual behaviors predispose patients to unusual pathogens
D. Pathophysiology
   1. In most cases, highly vascular synovium is infected through hematogenous spread
   2. Other mechanisms: invasion of organisms from nearby infection (osteomyelitis) or penetrating injuries into joint space that allow direct inoculation
E. Clinical features
   1. Historical findings (symptoms)
      a. Pain is most common presenting complaint with history of fever
      b. Younger child may present with limp; older child will localize pain better
      c. Refusal to ambulate or move affected area (pseudoparalysis)
   2. Physical exam findings (signs)
      a. Fever, sick-appearing child
      b. More subtle in neonate and young infant: septic appearance, irritability, unilateral swelling of extremity

QUICK HIT

Neonates and infants age <1 year with septic arthritis should have an MRI to detect concomitant osteomyelitis. Transphyseal vessels connecting the bone or the joint space recede after the 1st year of life.

QUICK HIT

Referred pain from the hip may be reported as groin, thigh, or knee pain.

TABLE 10-12 **Common Causes of Septic Arthritis by Age and Risk Factors**

Age/Risk Factors	Common Bacterial Etiology
Neonate to <2 months	*Staphylococcus aureus* Group B *Streptococcus* Gram-negative bacilli
>2 months to 5 years	*Staphylococcus aureus* Group A β-hemolytic *Streptococcus* *Streptococcus pneumoniae* *Kingella kingae**
>5 years	*Staphylococcus aureus* Group A β-hemolytic *Streptococcus* *Streptococcus pneumoniae*
Sickle cell disease	*Salmonella* *Staphylococcus aureus*
Foot puncture wound	*Pseudomonas aeruginosa* *Staphylococcus aureus*
History of IV drug usage	*P. aeruginosa*
History of sexual activity	*Neisseria gonorrhoeae*

*Typically in those age <36 months.

c. Involved joint will have obvious erythema, warmth, swelling *except* in hip joint due to deep location of joint, and significant pain with movement or weight bearing

d. Limited range of motion (ROM) of affected joint with positioning of affected limb to optimize intracapsular volume and minimize pain

F. Diagnosis

1. Differential diagnosis
   a. Transient synovitis
   b. Other common causes of single-joint inflammation include reactive arthritis, Lyme arthritis, rheumatoid arthritis, SLE, cellulitis, traumatic synovitis, and sympathetic effusion from adjacent osteomyelitis
2. Laboratory findings
   a. Elevated WBC count, ESR, and CRP (septic arthritis has elevated CRP at presentation in 90% of cases)
   b. Arthrocentesis for synovial fluid if septic arthritis suspected
      i. WBC count >100,000/mm^3 with neutrophil predominance
      ii. Positive Gram stain
      iii. Synovial fluid culture is positive in 50% of cases
   c. Blood culture can identify organism; helpful when organism is not isolated from synovial fluid
3. Radiology findings
   a. Plain x-rays may show effusion, rule out fracture or osteomyelitis; however, normal x-ray does not rule out septic arthritis
   b. Ultrasound most useful in identification and quantification of joint fluid
   c. MRI with contrast is sensitive for early detection and can identify cartilaginous involvement

G. Treatment

1. Therapy
   a. Early and effective therapy in collaboration with orthopedic surgeons and infectious disease specialists is essential to prevent permanent destruction of cartilage and ischemic injury to bone
   b. Immediate aspiration of synovial fluid to decompress intracapsular space, remove infected fluid, and provide specimens to be studied

QUICK HIT

It is important to distinguish arthritis from arthralgia; patients with arthralgia have joint paint *without* inflammatory findings of warmth, erythema, tenderness, and swelling.

QUICK HIT

Hip pain or limp in a child with a recent history of URI may suggest transient synovitis as the diagnosis in a relatively well-appearing child.

QUICK HIT

Inoculating joint fluid into a blood culture bottle increases yield of joint fluid culture from 50% to 75%.

c. Empiric IV antibiotic therapy based on most likely organism for age, local sensitivities, and results of synovial fluid Gram stain
   i. Gram-negative coverage should be used in neonates and adolescents
   ii. Antibiotics should be given for 3–4 weeks depending on organism and location; can switch from IV to PO antibiotics once clinical improvement occurs and CRP has declined (some centers use >50% CRP decline to guide switch to PO)
d. Surgical intervention including irrigation and drainage of joint typically required for hip or shoulder joint infections or when patient does not improve with IV antibiotics

2. Complications are associated with
   a. Delay in diagnosis and treatment of 4 days or longer
   b. Age <6 months
   c. Infection with *S. aureus* or gram-negative bacteria
   d. Osteomyelitis of adjacent bone
   e. Involvement of hip or shoulder
3. Prognosis
   a. Timely diagnosis and treatment provide best outcome
   b. Long-term sequelae due to complications may occur
      i. Avascular necrosis of femoral head in septic arthritis of hip
      ii. Limb-length disparities
      iii. Pseudoarthrosis, joint dislocations, and other bony/joint malformations

XXIII. Acute Osteomyelitis

A. General characteristics
   1. Bacterial infection of bone that can occur via 3 mechanisms: hematogenous, direct inoculation, or local spread by adjacent infection
   2. Most cases in pediatrics are hematogenous
   3. Younger children (age <5 years) are most often affected; much more common in pediatrics than in adults
   4. Boys are affected twice as often as girls
   5. Often associated with minor trauma
   6. 80% of infections are in tubular bones and 50% involve femur, tibia, or fibula
   7. Discitis and vertebral osteomyelitis = small percentage of cases
   8. Risk factors include sickle cell disease, immunodeficiency, bacteremia, and indwelling catheters
   9. *S. aureus* is most common organism (>50% of culture-positive cases); other causes are described in Box 10-14
B. Pathophysiology
   1. Children are often transiently bacteremic, and bacteria enter bone through metaphysis
C. Clinical features
   1. Historical findings (symptoms)
      a. Early symptoms are nonspecific and include low-grade fever and malaise
      b. Gradual onset with symptoms developing over days to weeks

QUICK HIT

CA-MRSA is increasingly identified as a cause of osteomyelitis.

BOX 10-14

Causes of Acute Hematogenous Osteomyelitis Other Than *Staphylococcus aureus*

- Group A *Streptococcus*
- *Streptococcus pneumoniae*
- *Kingella kingae*
- *Haemophilus influenzae* type b in the unvaccinated patient
- *Salmonella* (sickle cell disease)
- Atypical *Mycobacterium*
- *Bartonella henselae* (cat-scratch disease)
- *Brucella* species
- Group B *Streptococcus* (neonates)
- *Escherichia coli* or other gram-negative organisms (neonates)

c. Eventually localized pain and swelling
d. Child may develop limp if lower extremity or hip affected
2. Physical exam findings (signs)
a. Redness, swelling, pain at infection site
b. Loss of function or limited ROM

D. Diagnosis
1. Differential diagnosis: leukemia, tumor, fracture, septic arthritis
2. Labs: CBC with differential, blood culture, ESR, and CRP
3. Radiology
a. Plain films
i. Usually negative early in infection
ii. Later (2–4 weeks) findings include lytic sclerosis, periosteal new bone formation, and periosteal elevation
b. MRI confirms diagnosis and evaluates for bone abscess formation; can also guide surgical intervention
c. Bone scan can be useful if osteomyelitis is suspected but there are no localizing symptoms (e.g., neonates, vertebral or pelvic osteomyelitis)

E. Treatment
1. Debridement and evacuation of abscess should be done as soon as possible
2. Surgery can be diagnostic and therapeutic (by yielding organism)
3. Immobilization can treat pain and help prevent pathologic fractures
4. Empiric antibiotic treatment should cover CA-MRSA
5. Antibiotics may be deferred until after bone biopsy in clinically stable patients
a. Neonates: vancomycin and cefotaxime
b. Older children: clindamycin
c. Exceptions: clinically ill patients should receive vancomycin with or without clindamycin or oxacillin; linezolid may be used for vancomycin or clindamycin intolerance
6. Total duration of antibiotics is usually 4–6 weeks; initially, antibiotics are given parenterally
7. Transition to oral antibiotics is reasonable for patients with prompt clinical response, substantive decline in CRP, and no barriers to antibiotic absorption
8. ESR and CRP are followed during treatment to monitor response
a. CRP starts to decrease 2–3 days after treatment and is normal by 7–10 days
b. ESR starts to decrease 5–7 days after treatment and is normal by 3–4 weeks
9. Prognosis is excellent with virtually all cases resulting in complete resolution of symptoms; chronic osteomyelitis may require surgical debridement and >3 months of antibiotics

QUICK HIT

Children with osteomyelitis will generally tolerate passive ROM, whereas children with septic arthritis will have significant pain with passive ROM.

QUICK HIT

Nonspecific abdominal pain may be the most prominent complaint in children with pelvic or lumbar vertebral osteomyelitis.

QUICK HIT

Approximately 1/3–1/2 of all cases of osteomyelitis are culture-negative and no organism is ever identified.

XXIV. Human Immunodeficiency Virus Infection

A. Characteristics
1. Positive single-stranded RNA retrovirus that primarily infects humans; can progress to AIDS if not treated
2. Transmitted from mother to infant via 3 routes: transplacental, intrapartum (most common), and postpartum (via breastfeeding); also transmitted sexually or by shared needles in older children and adolescents
3. Mother-to-child transmission (vertical transmission) in U.S. has declined and is currently <200 infants born annually nationwide
4. Transmission among adolescents and young adults is rising; 50% of new HIV patients are ages 13–29 years in U.S.
5. HIV infects CD4 T cells of immune system, which help coordinate and direct entire immune response; when number of CD4 cells falls below set thresholds for age, immune system weakens and becomes susceptible to opportunistic infections signaling AIDS development
6. Genetics: no clear genetic predisposition; however, individuals with mutations in *CCR5* (coreceptor for HIV entry into cells) are less likely to become infected with HIV, and they also have slower progression of disease if they do become infected

QUICK HIT

Fluids that can transmit HIV are blood, vaginal secretions, semen, and breast milk.

QUICK HIT

Untreated mothers transmit HIV to their infants in 25%–50% of cases; risk depends on maternal viral load, timing of maternal HIV infection, and maternal CD4 count, among other factors.

QUICK HIT

Treatment of the HIV-exposed infant with zidovudine (AZT) for 6 weeks + 3 doses of nevirapine *or* AZT for 6 weeks + nelfinavir and lamivudine for 2 weeks decreases peripartum transmission of HIV to <3%.

7. Traditional risk factors for HIV acquisition of homosexual sex and shared needles are out of date given rise in heterosexual transmission in U.S.; >80% of women acquire HIV through heterosexual sex in U.S.

B. Clinical progression
1. HIV-infected children progress more rapidly than adults in development of immune dysfunction and resultant illness
2. Vertically acquired HIV can be divided into 3 categories
   a. **Rapid progressors** (80%–85%): present with opportunistic infections, failure to thrive (FTT), and encephalopathy at median age of 4 months; without treatment, they may survive 2–4 years
   b. **Slow progressors** (15%): more indolent course with median age of onset of symptoms and evidence of immune compromise at age 6 years; without treatment, they can live to adolescence
   c. **Nonprogressors** (<5%): clinically asymptomatic and have normal CD4 counts with low-level viral loads without therapy

C. Historical findings (symptoms)
1. Infants: poor weight gain, developmental delay, frequent infections including severe thrush, bacterial infection (otitis, pneumonias, skin infections, etc.), chronic diarrhea, and recurrent fevers (and FUO)
2. Adolescents (who acquire HIV behaviorally): asymptomatic until CD4 counts decline when they present with opportunistic infections such as oral thrush
   a. ~50% may present with primary HIV infection 2–4 weeks after acquiring infection, which mimics nonspecific viral illness such as mononucleosis with fever, sore throat, malaise, rash, painful adenopathy, and weight loss
   b. Acute symptoms usually resolve after 2 weeks
3. Screen for symptoms consistent with opportunistic infections when considering diagnosis of HIV in patient of any age

D. Physical exam findings
1. Infants: FUO, poor growth, developmental delay, oral thrush, hepatosplenomegaly, lymphadenopathy, chronic parotitis
2. Adolescents: present with findings consistent with opportunistic infections such as thrush; in acute HIV, they may have fever, pharyngitis, maculopapular rash, diffuse lymphadenopathy, and hepatosplenomegaly
3. Also assess for findings consistent with opportunistic infections, such as fever, thrush, respiratory distress, rash, and any localizing findings

E. Diagnosis
1. Differential diagnosis
   a. Infant
      i. Primary immune deficiencies (e.g., severe combined immune deficiency)
      ii. Congenital infections (e.g., syphilis)
      iii. Other infections (e.g., disseminated histoplasmosis, TB)
   b. Adolescents: may present with acute HIV, which can mimic mononucleosis caused by EBV or CMV, other viral infections such as influenza, hepatitis A and B, toxoplasmosis, and secondary syphilis
2. Laboratory findings
   a. Diagnosis of HIV is usually done by serologic testing (HIV enzyme-linked immunosorbent assay [ELISA])
      i. Until recently, recommended confirmatory testing had been Western blot (protein immunoassay)
      ii. Newer HIV ELISA tests have increased in sensitivity and will detect infection before Western blot becomes positive
      iii. Preferred confirmatory test is separate HIV1/HIV discriminatory immunoassay to confirm ELISA result and PCR testing for individuals who are screen positive but are negative on second screen
      iv. In infants age <18 months, HIV ELISA reflects maternal antibody, so PCR-based testing for presence of virus in blood must be used to make diagnosis

QUICK HIT

The highest incidence of progression to AIDS occurs in HIV-infected infants age <1 year; young children may also develop opportunistic infections despite relatively higher CD4 counts.

QUICK HIT

The most common opportunistic infection in infants >1 year of age is *P. jiroveci* (formerly *P. carinii*) pneumonia.

QUICK HIT

Primary HIV infection should be considered in any acute unexplained febrile illness in sexually active patients or patients with other high-risk behaviors.

QUICK HIT

HIV ELISA testing is designed to be very sensitive but is not very specific; therefore, confirmatory testing is needed to weed out false positives, which can be due to other viral infections, collagen vascular disease, pregnancy, and other causes.

b. HIV infection can cause a number of laboratory abnormalities
   i. CBC: leukopenia, lymphopenia, anemia, thrombocytopenia
   ii. Urinalysis: proteinuria
   iii. LFTs: elevated AST and ALT
3. Radiology findings in HIV are usually due to opportunistic infections

F. Treatment
1. Combination antiretroviral therapy (cART, or HAART) usually comprising 3 active antiretroviral medications from at least 2 classes of HIV medications
   a. cART is highly effective at suppressing viral replication and maintaining normal CD4 count and immune function
   b. HIV resistance to cART drugs can emerge, especially with poor medication adherence
2. Complications
   a. Untreated HIV infection: opportunistic infections including *P. jiroveci* pneumonia, CMV, HSV, recurrent bacterial infections (otitis, pneumonias, meningitis, osteomyelitis, sepsis), fungal infections (candidiasis, cryptococcal infections, histoplasmosis), and TB among others
   b. Treated HIV: side effects of medications including short-term effects, such as GI side effects (diarrhea, nausea), rash, hypersensitivity reactions, neuropsychiatric symptoms, and long-term effects, such as hyperlipidemia, metabolic syndrome, neuropathy, lipodystrophy, and viral resistance in nonadherent patients

G. Prognosis
1. Currently no cure for HIV; therapy must be lifelong
2. On effective therapy, patients can do very well and live for decades with normal immune function
3. Survival correlates with degree of immune compromise and viral replication
   a. More immunosuppressed individuals have significantly shorter survival
   b. Individuals with ongoing viral replication also have shorter survival due to complications of chronic inflammation

H. Prevention
1. Prevention of vertical transmission
   a. Maternal antiretroviral therapy during pregnancy
   b. IV zidovudine (AZT) during labor
   c. To reduce peripartum transmission to <3%, infant receives
      i. AZT for 6 weeks OR
      ii. Nevirapine (3 doses) and then AZT for 6 weeks OR
      iii. Nelfinavir and lamivudine for 2 weeks and AZT for 6 weeks
2. Educating youth regarding safer sex practices and condom use is key to prevention of behavioral transmission
3. Strong evidence to support successful cART treatment of HIV+ individuals decreases transmission by them to others

XXV. Toxic Shock Syndrome

A. Definition: toxin-mediated illness that occurs with infection with strain of ***S. aureus*** that produces TSST-1 toxin, along with other toxins

B. Cause/pathophysiology
1. Bacterial exotoxins cause cellular death or dysfunction
2. Exotoxins act as **superantigens**, which activate T cells and lead to massive release of proinflammatory cytokines
3. Often cause effects distant to site of bacterial growth.
4. ~50% of TSS cases in U.S. are related to **tampon use during menstruation**; use of superabsorbent tampons or infrequent changing of tampons increases risk by allowing *S. aureus* to multiply and release toxin
5. Other 50% caused by wide variety of conditions that allow toxin-producing strains of *S. aureus* to multiply (e.g., postsurgical wound infections and other invasive *S. aureus* infections)

6. **Streptococcal TSS** is similar syndrome caused by exotoxin-producing strain of **GABHS**
   a. Patients typically develop symptoms in midst of streptococcal skin or soft tissue infection
   b. Clinically similar to TSS but not associated with tampon use

C. Clinical presentation
1. Defined by Centers for Disease Control and Prevention (CDC) as
   a. Fever >38.9°C (102.2°F)
   b. Blood pressure <90 mm Hg in adults (or <5th percentile for age in children)
   c. **Blanching erythematous rash or erythroderma** (resembling a diffuse sunburn) with subsequent desquamation
   d. Patient must have involvement in 3 or more organ systems
      i. GI (vomiting or diarrhea at illness onset)
      ii. Muscular involvement (creatine phosphokinase >2× upper limits of normal or severe myalgias)
      iii. Mucous membrane hyperemia (vaginal, oral, conjunctival mucosa)
      iv. Renal involvement (serum Cr >2× normal or urine microscopy ≥5 WBC per HPF)
      v. Hepatic (transaminases >2× normal)
      vi. Thrombocytopenia (<100,000/mm^3)
      vii. CNS involvement (altered level of consciousness when fever or hypertension is not present)
2. Negative results of following tests
   a. Throat culture, CSF culture, or blood culture (other than blood culture showing *S. aureus*)
   b. Serologic test for RMSF, leptospirosis, measles

D. Testing
1. CBC: leukocytosis with neutrophil predominance and immature band forms, thrombocytopenia, and anemia
2. DIC may be present
3. Blood urea nitrogen/Cr and creatine phosphokinase may be elevated
4. In staphylococcal TSS, cultures for *S. aureus* are more likely to be positive from site of infection rather than blood, whereas 70% of blood cultures are positive in streptococcal TSS

E. Therapy
1. Supportive care: aggressive fluid resuscitation and blood pressure support
2. Identify location of toxin production: remove any retained tampons and drain any focus of infection or abscess
3. Prompt initiation of IV antistaphylococcal antibiotics such as **vancomycin**
4. **Clindamycin**, a protein synthesis inhibitor, should be added to antimicrobial regimen in both staphylococcal and streptococcal TSS to decrease organism's ability to produce toxin
5. With improvement, patient can be switched to PO antistaphylococcal antibiotic, such as clindamycin or cephalexin
6. Intravenous immunoglobulin (IVIG) should be considered for children who do not respond to above-mentioned therapy

XXVI. Ventricular Shunt Infections

A. General characteristics
1. Definition
   a. CSF shunts divert CSF from brain to another part of body in hydrocephalus
   b. Proximal portion is placed in cerebral ventricle, and distal portion drains to peritoneum (VP shunt) or atrium (VA shunt)
      i. Externalized shunts, also known as **external ventricular drains (EVDs)**, are typically short-term devices to acutely divert CSF to allow clinician to monitor ICP

ii. Other externalized CNS devices (e.g., Ommaya reservoir) deliver antimicrobials or chemotherapy agents directly into abscess cavity or tumor (distal portion of Ommaya reservoir, which is typically placed under scalp and accessed with needle, can become infected)

B. Epidemiology
1. ~5%–15% of CSF shunts become infected
2. Children most at risk in 1st month after placement

C. Cause
1. Proximal shunt infections (Table 10-13)
   a. Proximal portion of shunt becomes colonized with **skin flora**, usually intraoperatively
   b. Most occur in 1st 2 weeks after placement
   c. May occur with or without ventriculitis
2. Distal shunt infections
   a. Occur when portion of shunt in peritoneum becomes colonized with bowel flora with peritonitis or hematogenous seeding
   b. Caused by wide range of pathogens: gram-negative, gram-positive, anaerobic, and fungal organisms

D. Risk factors
1. Multiple revisions of shunt
2. Previous shunt infection, especially with *S. aureus*
3. Premature birth
4. Craniotomy
5. Cranial fracture with CSF leak
6. Intraventricular or subarachnoid hemorrhage

E. Pathophysiology
1. Infection of shunt increases risk of CSF obstruction due to inflammation and cellular debris within shunt
2. Shunt placement requires break in cutaneous barrier, which allows skin flora to form infection on foreign material
3. Biofilm formation on shunt material allows organisms to evade host defenses and antibiotics
4. Distal shunt infections occur when tip of peritoneal shunt becomes contaminated with bowel flora

F. Clinical features
1. Catheter malfunction is most frequent manifestation of infection
2. Leads to increased ICP, causing many symptoms and signs
3. Historical findings (symptoms)
   a. Can have subtle presentation, sometimes with few or no symptoms
   b. Initial symptoms can result from increased ICP, such as **headache**, **vomiting**, and **lethargy**

QUICK HIT

A **CSF pseudocyst** (also known as a "CSFoma") is the result of inflammation around the distal tip of the VP shunt. Its walls consist of intestinal serosa and peritoneum. It is a known cause of shunt obstruction and can be associated with infection.

Table 10-13 Organisms Responsible for Ventricular Shunt Infections

Common organisms
Coagulase-negative staphylococci
Staphylococcus aureus
Less common organisms
Propionibacterium acnes
Corynebacterium jeikeium
Enterococcus faecalis
Gram-negative rods
Pseudomonas aeruginosa
Candida species
Viridans group streptococci

QUICK HIT

Signs and symptoms of ventricular shunt infection are often related to increased ICP.

QUICK HIT

The "shampoo clue" is the presence of fever and chills with shunt compression (as may occur with shampooing) as bacteria are released into the bloodstream by an infected VA shunt.

QUICK HIT

LP alone is not sufficient to rule out a ventricular shunt infection because ventricular fluid may not communicate with lumbar spinal fluid.

QUICK HIT

Common causes of VP shunt infection include coagulase-negative staphylococci; *S. aureus*; and, in teenagers, *Propionibacterium acnes*.

c. Presence of fever is variable
d. Because distal end of VP shunt is typically in abdomen, patient may develop evidence of peritonitis with **fever**, **poor feeding**, and **abdominal pain**

G. Exam findings (signs)
1. Meningeal signs may be absent; may be ventriculitis without meningeal inflammation
2. Other exam findings may include **papilledema**, **bulging fontanel** (in those <1 year), increased deep tendon reflexes, 4th or 6th cranial nerve palsy, seizure, or respiratory compromise
3. **Cushing triad** (hypertension, bradycardia, and abnormal respiratory pattern) is sign of significantly increased ICP
4. External shunt infections may present as soft tissue swelling, erythema, or purulent drainage
5. Patients with ventriculoatrial (VA) shunts are more likely to have bacteremia with shunt infection

H. Diagnosis
1. No clear case definition, but diagnosis is usually made using clinical and laboratory data
2. CSF shunt infection is likely if pathogen is isolated from cultures of CSF, ventricular fluid, or blood *or* patient has CSF pleocytosis (>50 WBC/mm^3) *plus* at least 1 of the following:
   a. Fever
   b. Evidence of shunt malfunction
   c. Neurologic symptoms
   d. Peritonitis
3. Differential
   a. Mechanical shunt obstruction
   b. Bacterial or viral meningitis
   c. Encephalitis or encephalopathy
   d. Brain abscess
   e. Intracranial mass
4. Laboratory tests
   a. CBC, CSF analysis, blood culture
      i. CSF should be sampled from ventricular shunt
      ii. CSF should be sent for bacterial culture, Gram stain, protein, glucose, cell count, and differential
         (a) CSF WBC counts typically are <150 cells/mm^3
         (b) Pleocytosis is common but may be absent
   b. With pleocytosis, often difficult to differentiate infection from postsurgical inflammation; elevation in CSF protein is more common than decrease in CSF glucose

I. Radiology
1. Imaging is important to evaluate for increased ICP, shunt malfunction or obstruction, and evidence of infection
2. Often includes **head CT** and **x-ray shunt series**, which consists of anteroposterior and lateral views of skull, chest, and abdomen to evaluate shunt catheter for kinking or discontinuity
3. Distal tip should be evaluated for pseudocyst

J. Management
1. Therapy
   a. Removal of shunt
   b. Placement of **EVD** (if needed)
   c. IV antibiotics (vancomycin and 3rd-generation cephalosporin empirically)
   d. Daily CSF Gram stain and culture
   e. Replacing shunt after CSF cultures are negative for 7–14 days
2. Alter antibiotic therapy based on culture results
3. **Intraventricular antibiotics** are sometimes used when parental therapy fails to sterilize CSF or patient has resistant organism

K. Complications
  1. Brain injury and decrease in IQ (severity correlates with number of shunt infections)
  2. Complications of peritonitis include obstruction or bowel adhesions

L. Duration/prognosis
  1. Antibiotics are usually discontinued after shunt is replaced
  2. Prognosis depends on age of onset, severity of infection, degree of ventricular expansion, and extent of neurologic damage prior to treatment

M. Prevention
  1. Careful adherence to sterile technique *or* perioperative prophylaxis with vancomycin
  2. Antibiotic-impregnated shunts

XXVII. Catheter-Related Bloodstream Infection (CRBSI)

A. Characteristics
  1. Bacterial bloodstream infection associated with presence of central catheter or umbilical catheter; typically, central venous catheter
     a. Occurs in patients with an indwelling central venous catheter currently or during 48 hours preceding infection
     b. Symptoms and laboratory results indicate infection is *not* related to infection at another site on body
  2. Predominant cause of hospital-acquired infection
  3. Rates higher for central venous catheters when compared to peripherally inserted catheters and arterial catheters
  4. Most CRBSIs are caused by coagulase-negative staphylococci and *S. aureus* (Table 10-14)
  5. Risk factors
     a. Extended use of central catheter, primarily venous type
     b. Multiple intravascular access catheters in place
     c. Lack of antibiotic or antiseptic coating on central line
     d. Extremely low birth weight (1,000–1,500 g)
     e. Lipids or total parenteral nutrition infused through catheter, especially in neonates
     f. Host factors: presence of acquired or congenital immunodeficiency, short-gut syndrome, or burn patient

B. Pathophysiology
  1. Infectious agent may be introduced at catheter insertion
  2. Short-term catheters (<1 week) most commonly colonized by skin microorganisms that gain access to bloodstream by migration along external surface of catheter
  3. Long-term catheters (>1 week) colonized by microorganisms that gain access to bloodstream by intraluminal spread from catheter hub

Infectious Diseases

Table 10-14 Other Causes of Catheter-Related Bloodstream Infection

Neonates	*Candida* spp. Enterococci Gram-negative bacilli
Infants with short-gut syndrome	Gram-negative bacilli
Other organisms seen in patients	*Enterobacter* spp. *Pseudomonas aeruginosa* *Klebsiella pneumoniae* *Escherichia coli* *Candida* spp.
Other *less common* organisms seen in all patients	*Corynebacterium Bacillus* spp. Nontuberculous mycobacteria Other gram-negative bacilli including *Acinetobacter* spp. and *Citrobacter* spp.

> **QUICK HIT**
> All febrile episodes in children with central venous catheters must be investigated for CRBSI.

C. Clinical features
  1. Symptoms are typically nonspecific and may appear similar to those encountered in septic patient
  2. Physical exam findings
     a. Fever is most common clinical sign
  3. Most cases lack focal signs of infections but may see erythema, induration, or pus at insertion/exit site or along tunneled catheter
  4. Chills, fever, or hypotension associated with catheter flushing or catheter malfunction may indicate infection

D. Diagnosis
  1. Differential includes sepsis and septic shock due to other infections unrelated to catheter, local cellulitis, or abscess
  2. CRBSI diagnosis requires signs of infection (but not related to another identifiable focus) plus positive blood culture (>1 positive blood culture if skin flora such as coagulase-negative staphylococci are isolated)

E. Laboratory findings
  1. WBC count may be normal or elevated with left shift
  2. If central catheter is left in place, paired blood cultures should be obtained from both central catheter (all lumens) and peripheral vein for comparison
     a. Cultures diagnostic of CRBSI when colony counts are at least 3× higher in catheter culture than peripheral culture; this approach is not practical in children, so quantitative cultures are rarely performed
     b. Differential time to positivity more commonly used; CRBSI likely if catheter culture is positive before peripheral culture
  3. If catheter is removed due to suspected CRBSI, tip can be submitted for Gram stain and culture
     a. Diagnostic if >15 colony-forming units (CFUs) on semiquantitative culture (tip is rolled across surface of an agar plate and CFUs counted)
     b. Diagnostic if >100 CFUs in quantitative broth culture
     c. If organisms on catheter tip have also been isolated from peripheral blood culture, then CRBSI can be confirmed
  4. Purulent material from area near catheter entrance/exit should be submitted for Gram stain and culture

F. Treatment
  1. Therapy
     a. Blood cultures from central catheter and peripheral vein should be obtained prior to starting antibiotics
     b. Empiric antibiotic therapy regimen for suspected CRBSI should be started based on commonly isolated organisms and those associated with special patient populations (see Table 10-14)
        i. In general, coverage for both gram-positive and gram-negative organisms should be provided with vancomycin and 4th-generation cephalosporin (e.g., cefepime) with activity against *Pseudomonas* species
        ii. Antibiotics should be given through involved catheter for 7–10 days if catheter was removed; 14 days or longer if catheter retained
     c. **Antibiotic lock therapy** (concentrated antibiotic solution placed in catheter) may be given in addition to IV antibiotics
     d. Unlike in adults, catheters are not routinely removed in children with CRBSI because of difficulty with catheter placement
     e. Central catheter should be removed in the following cases:
        i. No longer required
        ii. *Candida* spp., *S. aureus*, or mycobacteria isolated
        iii. Bacteremia >72 hours
        iv. Endocarditis or septic lung emboli

> **QUICK HIT**
> Patients with persistent *S. aureus* bacteremia should be evaluated for endocarditis.

G. Complications
  1. Treatment of fungemia without removal of catheter increases overall morbidity and may lead to disseminated infection

2. Endocarditis, sepsis syndrome, septic thrombophlebitis, and spread to solid organs (especially lungs, liver, kidneys, and spleen)
3. Relapse of infection is unusual, but reinfection with different organism is more common in catheters that have previously been infected

H. Prognosis
1. Related to pathogen, host, and therapy; most patients who are recognized early and treated appropriately have high cure rate
2. Delayed recognition or therapy is associated with increased morbidity and mortality

I. Prevention
1. Primarily by consistent use of principles and practices known to decrease CRBSI (also called **catheter care bundles**), such as use of sterile barrier precautions for catheter insertion, optimal hand hygiene practices, daily assessment of need for continuing central venous catheters, and use of chlorhexidine gluconate for skin antisepsis
2. **Ethanol lock therapy** also gaining popularity

XXVIII. Varicella

A. General characteristics
1. Definition: varicella-zoster virus (VZV) causes 2 distinct illnesses
2. Primary infection with VZV causes **varicella (chickenpox)**; reactivation of latent VZV causes **herpes zoster (shingles)**

B. Epidemiology
1. Varicella
   a. VZV can be spread person to person via respiratory secretions (including aerosolized droplets) and fluid from vesicular lesions
   b. VZV enters human host after virus comes in contact with mucous membranes of eyes or is inhaled into respiratory tract
   c. Virus is highly contagious, and ~90% of unimmunized household contacts will contract varicella
   d. Incubation period is usually 14–16 days but can be as short as 10 days and as long as 21 days after contact
   e. Person considered infectious from 48 hours prior to development of skin lesions to when skin lesions have fully crusted over
   f. In utero transmission (rare) occurs from transplacental passage during maternal varicella infection
   g. Varicella vaccine has dramatically reduced number of children seen with varicella and its complications
2. Zoster
   a. Zoster reactivation of varicella in a dermatome distribution occurs in immunocompromised children but is rare in healthy children
   b. Immunocompetent people with zoster can transmit virus through contact with vesicular lesions, but VZV is not found in their respiratory secretions, whereas immunocompromised people can transmit virus to others through respiratory secretions

QUICK HIT

Varicella vaccine is given to children in a 2-dose series, the first between ages 12 and 15 months and the second between ages 4 and 6 years.

3. Cause: double-stranded DNA virus with humans only known source of infection
4. Risk factors
   a. Varicella is usually a benign, self-limited illness but can cause severe or life-threatening illness in otherwise healthy children
   b. Newborns, adolescents, and pregnant women: higher risk of complications
   c. Immunocompromised hosts (e.g., HIV, chronic steroid use, malignancy, immunosuppressive drugs): higher risk of severe varicella-related complications, such as hemorrhagic skin lesions and pneumonia

C. Pathophysiology
1. After replication in lymph nodes 4–6 days after entry, initial viremic phase with seeding of reticuloendothelial system
2. Followed by 2nd viremic phase ~9 days after infection that continues until skin lesions are seen (10–21 days after initial infection)

QUICK HIT

The varicella vaccine prevents >80% of all varicella infection and >98% of serious varicella infections.

QUICK HIT

Breakthrough varicella cases usually have a mild clinical course with lesions that often do not have the classic vesicular appearance of chickenpox.

QUICK HIT

Unvaccinated children with varicella have >300 lesions compared with <50 lesions for vaccinated children with "breakthrough" disease.

QUICK HIT

The rash of varicella occurs in crops of vesicles, so that lesions in the same area are in various states of progression from vesicle to crusted lesions.

3. Virus establishes latency in dorsal root ganglia during primary infection
4. Reactivation results in herpes zoster, which consists of vesicular lesions in distribution of 1–3 sensory dermatomes
5. Immunocompromised children may have disseminated zoster

D. Clinical features
1. Historical findings (symptoms): in immunocompetent hosts: primary uncomplicated varicella typically causes fever, pharyngitis, malaise, and generalized vesicular rash, which appear in successive crops over multiple days
   a. Rash is very pruritic
   b. Lesions start to crust over in 24–48 hours
   c. Zoster is usually preceded by pain, burning, and pruritus in affected dermatomes
2. Exam findings (signs)
   a. Skin lesions begin as macules, which then progress to papules, with final progression into clear, fluid-filled vesicles with erythematous irregular margin ("dew drops on a rose petal")
   b. Rash starts on scalp, face, and trunk and spreads to extremities
   c. Individual lesions start to crust over in 1–2 days
   d. Hallmark of varicella is that different areas of body have lesions at different stages of development
   e. Children who receive vaccine sometimes develop varicella, although clinical course is usually mild with <50 vesicles (**breakthrough varicella**)

E. Diagnosis
1. Differential
   a. Insect bites
   b. Measles
   c. Meningococcemia (hemorrhagic varicella)
   d. Enterovirus

F. Laboratory
1. Diagnosis usually based on clinical appearance of lesions
2. If laboratory confirmation is desired (e.g., immunocompromised children) or if diagnosis is uncertain, a VZV PCR may be obtained from fluid collected from ruptured vesicle
3. Direct fluorescent antibody may be used but has less sensitivity than PCR
4. Tzanck smear and viral culture have low sensitivity for diagnosis of VZV and are rarely performed

G. Radiology
1. Brain imaging may be helpful when VZV encephalitis is being considered to help evaluate other causes of symptoms as well as infarction or hemorrhage
2. Chest radiograph may be helpful when VZV pneumonitis is being considered

H. Management
1. Therapy
   a. Supportive care: sufficient for most immunocompetent hosts
      i. Antihistamines: reduce pruritus
      ii. Acetaminophen: reduces fever
      iii. Fingernails should be clipped to reduce skin breakdown from itching, thereby minimizing risk of secondary bacterial skin infection
   b. Acyclovir
      i. Modest decrease in illness severity if started early in illness (ideally in 1st 24–72 hours)
      ii. IV or PO acyclovir should be considered for groups that are at increased risk of complications from varicella (**Table 10-15**)
      iii. In zoster: reduces pain, duration of illness, and new lesion formation in children if started within 72 hours of infection
2. Care of nonimmune children exposed to varicella
   a. **Varicella vaccine**: as soon as possible after exposure; can prevent or modify disease

Table 10-15 Indications for Oral and Intravenous Acyclovir in Children with Varicella

Indications for PO acyclovir
Older children (>12 years of age)
History of chronic cutaneous, diabetes, or pulmonary disorder (IV may also be appropriate, depending on severity)
Those taking steroids (systemic or inhaled) or chronic salicylates
Secondary household cases (because varicella can be more severe)
Indications for IV acyclovir
Children with severe complications of varicella such as pneumonia, hepatitis, or encephalitis
Immunocompromised children with varicella (complicated or uncomplicated)
Infants with varicella

IV, intravenous; PO, oral.

b. **Varicella-zoster immune globulin (VariZIG)**: nonimmune children at high risk of complications from varicella *and* who had significant exposure may benefit
   i. Human Ig containing high levels of antivaricella antibodies
   ii. Should be given as soon as possible after exposure (up to 96 hours)
   iii. Unimmunized, immunocompromised, and premature infants <28 weeks' gestation may benefit from VariZIG

c. **Acyclovir postexposure prophylaxis**: some experts recommend acyclovir as postexposure prophylaxis if VariZIG and/or vaccine cannot be used (limited supporting data)

I. Complications (Table 10-16)

J. Duration/prognosis
1. In routine varicella, lesions start to crust over in 24–48 hours
2. New lesions continue to appear for 1–7 days
3. Prognosis is good in otherwise healthy children, but complications and death do rarely occur in this population
4. Significant morbidity and mortality in children with comorbidities

Table 10-16 Complications of Varicella-Zoster Virus

Complications of varicella in otherwise healthy children
Secondary bacterial infection (e.g., cellulitis, necrotizing fasciitis), most commonly with *Streptococcus pyogenes*
Pneumonia (more common in older children and adults)
Encephalitis/aseptic meningitis
Acute cerebellar ataxia
Reye syndrome (associated with concurrent varicella and salicylate use)
Complications of varicella in high-risk populations
Fetus—congenital varicella syndrome if acquired in first 20 weeks of gestation
Newborn—neonatal varicella if mother develops varicella 5 days before to 2 days after delivery (30% mortality if untreated)
Immunocompromised hosts—severe disseminated varicella associated with hemorrhagic skin lesions, severe pneumonia, and disseminated intravascular coagulation
Complications of zoster
Otherwise healthy host—may cause complications related to affected nerve (e.g., conjunctivitis, keratitis, facial palsies)
Postherpetic neuralgia—pain that persists after resolution of the zoster rash
Immunocompromised hosts—visceral dissemination

K. Prevention
   1. Vaccine
      a. Live attenuated virus licensed by U.S. in 1995
      b. 85% develop immunity after 1 dose; ~100% develop immunity after 2 doses
      c. Introduction associated with large decrease in cases in U.S.
   2. Infection control
      a. Infected child should be placed on airborne (N-95 mask) and contact precautions
      b. Immunocompetent children with localized zoster should be on contact precautions only
      c. Immunocompromised children with zoster should be on airborne (N-95) and contact precautions

QUICK HIT

VariZIG's main role is to prevent or attenuate disease in children who are at high risk of complications of varicella. It has little to no benefit after the patient has become symptomatic with varicella disease.

XXIX. Vaccines

A. Overview
   1. National vaccine immunization program is dramatic example of very effective preventive health care in drastically reducing disease rates in U.S. children over past few decades
   2. CDC and American Association of Pediatrics regularly update guidelines to reflect changes
   3. State requirements for school entry and exemption criteria differ
   4. Unvaccinated children (and even vaccinated children exposed to unvaccinated children) more likely to be infected

B. Dosing schedule recommendations (Table 10-17)

C. Contraindications
   1. Allergy to prior vaccine or any component of specific vaccine
      a. Hepatitis B vaccine: yeast
      b. Some DTaP vaccines (diphtheria, tetanus, acellular pertussis) and some rotavirus vaccines (RV1 but not RV5): latex
      c. MMR vaccine (measles, mumps, rubella): gelatin, neomycin
      d. LAIV (live attenuated influenza vaccine, nasal): egg, chicken, gentamicin, gelatin, arginine
      e. TIV (trivalent inactivated influenza vaccine, injection): egg, chicken, thimerosal (in some, but not all, TIV)
   2. Moderate or severe illness: pertussis, MMR, VZV, pneumococcal conjugate vaccine, influenza, rotavirus, meningococcal
   3. Live attenuated vaccines
      a. MMR, VZV, LAIV, rotavirus: immunodeficiency, pregnancy
      b. Pertussis: encephalopathy within 7 days of prior pertussis vaccine without identifiable cause, progressive neurologic disorder
      c. LAIV (in addition to above): age <2 years, asthma/recurrent wheezing, underlying medical conditions that increase risk for severe influenza infection, close contact with severely immunocompromised individuals, long-term salicylate therapy

QUICK HIT

Thimerosal, a mercury-containing preservative, was used in many different vaccines in the past with no evidence of harm in the small amounts used, but thimerosal-free vaccines are now available and more commonly used.

QUICK HIT

Mild illness, even with fever, is usually not a contraindication to vaccination.

D. Precautions: may increase risk of serious reaction; risk/benefit ratio needs to be considered
   1. Pertussis: seizure, fever >105°F or change in neurologic status following prior dose and neurologic disease that increases risk of seizures or may be progressive
   2. Diphtheria/tetanus and influenza: Guillain-Barré syndrome, especially within 6 weeks of prior dose
   3. MMR: thrombocytopenia after prior MMR, personal or family history of seizures (MMRV?)
   4. Live attenuated vaccines: MMR, VZV, LAIV, rotavirus: close contact with immunocompromised individuals
   5. VZV: high-dose glucocorticoid therapy, blood product therapy

TABLE 10-17 Recommended Immunization Schedule for Persons Aged 0 through 18 Years – 2013

These recommendations must be read with the footnotes that follow. For those who fall behind or start late, provide catch-up vaccination at the earliest opportunity as indicated by the green bars in Figure 1. To determine minimum intervals between doses, see the catch-up schedule (Figure 2). School entry and adolescent vaccine age groups are in bold.

Vaccines	Birth	1 mo	2 mos	4 mos	6 mos	9 mos	12 mos	15 mos	18 mos	19–23 mos	2-3 yrs	**4-6 yrs**	7-10 yrs	**11-12 yrs**	13–15 yrs	16–18 yrs
Hepatitis B[1] (HepB)	←1st dose→	←2nd dose→					←3rd dose→									
Rotavirus[2] (RV) RV-1 (2-dose series); RV-5 (3-dose series)			←1st dose→	←2nd dose→	See footnote 2											
Diphtheria, tetanus, & acellular pertussis[3] (DTaP: <7 yrs)			←1st dose→	←2nd dose→	←3rd dose→			←4th dose→				←5th dose→				
Tetanus, diphtheria, & acellular pertussis[4] (Tdap: ≥7 yrs)														(Tdap)		
Haemophilus influenzae type b[5] (Hib)			←1st dose→	←2nd dose→	See footnote 5		←3rd or 4th dose, see footnote 5→									
Pneumococcal conjugate[6a,c] (PCV13)			←1st dose→	←2nd dose→	←3rd dose→		←4th dose→									
Pneumococcal polysaccharide[6b,c] (PPSV23)																
Inactivated Poliovirus[7] (IPV) (<18years)			←1st dose→	←2nd dose→			←3rd dose→					←4th dose→				
Influenza[8] (IIV; LAIV) 2 doses for some: see footnote 8							Annual vaccination (IIV only)						Annual vaccination (IIV or LAIV)			
Measles, mumps, rubella[9] (MMR)							←1st dose→					←2nd dose→				
Varicella[10] (VAR)							←1st dose→					←2nd dose→				
Hepatitis A[11] (HepA)							←2 dose series, see footnote 11→									
Human papillomavirus[12] (HPV2: females only; HPV4: males and females)														(3-dose series)		
Meningococcal[13] (Hib-MenCY ≥ 6 weeks; MCV4-D≥9 mos; MCV4-CRM ≥ 2 yrs.)							see footnote 13							←1st dose→		booster

Range of recommended ages for all children | Range of recommended ages for catch-up immunization | Range of recommended ages for certain high-risk groups | Range of recommended ages during which catch-up is encouraged and for certain high-risk groups | Not routinely recommended

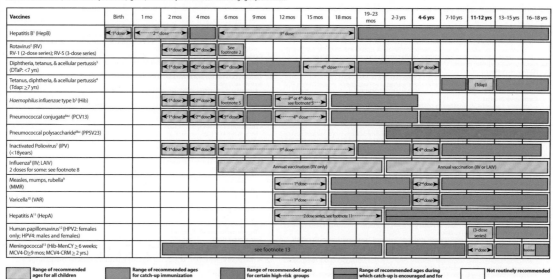

This schedule includes recommendations in effect as of January 1, 2013. Any dose not administered at the recommended age should be administered at a subsequent visit, when indicated and feasible. The use of a combination vaccine generally is preferred over separate injections of its equivalent component vaccines. Vaccination providers should consult the relevant Advisory Committee on Immunization Practices (ACIP) statement for detailed recommendations, available online at http://www.cdc.gov/vaccines/pubs/acip-list.htm. Clinically significant adverse events that follow vaccination should be reported to the Vaccine Adverse Event Reporting System (VAERS) online (http://www.vaers.hhs.gov) or by telephone (800-822-7967).Suspected cases of vaccine-preventable diseases should be reported to the state or local health department. Additional information, including precautions and contraindications for vaccination, is available from CDC online (http://www.cdc.gov/vaccines) or by telephone (800-CDC-INFO [800-232-4636]).

This schedule is approved by the Advisory Committee on Immunization Practices (http://www.cdc.gov/vaccines/acip/index.html), the American Academy of Pediatrics (http://www.aap.org), the American Academy of Family Physicians (http://www.aafp.org), and the American College of Obstetricians and Gynecologists (http://www.acog.org).

NOTE: The above recommendations must be read along with the footnotes of this schedule.

Footnotes — Recommended immunization schedule for persons aged 0 through 18 years—United States, 2013

For further guidance on the use of the vaccines mentioned below, see: http://www.cdc.gov/vaccines/pubs/acip-list.htm.

1. **Hepatitis B (HepB) vaccine. (Minimum age: birth)**
   Routine vaccination:
   At birth
   - Administer monovalent HepB vaccine to all newborns before hospital discharge.
   - For infants born to hepatitis B surface antigen (HBsAg)–positive mothers, administer HepB vaccine and 0.5 mL of hepatitis B immune globulin (HBIG) within 12 hours of birth. These infants should be tested for HBsAg and antibody to HBsAg (anti-HBs) 1 to 2 months after completion of the HepB series, at age 9 through 18 months (preferably at the next well-child visit).
   - If mother's HBsAg status is unknown, within 12 hours of birth administer HepB vaccine to all infants regardless of birth weight. For infants weighing <2,000 grams, administer HBIG in addition to HepB within 12 hours of birth. Determine mother's HBsAg status as soon as possible and, if she is HBsAg-positive, also administer HBIG for infants weighing ≥2,000 grams (no later than age 1 week).

   Doses following the birth dose
   - The second dose should be administered at age 1 or 2 months. Monovalent HepB vaccine should be used for doses administered before age 6 weeks.
   - Infants who did not receive a birth dose should receive 3 doses of a HepB-containing vaccine on a schedule of 0, 1 to 2 months, and 6 months starting as soon as feasible. See Figure 2.
   - The minimum interval between dose 1 and dose 2 is 4 weeks and between dose 2 and 3 is 8 weeks. The final (third or fourth) dose in the HepB vaccine series should be administered no earlier than age 24 weeks, and at least 16 weeks after the first dose.
   - Administration of a total of 4 doses of HepB vaccine is recommended when a combination vaccine containing HepB is administered after the birth dose.

   Catch-up vaccination:
   - Unvaccinated persons should complete a 3-dose series.
   - A 2-dose series (doses separated by at least 4 months) of adult formulation Recombivax HB is licensed for use in children aged 11 through 15 years.
   - For other catch-up issues, see Figure 2.
2. **Rotavirus (RV) vaccines. (Minimum age: 6 weeks for both RV-1 [Rotarix] and RV-5 [RotaTeq]).**
   Routine vaccination:
   - Administer a series of RV vaccine to all infants as follows:
     1. If RV-1 is used, administer a 2-dose series at 2 and 4 months of age.
     2. If RV-5 is used, administer a 3-dose series at ages 2, 4, and 6 months.
     3. If any dose in series was RV-5 or vaccine product is unknown for any dose in the series, a total of 3 doses of RV vaccine should be administered.

   Catch-up vaccination:
   - The maximum age for the first dose in the series is 14 weeks, 6 days.
   - Vaccination should not be initiated for infants aged 15 weeks 0 days or older.
   - The maximum age for the final dose in the series is 8 months, 0 days.
   - If RV-1(Rotarix) is administered for the first and second doses, a third dose is not indicated.
   - For other catch-up issues, see Figure 2.
3. **Diphtheria and tetanus toxoids and acellular pertussis (DTaP) vaccine. (Minimum age: 6 weeks)**
   Routine vaccination:
   - Administer a 5-dose series of DTaP vaccine at ages 2, 4, 6, 15–18 months, and 4 through 6 years. The fourth dose may be administered as early as age 12 months, provided at least 6 months have elapsed since the third dose.

   Catch-up vaccination:
   - The fifth (booster) dose of DTaP vaccine is not necessary if the fourth dose was administered at age 4 years or older.
   - For other catch-up issues, see Figure 2.
4. **Tetanus and diphtheria toxoids and acellular pertussis (Tdap) vaccine. (Minimum age: 10 years for Boostrix, 11 years for Adacel).**
   Routine vaccination:
   - Administer 1 dose of Tdap vaccine to all adolescents aged 11 through 12 years.
   - Tdap can be administered regardless of the interval since the last tetanus and diphtheria toxoid-containing vaccine.
   - Administer one dose of Tdap vaccine to pregnant adolescents during each pregnancy (preferred during 27 through 36 weeks gestation) regardless of number of years from prior Td or Tdap vaccination.

   Catch-up vaccination:
   - Persons aged 7 through 10 years who are not fully immunized with the childhood DTaP vaccine series, should receive Tdap vaccine as the first dose in the catch-up series; if additional doses are needed, use Td vaccine. For these children, an adolescent Tdap vaccine should not be given.
   - Persons aged 11 through 18 years who have not received Tdap vaccine should receive a dose followed by tetanus and diphtheria toxoids (Td) booster doses every 10 years thereafter.
   - An inadvertent dose of DTaP vaccine administered to children aged 7 through 10 years can count as part of the catch-up series. This dose can count as the adolescent Tdap dose, or the child can later receive a Tdap booster dose at age 11–12 years.
   - For other catch-up issues, see Figure 2.
5. ***Haemophilus influenzae* type b (Hib) conjugate vaccine. (Minimum age: 6 weeks)**
   Routine vaccination:
   - Administer a Hib vaccine primary series and a booster dose to all infants. The primary series doses should be administered at 2, 4, and 6 months of age; however, if PRP-OMP (PedvaxHib or Comvax) is administered at 2 and 4 months of age, a dose at age 6 months is not indicated. One booster dose should be administered at age 12 through15 months.
   - Hiberix (PRP-T) should only be used for the booster (final) dose in children aged 12 months through 4 years, who have received at least 1 dose of Hib.

   Catch-up vaccination:
   - If dose 1 was administered at ages 12-14 months, administer booster (as final dose) at least 8 weeks after dose 1.
   - If the first 2 doses were PRP-OMP (PedvaxHIB or Comvax), and were administered at age 11 months or younger, the third (and final) dose should be administered at age 12 through 15 months and at least 8 weeks after the second dose.
   - If the first dose was administered at age 7 through 11 months, administer the second dose at least 4 weeks later and a final dose at age 12 through 15 months, regardless of Hib vaccine (PRP-T or PRP-OMP) used for first dose.
   - For unvaccinated children aged 15 months or older, administer only 1 dose.

(continued)

TABLE 10-17 Recommended Immunization Schedule for Persons Aged 0 through 18 Years – 2013 *(Continued)*

For further guidance on the use of the vaccines mentioned below, see: http://www.cdc.gov/vaccines/pubs/acip-list.htm.

- For other catch-up issues, see Figure 2.

Vaccination of persons with high-risk conditions:

- Hib vaccine is not routinely recommended for patients older than 5 years of age. However one dose of Hib vaccine should be administered to unvaccinated or partially vaccinated persons aged 5 years or older who have leukemia, malignant neoplasms, anatomic or functional asplenia (including sickle cell disease), human immunodeficiency virus (HIV) infection, or other immunocompromising conditions.

6a. Pneumococcal conjugate vaccine (PCV). (Minimum age: 6 weeks)

Routine vaccination:

- Administer a series of PCV13 vaccine at ages 2, 4, 6 months with a booster at age 12 through 15 months.
- For children aged 14 through 59 months who have received an age-appropriate series of 7-valent PCV (PCV7), administer a single supplemental dose of 13-valent PCV (PCV13).

Catch-up vaccination:

- Administer 1 dose of PCV13 to all healthy children aged 24 through 59 months who are not completely vaccinated for their age.
- For other catch-up issues, see Figure 2.

Vaccination of persons with high-risk conditions:

- For children aged 24 through 71 months with certain underlying medical conditions (see footnote 6c), administer 1 dose of PCV13 if 3 doses of PCV were received previously, or administer 2 doses of PCV13 at least 8 weeks apart if fewer than 3 doses of PCV were received previously.
- A single dose of PCV13 may be administered to previously unvaccinated children aged 6 through 18 years who have anatomic or functional asplenia (including sickle cell disease), HIV infection or an immunocompromising condition, cochlear implant or cerebrospinal fluid leak. See MMWR 2010;59 (No. RR-11), available at http://www.cdc.gov/mmwr/pdf/rr/rr5911.pdf.
- Administer PPSV23 at least 8 weeks after the last dose of PCV to children aged 2 years or older with certain underlying medical conditions (see footnotes 6b and 6c).

6b. Pneumococcal polysaccharide vaccine (PPSV23). (Minimum age: 2 years)

Vaccination of persons with high-risk conditions:

- Administer PPSV23 at least 8 weeks after the last dose of PCV to children aged 2 years or older with certain underlying medical conditions (see footnote 6c). A single revaccination with PPSV should be administered after 5 years to children with anatomic or functional asplenia (including sickle cell disease) or an immunocompromising condition.

6c. Medical conditions for which PPSV23 is indicated in children aged 2 years and older and for which use of PCV13 is indicated in children aged 24 through 71 months:

- Immunocompetent children with chronic heart disease (particularly cyanotic congenital heart disease and cardiac failure); chronic lung disease (including asthma if treated with high-dose oral corticosteroid therapy), diabetes mellitus; cerebrospinal fluid leaks; or cochlear implant.
- Children with anatomic or functional asplenia (including sickle cell disease and other hemoglobinopathies, congenital or acquired asplenia, or splenic dysfunction);
- Children with immunocompromising conditions: HIV infection, chronic renal failure and nephrotic syndrome, diseases associated with treatment with immunosuppressive drugs or radiation therapy, including malignant neoplasms, leukemias, lymphomas and Hodgkin disease; or solid organ transplantation, congenital immunodeficiency.

7. Inactivated poliovirus vaccine (IPV). (Minimum age: 6 weeks)

Routine vaccination:

- Administer a series of IPV at ages 2, 4, 6–18 months, with a booster at age 4–6 years. The final dose in the series should be administered on or after the fourth birthday and at least 6 months after the previous dose.

Catch-up vaccination:

- In the first 6 months of life, minimum age and minimum intervals are only recommended if the person is at risk for imminent exposure to circulating poliovirus (i.e., travel to a polio-endemic region or during an outbreak).
- If 4 or more doses are administered before age 4 years, an additional dose should be administered at age 4 through 6 years.
- A fourth dose is not necessary if the third dose was administered at age 4 years or older and at least 6 months after the previous dose.
- If both OPV and IPV were administered as part of a series, a total of 4 doses should be administered, regardless of the child's current age.
- IPV is not routinely recommended for U.S. residents aged 18 years or older.
- For other catch-up issues, see Figure 2.

8. Influenza vaccines. (Minimum age: 6 months for inactivated influenza vaccine [IIV]; 2 years for live, attenuated influenza vaccine [LAIV])

Routine vaccination:

- Administer influenza vaccine annually to all children beginning at age 6 months. For most healthy, nonpregnant persons aged 2 through 49 years, either LAIV or IIV may be used. However, LAIV should NOT be administered to some persons, including 1) those with asthma, 2) children 2 through 4 years who had wheezing in the past 12 months, or 3) those who have any other underlying medical conditions that predispose them to influenza complications. For all other contraindications to use of LAIV see MMWR 2010; 59 (No. RR-8), available at http://www.cdc.gov/mmwr/pdf/rr/rr5908.pdf.
- Administer 1 dose to persons aged 9 years and older.

For children aged 6 months through 8 years:

- For the 2012–13 season, administer 2 doses (separated by at least 4 weeks) to children who are receiving influenza vaccine for the first time. For additional guidance, follow dosing guidelines in the 2012 ACIP influenza vaccine recommendations, MMWR 2012; 61: 613–618, available at http://www.cdc.gov/mmwr/pdf/wk/mm6132.pdf.
- For the 2013–14 season, follow dosing guidelines in the 2013 ACIP influenza vaccine recommendations.

9. Measles, mumps, and rubella (MMR) vaccine. (Minimum age: 12 months for routine vaccination)

Routine vaccination:

- Administer the first dose of MMR vaccine at age 12 through 15 months, and the second dose at age 4 through 6 years. The second dose may be administered before age 4 years, provided at least 4 weeks have elapsed since the first dose.
- Administer 1 dose of MMR vaccine to infants aged 6 through 11 months before departure from the United States for international travel. These children should be revaccinated with 2 doses of MMR vaccine, the first at age 12 through 15 months (12 months if the child remains in an area where disease risk is high), and the second dose at least 4 weeks later.
- Administer 2 doses of MMR vaccine to children aged 12 months and older, before departure from the United States for international travel. The first dose should be administered on or after age 12 months and the second dose at least 4 weeks later.

Catch-up vaccination:

- Ensure that all school-aged children and adolescents have had 2 doses of MMR vaccine; the minimum interval between the 2 doses is 4 weeks.

10. Varicella (VAR) vaccine. (Minimum age: 12 months)

Routine vaccination:

- Administer the first dose of VAR vaccine at age 12 through 15 months, and the second dose at age 4 through 6 years. The second dose may be administered before age 4 years, provided at least 3 months have elapsed since the first dose. If the second dose was administered at least 4 weeks after the first dose, it can be accepted as valid.

Catch-up vaccination:

- Ensure that all persons aged 7 through 18 years without evidence of immunity (see MMWR 2007;56 [No. RR-4], available at http://www.cdc.gov/mmwr/pdf/rr/rr5604.pdf) have 2 doses of varicella vaccine. For children aged 7 through 12 years the recommended minimum interval between doses is 3 months (if the second dose was administered at least 4 weeks after the first dose, it can be accepted as valid); for persons aged 13 years and older, the minimum interval between doses is 4 weeks.

11. Hepatitis A vaccine (HepA). (Minimum age: 12 months)

Routine vaccination:

- Initiate the 2-dose HepA vaccine series for children aged 12 through 23 months; separate the 2 doses by 6 to 18 months.
- Children who have received 1 dose of HepA vaccine before age 24 months, should receive a second dose 6 to 18 months after the first dose.
- For any person aged 2 years and older who has not already received the HepA vaccine series, 2 doses of HepA vaccine separated by 6 to 18 months may be administered if immunity against hepatitis A virus infection is desired.

Catch-up vaccination:

- The minimum interval between the two doses is 6 months.

Special populations:

- Administer 2 doses of Hep A vaccine at least 6 months apart to previously unvaccinated persons who live in areas where vaccination programs target older children, or who are at increased risk for infection.

12. Human papillomavirus (HPV) vaccines. (HPV4 [Gardasil] and HPV2 [Cervarix]). (Minimum age: 9 years)

Routine vaccination:

- Administer a 3-dose series of HPV vaccine on a schedule of 0, 1-2, and 6 months to all adolescents aged 11-12 years. Either HPV4 or HPV2 may be used for females, and only HPV4 may be used for males.
- The vaccine series can be started beginning at age 9 years.
- Administer the second dose 1 to 2 months after the **first** dose and the third dose 6 months after the **first** dose (at least 24 weeks after the first dose).

Catch-up vaccination:

- Administer the vaccine series to females (either HPV2 or HPV4) and males (HPV4) at age 13 through 18 years if not previously vaccinated.
- Use recommended routine dosing intervals (see above) for vaccine series catch-up.

13. Meningococcal conjugate vaccines (MCV). (Minimum age: 6 weeks for Hib-MenCY, 9 months for Menactra [MCV4-D], 2 years for Menveo [MCV4-CRM]).

Routine vaccination:

- Administer MCV4 vaccine at age 11–12 years, with a booster dose at age 16 years.
- Adolescents aged 11 through 18 years with human immunodeficiency virus (HIV) infection should receive a 2-dose primary series of MCV4, with at least 8 weeks between doses. See MMWR 2011; 60:1018–1019 available at: http://www.cdc.gov/mmwr/pdf/wk/mm6030.pdf.
- For children aged 2 months through 10 years with high-risk conditions, see below.

Catch-up vaccination:

- Administer MCV4 vaccine at age 13 through 18 years if not previously vaccinated.
- If the first dose is administered at age 13 through 15 years, a booster dose should be administered at age 16 through 18 years with a minimum interval of at least 8 weeks between doses.
- If the first dose is administered at age 16 years or older, a booster dose is not needed.
- For other catch-up issues, see Figure 2.

Vaccination of persons with high-risk conditions:

- For children younger than 19 months of age with anatomic or functional asplenia (including sickle cell disease), administer an infant series of Hib-MenCY at 2, 4, 6, and 12-15 months.
- For children aged 2 through 18 months with persistent complement component deficiency, administer either an infant series of Hib-MenCY at 2, 4, 6, and 12 through 15 months or a 2-dose primary series of MCV4-D starting at 9 months, with at least 8 weeks between doses. For children aged 19 through 23 months with persistent complement component deficiency who have not received a complete series of Hib-MenCY or MCV4-D, administer 2 primary doses of MCV4-D at least 8 weeks apart.
- For children aged 24 months and older with persistent complement component deficiency or anatomic or functional asplenia (including sickle cell disease), who have not received a complete series of Hib-MenCY or MCV4-D, administer 2 primary doses of either MCV4-D or MCV4-CRM. If MCV4-D (Menactra) is administered to a child with asplenia (including sickle cell disease), do not administer MCV4-D until 2 years of age and at least 4 weeks after the completion of all PCV13 doses. See MMWR 2011;60:1391–2, available at http://www.cdc.gov/mmwr/pdf/wk/mm6040.pdf.
- For children aged 9 months and older who are residents of or travelers to countries in the African meningitis belt or to the Hajj, administer an age appropriate formulation and series of MCV4 for protection against serogroups A and W-135. Prior receipt of Hib-MenCY is not sufficient for children traveling to the meningitis belt or the Hajj. See MMWR 2011;60:1391–2, available at http://www.cdc.gov/mmwr/pdf/wk/mm6040.pdf.
- For children who are present during outbreaks caused by a vaccine serogroup, administer or complete an age and formulation-appropriate series of Hib-MenCY or MCV4.
- For booster doses among persons with high-risk conditions refer to http://www.cdc.gov/vaccines/pubs/acip-list.htm#mening.

Additional information

- For contraindications and precautions to use of a vaccine and for additional information regarding that vaccine, vaccination providers should consult the relevant ACIP statement available online at http://www.cdc.gov/vaccines/pubs/acip-list.htm.
- For the purposes of calculating intervals between doses, 4 weeks = 28 days. Intervals of 4 months or greater are determined by calendar months.
- Information on travel vaccine requirements and recommendations is available at http://wwwnc.cdc.gov/travel/page/vaccinations.htm.
- For vaccination of persons with primary and secondary immunodeficiencies, see Table 13, "Vaccination of persons with primary and secondary immunodeficiencies," in General Recommendations on Immunization (ACIP), available at http://www.cdc.gov/mmwr/preview/mmwrhtml/rr6002a1.htm; and American Academy of Pediatrics. Immunization in Special Clinical Circumstances. In: Pickering LK, Baker CJ, Kimberlin DW, Long SS eds. Red book: 2012 report of the Committee on Infectious Diseases. 29th ed. Elk Grove Village, IL: American Academy of Pediatrics.

U.S. Department of Health and Human Services
Centers for Disease Control and Prevention

6. TIV: high-dose glucocorticoid or chemotherapy (safe but may not have good antibody response)
7. LAIV: congestion that may inhibit nasal absorption
8. Rotavirus: moderate to severe gastroenteritis, chronic underlying GI disease, history of intussusception

E. Adverse reactions
1. General: local swelling, erythema, pain; low-grade fever; fussiness
2. Hepatitis A: headache
3. DTaP: limb swelling, hypotonic or hyporesponsive episode (not associated with long-term sequelae), high fever
4. MMR: joint pain, inactivated poliovirus vaccine (ITP) (rare; some studies show no increased risk over baseline), febrile seizures, transient rashes
5. VZV: transmission of VZV (very rare, extremely mild cases)
6. Meningococcal: higher rate of Guillain-Barré syndrome above baseline in 6 weeks after vaccination with Menactra
7. TIV: rash, febrile seizure (more so in those who received pneumococcal vaccine concurrently), mild URI symptoms, Guillain-Barré syndrome (very rare in children)
8. LAIV: mild URI symptoms
9. Rotavirus: mild vomiting or diarrhea

F. Special considerations
1. Increasing trend to use DTaP (with pertussis) over Td booster in older children and adults in order to help maintain pertussis immunity over time; this helps protect young infants who are not yet fully immunized and at greatest risk for severe infection by decreasing their exposure
2. Special recommendations for those traveling internationally, those at increased risk for certain illnesses or adverse effects, and those who have not received prior vaccines on recommended schedule

QUICK HIT

Live attenuated oral poliovirus vaccine (OPV) can rarely cause paralytic poliomyelitis, and OPV is no longer used in the United States. IPV does not carry this risk.

QUICK HIT

There is lack of evidence for a vaccine–autism association.

11 Allergic and Immunologic Disorders

SYMPTOM SPECIFIC: ALLERGIC

I. Approach to Anaphylaxis

A. General characteristics
  1. Definition: acute, potentially life-threatening **type I (immediate) hypersensitivity reaction** (Table 11-1)
    a. Requires previous exposure to specific antigen
    b. Initial exposure: production of antigen-specific immunoglobulin (Ig) E antibodies that bind to mast cells
    c. Subsequent exposure: antigen binds to mast cells causing release of chemical mediators
  2. Signs and symptoms: most commonly sudden onset of cutaneous and respiratory symptoms
    a. May also include
      i. Constitutional: watery eyes, sweating, flushing, anxiety
      ii. Dermatologic: hives, pruritus
      iii. Respiratory: nasal congestion, hoarseness, chest tightness, **stridor**, wheezing, shortness of breath
      iv. Cardiovascular: tachycardia, dizziness, syncope
      v. Gastrointestinal (GI): abdominal pain, vomiting, diarrhea
      vi. Genitourinary (GU) symptoms: urinary urgency, incontinence
      vii. Neurologic: headache, seizure
    b. Reaction occurs typically within minutes but can occur up to 1 hour after exposure to allergen

> **QUICK HIT**
> Wheezing, GI, and GU symptoms are due to smooth muscle contraction.

> **QUICK HIT**
> Anaphylactic shock is a "warm" shock with flushed skin, bounding pulses, tachycardia, and hypotension.

> **QUICK HIT**
> Cardiac arrhythmias may accompany anaphylactic shock

TABLE 11-1 **Classification of Hypersensitivity Reactions**

Type	Name	Description	Clinical Example
I	Immediate	IgE-mediated mast cell release of histamine and other mediators	Severe allergic reaction to a precipitant (e.g., peanuts) that results in anaphylaxis, angioedema, or urticaria
II	Cytotoxic	IgG or IgM antibodies bind to cell surface antigens	Autoimmune diseases such as rheumatic fever and hemolytic disease of the newborn
III	Immune-complex	Circulating antigen–antibody immune complexes deposit in postcapillary venules	Subacute bacterial endocarditis and poststreptococcal glomerulonephritis
IV	Delayed	T-cell–mediated immunity (as opposed to antibody mediated)	Positive tuberculin skin test and allergic bronchopulmonary aspergillosis

Ig, immunoglobulin.

TABLE 11-2 **Common Causes for Anaphylaxis**

Foods	Medications	Environmental
Additives containing sulfite	Penicillins	Insect venom
Legumes	Sulfonamides	Exercise
Nuts	Salicylates	Cold weather
Berries	Local anesthetics	Heat
Seafood	Enzymes (L-asparaginase)	Latex
Eggs	Vaccines	
Dairy		
Shellfish		

c. Severe reaction may precipitate vascular collapse, leading to shock
d. Variable course of symptoms
    i. **Uniphasic**: lasts 1–2 hours and resolves with treatment
    ii. **Biphasic**: relapse may occur after hours to days
    iii. **Protracted**: lasts for days despite aggressive therapy
3. Causes of anaphylaxis (Table 11-2)

B. Historical questions
1. Characteristics of episode: timing, symptoms, duration
2. Possible triggers: recent medications, insect bites, foods
3. Past history: known allergies, previous anaphylactic reactions, presence of atopic conditions (eczema, asthma), family history

C. Physical exam findings
1. Vital signs: tachycardia, tachypnea, hypotension (late finding)
2. General: diaphoresis, anxiety, pruritus
3. Skin: warm to touch, generalized flushing, hives (**urticaria**)
4. Respiratory exam: stridor or wheeze may be auscultated, retractions, flaring
5. Ear, nose, and throat: "boggy" nasal mucosa; rhinorrhea; lips, tongue, and/or periorbital edema (Figure 11-1)
6. Extremities: warm extremities with bounding pulses

D. Laboratory testing and radiologic imaging
1. **Diagnosed clinically** by symptoms and response to treatment
2. Elevated, but generally not checked: tryptase level, IgE level
3. Allergy testing to identify possible trigger
    a. Skin-prick tests for specific antigens
    b. Serum radioallergosorbent test (RAST) for antigen-specific IgE levels

FIGURE 11-1 Angioedema of lip.

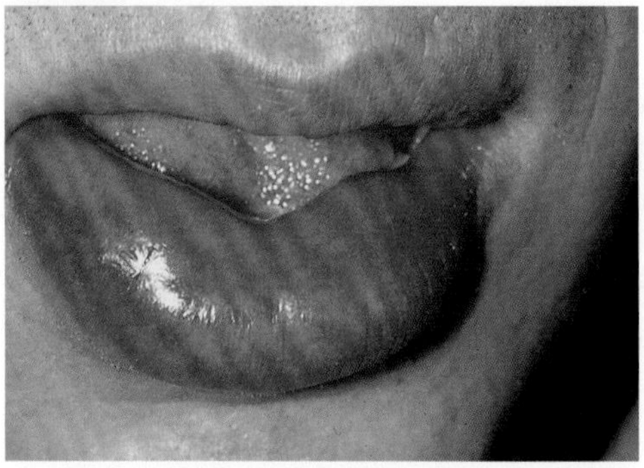

Angioedema is a diffuse, nonpitting, tense swelling of the dermis and subcutaneous tissue. It develops rapidly and typically disappears over subsequent hours or days. It may be associated with food allergies. (From Neville B, et al. *Color Atlas of Clinical Oral Pathology*. Philadelphia: Lea & Febiger; 1991. Used with permission.)

QUICK HIT

Increased risk of biphasic reactions occurs with food allergies, patients receiving more than 1 dose of epinephrine, and delay in initial epinephrine administration.

QUICK HIT

With anaphylaxis, ⅓ of cases are idiopathic with no identifiable trigger.

QUICK HIT

Breastfeeding mothers of infants with food allergies must also eliminate the triggering food from their diet.

QUICK HIT

Children with spina bifida have increased risk for latex allergy.

QUICK HIT

Peanuts, tree nuts, dairy, citrus, eggs, and shellfish are common causes of food-related anaphylaxis.

QUICK HIT

Children with shellfish allergy are often also allergic to radiocontrast dye.

QUICK HIT

Hives are raised, blanchable (i.e., will disappear with light finger pressure) skin eruptions.

QUICK HIT

RAST testing is highly sensitive, which makes it a good screening test, whereas skin-prick tests are more specific for a particular antigen, making them good confirmatory tests.

QUICK HIT

All patients at risk for anaphylaxis should carry an epinephrine autoinjector with them at all times because it can be a life-saving treatment.

QUICK HIT

Parents should be taught how to use an epinephrine autoinjector with instructions to give the injection if the child has any other symptoms (i.e., respiratory or GI) in addition to hives.

QUICK HIT

Always think "ABCs": address **a**irway, **b**reathing, and **c**irculation issues during acute episodes.

QUICK HIT

Patients are usually admitted to the hospital to monitor for a biphasic reaction.

QUICK HIT

Baseline asthma severity is categorized as intermittent or persistent (mild, moderate, or severe) based on impairment and risk.

QUICK HIT

Status asthmaticus is an asthma exacerbation unresponsive to usual therapies with risk for respiratory failure.

QUICK HIT

In patients with status asthmaticus, wheezing might not be heard if the patient has severely limited air movement—*this represents a medical emergency!*

E. Treatment
   1. Immediate dose of epinephrine via intramuscular (IM) injection; may repeat as needed
   2. Antihistamines: diphenhydramine (H_1 antagonist) and ranitidine (H_2)
   3. Systemic corticosteroids
   4. Albuterol nebulizer treatment may be given for bronchospasm
   5. Severe cases with shock require intubation and vasoactive infusion support

DISEASE SPECIFIC: ALLERGIC

II. Asthma

A. Characteristics
   1. Definition: chronic respiratory disease with recurrent, reversible symptoms of bronchoconstriction and airway edema
   2. Risk factors: family history of asthma, male sex, airway hyperreactivity, history of atopy and allergies, history of prematurity, and exposure to environmental tobacco smoke

B. Clinical features
   1. Historical findings
      a. Acute symptoms
         i. Ask about wheezing, cough, work of breathing, duration of symptoms, and treatment prior to seeking medical attention
         ii. Ask about risk factors for death (Table 11-3)
      b. Chronic symptoms: assess baseline asthma control (Table 11-4)
         i. Ask about **impairment**: daytime symptoms, use of short-acting β_2-agonist medications for rescue therapy, interruption of activity including missed school and work, and nighttime awakenings
         ii. Ask about **risk**: number of exacerbations requiring oral steroids, frequency and severity of previous exacerbations
   2. Physical exam findings
      a. Focus on general assessment including hydration status, vital signs, and pulmonary and cardiac exam
      b. Acute asthma exacerbation: tachypnea, tachycardia, retractions, decreased air entry, prolonged expiration, and **expiratory wheezing**

TABLE 11-3 **Risk Factors for Death from Asthma**

Severe asthma history	Previous severe exacerbation requiring intubation ≥2 hospitalizations for asthma in the past year ≥3 ED visits for asthma in the past year Hospitalization or ED visit for asthma in the past month Use of >2 canisters of short-acting β_2-agonists per month Difficulty perceiving asthma symptoms
Social issues	Low socioeconomic status or inner city residence Illicit drug use Major psychosocial problems
Comorbid conditions	Cardiovascular disease Other chronic lung disease Chronic psychiatric disease

ED, emergency department.

TABLE 11-4 **National Heart, Lung, and Blood Institute Classification of Asthma Baseline Severity and Therapy Initiation**

	Intermittent	Mild Persistent	Moderate Persistent	Severe Persistent
Daytime symptoms	≤2 days/week	>2 days/week but not daily	Daily	Throughout day
Short-acting β-agonist use for rescue therapy	≤2 days/week	>2 days/week but not daily	Daily	Several times a day
Interference with normal activity	None	Minor limitation	Some limitation	Extremely limited
Nighttime awakenings	None	≤2× month	≤4× month	>1× weekly
Risk (number of exacerbations requiring oral steroids)	≤1×/year	≥2×/year	≥2×/year	≥2×/year
Recommended therapy	Albuterol alone as needed for symptomatic relief	Low-dose ICS	Low-dose ICS plus LABA or LTRA **OR** medium-dose ICS	Medium-dose ICS ± LABA or LTRA

ICS, inhaled corticosteroid; LABA, long acting β_2-agonist; LTRA, leukotriene receptor antagonist.

c. Other pertinent findings include **signs of atopy** (atopic dermatitis, **allergic stigmata**)

C. Diagnosis
1. Differential diagnosis of wheeze (Box 11-1)
2. Laboratory findings
   a. Asthma is a clinical diagnosis; laboratory tests are rarely indicated
   b. Pulse oximetry is used to assess oxygen saturation in acute asthma exacerbation
3. Radiology findings: chest radiograph
   a. Should not be obtained routinely
   b. Consider in patients with diagnostic uncertainty or any patient with status asthmaticus not improving as expected or deteriorating
   c. Typical findings: increased lung volumes with hyperexpansion and diffuse atelectasis
   d. May reveal pneumothorax or pneumomediastinum
4. Other evaluation
   a. Pulmonary function tests (PFTs): not indicated in acute asthma exacerbation but recommended for chronic management in children age 5 years or older
   b. Peak expiratory flow monitoring: used to measure airflow in acute and chronic management for children age 5 years or older

QUICK HIT

Allergic stigmata include **Dennie lines** (folds or lines in the skin beneath the lower eyelid), allergic shiners, nasal crease, and bilateral conjunctival injection.

QUICK HIT

Not all that wheezes is asthma.

QUICK HIT

In patients with moderate to severe acute asthma exacerbations, oxygen saturation may be decreased to <95%.

BOX 11-1

Differential Diagnosis of Wheezing by Age

Infants	Bronchiolitis Bronchopulmonary dysplasia Foreign body aspiration Aspiration Cystic fibrosis Anatomic abnormalities such as laryngotracheomalacia or vascular rings Congestive heart disease
Children and adolescents	Viral lower airways disease Foreign body aspiration Allergic rhinitis and sinusitis Vocal cord dysfunction Congestive heart failure

D. Treatment
1. Medications: 2 major classes
   a. **Rescue medications**: for symptomatic use or can be used prior to activity with exercise-induced component (short-acting β_2-agonists, such as albuterol or levalbuterol)
   b. **Controller medications**: control or prevent airway inflammation and hyperresponsiveness (inhaled corticosteroids, long-acting β_2-agonists, leukotriene-receptor antagonist [LTRA]) in patients with persistent asthma
2. Acute asthma exacerbations
   a. Outpatient
      i. In health care facility: administer up to 3 doses of short-acting β_2-agonists within 1st hour
      ii. Systemic corticosteroids (prednisone or prednisolone 1–2 mg/kg/dose): indicated for any acute asthma exacerbation
   b. Inpatient
      i. 1st-line therapies
         (a) Supplemental oxygen to keep O_2 saturations >90%
         (b) Intermittent short-acting β_2-agonists based on symptom severity
         (c) Systemic steroids (prednisone or prednisolone 1–2 mg/kg/day with maximum 60 mg/day)
      ii. 2nd-line therapies
         (a) Continuous short-acting β_2-agonists
         (b) Intravenous (IV) magnesium sulfate or terbutaline
3. Chronic asthma control
   a. Controller therapy: based on patient's level of baseline asthma severity (see Table 11-4)
      i. 1st-line therapy: inhaled corticosteroid
      ii. Treatment is stepwise based on response to therapy and in addition to inhaled steroids may include
         (a) Long-acting β_2-agonist
         (b) LTRA
   b. **Asthma action plan** (home management): directions for actions based on symptoms for
      i. Trigger avoidance
      ii. Symptom recognition and danger signs
      iii. Timing of controller and rescue medication use
      iv. Device use (including metered-dose inhaler [MDI] and aerochamber)
4. Duration/prognosis
   a. Generally excellent with appropriate treatment and control
   b. Wide racial and socioeconomic discrepancies in outcomes
5. Prevention
   a. Largely focused on asthma action plan
   b. Avoid known triggers if possible for asthma exacerbations

QUICK HIT

Indications for hospitalization include persistent hypoxemia (<92%), moderate to severe wheezing, increased work of breathing, or tachypnea not responsive to initial management.

QUICK HIT

Asthma is a chronic disease and requires a family-centered care approach with communication between the inpatient and outpatient providers.

QUICK HIT

An MDI is a device that delivers an aerosolized burst of medication to be inhaled by the patient.

QUICK HIT

Proven strategies to reduce asthma readmissions include (1) classifying asthma severity and prescribing controller medications to those with persistent symptoms and (2) providing the family with a 30-day medication supply at hospital discharge.

III. Allergic Rhinitis

A. Definition
1. Inflammation of nasal mucosa caused by allergen
2. Classified as either **seasonal** or **perennial**

B. Cause/pathophysiology
1. After exposure to antigen, IgE is released
2. Mast cells release histamine, prostaglandins, leukotrienes, and other chemical mediators that cause symptoms of allergic rhinitis

C. Clinical presentation
1. Symptoms of upper airway inflammation: rhinorrhea; congestion; sneezing; and itchy nose, throat, and eyes
2. Transverse nasal crease (from rubbing nose)
3. "**Allergic salute**" (pushing nose up with hand)

QUICK HIT

Common asthma triggers include environmental exposures such as tobacco smoke, weather changes, viral illnesses, and allergens.

4. Bluish or boggy nasal turbinates and **cobblestoned pharynx**
5. "**Allergic shiners**" (infraorbital edema and darkening)

D. Testing: allergen-specific RAST or skin-pinprick test for patients with severe reactions without obvious cause to avoid future triggers

E. Therapy
1. Allergen avoidance
2. Medications
    a. Intranasal glucocorticoids (1st-line therapy): beclomethasone, flunisolide, budesonide, fluticasone, mometasone
    b. Antihistamines
        i. 2nd generation (e.g., loratadine)
            (a) Less sedating and fewer side effects
        ii. 1st generation (e.g., diphenhydramine, hydroxyzine)
            (a) 1st line for severe allergic reactions, more anticholinergic side effects, available in oral and IV forms
3. Allergen subcutaneous injection immunotherapy: variable efficacy and results
4. Referral to allergy-immunology specialist: if symptoms are severe or persistent despite appropriate medical management

> **QUICK HIT**
>
> The most common IgE-mediated food allergies in children are caused by milk protein allergy, affecting 2%–3% of children age >12 months, followed by egg allergy, affecting 1%–2% of children.

IV. Food Allergies

A. Cause/pathophysiology: adverse immune reactions to proteins in food; divided into
1. IgE-mediated reactions
2. Non–IgE-mediated reactions
3. Eosinophilic GI disorders

B. Clinical presentation
1. IgE-mediated reactions can present as urticaria and angioedema, rhinoconjunctivitis, GI upset, and anaphylaxis
2. Non–IgE-mediated reactions include food protein–induced enterocolitis and celiac disease; can present with GI symptoms such as vomiting and/or diarrhea
3. Eosinophilic esophagitis and gastroenteritis often present with pain, dysphasia, or nausea

C. Testing
1. Thorough history and physical exam and keep a detailed food diary
2. Confirmatory tests
    a. Skin and serum allergy testing: pinprick test, RAST
    b. Trial elimination of suspected food items
    c. Food challenges

D. Therapy
1. Avoid offending allergen
2. Refer to allergy-immunology specialist if symptoms are severe or persistent despite appropriate medical management

V. Urticaria

A. Definition
1. Transient, edematous, pruritic, well-delineated pink to red papules or plaques; range in size from 1 mm to 10 cm; also referred to as **wheals** or **hives**
    a. **Acute urticaria**: new and present for <6 weeks
    b. **Chronic urticaria**: recurrent and occurs intermittently (but present on most days) for >6 weeks
2. Sometimes associated with **angioedema**, or severe allergic reactions
3. Triggers include environmental allergens, insect bites, and foods

B. Cause/pathophysiology
1. Occurs due to mast cell activation by allergen or irritant
2. Several etiologies exist but often specific cause cannot be identified
    a. Insect bites/stings, latex, foods
    b. Medications: narcotics, antibiotics, antiepileptics, radiocontrast
    c. Viral, bacterial, and parasitic infections

> **QUICK HIT**
>
> Viral infections are the most common cause of acute urticaria in children.

FIGURE 11-2 **Urticaria lesions are erythematous and irregular.**

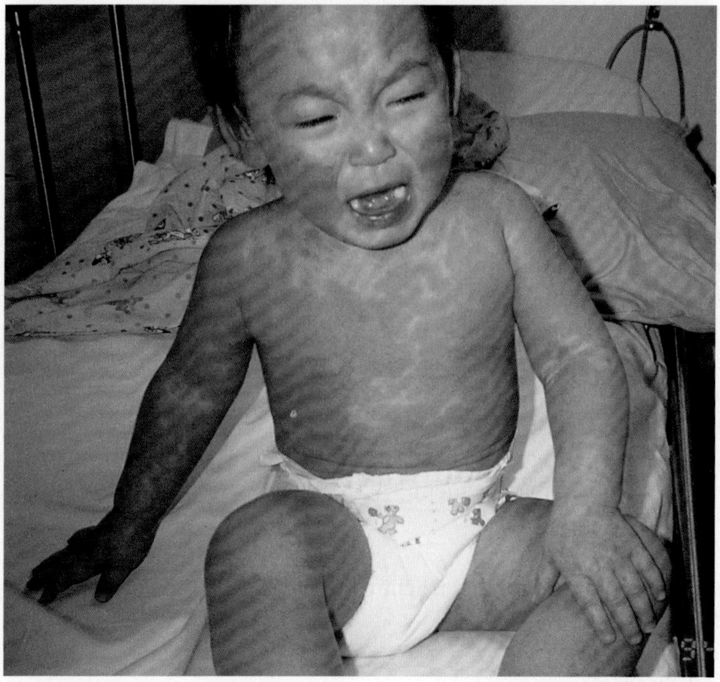

(From Fleisher GR, Ludwig S, Baskin MN. *Atlas of Pediatric Emergency Medicine*. Philadelphia: Lippincott Williams & Wilkins; 2004.)

C. Clinical presentation: appears as pruritic and painless raised red plaques on skin (Figure 11-2)

D. Testing
   1. No specific test confirms urticaria other than physical exam
   2. Can consider RAST or skin-pinprick testing

E. Therapy
   1. 1st-generation antihistamines—1st-line agents
   2. H_2 antihistamines for mild disease: ranitidine, famotidine, cimetidine
   3. Glucocorticoids for refractory cases: prednisolone, prednisone
   4. If allergic reaction is severe, patients should receive epinephrine autoinjector

VI. Angioedema

A. Definitions: localized subcutaneous/submucosal swelling that occurs when fluid moves into interstitial tissues

B. Cause/pathophysiology
   1. Allergic reactions
   2. Drug induced
      a. Aspirin and nonsteroidal anti-inflammatory drugs
      b. Angiotensin-converting enzyme inhibitors, angiotensin II receptor blockers
      c. Calcium channel blockers
   3. Other
      a. Chronic urticaria with or without angioedema
      b. Hereditary and acquired angioedema

C. Clinical presentation
   1. Most commonly affects loose connective tissue (edema of face, lips, throat, larynx, genitalia, and/or extremities)
   2. Can also affect bowel wall, leading to colicky abdominal pain
   3. Onset: minutes to hours
   4. Associated with other signs and symptoms of allergic reactions

QUICK HIT

Angioedema often occurs with urticaria or anaphylaxis.

Allergic and Immunologic Disorders

D. Therapy
  1. Treatment depends on severity and underlying mechanism involved
  2. Life-threatening situations (ABCs)
    a. Airway stabilization
    b. Ensure hemodynamic stability: fluids, pressors
    c. IM/IV epinephrine early if suspicion for developing respiratory compromise
  3. General treatment similar to anaphylaxis or allergic reactions (see sections 11-I and 11-VI)

SYMPTOM SPECIFIC: IMMUNOLOGIC

VII. Approach to Suspected Immunodeficiencies

A. Background information: immunodeficiencies may be primary or secondary
  1. Primary
    a. Inherited, typically present early in life
    b. Severity and types of infection depend on which component of immune system is involved
  2. Secondary: due to underlying disease (e.g., HIV, sickle cell disease, malignancies), medications (e.g., immunosuppressive/chemotherapeutic drugs)

B. Symptoms: when to suspect immunodeficiency
  1. When child has recurrent, severe, prolonged, or unusual infections
    a. Average child has 4–8 respiratory infections per year (up to 12 can be normal); average duration of symptoms is 8 days (up to 14 days can be normal)
    b. Most respiratory infections are viral; recurrent otitis media (>3) or pneumonia (>1) should raise suspicion
    c. Any opportunistic infection should prompt evaluation for immunodeficiency
  2. Nonimmunologic causes of recurrent infections
    a. Anatomic defects: skin anomaly or asplenia
    b. Inadequate clearing of secretions: ciliary dysfunction (e.g., primary ciliary dyskinesia), abnormal mucus production (e.g., cystic fibrosis [CF])
    c. Indwelling devices: shunts, central lines, catheters
    d. Recurrent exposures to contaminated sources

C. Important historical questions
  1. Growth and development: monitoring of height, weight, head circumference, and developmental milestones over time
  2. Immunization history
    a. General vaccination history important when testing antibody titers to evaluate humoral immune system (see Diagnostic Workup)
  3. Medications
    a. Number of courses, duration, effectiveness
    b. Note any immunosuppressive drugs
  4. Medical history
    a. Underlying or chronic illnesses, hospitalizations, surgeries, or prolonged school absences
    b. Evidence for nonimmunologic causes of recurrent infections
  5. Family history: recurrent infections, autoimmune disorders, unexplained deaths, or consanguinity (Table 11-5)
  6. Social history
    a. Home, daycare, school, parental work, travel exposures
    b. Allergens, toxins, tobacco smoke, contaminated water, farm animals, industrial solvents or toxins
  7. Infection history
    a. Age of onset (Table 11-6), duration, and frequency of infections
    b. Types of infections and organisms involved (Table 11-7)

QUICK HIT

B-cell and combined B- and T-cell deficiencies account for 75% of the primary immunodeficiencies.

QUICK HIT

Remember that 10% of children with recurrent infections have an underlying immunodeficiency.

QUICK HIT

Delayed umbilical cord detachment (after 30 days) can be seen in leukocyte adhesion defects.

QUICK HIT

Failure to thrive (FTT) is 1 of the 10 warning signs of an immunodeficiency.

QUICK HIT

Congenital antibody deficiencies often manifest after age 6 months as maternally transmitted antibodies wane.

QUICK HIT

Absent tonsils or lymph nodes during respiratory illnesses may indicate antibody deficiencies.

QUICK HIT

Eczema may be associated with several immunodeficiency syndromes, including Wiskott-Aldrich and Job syndromes as well as severe combined immunodeficiency (SCID).

TABLE 11-5 Mendelian Inheritance of Primary Immunodeficiencies

X-linked	Chronic granulomatous disease Wiskott-Aldrich syndrome X-linked agammaglobulinemia X-linked hyper-IgM syndrome X-linked SCID (more common)
Autosomal recessive	Ataxia telangiectasia Leukocyte adhesion defect Chédiak-Higashi syndrome Shwachman-Diamond syndrome Autosomal recessive SCID
Autosomal dominant	Job (hyper-IgE) syndrome Hereditary angioedema
Sporadic	DiGeorge syndrome Common variable immunodeficiency

Ig, immunoglobulin; SCID, severe combined immunodeficiency.

TABLE 11-6 Typical Age of Onset of Primary Immunodeficiencies

0–6 months	SCID DiGeorge syndrome Leukocyte adhesion defects
6 months–2 years	Antibody deficiencies (X-linked agammaglobulinemia and hyper-IgM syndrome)
2–6 years	Less severe antibody deficiencies (IgA deficiency and selective IgG antibody deficiency)
6–18 years	Common variable immunodeficiency Secondary immunodeficiencies

Ig, immunoglobulin; SCID, severe combined immunodeficiency.

TABLE 11-7 Types of Infections Associated with Specific Immune Cell Deficiencies

	Cell Type	Types of Infections	Typical Infectious Organisms
Adaptive immune system	B cell	Sinopulmonary infections	*Streptococcus pneumoniae, Haemophilus influenzae, Staphylococcus aureus, Pseudomonas, Enterovirus, Giardia*
	T cell	Opportunistic infections	*Candida, Pneumocystis, Mycobacteria, cytomegalovirus*
Innate immune system	Phagocyte	Abscesses, soft tissue infections	*Aspergillus, Staphylococcus aureus, coagulase-negative staphylococci, Serratia marcescens*
	Complement	Sepsis, meningitis	*Neisseria meningitidis*

TABLE 11-8 Immunologic Tests for Primary Immunodeficiencies

	Cell Type	Qualitative	Quantitative
Adaptive immune system	B cell	Vaccine antibody titers Vaccine response challenge	Quantitative immunoglobulin levels Flow cytometry (CD19) IgG subclass levels
	T cell	Delayed cutaneous hypersensitivity Lymphoproliferative assays	Flow cytometry - lymphocyte subset analysis (CD3, CD4, CD8)
Innate immune system	Phagocyte		
	LAD		Flow cytometry - cell surface marker expression (CD11, CD18, CD15)
	CGD	Oxidative burst: Dihydrorhodamine (DHR) or Nitroblue tetrazolium (NBT)	
	Complement	CH50	Complement assays

CGD, chronic granulomatous disease; Ig, immunoglobulin; LAD, leukocyte adhesion deficiency.

D. Diagnostic workup
   1. Testing for specific immune disorders (Table 11-8)
   2. Imaging: chest x-ray (CXR): evaluate for pneumonia, congenital lung abnormalities in patients with cough, and thymic shadow in newborns
E. Management of primary immunodeficiencies
   1. General principles (should be managed by an immunologist)
      a. Prompt recognition and aggressive treatment of infections
      b. Intravenous immunoglobulin (IVIG) for some humoral deficiencies
      c. Avoidance of live vaccines

QUICK HIT

Lymphopenia is an absolute lymphocyte count <2,500/mm^3 in children younger than age 5 years and <1,500/mm^3 in children older than age 5 years, whereas **neutropenia** is an absolute neutrophil count <1,500/mm^3.

QUICK HIT

Live vaccines include bacillus Calmette-Guérin, oral poliovirus, measles-mumps-rubella, varicella, intranasal influenza, and smallpox vaccines.

VIII. Classification of Primary Immunodeficiency

A. Immunodeficiency can occur in any of 4 major cellular components of immune system: B cells, T cells, complement, and phagocytes
B. Present with different types of infection by type (see Table 11-7)
C. Primary B-cell disorders
   1. Congenital agammaglobulinemia
   2. Hypogammaglobulinemia
   3. Common variable immunodeficiency
   4. Selective IgA deficiency
   5. IgG subclass deficiencies
D. Primary T-cell or combined defects
   1. Isolated defects of T lymphocytes are unusual
   2. Patients with T-cell defects have abnormal T-cell function and therefore also problems with antibody production
   3. Examples include
      a. Severe combined immunodeficiency (SCID)
      b. DiGeorge syndrome
      c. Ataxia telangiectasia
      d. Wiskott-Aldrich syndrome

QUICK HIT

Encapsulated organisms are the most common pathogens in B-cell disorders and include *Streptococcus pneumoniae, Haemophilus influenzae*, and *Neisseria meningitidis*.

QUICK HIT

B-cell maturation requires antigen stimulation with T-helper cells; therefore, severe defects in cellular immunity such as SCID can also lead to humoral immunodeficiency.

QUICK HIT

Because antibodies are important in the opsonization of encapsulated bacteria and viruses, X-linked agammaglobulinemia patients are most susceptible to those organisms, particularly **enteroviruses**.

QUICK HIT

The key physical exam finding is absence of peripheral lymphoid tissue, due to the absence of B-cell maturation, proliferation, class switching, and antigen stimulation in lymph nodes.

QUICK HIT

Absent B cells are a hallmark of X-linked agammaglobulinemia; B-cell levels are typically normal in other primary antibody immunodeficiencies.

QUICK HIT

Selective IgA deficiency is the most common immunologic defect (affecting ~1 in 500 people).

QUICK HIT

IgA is secreted in mucosal linings (GI, GU, sinopulmonary tracts) and is important in mucosal immunity by preventing microorganism penetration of mucosal surfaces.

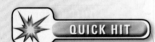

E. Phagocytic cells
   1. Neutrophils constitute 1st line of defense against microbial invasion and protect skin, GI tract, respiratory tract, and mucous membranes
   2. Sufficient neutrophils are necessary to rapidly eliminate microorganisms invading natural barriers
   3. Otherwise, infection can quickly disseminate locally and systemically
   4. Examples are
      a. Leukocyte adhesion defect
      b. Chronic granulomatous disease
      c. Chédiak-Higashi syndrome
      d. Cyclic neutropenia
      e. Kostmann syndrome

F. Complement deficiency
   1. Complement system is essential component of innate immunity by defending against pyogenic organisms
      a. Enhances phagocytosis (**opsonization**)
      b. Mediates inflammation via chemotaxis
      c. Cell lysis by insertion of complement proteins into cell membrane called **membrane attack complex**

DISEASE SPECIFIC: IMMUNOLOGIC

IX. X-Linked (Bruton) Agammaglobulinemia (XLA)

A. Characterized by **agammaglobulinemia** (absence of Ig in blood) and increased susceptibility to infections

B. Cause/pathophysiology: mutation in *BTK* gene (signal transduction critical for B-cell maturation) → inability of B cells to mature → defective antibody response

C. Clinical presentation
   1. **Failure to thrive (FTT)** and **recurrent** (otitis media, pneumonia, sinusitis) or **severe** (sepsis, osteomyelitis, meningoencephalitis) **infections**
   2. Symptoms typically present after 6 months when maternally transferred IgG disappears

D. Testing
   1. Complete blood count (CBC) with differential and flow cytometry to evaluate lymphocyte subsets
   2. Quantitative Ig levels
   3. Humoral immune panel (to test for immune response to vaccines)
   4. Genetic testing available

E. Therapy
   1. Regular (usually every 2–4 weeks) IVIG or subcutaneous Ig (SCIG): lowers rates of infection, hospitalization, complications, and overall morbidity/mortality
   2. Antibiotics: prolonged therapy for suspected infections
   3. Avoidance of live vaccines

X. Selective Immunoglobulin A (IgA) Deficiency

A. Definitions: isolated serum IgA deficiency in patient age >4 years without other immunodeficiencies

B. Cause/pathophysiology
   1. Heterogeneous, multifactorial disorder with genetic component
   2. Most significant risk factor is family history of immunodeficiency
   3. B cells cannot differentiate into plasma cells that secrete IgA

C. Testing: quantitative immunoglobulins (demonstrates low IgA)

D. Clinical presentation
   1. Most patients (85%–90%) are asymptomatic
   2. Of remaining 15%–20% of symptomatic patients, 4 possible presentations
      a. Recurrent sinopulmonary infections with encapsulated organisms (otitis media, pneumonia, sinusitis)

b. GI disorders (*Giardia* infections, celiac disease, inflammatory bowel disease [IBD])
c. Autoimmune disorders (systemic lupus erythematosus [SLE] and juvenile rheumatoid arthritis [JRA])
d. Anaphylactic transfusion reactions (to blood and IVIG)

E. Therapy
1. Asymptomatic: no need for therapy, just frequent monitoring
2. Recurrent infections: treat infections with antibiotics (e.g., metronidazole for *Giardia*); consider IVIG for severe or recurrent infections
3. Autoimmune disorders: steroids, immune modulators
4. Anaphylactic transfusion reactions: desensitization to blood products

XI. Transient Hypogammaglobulinemia of Infancy

A. Definition
1. IgG levels 2 or more standard deviations (SDs) below mean in patients age >6 months in whom other immunodeficiencies are excluded; **diagnosis of exclusion**
2. Cause unknown; may be extreme of **physiologic nadir**

B. Clinical presentation: recurrent or severe infections beginning early in life
1. Many cases are asymptomatic
a. Recurrent upper respiratory infections (URIs), otitis media, pneumonia, gastroenteritis, oral thrush
b. Severe or invasive infections, such as sepsis or meningitis

C. Testing
1. Quantitative Ig levels
2. Repeat lab testing every 6–12 months to monitor for normalization of IgG levels or progression to other immunodeficiencies

XII. Disorders of T-Cell Function

A. Definitions
1. Dysfunction impairs T-cell ability to destroy intracellular and other bacteria, viruses, fungi, parasites, and mycobacteria
2. T-cell to B-cell communication is defective, causing defects in antibody production and increased incidence of atopy and autoimmune disorders
3. Examples include
a. Thymic aplasia (DiGeorge syndrome, 22q deletion syndrome)
b. Chronic mucocutaneous candidiasis
c. Hyper-IgM syndrome
d. Wiskott-Aldrich syndrome
e. Ataxia telangiectasia

B. Clinical presentation
1. Age at onset of infection: usually ages 2–6 months
2. Specific pathogens involved
a. Common viral infections
b. Mycobacteria
c. Mucocutaneous candidiasis
d. *Pneumocystis*

C. Testing
1. Reduced absolute lymphocyte count and abnormal morphology (normal result indicates T-cell defect unlikely)
2. Flow cytometry to enumerate T cell and T-cell subpopulations
3. CXR examination for thymic size
4. Delayed-type hypersensitivity reaction by skin test (e.g., *Candida albicans*, tetanus toxoid)

D. Therapy
1. Bone marrow transplantation for patients with Wiskott-Aldrich syndrome or complete DiGeorge syndrome

QUICK HIT

Absolute serum IgA levels correlate with certainty of diagnosis but do not correlate with presence or severity of symptoms.

QUICK HIT

Live vaccines should be avoided until other immunodeficiencies have been excluded.

QUICK HIT

IVIG provides pathogen-specific donor IgG but does not actually replete IgA levels. It should be given only to patients with severe, recurrent infections.

QUICK HIT

The transplacental transfer of maternal IgG that comprises the Igs present at birth occurs in the 3rd trimester.

QUICK HIT

Transient hypogammaglobulinemia of infancy patients usually have normal lymphocyte subpopulations, cellular immune function, memory B-cell levels, and antibody responses to immunizations.

QUICK HIT

IVIG is not indicated for low IgG levels in the absence of infection.

QUICK HIT

Lymphopenia is an absolute lymphocyte count ≤2,500/mm^3 (birth), ≤4,000/mm^3 (age >6 months), or ≤1,000/mm^3 (adult).

QUICK HIT

If the *Candida* skin test result is positive, all primary T-cell defects are precluded, and there is no need to do more expensive in vitro tests.

QUICK HIT

C. albicans intradermal skin test is the most cost-effective test to exclude T-cell disorders.

QUICK HIT

The leading cause of SCID is mutation in the gene for the γ chain, and the 2nd most common cause is adenosine deaminase (ADA) enzyme deficiency.

QUICK HIT

Four or more new ear infections in 1 year may be a sign of immunodeficiency.

QUICK HIT

Two or more serious sinus infections or pneumonias within 1 year may be a sign of immunodeficiency.

QUICK HIT

SCID patients and household members should not receive live vaccines!

QUICK HIT

All blood products administered to SCID patients must be irradiated and cytomegalovirus negative to prevent infection.

2. Prophylaxis with trimethoprim-sulfamethoxazole to prevent *Pneumocystis* pneumonia
3. Avoidance of live viral vaccines

XIII. Severe Combined Immunodeficiency

A. Definitions
1. Both **cell-mediated** (**T-cell**) and **humoral** (**B-cell**) **immunity** deficient; therefore, susceptible to infection from all classes of microorganisms
2. Inheritance most commonly is **autosomal recessive**, but it may also be **X-linked**

B. Cause/pathophysiology: failure of stem cell to differentiate into T and B lymphocytes

C. Clinical presentation
1. Extreme susceptibility to infection presenting in infancy
2. Severe presentation of common infections and opportunistic infections: **chronic otitis**, **sepsis**, **diarrhea** (frequently *Salmonella* or *Escherichia coli*), **recurrent pulmonary infections**, **persistent thrush**
3. Opportunistic infections: ***Pneumocystis* pneumonia**, invasive fungal and viral infections (e.g., chickenpox)
4. **FTT** due to recurrent infections
5. Small or absent lymphoid tissues
6. Graft-versus-host disease (GVHD) reactions from engrafted maternal T cells, resulting in severe cutaneous, GI, and hematologic disease and hepatosplenomegaly; **morbilliform erythroderma** can progress to necrosis

D. Testing
1. CBC shows **lymphopenia**
2. Flow cytometry shows decreased T cells
3. Quantitative Ig reveals **absent IgG and IgM**
4. Mitogen-stimulation test shows absence of T- and B-cell function
5. Exclude HIV as acquired cause of immunodeficiency

E. Therapy
1. Bone marrow transplant before age 3 months improves survival
2. If not transplant candidate, alternative therapies include
   a. ADA enzyme replacement
   b. Gene therapy
3. **IVIG** infusions
4. Preventative therapy/precautions
   a. Avoid public exposure before transplantation
   b. ***Pneumocystis* prophylaxis** with trimethoprim-sulfamethoxazole

XIV. Ataxia Telangiectasia

A. Definitions
1. Combined T-lymphocyte and Ig deficiency with neurocutaneous findings
2. Autosomal recessive inheritance
3. Predisposition to malignancy

B. Cause/pathophysiology: **ataxia telangiectasia–mutated (ATM) protein** (DNA repair protein)

C. Clinical presentation
1. Progressively worsening ataxia
   a. Truncal ataxia by ages 1–2 years
   b. Appendicular ataxia worsening in school-age years
   c. Wheelchair bound by teenage years
2. Bulbar telangiectasias at ages 3–5 years; telangiectasias spread to rest of body from ages 3–7 years
3. Ig deficiencies predispose to recurrent respiratory infections in most patients
4. Leukemia (T cell) or lymphomas (B cell) occur in 10%–15%

D. Testing
1. Diagnosis usually made by clinical presentation and exam
2. Serum α-fetoprotein (elevated in >99%)
3. Quantitative Ig levels and IgG subclasses

XV. Wiskott-Aldrich Syndrome

A. Definitions
1. Defective B- and T-cell functions
2. X-linked recessive inheritance

B. Cause/pathophysiology
1. Defective B- and T-cell functions make susceptible to infection
2. Defect in platelet synthesis causes production of small, short-lived platelets, resulting in thrombocytopenia

C. Clinical presentation
1. Average age at diagnosis is 8 months
2. 30% with classic triad: **thrombocytopenia**, **eczema**, and **chronic otitis media**
3. Other infections may include sinusitis, pneumonia, sepsis, meningitis, severe viral infections, and opportunistic infections
4. Neonates usually present with symptoms related to thrombocytopenia (i.e., bloody stools, bleeding from circumcision site, petechiae, and purpura)
5. 20% prone to **lymphoreticular malignancies** (i.e., B-cell lymphoma)
6. 40% with autoimmune disease (e.g., anemia, vasculitis, colitis)
7. **Average age of death is 8 years**, usually from bleeding or infection

D. Testing
1. Platelet count $<70{,}000/\text{mm}^3$ with small platelets (mean platelet volume [MPV] 50% of normal)
2. **Lymphopenia** (mostly T cells) is common
3. Quantitative Igs: normal IgG, low IgM, and high IgA and IgE
4. Flow cytometry to evaluate T and B cells and rule out SCID

E. Therapy
1. Peripheral blood stem cell or bone marrow transplantation
2. Splenectomy is an option if thrombocytopenia is severe

XVI. Chronic Granulomatous Disease (CGD)

A. Definition: immune deficiency characterized by granuloma development and recurrent infections due to inability of phagocytic cells to kill certain ingested pathogens

B. Cause/pathophysiology: defect in nicotinamide adenine dinucleotide phosphate → no superoxide free radical → no microbial death

C. Clinical presentation
1. Early (age <2 years) onset of severe, recurrent bacterial and fungal infections
   a. Pneumonia, abscesses, osteomyelitis, bacteremia, fungemia
2. Granulomas in skin and GI and GU tracts

D. Testing
1. DHR (dihydrorhodamine) test: fluorescence = normal phagocytes
2. Older test: **nitroblue-tetrazolium (NBT)**
3. Genetic testing to specify which mutation, if NBT or DHR positive

E. Therapy
1. Treat infections
2. High-dose interferon (IFN)-γ during severe infections and for prophylaxis
3. Daily prophylaxis with trimethoprim-sulfamethoxazole and/or antifungals

XVII. Hyper-IgE Syndrome (Job Syndrome)

A. Definitions: immunodeficiency syndrome characterized by dermatitis, recurrent abscesses, distinctive facial features, fractures, and high levels of serum IgE

B. Cause/pathophysiology: unknown

C. Clinical presentation
1. Recurrent staphylococcal abscesses of skin, lungs, and joints
2. Pruritic dermatitis: due to histamine release by mast cells
3. Distinctive coarse facial features
4. Recurrent fractures from minor trauma due to osteopenia

QUICK HIT

T cells usually act as immune surveillance against malignant transformation.

QUICK HIT

Heterozygote carriers for the *ATM* gene will not have classic symptoms, but may have a higher incidence of solid tumor malignancies such as breast cancer.

QUICK HIT

Variant ataxia telangiectasia is a milder form, in which patients may have delayed development of ataxia and may never develop classic telangiectasias.

QUICK HIT

Eczema in Wiskott-Aldrich syndrome is usually focused in the scalp and flexural areas.

QUICK HIT

Consider Wiskott-Aldrich syndrome in any patient with thrombocytopenia and small platelets.

QUICK HIT

The 5-year survival post-transplant is 70%. Survival improved in transplants with human leukocyte antigen–identical siblings.

MNEMONIC

Catalase-positive organisms = **BEANS**
***B**urkholderia cepacia*
***E**nterobacteriaceae*
***A**spergillus*
***N**ocardia*
***S**taphylococcus aureus*

MNEMONIC

Think: Job's nickname was **FREDD**
Fractures (recurrent)
Recurrent staphylococcal abscesses
Eosinophilia and high IgE
Dermatitis
Distinctive coarse facial features

D. Testing
  1. Diagnosis based on clinical features
  2. Laboratory findings: exceptionally high serum IgE and IgD
E. Therapy
  1. Treat infections
  2. Hydration and emollients for affected skin
  3. Prophylaxis with trimethoprim-sulfamethoxazole

XVIII. Chédiak-Higashi Syndrome

A. Definition: autosomal recessive immune disorder characterized by recurrent bacterial infections, partial oculocutaneous albinism, coagulation defects, and progressive neurologic abnormalities
B. Cause/pathophysiology: no phagolysosome formation and impaired killing of phagocytosed bacteria
C. Clinical presentation
  1. Recurrent pyogenic infections of skin
  2. **Albinism**: abnormal distribution of melanosomes in hair, skin, and retina
  3. Coagulation defects
  4. Peripheral neuropathy and/or autonomic dysfunction
  5. Accelerated phase: lymphoma-like aggressive phase in adolescents leading to diffuse organ infiltration and death
D. Testing: peripheral smear
  1. Giant lysosomes and microscopic examination of hair
  2. Melanin clumps
E. Therapy
  1. Infection: aggressively treat with granulocyte colony-stimulating factor (G-CSF) for neutropenia during infection
  2. Accelerated phase
    a. High-dose systemic glucocorticoids
    b. Bone marrow transplantation

XIX. Shwachman-Diamond Syndrome

MNEMONIC

Shwachman found **Diamonds** while searching for **bone** (marrow disruption)s. His friend **Luke** (leukemia) found **abnormal skeletons** while **pan**(creatic insufficiency)ning for gold.

A. Definition: autosomal recessive syndrome characterized by bone marrow dysfunction, exocrine pancreatic insufficiency, predisposition for leukemia, skeletal abnormalities, and recurrent infections
B. Cause/pathophysiology: impaired chemotaxis and migration of neutrophils
C. Clinical presentation
  1. **Pancytopenia**
  2. Exocrine pancreatic insufficiency: large stools in infancy, FTT
  3. Skeletal abnormalities
  4. Recurrent pneumonia, otitis media, and skin and soft tissue infections
D. Testing
  1. CBC
    a. Neutropenia > anemia > thrombocytopenia
    b. 5%–10% develop leukemia
  2. 72-hour fecal fat measurement and sweat test to rule out CF
E. Therapy
  1. Treat bacterial infections
  2. Pancreatic enzymes, ADEK vitamins, low-fat diet for exocrine pancreatic insufficiency
  3. Transfusions, G-CSF

XX. Disorders of Complement

QUICK HIT

All classical pathway deficiencies are autosomal recessive.

A. Definition: any disruption in complement cascade that leads to
  1. Deficiency in opsonization and phagocytosis of encapsulated microorganisms
  2. Clearance of immune complexes from circulation
B. Cause/pathophysiology
  1. **Primary disorders** = hereditary or acquired complement deficiencies; most are autosomal recessive

2. **Secondary disorders** = mediated by immune complexes causing consumption of complement

C. Clinical presentation
  1. Infectious
    a. Recurrent pyogenic infections
    b. Disseminated gonococcal infections
    c. *Neisseria meningitidis*
    d. Septicemia (consider when 2 or more episodes)
  2. Renal: chronic nephritis
  3. Connective tissue: patients with collagen vascular disease or recurrent angioedema

D. Testing
  1. Total hemolytic complement activity (CH_{50})
  2. Complement levels

E. Therapy
  1. No specific therapy for most disorders, except hereditary angioedema
  2. Fever should prompt blood cultures and initiation of broad-spectrum antibiotics
  3. Immunize patient and household contacts for pneumococci, *Haemophilus influenzae,* and *N. meningitidis*

QUICK HIT

Suspect complement deficiency when there is a family history of recurrent infections with encapsulated organisms, especially *N. meningitidis*.

12 Dermatologic Conditions

SYMPTOM SPECIFIC

I. Classification of Rashes

A. Historical questions (Box 12-1)

B. Physical examination findings

1. Full physical exam, especially
   a. Entire body surface, mucous membranes, conjunctiva, hair, and nails
   b. Look for signs of systemic disease
2. Examine rash: primary lesion, secondary changes, distribution (location of rash), pattern (e.g., flexural areas, sun-exposed areas)
   a. Describe the rash (Table 12-1)
   b. Note secondary lesions/changes (Table 12-2)
   c. Note distribution/pattern (Table 12-3)

C. Laboratory testing: diagnostic procedures are not required for diagnosis of most pediatric rashes

1. Wood's lamp: ultraviolet (UV) light to detect hyperpigmented or hypopigmented macules; also useful for tinea capitis
2. Potassium hydroxide (KOH) prep: microscopic examination for fungal elements
3. Scraping of burrow for scabies mites
4. Immunofluorescence studies on skin biopsy

> **QUICK HIT**
> Easy visibility of rashes commonly results in a cursory exam and hasty diagnosis. A thorough history and exam are warranted.

> **QUICK HIT**
> Primary lesions are usually more helpful for diagnostic purposes than secondary lesions.

II. Approach to Purpura

A. General characteristics

1. Reddish/bluish/purplish skin lesions
2. Result from leakage of blood from vessel into surrounding tissues (can be skin or mucosal membranes)
3. Because blood is outside vessel, lesions are **nonblanching** (do not change color with external pressure)

> **QUICK HIT**
> Potentially serious causes of purpura include meningococcemia, Henoch-Schönlein purpura, and idiopathic thrombocytopenic purpura.

BOX 12-1

Questions to Ask on History for Rashes

When did the rash start?
How did it look when it started, and how has it changed?
Where is the rash?
Any associated symptoms (pain, itching)?
Any systemic symptoms (fever)?
What treatments have you tried, and how have they helped?
Have you had this before?
Does anyone else in the family have a rash like this?
Any inciting factors (lotion, soap, swimming, medications, immunizations, travel, recent illness, injury)?
What is your past medical history?
Do you take any prescription or over-the-counter medications or supplements?

TABLE 12-1 Description of Primary Lesion

Macule	Flat alteration in skin color, without elevation or depression, <1 cm
Patch	Flat alteration in skin color, larger than macule, >1 cm
Papule	Palpable, elevated, nonvesicular, nonpustular, solid lesions <0.5–1 cm
Nodule	Palpable, circumscribed, solid lesions larger than papule (1–2 cm)
Tumor	Palpable solid mass larger than nodule; vary in mobility and consistency
Plaque	Broad, elevated lesion; frequently a confluence of papules or pustules
Urticaria	Solid elevation formed by local, superficial, transient edema; vary in size and configuration; can change over hours
Vesicle	Sharply circumscribed, elevated, fluid-containing lesions <0.5 cm
Bulla	Larger circumscribed, elevated, fluid-containing lesions >0.5 cm
Pustule	Circumscribed elevations containing a purulent exudate
Telangiectasia	Relatively permanent dilation of superficial venules, capillaries, or arterioles of the skin
Cyst	Circumscribed, thick-walled lesion located deep in the skin, covered by normal epidermis
Petechiae	Nonblanching red/purple hemorrhage in the skin or mucous membranes <2 mm
Purpura	Larger nonblanching red/purple hemorrhage in the skin or mucous membranes >2 mm; if raised, called "palpable purpura"

4. Vary in size
   a. **Petechiae**: <2 mm
   b. **Ecchymoses**: >2 mm (often called **bruises**)
5. Can be palpable or nonpalpable: palpable caused by inflammation/destruction of vessel walls (i.e., vasculitis)
6. Causes range from benign to true emergency

B. History
1. Establish time course and progression
2. Presence of fever (makes infectious etiology more likely)
3. Age (younger ages make bleeding disorders more likely)
4. Location and type of lesion
   a. Palpable purpura in areas of pressure (e.g., waistband or sock line) or dependency (e.g., over buttocks and lower extremities) is classic for Henoch-Schönlein purpura (HSP)

TABLE 12-2 Secondary Skin Changes

Crust	Dried remains of serum, blood, pus, or exudate overlying areas of lost or damaged epidermis
Scale	Accumulation of compact desquamation layers of stratum corneum
Fissure	Splitting or cracking
Erosion	Superficial, focal loss of epidermis
Ulcerations	Focal loss extending to dermis; tend to heal with scarring
Excoriation	Ulcerated lesions inflicted by scratching; often linear
Scar	Fibrous connective tissue
Lichenification	Thickening of skin with accentuation of normal skin lines caused by chronic rubbing, scratching, or inflammation
Atrophy	Loss of skin tissue resulting in thinness, depression

TABLE 12-3 **Configuration of Lesions**

Term	Definition	Example
Annular	Ring shaped	Tinea corporis, granuloma annulare
Clustering	Lesions group together	Contact dermatitis
Confluent	Lesions that tend to join together	Viral exanthems
Dermatomal	Localizing into a dermatome supplied by ≥1 dorsal ganglia	Herpes zoster
Discoid	Solid, raised, disk shaped	Lupus
Discrete	Individual lesions remain separate	Insect bites
Eczematoid	Inflammation with thickening of skin, oozing	Eczema, psoriasis
Guttate	Drop-like lesions	Psoriasis
Keratotic	Horny thickening	Keratosis pilaris
Linear	Lesions in a line or band	Striae, poison ivy
Multiform	More than 1 variety or shape of lesions	Erythema multiforme
Nummular	Coin-like	Nummular eczema
Polycyclic	Oval lesions containing more than 1 ring	Urticaria
Reticular	Net-like pattern	Cutis marmorata, fifth disease
Serpiginous	Snake-like configuration	Cutaneous larva migrans
Umbilicated	Depressed center	Molluscum contagiosum
Universal	Widespread, throughout	Alopecia universalis

b. Ecchymoses on ears, buttocks, perineum, and upper arms are concerning for child abuse, particularly when a reasonable mechanism of injury is not provided

5. Prior bleeding history (including losing teeth and surgeries like circumcision)
6. History of "easy bruising" (ecchymoses in unusual distributions are concerning for child abuse)
7. Family bleeding history (look for inheritance patterns like X-linked hemophilia)
8. Tick exposure (e.g., Rocky Mountain spotted fever [RMSF])

C. Physical examination

1. Critical to establish child's level of illness/toxicity: altered mental status = emergency
    a. Purpura with shock is concerning for **purpura fulminans** (caused by *Neisseria meningitidis*)
2. Skin
    a. Determine size, location, and distribution
        i. Buttock/lower extremity is consistent with HSP
        ii. Petechiae on chest/face can occur with coughing/vomiting
    b. Distinguish between palpable or nonpalpable lesions
3. Abdomen
    a. Hepatomegaly can indicate liver dysfunction
    b. Splenomegaly with infection or malignancy
4. Extremities
    a. Arthritis/arthralgias more common with etiology like HSP
    b. **Hemarthrosis** (bleeding into a joint) is common with hemophilia
5. Neurologic: altered mental status can be related to intracranial bleeding in children bruised from child abuse

FIGURE 12-1 The approach to the child with purpura.

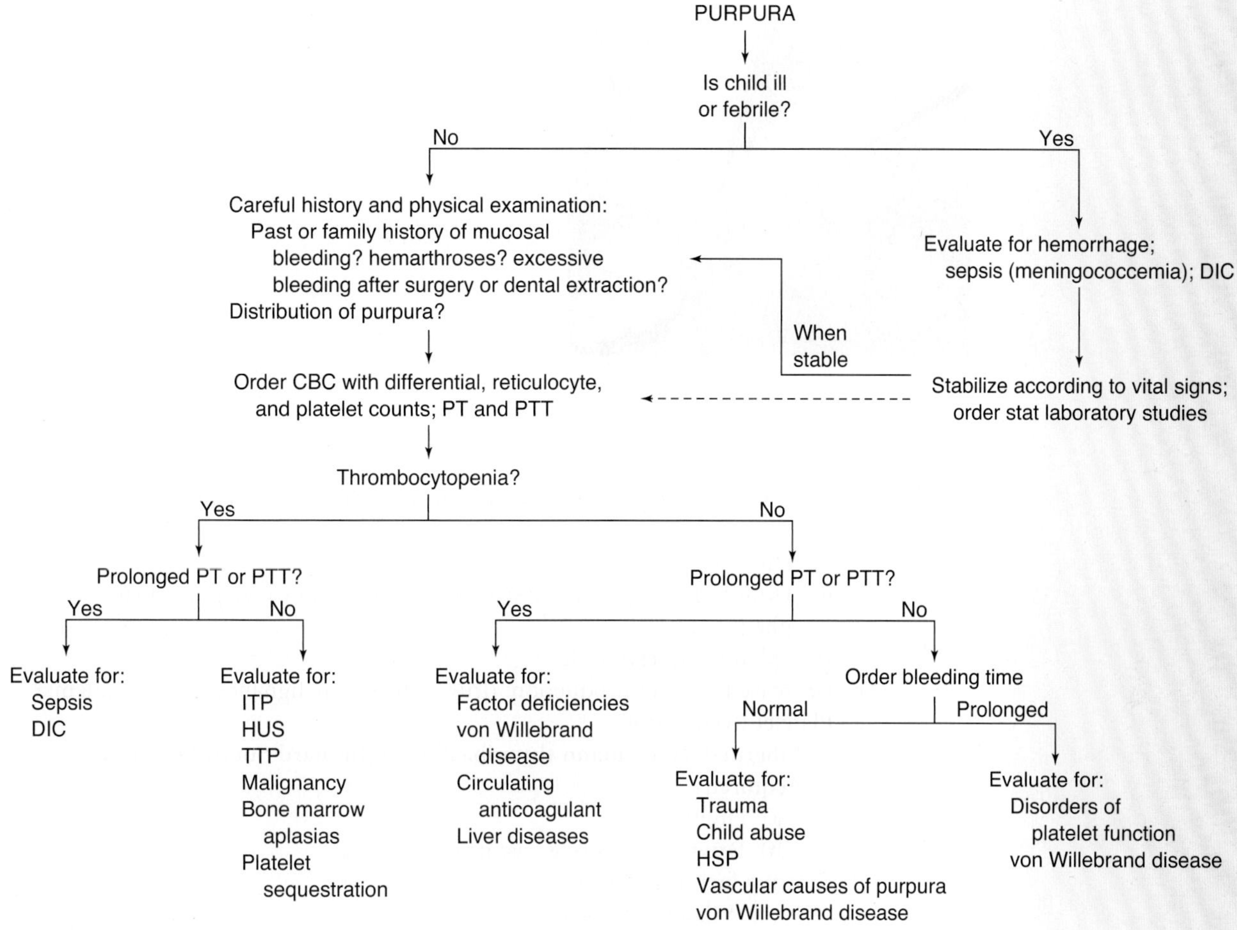

CBC, complete blood count; DIC, disseminated intravascular coagulation; HSP, Henoch-Schönlein purpura; HUS, hemolytic-uremic syndrome; ITP, idiopathic thrombocytopenic purpura; PT, prothrombin time; PTT, partial thromboplastin time; TTP, thrombotic thrombocytopenic purpura.

D. Differential diagnosis (Figure 12-1)
  1. Disruptions in vascular integrity
    a. Trauma (bruising)
      i. Can be accidental or nonaccidental (child abuse)
        (a) Accidental pattern of lesions classically over lower extremities, knees, elbows, forehead
        (b) Bruising patterns concerning for child abuse include ears, neck, buttocks, genitals, upper thighs, and back
    b. Vasculitis (**palpable purpura**)
      i. HSP (Figure 12-2): lesion classically over buttocks and lower extremities
    c. Infectious diseases
      i. Purpura fulminans
        (a) Rapid presentation and progression to life-threatening condition
        (b) Purpura seemingly develops or progresses "before your eyes"
        (c) Purpuras are often large; coalesce together rapidly
        (d) Disseminated intravascular coagulation (DIC)
        (e) Infection with *N. meningitidis* (can occur with sepsis from other gram-negative and gram-positive bacteria as well)
      ii. Viral infections: parvovirus, adenovirus, enterovirus
      iii. Rickettsial disease: RMSF
    d. Collagen vascular diseases
      i. Systemic lupus erythematosus (SLE)
      ii. Ehlers-Danlos syndrome

QUICK HIT

Purpura in HSP follows a waist-down distribution. This can include the hands and lower arms, which hang below the waist.

FIGURE 12-2 Henoch-Schönlein purpura (HSP).

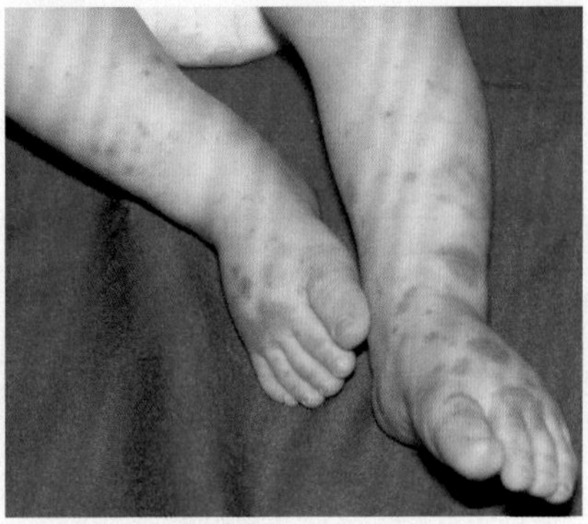

2. Abnormal hemostasis
   a. Increased platelet destruction
      i. **Idiopathic thrombocytopenic purpura (ITP)** (see Chapter 9, Hematologic Diseases)
      ii. DIC (see Chapter 9)
      iii. Drug-induced platelet destruction: sulfonamides, valproic acid, phenytoin
      iv. Splenic sequestration
   b. Decreased platelet production: drug induced, malignancy, aplastic anemia
   c. Platelet dysfunction
      i. Inherited: **Glanzmann thrombasthenia, Bernard-Soulier syndrome**
      ii. Acquired
         (a) Uremia
         (b) Drug induced (e.g., aspirin)
   d. Clotting factor deficiency (see Chapter 9)
      i. von Willebrand disease (VWD)
      ii. Hemophilia
      iii. Vitamin K deficiency
   e. Clotting factor dysfunction

E. Laboratory evaluation
1. Complete blood count (CBC) with peripheral smear
2. Coagulation studies
   a. Prothrombin time (PT)/international normalized ratio (INR)
   b. Activated partial thromboplastin time (aPTT)
3. DIC: D-dimer, fibrinogen, fibrinogen-split products

F. Management
1. Specific etiology-driven therapies
   a. Purpura fulminans
      i. Fluid resuscitation, broad-spectrum antibiotics
   b. ITP: administer intravenous immunoglobulin (IVIG)
   c. DIC: identify trigger; administer fresh frozen plasma (FFP), cryoprecipitate, and/or platelets
   d. Hemophilia: administer recombinant factor VIII or factor IX
   e. Uremia: therapy to improve renal function such as dialysis

Dermatologic Conditions

QUICK HIT

Varicella lesions will be present in all stages at 1 time and in 1 place from vesicles ("dewdrop on a rose petal") to crusted areas.

III. Approach to Vesicular Rashes

A. Differential diagnosis (Table 12-4)

B. Historical questions
1. Evolution of lesions over time
2. Past history of similar lesions
   a. Herpes zoster occurs in patients who have had prior varicella infection
   b. Recurrent herpes simplex virus (HSV) infections are generally less severe than initial presentation

TABLE 12-4 **Differential Diagnosis of Vesicles**

Infectious	Congenital/Immune Related	Acquired
Herpes simplex virus Varicella Herpes zoster Hand, foot, and mouth disease Impetigo Syphilis	Acropustulosis of infancy Epidermolysis bullosa Juvenile spring eruption	Contact dermatitis Rhus dermatitis (poison ivy, poison oak, poison sumac) Pompholyx Friction blister

c. Acropustulosis of infancy presents as recurrent episodes of pruritic lesions on palms and soles
d. **Pompholyx** (dyshidrotic eczema) presents with frequent relapses of symmetric, bilateral deep lesions on palms, soles, and lateral fingers
3. Recent contact with sick individuals
4. Recent exposures to possible allergens
5. Associated itching or pain
   a. Herpes zoster is often preceded by pain, tingling, or burning
   b. Itching: contact dermatitis, bites, other rashes
6. Associated systemic symptoms
   a. Neonatal herpes simplex virus (HSV) infection: hepatitis, meningitis
   b. Varicella: prodrome of cold symptoms/fever
   c. Hand, foot, and mouth disease: fever and drooling

> **QUICK HIT**
> Herpes zoster, also known as *shingles*, is caused by varicella-zoster virus, a virus in the family Herpesviridae.

C. Physical exam
1. Assess patient's condition; inspect all skin areas
2. Distribution of lesions may be clue to diagnosis
   a. Hand, foot, and mouth lesions: posterior mouth, hands, feet
   b. Dermatome distribution: herpes zoster
   c. Primary oral HSV presents with lesions in anterior mouth; recurrent infections on lips
   d. Contact dermatitis lesions will reflect specific exposure; may see **koebnerization** (spread of lesions along lines of scratching)
   e. Bed bug bites may appear in linear clusters of 3 or 4 lesions: "**breakfast, lunch, and dinner**" **sign**

D. Laboratory testing
1. Rarely needed because most diagnoses are made clinically
2. Direct fluorescent antibody (DFA) of bottom of blister
3. Polymerase chain reaction (PCR) for varicella-zoster virus (VZV) and HSV
4. **Tzanck smear** to diagnose HSV lesions is outdated
5. Viral culture of lesions for HSV or VZV: growth takes 2–3 days

IV. Approach to Bullae

A. Definition: fluid-filled (clear or bloody) lesion measuring >0.5 cm
B. Pathophysiology
1. Tense: deeper process where split is below lamina lucida
2. Flaccid: superficial process
   a. **Nikolsky sign**: shearing or blistering of skin by rubbing normal-appearing skin

> **QUICK HIT**
> Nikolsky sign is a classic feature of toxic epidermal necrolysis.

C. Clinical presentation
1. Neonatal
   a. Infectious: syphilis, candidiasis, HSV, VZV, scabies
   b. Genetic: epidermolysis bullosa (EB), ectodermal dysplasia, acrodermatitis enteropathica

TABLE 12-5 **Testing**

Direct Preps	
Tzanck smear	Herpesviruses
Gram stain	Bacteria, white blood cells/eosinophils
KOH	Fungal elements
Mineral oil	Scabies
Giemsa or Wright stain	Inflammatory cell types
Dark field	Syphilis
Fluorescent Ab testing	HSV, VZV, syphilis
Laboratory Tests	
CBC with differential	Infectious and incontinentia pigmenti (eosinophils)
Zinc, alkaline phosphatase	Acrodermatitis enterohepatica
PCR	HSV, VZV, enterovirus
ANA	Lupus erythematosus

Ab, antibody; ANA, antinuclear antibody; CBC, complete blood count; HSV, herpes simplex virus; KOH, potassium hydroxide; PCR, polymerase chain reaction; VZV, varicella-zoster virus.

QUICK HIT

Second-degree burns should be included in the differential for bullae and could represent child abuse.

2. Infantile/childhood vesiculobullous disorders
   a. Acquired: psoriasis, Stevens-Johnson syndrome (SJS)
   b. Autoimmune: pemphigus, EB, bullous pemphigoid
   c. Infectious: **impetigo**, **blistering distal dactylitis**, staphylococcal scalded skin syndrome (SSSS), scabies, bullous arthropod reaction, primary or breakthrough varicella, herpes zoster, coxsackie virus

D. Testing (Table 12-5)

QUICK HIT

Eczema is often referred to as the "itch that rashes," because scratching induces trauma, which causes inflammation, in turn, worsening pruritus.

DISEASE SPECIFIC

V. Atopic Dermatitis (AD)/Eczema

A. General characteristics
1. Chronic, itchy, inflammatory skin condition that usually begins in young childhood (Figure 12-3)
2. Affects ~5%–20% of children worldwide; incidence appears to be increasing
3. Both genetics and environment cause disease

FIGURE 12-3 **Atopic dermatitis in an older child. The crusting and lichenification involving the flexor crease were caused by repeated rubbing and scratching.**

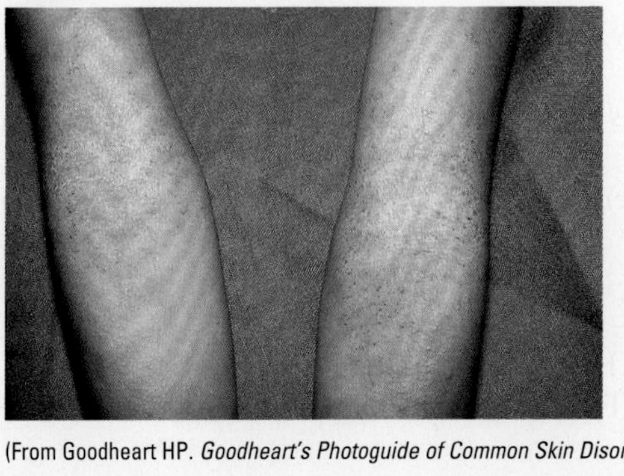

(From Goodheart HP. *Goodheart's Photoguide of Common Skin Disorders.* 2nd ed. Philadelphia: Lippincott Williams & Wilkins; 2003.)

B. Clinical presentation: dry, itchy papules and plaques with scale, crust, and secondary changes to skin (e.g., **lichenification**) due to chronic rubbing or scratching
   1. **Infantile** (infancy to age 2 years)
      a. Pruritic, red, scaly, crusted lesions: extensor surfaces, cheeks, scalp
      b. Usually spares diaper area
      c. Acute lesions can include vesicles; serous exudates/crusting in severe cases or with bacterial superinfection
   2. **Childhood** (ages 2–12 years): less exudates; lichenified (thickened with increased skin markings) plaques on flexural areas (antecubital and popliteal fossae; volar aspect of wrists, ankles, and neck)
   3. **Adult stage** (age >12 years)
      a. More localized and lichenified; excoriated and fibrotic papules
      b. Similar distribution to childhood stage

C. Diagnosis/testing: clinical diagnosis; no testing is necessary
   1. Differential diagnosis: seborrheic dermatitis, contact dermatitis, psoriasis, scabies

D. Treatment
   1. Therapy focuses on repair of epidermal barrier
      a. Maintain skin hydration with emollients
      b. Topically applied corticosteroids
      c. Antihistamines to treat itching
      d. Other treatments are limited due to side effects and risks
         i. Topical calcineurin inhibitors (i.e., tacrolimus, pimecrolimus) do not cause skin atrophy (unlike topical steroids)
         ii. Oral cyclosporine can cause hypertension and renal dysfunction
         iii. Oral glucocorticoids are limited due to side effects
         iv. UV light therapy ± psoralens is effective but may lead to increased risk of skin cancer
   2. Complications are primarily infectious
      a. Cellulitis
         i. Obtain bacterial cultures in patients with exudate
         ii. Extensive infections should be treated with oral antibiotics
         iii. Bathing in very dilute bleach solution may decrease colonization with *Staphylococcus aureus*
      b. HSV (i.e., eczema herpeticum/Kaposi varicelliform eruption) (Figure 12-4)
         i. Skin with punched-out erosions, hemorrhagic crusts, and/or vesicles
         ii. Pruritic or painful
         iii. Treated immediately, high rate of viremia: consider admission on intravenous (IV) acyclovir; need ophthalmologic exam if around eye: leads to keratitis/blindness

QUICK HIT

Lotions that have a high water and low oil content can worsen **xerosis** (dry skin) via evaporation and trigger a flare of the disease. Thick creams (e.g., Eucerin, Cetaphil) that have a low water content or ointments (e.g., petroleum jelly) that have zero water content better protect against xerosis.

QUICK HIT

Nummular (discoid) eczema can resemble ringworm, leading to diagnostic confusion and "treatment failure" when antifungal agents are presented.

QUICK HIT

Eczema herpeticum may be life or vision threatening!

FIGURE 12-4 **Eczema herpeticum. Ulcers and excoriation.**

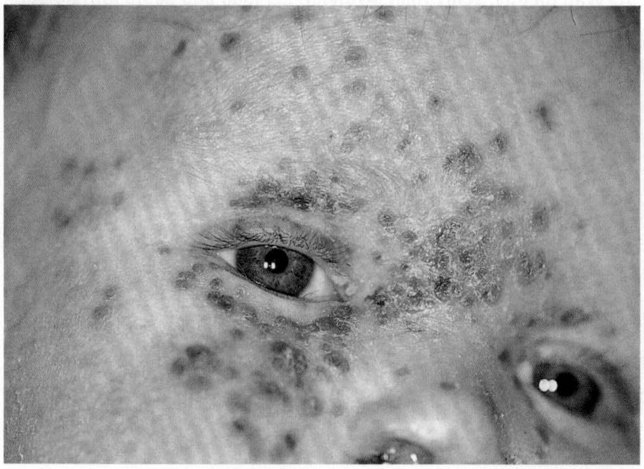

(From Fleisher GR, Ludwig S, Baskin MN. *Atlas of Pediatric Emergency Medicine*. Philadelphia: Lippincott Williams & Wilkins; 2004.)

Dermatologic Conditions

c. Molluscum contagiosum and dermatophyte infections are more common in patients with AD due to breakdown of skin barrier
3. Prognosis: 2/3 of children improve by preschool age
4. Flare-ups are preventable
a. Avoid low-humidity environments, overheating of skin, perspiration
b. Avoid harsh soaps and itchy fabrics like wool
c. Frequent water or bleach baths without soap; emollients or topical medications applied afterward
d. Manage emotional stress
e. Routine topical therapy and treat skin infections

VI. Keratosis Pilaris

A. A common benign rash on upper arms (or cheeks and upper thighs/buttocks)
B. Cause: failure of keratin to exfoliate, resulting in plugging of hair follicle
C. Clinical presentation
1. Flesh-colored papules that look similar to "goose bumps"
2. Worse in winter
D. Diagnosis/testing: clinical diagnosis; no testing indicated
E. Therapy: emollients, lactic acid solutions, topical retinoids

VII. Seborrheic Dermatitis

A. Definition: greasy, flaky, yellowish scale known as "**cradle cap**" (Figure 12-5)
1. Typically involves scalp and face of infants at ages 3 weeks to 12 months
2. Second peak in adolescence
B. Unknown etiology; may be related to growth of sebaceous gland due to maternal androgens and/or fungus *Malassezia*; affects ~10% of infants, 2%–5% of adolescents
C. Clinical presentation
1. Infants: usually asymptomatic; can be mildly pruritic
2. Adolescents/adults
a. Scalp: can be mild with white flakes (i.e., **dandruff**)
b. Periocular redness and crusting alone or with other involvement
D. Diagnosis
1. Clinical diagnosis; no testing necessary
2. Differential includes eczema, irritant, psoriasis, fungal infections
E. Treatment
1. Infants
a. Cosmetic only: mineral oil to scalp, lift off scale with fine comb
b. Face and/or diaper area: creams with ketoconazole are helpful

FIGURE 12-5 **Seborrhea typically manifests with an oily, scaly rash involving the face and scalp (cradle cap).**

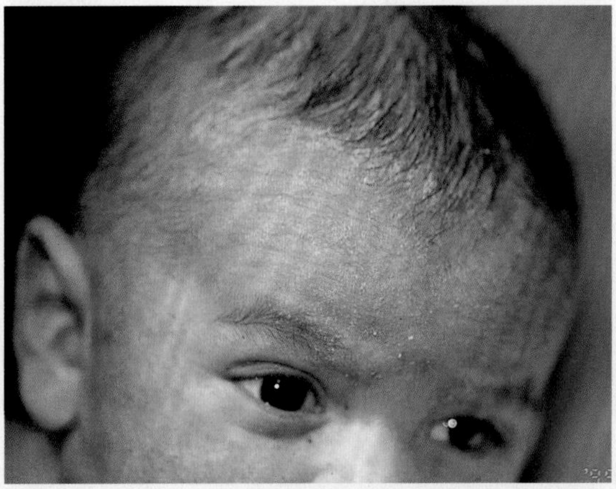

(From Fleisher GR, Ludwig S, Baskin MN. *Atlas of Pediatric Emergency Medicine*. Philadelphia: Lippincott Williams & Wilkins; 2004.)

Dermatologic Conditions

2. Adolescents
   a. Can clear spontaneously but may be recurrent
   b. Scalp: shampoos containing selenium sulfide, tar, or ketoconazole
   c. Other areas: creams with ketoconazole or topical steroids

VIII. Psoriasis Vulgaris

A. Definition: hereditary disorder characterized by chronic erythematous plaques with silvery white scale in characteristic distribution
B. Cause
   1. Multifactorial inheritance: several human leukocyte antigen (HLA) types
   2. Triggers include minor trauma, upper respiratory infections (URIs), stress, cold, low sunlight, some drugs
   3. Pathophysiology: defective inhibitor of epidermal cell proliferation with shortening of cell cycle: accumulated dead cells appear as silvery white scale
   4. Affects 1%–5% of adults; 10% of patients affected before age 10 years
C. Clinical presentation diagnostic (Figure 12-6)
   1. Usually chronic but can be acute onset
   2. Itching common
   3. Bilateral distribution in unexposed or traumatized areas (elbows, knees, face, scalp, intertriginous areas) or generalized
   4. Nails affected in 25%; pitting, onycholysis, yellow spots under nail plate
   5. Psoriasis vulgaris; guttate (drop-like lesions) type is relatively rare
      a. Can appear acutely following streptococcal pharyngitis
      b. 2 mm–1 cm pink, discrete, scattered papules (often droplet shaped) that are generalized and concentrate on trunk
D. Diagnosis/testing: clinical diagnosis; no testing necessary
E. Therapy
   1. Avoid rubbing/scratching because trauma can stimulate psoriatic plaques
   2. Emollients: petrolatum or moisturizers to keep skin well hydrated
   3. Sunlight exposure helps: sunscreen should be used; worsened by sunburn
   4. Baths soothe itching and remove scales
   5. Tar preparations can reduce skin inflammation
   6. Children: topical steroids, vitamin D analogs
   7. Adults: retinoids, anthralin
   8. Oral antibiotics if triggered by strep throat or signs of bacterial infection
   9. UV light treatments for severe, refractory cases
   10. Tar, selenium, zinc, or ketoconazole shampoos for scalp scaling

QUICK HIT

Of psoriasis cases, 5% can be associated with arthritis or fever.

QUICK HIT

Scale removal results in the appearance of miniscule blood droplets.

QUICK HIT

Nail pitting is common in patients with psoriasis.

FIGURE 12-6 **Psoriasis. These lesions with whitish, micaceous scale are seen in a typical location.**

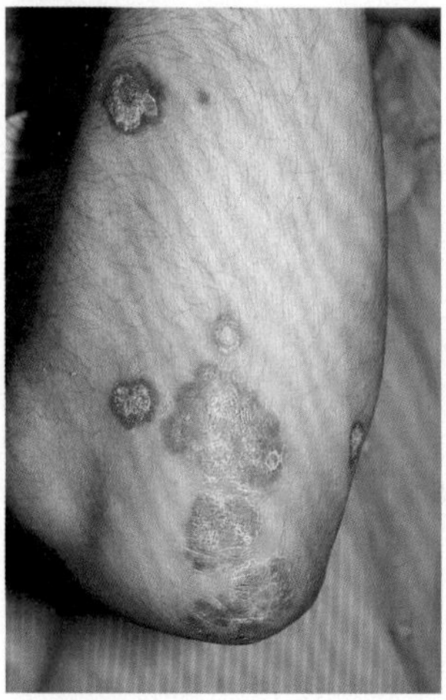

(From Goodheart HP. *Goodheart's Photoguide of Common Skin Disorders.* 2nd ed. Philadelphia: Lippincott Williams & Wilkins; 2003.)

QUICK HIT

Diaper dermatitis that is refractory to treatment or associated with periorificial and acral findings should lead clinician to suspect acrodermatitis enteropathica.

QUICK HIT

Patients with Epstein-Barr virus or cytomegalovirus mononucleosis syndrome develop an exanthematous drug reaction when given ampicillin or amoxicillin. Although this can be confused with a drug reaction, it is actually virally mediated.

QUICK HIT

Less than 10% of patients allergic to penicillins will exhibit cross-reactivity with cephalosporins; additionally, most patients (85%–90%) who report penicillin allergy are found not to be allergic.

QUICK HIT

Vancomycin's most frequent adverse reaction, the "red man syndrome," is a rate-dependent infusion reaction and not a true allergic reaction. It can be treated by infusing the medication more slowly (i.e., over 1–2 hours).

QUICK HIT

Unlike urticaria, EM lesions are not transient. If a lesion circled in ink subsequently disappears, it is likely urticarial rather than EM.

IX. Acrodermatitis Enteropathica

A. Definition: vesiculobullous eczematous dermatitis caused by poor intestinal zinc absorption
B. Etiology: can be hereditary (congenital) or acquired (from gastrointestinal [GI] disease or malnutrition)
C. Clinical presentation: scaly, erythematous plaques, may progress to bullae or erosions
   1. Rash is in a typical distribution: acral, perioral (with ulcers), buttocks, extensor surfaces
   2. May have diarrhea, weight loss, alopecia, behavioral symptoms
D. Testing: low serum zinc level <50 μg/dL
E. Therapy: if untreated, progresses to infection and disability; dietary supplement of zinc is curative

X. Drug-Associated Rashes

A. Definition: drug hypersensitivity/morbilliform drug eruption is an allergic response to administered drug; may mimic viral exanthem
B. Cause/pathophysiology: likely to be type III or type IV immune response; most common type of cutaneous drug reaction
C. Clinical presentation
   1. Pink or red at onset, fading to purple/brown; macules and/or papules
   2. Usually begins on trunk and spreads to face and extremities
   3. Lesions are persistent, in contrast to urticaria, which are transient
   4. Timing
      a. Occurs at any time between days 1 and 21 after starting treatment
      b. After prior sensitization, re-exposure to drug will elicit allergic response 2–3 days after initiating treatment
D. Diagnosis/testing: clinical diagnosis; no testing necessary
E. Therapy: clears 2–3 days after drug is stopped

XI. Erythema Multiforme (EM)

A. Definition: acute, immune-mediated condition characterized by distinctive target-like lesions on skin (Figure 12-7)
   1. Histopathology similar to mild SJS
   2. EM and SJS are distinct diseases; some consider SJS to be on severe end of EM spectrum
   3. EM tends to be milder, with less mucosal involvement and better prognosis
B. Cause/pathophysiology: most commonly unclear, possibly induced by infection
   1. Especially HSV and *Mycoplasma pneumoniae*
   2. Less common: induced by medications, autoimmune disease, malignancy
C. Clinical presentation
   1. Classic lesion: target-like papules with erythematous outer ring, pale inner ring
   2. Initial lesion: red macules or urticarial plaques that expand over 2–3 days
   3. Can have numerous morphologic manifestations
   4. Abrupt, symmetric, widely distributed
   5. Usually asymptomatic, although can have itching or burning
D. Diagnosis/testing: clinical diagnosis, no testing necessary
E. Treatment: supportive (e.g., antihistamines for itching)
F. Prognosis: usually self-limited, resolving within 2 weeks; recurs in minority of cases

XII. Stevens-Johnson Syndrome and Toxic Epidermal Necrolysis (TEN)

A. General characteristics
   1. Rare, but serious dermatologic condition
   2. Can occur at any age
   3. Characterized by **skin necrosis and sloughing**
   4. Commonly triggered by medication or infectious exposure

FIGURE 12-7 **Erythema multiforme. Target lesions, which consist of a red ring around a clear area (sometimes with a central bull's eye), characterize erythema multiforme.**

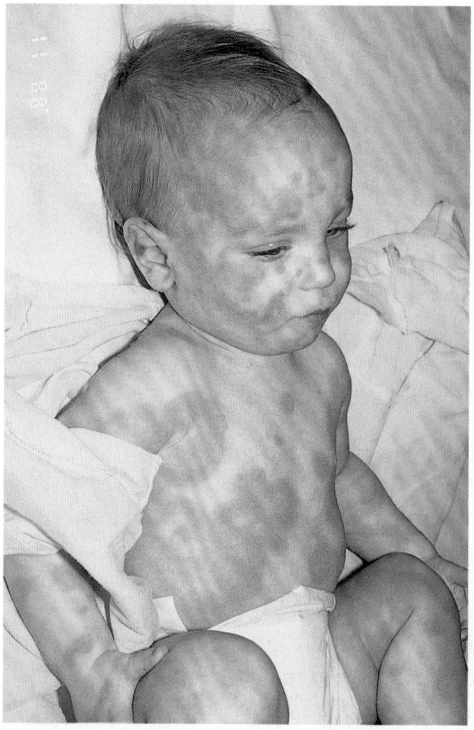

(From Fleisher GR, Ludwig S, Baskin MN. *Atlas of Pediatric Emergency Medicine.* Philadelphia: Lippincott Williams & Wilkins; 2004.)

B. Clinical presentation
  1. Prodrome
    a. Fever, malaise, URI symptoms
    b. Typically begins several days prior to skin changes
    c. May have associated skin tenderness/pain
  2. Rash
    a. Often begins with erythema of skin
    b. Irregular erythematous macules/purpura develop
    c. Often starts on face/thorax and spreads outward
    d. Usually with **mucosal membrane** involvement
  3. Rash progression
    a. Macules/purpura lead to subsequent sloughing
    b. Progression is often rapid
    c. Progression may be fulminant in cases of TEN
    d. Mucosal involvement with >90% of cases
      i. Ophthalmic
        (a) Occurs in >85% of cases
        (b) Varying severity including corneal scarring
      ii. Oral
        (a) Includes severe blistering of lips/tongue
        (b) Can lead to airway compromise
      iii. Genitourinary: urethritis—dysuria and/or urinary retention
      iv. Pulmonary
        (a) Can vary markedly in severity
        (b) Most severe: **bronchiolitis obliterans**
C. Clinical spectrum
  1. SJS
    a. Less severe end of continuum
    b. Involves <10% body surface area (BSA)

c. More likely to include targetoid lesions
d. Mucosal involvement >90% of time
2. SJS–TEN overlap syndrome
a. Middle of severity continuum
b. Involves 10%–30% BSA
3. TEN
a. Most severe form
b. Involves >30% BSA
c. Skin pain is "out of proportion" to clinical exam

D. Differential diagnosis: EM, drug eruption, toxic shock, SSSS
E. Risk factors: HIV, certain HLA subtypes, *Mycoplasma* infection, HSV, SLE
F. Pathophysiology: controversial and unclear
G. Diagnostic evaluation
1. Diagnosis is clinical
2. Skin biopsy can be helpful to support diagnosis
a. Lymphocytic predominance
b. Progression to full-thickness epidermal necrosis

H. Management
1. Removal of offending agent if present: more rapid cessation/removal associated with improved prognosis
2. Supportive care
a. **Wound management** is crucial
i. Treat like a burn; consider burn unit transfer
ii. Success with debridement and active wound management
iii. Dressings with silver products decrease risk of infection
b. Fluid and nutrition
i. Significantly increased insensible fluid losses
ii. Warm environment decreases insensible losses
c. Analgesia
d. Eye care by ophthalmology: moistening drops/ointments, barrier methods, serial exams
e. Monitoring for superinfection
i. Avoidance of empiric systemic antibiotics
ii. Surveillance cultures
iii. Observe for signs of developing infection
3. Potential adjunctive therapies
a. Glucocorticoids are not recommended
b. IVIG daily for 3 days may be useful; limited data

I. Prognosis/long-term sequelae
1. Overall survival is good
2. Affected patients can develop long-term sequelae
a. Dermatologic: scarring, skin discoloration, nail changes, hair loss
b. Ophthalmologic: dry eyes, photophobia, in severe cases blindness
c. Pulmonary
i. Chronic bronchiolitis/bronchiectasis
ii. Bronchiolitis obliterans

> **QUICK HIT**
> Ibuprofen is commonly identified as the inciting medication in SJS–TEN overlap syndrome.

> **QUICK HIT**
> SJS mortality is 1%–3%, whereas TEN mortality can be as high as 25%–35%.

XIII. Serum Sickness

A. General characteristics
1. **Classic triad**: fever, rash, and arthralgias/arthritis
2. Related to exposure to foreign protein (e.g., animal-derived antitoxin), drug (e.g., amoxicillin), or infection
3. Immune-mediated reaction, usually 1–3 weeks after exposure
4. Self-limited condition with excellent prognosis
5. Repeat exposure may lead to more rapid and more severe reactions

B. Clinical presentation: fever, rash, and arthritis
1. Rash: variable skin findings, although typically urticarial, pruritic, lasts 1–14 days

2. Arthralgias/arthritis
   a. Develops after rash; present in 2/3 of patients
   b. Typically involves, in decreasing order, knees, ankles, shoulders, wrists, spine, and temporomandibular joint
3. Other associated features include central nervous system (CNS), facial/peripheral edema, or GI symptoms

C. Differential diagnosis: EM, viral exanthema, hypersensitivity vasculitis, juvenile idiopathic arthritis (JIA), Kawasaki disease

D. Pathophysiology
1. Type III (immune complex–mediated reaction)
2. Foreign protein, drug, or infection serves as triggering antigen, which leads to antibody production.
3. Circulating antigen–antibody complexes activate complement cascade, leading to activation of neutrophils and mast cell degranulation/histamine release

E. Diagnosis is clinical

F. Management
1. Remove offending agent; provide supportive care (fever and pain control, diphenhydramine for itching)
2. Prevention of recurrence by avoiding offending agent

XIV. Drug Reaction with Eosinophilia and Systemic Symptoms (DRESS) Syndrome

A. Severe idiosyncratic drug reaction with mortality of 8%–10%

B. Clinical presentation
1. Fever (usually precedes and continues through rash)
2. Rash
   a. Widespread/variable rash
      i. Most commonly morbilliform
      ii. Often includes erythroderma
      iii. Can have erythematous macules
      iv. Can include papules, pustules, vesicles, bullae, purpura
   b. Pruritic rash, starts centrally, progresses to extremities
   c. Facial edema usually present
   d. Delayed onset of rash 2–8 weeks after drug exposure
3. Lymphadenopathy (75% of patients)
4. Hematologic abnormalities: eosinophilia, atypical lymphocytes, may have aplastic anemia
5. Organ involvement
   a. Liver: range of simple transaminitis through fulminant hepatic necrosis
   b. Kidneys: mild hematuria through renal failure
   c. Cardiopulmonary: pneumonitis, pericarditis, myocarditis
   d. Thyroiditis

C. Differential diagnosis: SJS, TEN, Kawasaki disease, JIA, viral infection (e.g., Epstein-Barr virus, cytomegalovirus, HIV, hepatitis)

D. Risk factors
1. Drug exposure
   a. Most commonly associated with aromatic antiepileptic drugs: phenytoin, carbamazepine, and phenobarbital
   b. Other medications have caused reaction: sulfonamides, allopurinol, antidepressants, nonsteroidal anti-inflammatory drugs, angiotensin-converting enzyme inhibitors, β-blockers

E. Pathophysiology: unknown

F. Management
1. Removal of offending agent; do not reuse, as DRESS will recur
2. Systemic glucocorticoids
   a. Administration often leads to rapid resolution
   b. Steroid cessation is often associated with return of symptoms
3. Supportive care (pain control, antihistamines for pruritus)

XV. Staphylococcal Scalded Skin Syndrome

A. General characteristics
   1. Caused by exotoxin-producing *S. aureus*
   2. Usually seen in infants and young children
   3. **Exfoliative desquamating rash** that leads to loss of large amounts of epidermis
   4. Severity can range from mild skin peeling to systemic toxicity

B. Clinical presentation
   1. Preceding mild infection on the face or skin
   2. Within hours or days: fever, irritability, and vomiting
   3. Diffuse erythroderma, **like sunburn**, spreads from head to toe
   4. Thin bullae form and subsequently rupture, sometimes large/diffuse
   5. **Nikolsky sign**: light traction leads to further separation of epidermis/dermis

C. Differential diagnosis: severe EM, SJS, TEN

D. Management
   1. Treat staphylococcal infection
      a. Appropriate systemic antibiotic therapy
         i. IV nafcillin or oxacillin (bactericidal) + clindamycin (ribosomal activity reduces toxic protein production by bacteria)
         ii. Consider adding vancomycin if high incidence of methicillin-resistant *S. aureus* (MRSA) and if severe disease
         iii. Switch to single oral antibiotic when improved
      b. Local debridement if focal infection found

XVI. Ecthyma Gangrenosum

A. General characteristics
   1. Ulcerative skin infection caused by *Pseudomonas*
   2. More common in immunocompromised individuals

B. Clinical presentation
   1. Lesions begin as erythematous macules, progress to **"punched out" ulcerative lesions** central to area of induration and erythema
   2. Hematogenous bacterial seeding may result in multiple lesions and/or signs of systemic illness, such as shock/sepsis

C. Management
   1. Antibiotic therapy targeted at causative bacterium (usually imipenem-cilastatin or cefepime empirically)
   2. Removal of any infected venous catheters or other focal sources

QUICK HIT

Bacterial culture of deep tissue (obtained by punch biopsy) usually reveals the causative bacterium, whereas a superficial culture cannot distinguish skin colonization from infection.

XVII. Epidermolysis Bullosa

A. Group of hereditary conditions presenting at birth that lead to blistering after minor trauma; may lead to eventual development of various skin cancers
   1. **EB simplex (most common form)**
      a. Autosomal dominant inheritance
      b. Gene defect leads to abnormal keratin formation
   2. **Junctional EB**
      a. Autosomal recessive inheritance
      b. More severe than EB simplex
      c. Gene defect leads to abnormal cell adhesion proteins
      d. Other features: dysplastic nails, teeth, oral lesions, pyloric stenosis
   3. **Dystrophic EB**
      a. Autosomal dominant or recessive inheritance
      b. Most severe and detrimental type of EB with extensive scarring
      c. Gene defect leads to abnormal collagen formation
      d. Often die in early adulthood; severe scarring and contractures

B. Management is supportive: prevent trauma, wound care, analgesia

QUICK HIT

Diagnosis of epidermolysis bullosa requires a skin biopsy.

XVIII. Vascular Malformations

A. Definitions
   1. Hemangiomas are benign, vascular proliferations and are most common neoplasm of childhood (Figure 12-8)

FIGURE 12-8 Cavernous hemangioma.

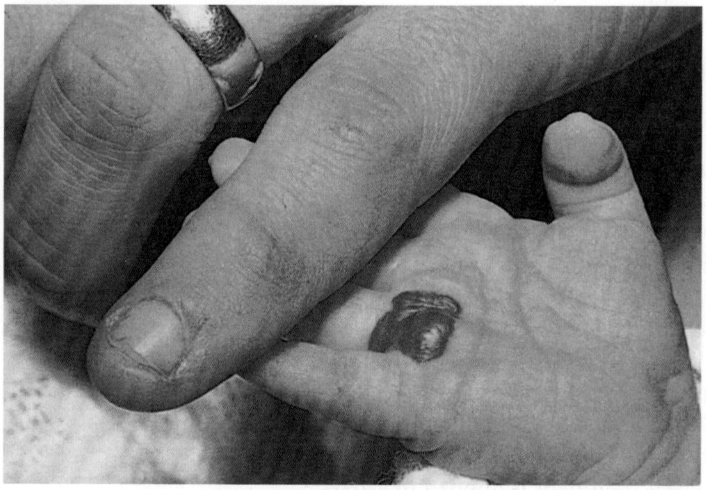

(From O'Doherty N. *Atlas of the Newborn.* Philadelphia: JB Lippincott; 1979:342–345, with permission.)

2. Other vascular malformations include port-wine stains, salmon patches, and arteriovenous malformations

B. Clinical presentation
1. Most lesions present soon after birth; may be very subtle at birth
2. Overlying skin is red; marked growth within first few months; many hemangiomas have both superficial and deep components
3. Spontaneous involution usually starts after 1st year of life
4. Cavernous hemangiomas: may have bluish discoloration, soft to touch (see Figure 12-8)
5. Port-wine stains: purplish red and do not enlarge over time; most commonly located on face, unilaterally and associated with
   a. Klippel-Trenaunay-Weber syndrome: hemihypertrophy
   b. **Sturge-Weber** syndrome: ophthalmic branch of trigeminal nerve with seizures, mental retardation, hemiplegia, and glaucoma
6. Salmon patch (often referred to as "stork bite"): normal variant seen in 40% of newborns on nape of neck, glabella, forehead, or upper eyelid
7. Pyogenic granuloma (red pedunculated lesion, bleeds easily)
   a. Vascular overgrowth of granulation tissue after injury; often on face
   b. Lesions often solitary, bright red, pedunculated, and bleed easily
8. Spider angioma (localized area of dilated capillaries): seen in hereditary hemorrhagic telangiectasia or CREST syndrome
9. Cherry angioma: small benign, red, dome-shaped lesions, usually on trunk

C. Therapy
1. Airway hemangiomas: clinical suspicion of presence if many other cutaneous hemangiomas (especially in neck/face region), stridor, hoarseness
   a. Systemic steroids, propranolol, laser ablation, tracheostomy
2. Hemangiomas near the eye may need treatment if vision is obstructed to prevent vision loss

QUICK HIT

Large hemangiomas may cause physical shearing of red blood cells and platelets, resulting in anemia and/or thrombocytopenia (**Kasabach-Merritt syndrome**).

MNEMONIC

CREST syndrome is the cutaneous form of systemic scleroderma:
Calcinosis
Raynaud syndrome
Esophageal dysmotility
Sclerodactyly
Telangiectasia

QUICK HIT

Most hemangiomas require no intervention other than education.

XIX. Scabies

A. General characteristics
1. Skin infestation caused by mite
2. Symptoms are due to hypersensitivity reaction to mite and feces
3. Infestation is highly infectious; spread by direct contact with infected individuals or contact with fomites such as bedding

B. Clinical features
1. Historical findings
   a. Intense pruritus, often worsening in evening (infants with irritability)
   b. Symptoms are usually present in multiple family members

QUICK HIT

The classic lesions of scabies are intensely pruritic burrows in the interdigital areas, wrists, ankles, waist, axillae, palms, and soles.

2. Physical exam findings
   a. Papules and vesiculopustules, often in webs of fingers
   b. Infants and toddlers often present with vesicles
   c. Lesions are typically excoriated
   d. Scabies nodules
      i. Red-brown nodules represent vigorous hypersensitivity reaction
      ii. Primarily seen in infants on trunk and axillary regions
      iii. May persist for months before resolving
   e. Norwegian or crusted scabies
      i. Presents as scaly papules or plaques, which mimic eczema or psoriasis
      ii. Seen in immunocompromised or incapacitated patients

C. Diagnosis is clinical, but if uncertain, scabies and eggs can be seen in scrapings under microscope (mineral oil prep)

D. Treatment
1. 5% permethrin cream
   a. Applied from neck down with attention to all creases and under nails; leave on overnight before rinsing
   b. Typically, repeat treatment is applied in 7 days
2. All close contacts should be treated even if asymptomatic
3. Environmental decontamination is critical
   a. Wash clothing/bed linens in hot water and dry in high heat
   b. Unwashables, such as stuffed animals, should be stored in bags for at least 1 week until mites have died

XX. Head Lice

A. General characteristics
1. Lice are small (1–4 mm), 6-legged, wingless, gray-white insects
2. Infestation is spread by head-to-head contact or by sharing combs, brushes, or hats
3. Usually affects children ages 3–12 years

B. Clinical features
1. Itchy scalp or asymptomatic
2. Physical exam findings
   a. Live lice in hair
   b. Viable lice egg cases (nits): specks stuck to hair 1–2 mm from scalp

QUICK HIT

Nits found more than 5 mm from the scalp represent old infestations only and do not warrant treatment.

C. Topical shampoo treatment: treat once, then again 7 days later to kill maturing nits
1. Insecticides
   a. 1% permethrin cream rinse (e.g., Nix); increasing resistance
   b. Pyrethrins (e.g., RID)
   c. Malathion 0.5% lotion (OVIDE)
2. Benzyl alcohol shampoo (Ulesfia)
   a. No resistance, not a pesticide
   b. Works through suffocation
3. Manual lice and nit removal
   a. Tedious task using nit combs (fine-toothed combs)
   b. Some schools mandate nit removal, but it is not effective
4. Other family members and close contacts should be examined and treated if any lice or nits are found
5. Environmental decontamination should also be performed
   i. Vacuum furniture
   ii. Wash bedding and clothing in hot water
   iii. Unwashables should be bagged for 2 weeks
   iv. Brushes, combs, and hats should not be shared

XXI. Tinea Infections

A. Definition/clinical presentation: fungal infections named based on location

B. Pathophysiology: caused by 3 main types of fungi including *Trichophyton*, *Microsporum*, and *Epidermophyton*

Dermatologic Conditions

FIGURE 12-9 **Tinea corporis (ringworm). Note the annular appearance, central clearing, and "active" scaly border that demonstrate hyphae on potassium hydroxide examination.**

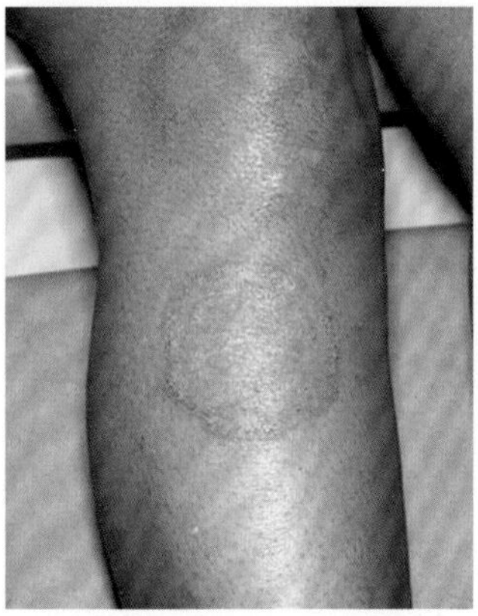

(From Goodheart HP. *Goodheart's Photoguide of Common Skin Disorders.* 2nd ed. Philadelphia: Lippincott Williams & Wilkins; 2003.)

C. Clinical presentation
   1. **Tinea corporis (body)**: small to large scaling plaques/pustules or vesicles, noted to have peripheral enlargement and central clearing (Figure 12-9)
   2. **Tinea faciei (face)**: asymptomatic papule enlarging to plaque; elevated borders
   3. **Tinea capitis (scalp ringworm)**: scaly, pruritic patches on scalp with hair loss (Figure 12-10)
   4. **Tinea cruris (jock itch)**: well-demarcated plaques/papules in upper thigh/groin area with central clearing
   5. **Tinea pedis (athlete's foot)**: scaling of feet with white scales or papules
   6. **Tinea manuum**: hand scaling often with tinea pedis or onychomycosis
   7. **Tinea unguium**: white or brown discoloration of nail, most often toes
   8. **Tinea versicolor**: macular rash with scales on trunk that are easily wiped off (from overgrowth of *Pityrosporum ovale*)

D. Diagnosis is most often clinical, based on appearance; can perform KOH prep, Wood's lamp (tinea capitis *Microsporum* may fluoresce), or fungal culture

E. Therapy
   1. Topical therapy (nystatin, clotrimazole [Lotrimin], etc.) used except tinea capitis and tinea unguium
      a. Tinea capitis: topical shampoo (e.g., selenium) plus oral griseofulvin
      b. Tinea unguium: fluconazole, itraconazole, or simply live with it

QUICK HIT

Tinea capitis will create broken hairs close to the skin with a "black dot" appearance.

XXII. Impetigo

A. Definition: contagious superficial infection from group A streptococci or staphylococci

FIGURE 12-10 **Tinea capitis. Scaly, alopecic patches mimic seborrheic dermatitis.**

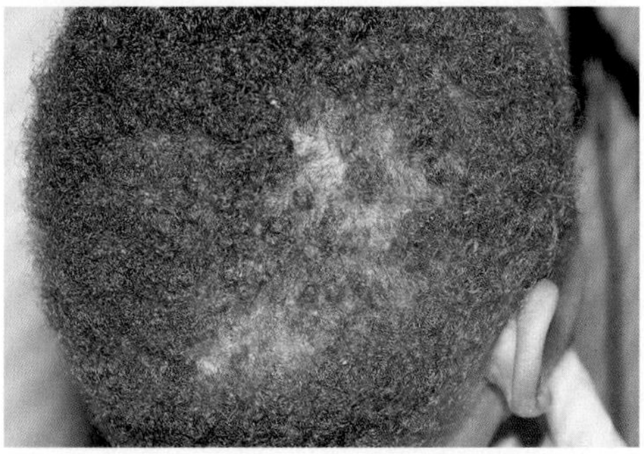

(From Goodheart HP. *Goodheart's Photoguide of Common Skin Disorders.* 2nd ed. Philadelphia: Lippincott Williams & Wilkins; 2003.)

FIGURE 12-11 **Staphylococcal scalded skin syndrome. The thin, yellow crusting around the mouth and nares of this boy characterizes this syndrome, which is most often secondary to impetigo in the perioral and nasal regions.**

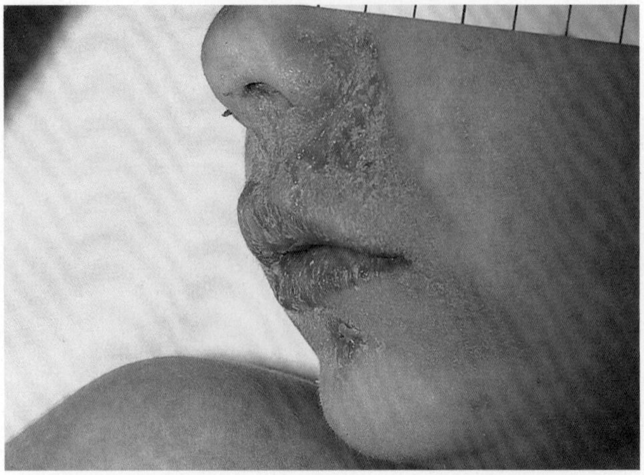

(From Fleisher GR, Ludwig S, Baskin MN. *Atlas of Pediatric Emergency Medicine.* Philadelphia: Lippincott Williams & Wilkins; 2004.)

B. Pathophysiology
   1. Infection is spread by autoinoculation by fingers or towels
   2. Reservoir for staphylococci in upper respiratory tract or groin
   3. Streptococcal infection spreads from lesions on other individuals
C. Clinical characteristics
   1. Nonbullous (crusting) impetigo (Figure 12-11): small papules/pustules easily rupture: release of thin yellow fluid, which dries leaving **honey-colored** crust
   2. Bullous impetigo: flaccid, thin-walled bullae or tender shallow erosions surrounded by remains of blister roof
   3. Associated symptoms and complications
      a. Fever, lymphadenopathy more common in nonbullous impetigo
      b. May evolve into sepsis, osteomyelitis, arthritis, and pneumonia
D. Treatment
   1. Untreated infections typically last for 2–3 weeks
   2. Gentle removal of crusts can help prevent localized spread
   3. Topical antibiotics
      a. Useful in mild infections due to *S. aureus*
      b. Mupirocin (Bactroban) has broad activity against both staphylococcal and streptococcal infections with few side effects
      c. Likely equally or more effective than oral antibiotics
   4. Oral antibiotics
      a. 1st-generation cephalosporin (cephalexin)
      b. If high rates of community-acquired MRSA are present, consider clindamycin
   5. Lesions typically heal without scarring

QUICK HIT

The classic appearance of impetigo is *honey-colored* crusted lesions around the nose of a young child with a URI.

XXIII. Pityriasis Rosea

A. Definition: benign, self-limited rash of unclear etiology
B. Clinical presentation
   1. 70% of patients present with "herald patch"
      a. Sharply defined oval patch of scaly dermatitis with fine scale
      b. Generally found on trunk, upper arm, neck, or thigh
      c. Patch starts as 2–5 cm in diameter and gradually expands
   2. 2–21 days later, more generalized eruption of smaller (0.2–1 cm) papules appears and peaks over a few days to a week in a "Christmas tree" pattern (Figure 12-12)
      a. Most papules are concentrated on trunk and spare face
      b. 25% of patients will experience pruritus of secondary eruption

QUICK HIT

Patients may not have noticed the "herald patch" of pityriasis rosea until asked about it by the physician. The herald patch may be confused with tinea corporis.

QUICK HIT

Pityriasis rosea often follows the lines of skin cleavage, leading to a "Christmas tree" appearance on the back.

FIGURE 12-12 **Pityriasis rosea causes a papulosquamous eruption that frequently involves the thorax and assumes a characteristic "Christmas tree" appearance.**

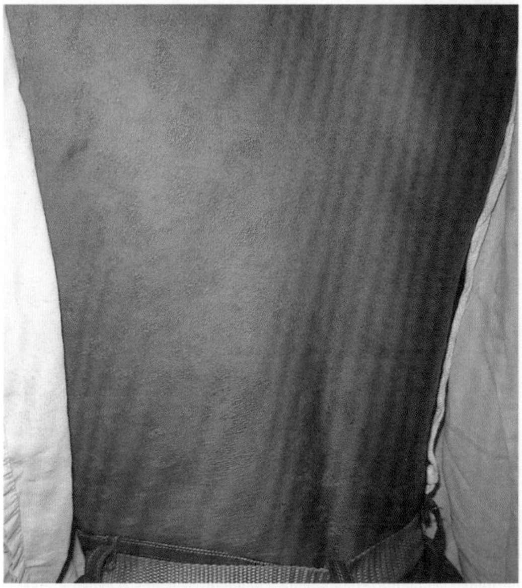

(From Fleisher GR, Ludwig S, Baskin MN. *Atlas of Pediatric Emergency Medicine*. Philadelphia: Lippincott Williams & Wilkins; 2004.)

3. Most patients are otherwise well
4. Warn families: rash clears over 6 weeks to 5 months
5. Postinflammatory hypo- or hyperpigmentation may occur

C. Treatment is generally unnecessary: reassurance to families

XXIV. Warts

A. Definition: cutaneous infection by human papillomavirus (HPV)

B. Pathophysiology: HPV is spread by skin-to-skin contact or contact with fomites

C. Clinical presentation
1. Incidence in children and young adults is high
2. Generally benign and self-involuting but can be painful or have social stigma
3. Found on hands, finger, elbows, and periungual areas; known as **verruca vulgaris**, or "common warts"
   a. Flesh-colored, rough papules: from dome shaped to filiform (stalked)
4. Flat warts (**verrucae plana**) are found on face and neck
   a. Flesh-colored or pink or brown flat-topped papules 2–5 mm
   b. From few lesions to hundreds
   c. Tend to spread in areas after shaving (face in men, legs in women)
5. Most symptomatic warts found on plantar surface of foot (**verrucae plantaris**): can be asymptomatic, but eventually sometimes painful (Figure 12-13)

> **QUICK HIT**
> A classic feature of warts is **koebnerization**, or the spread of warts in lines by autoinoculation by scratching.

D. Treatment
1. 2/3 of warts resolve spontaneously within 2 years, so watchful waiting is reasonable plan for many asymptomatic warts
2. Painful or cosmetically troubling warts are candidates for treatment
3. Debridement before treatment can increase effectiveness of treatment
4. Salicylic acid
   a. Available over the counter (OTC) as liquid, gel, impregnated pads
   b. Can lead to local skin irritation
5. Cryotherapy
   a. Highly effective but can be very painful
   b. Liquid nitrogen (–196°C) is applied to wart with cotton-tipped applicator or spray gun for 10–20 seconds, causing blister above dermal–epidermal junction
   c. Can be repeated every 2–4 weeks
   d. OTC products are available but do not achieve as low temperature and are less effective

FIGURE 12-13 **Plantar wart. As opposed to warts on other surfaces, those on the sole of the foot are flat.**

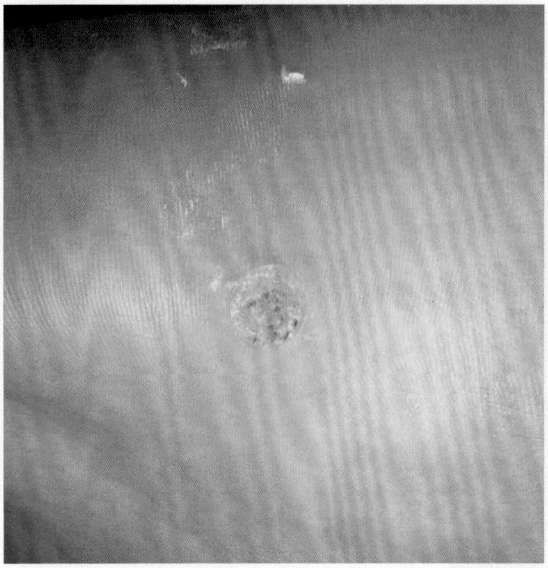

(From Fleisher GR, Ludwig S, Baskin MN. *Atlas of Pediatric Emergency Medicine.* Philadelphia: Lippincott Williams & Wilkins; 2004.)

6. Immunotherapy
   a. Induce host immune system to mount response against HPV infection
   b. Oral cimetidine
   c. Topical imiquimod (Aldara) induces interferon-α production
   d. Squaric acid dibutylester (SADBE)
7. Pulsed dye laser therapy
   a. Destruction of blood vessels within wart leads to regression
   b. Painless and effective but limited to recalcitrant lesions due to cost
8. Duct tape occlusion
   a. Cover wart for 7 days with duct tape, then rub with pumice stone/nail file, then re-cover
   b. About as effective as cryotherapy after about 3 weeks

XXV. Molluscum Contagiosum

A. Definition: cutaneous viral infection caused by member of poxvirus family
B. Pathophysiology
   1. Spread is via direct skin-to-skin contact and via fomites
   2. Children: usually nonsexual spread; adults: often sexually transmitted
C. Clinical presentation
   1. Pearly, flesh-colored, 2–8-mm papules (Figure 12-14)
   2. Lesions have umbilicated center, with/without white discharge

FIGURE 12-14 **Molluscum contagiosum.**

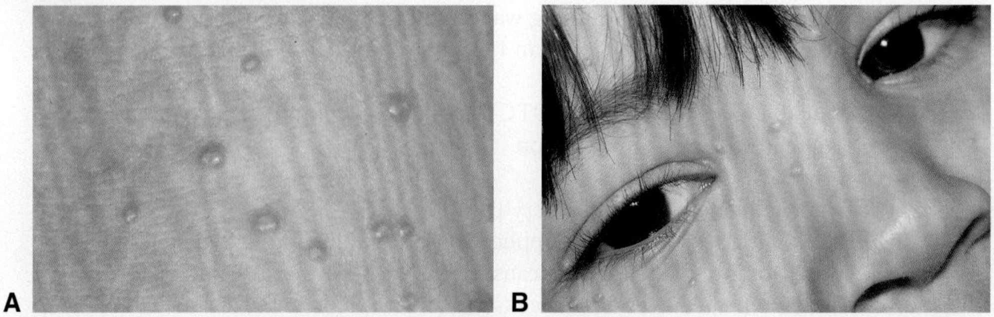

A. Characteristic dome-shaped, shiny, waxy papules have a central white core. **B.** This is a typical distribution of lesions on a child's face. Note the eyelid lesions. (From Goodheart HP. *Goodheart's Photoguide of Common Skin Disorders.* 2nd ed. Philadelphia: Lippincott Williams & Wilkins; 2003.)

3. Lesions occur in clusters, in areas of skin rubbing (antecubital fossa, popliteal fossa, axilla, groin)
4. Koebnerization does occur (linear spread due to scratching)
5. "Molluscum dermatitis" or surrounding dermatitis is common
6. Complications are rare, but secondary bacterial infections can occur

D. Treatment
1. No treatment may be necessary as spontaneous clearing occurs in most patients
2. Therapy relies on destruction: curettage, cryotherapy, or cantharidin
3. Secondary bacterial infections are possible

XXVI. Ichthyosis

A. Definition: group of hereditary skin disorders; excess accumulation of cutaneous scale

B. Types of disease
1. Ichthyosis vulgaris: autosomal dominant, common, generally mild course
2. X-linked ichthyosis: recessive, X-linked, seen only in boys, relatively common, mild course
3. Epidermolytic hyperkeratosis: autosomal dominant, rare, severe
4. Lamellar ichthyosis: autosomal recessive, very rare, can be fatal

C. History and clinical presentation/diagnosis
1. Worst during winter months
2. Diagnosis based on clinical findings

D. Therapy
1. Hydration of stratum corneum using Vaseline, hydrolated petrolatum, Aquaphor
2. Keratolytic agents (i.e., Epilyt, Keralyt, Camol, Lac-Hydrin)
3. Systemic retinoids reserved for severe cases

XXVII. Alopecia

A. Definition: hair loss secondary to broad etiologies
1. **Alopecia telogen effluvium**
2. **Alopecia anagen effluvium**
3. **Alopecia areata**
4. **Trauma-induced alopecia**

B. Cause/pathophysiology
1. Alopecia telogen effluvium: partial, temporary alopecia seen after stress
2. Alopecia anagen effluvium: sudden loss of growing hairs due to abnormal cessation of anagen phase
3. Alopecia areata: autoimmune disease with abrupt hair loss with well-circumscribed areas of nonscarring alopecia
4. Trauma-induced alopecia: friction alopecia, traction alopecia, and **trichotillomania** (compulsive urge to pull out one's own hair)

C. Diagnosis: clinical diagnosis, based on history and physical exam

D. Therapy
1. Variety of treatments: topical, systemic, injected into lesions
2. Psychosocial support should be offered

> QUICK HIT
>
> **Alopecia universalis** is thought to be an autoimmune disorder and involves rapid loss of all hair on the body.

XXVIII. Aplasia Cutis Congenita

A. Definition: congenital defect of growth of skin/subcutaneous tissue of scalp

B. Clinical presentation: asymptomatic ulceration of scalp at birth

C. Diagnosis/testing: clinical diagnosis; no testing necessary, heals with scarring

D. Therapy: local care: gentle cleansing, topical antibiotic creams, protective covering

XXIX. Nevi

A. Definition: group of congenital and acquired lesions of skin that may involve multiple tissue elements

B. Clinical presentation
1. **Congenital nevomelanocytic nevi (malignant potential)**
   a. Present at birth, often with associated hairs
   b. Recommend annual exam by dermatologist; removal if size permits

2. **Acquired nevomelanocytic nevi (common mole; most are benign)**: begin in early childhood; small, slowly enlarge and progress
3. **Melanomas (malignant potential)**: may occur in isolation or within giant congenital nevus
4. **Blue nevus (benign)**: acquired, benign, small, dark-blue to black papule
5. **Halo nevus (most benign)**: nevus that becomes surrounded by halo of depigmentation
6. **Nevus spilus (benign)**: flat, brown macule with smaller dark brown to black macules/papules often found on torso and extremities
7. **Spitz nevus (benign)**: benign, red, dome-shaped nodule typically on face of child
8. **Ephelides (freckles)**: light brown macules that occur most often on sun-exposed skin
9. **Nevus sebaceous of Jadassohn (malignant potential, but excision not mandatory)**: hairless, skin-colored plaque on scalp, face, or neck

MNEMONIC

Indications for melanoma excision are ABCDE:
Appearance: rapid change in size, shape, or outline
Borders: irregular borders
Color: change to different shades of black or brown or mixture of red, white, and blue
Discomfort: burning, itching, or tenderness
Elevation: change in surface elevation

13

Diseases Unique to Adolescent Medicine

SYMPTOM SPECIFIC

I. Approach to Adolescent History and Physical Examination

A. Overview
1. Definitions
    a. **Adolescence**: phase of human development involving transition from childhood to adulthood
        i. Physical growth and maturation
        ii. Identity formation and development of self-esteem
        iii. Developing sexuality, understanding self as sexual being
        iv. Establish own sense of right versus wrong (experimentation, testing boundaries)
        v. Assumption of self-responsibility (struggle for autonomy)
        vi. Establishing a vocational direction (moving from egocentrism to sense of self as part of larger society)
    b. **Puberty**: physical changes, particularly development of secondary sexual characteristics, involved in transition from childhood to adulthood
2. Characteristics of adolescent health
    a. Biologic, cognitive, and psychosocial changes influence health
    b. Morbidity and mortality often due to behavior and social environment
    c. Health and illness cannot be separated from psychosocial development
3. Features of adolescent visit
    a. Encourage emerging sense of autonomy and independence
        i. Interview adolescent alone for at least part of visit
        ii. Promote concept of confidentiality in adolescent care
    b. Cognitive development of individual patient should guide discussion
        i. Don't focus on long-term consequences with younger, "concrete" thinkers
        ii. Older, "abstract" thinkers do better than "concrete" thinkers with open-ended questions
    c. Optimize communication with teen
        i. Explain relevance and rationale for asking "sensitive" questions during social history
        ii. Direct questions/discussion to adolescent while attending to and validating parental input

B. Historical questions
1. Psychosocial interview is core component
    a. HEADDDSS guides history (Table 13-1)
    b. Should be conducted with patient alone
    c. Ensure teen (and parent) understands confidentiality and its limits
2. Start with nonthreatening topics (school, friends); work toward more sensitive issues (sexuality, suicidality)

QUICK HIT

The 3 leading causes of death in adolescents are preventable accidents, homicide, and suicide.

QUICK HIT

Confidentiality has limits within adolescent care. Confidentiality cannot be maintained if a patient is a threat to self or others or is being abused.

MNEMONIC

HEADDDSS guides adolescent patient assessment.
Home
Education
Activities
Diet
Drugs/alcohol/tobacco
Depression/suicidality
Sexuality
Safety

QUICK HIT

If a parent steadfastly refuses to leave a teen alone with the physician, consideration should be given that the parent and child may have an abusive or troubled relationship.

TABLE 13-1 **HEADDDSS: The Adolescent Psychosocial History**

Topic	Questions to Ask
Home	Family composition? Where do you live? How do you get along with parents and siblings?
Education	Grade, school, school performance, suspensions, goals
Activities	Hobbies/interests, exercise, TV watching, peer group
Diet	How do you feel about your weight? What do you typically eat? Any restrictive or purging behaviors?
Drugs/alcohol/tobacco	Have friends tried any? Has patient tried? Ask about specific substances. Praise resistance to peer pressure.
Depression/suicide	Describe mood. What does patient do when sad or stressed? Ever had thoughts of hurting or killing self?
Sexuality	In a relationship? Attracted to boys, girls, both? Ever had sex? Tell me about your partner(s). History of STIs?
Safety	Seat belts, bike helmets, weapons, bullying, sexual or physical abuse, riding with drunk drivers

STIs, sexually transmitted infections.

QUICK HIT

Remaining nonjudgmental is important when gathering history from an adolescent. Expressions of shock or dismay in response to answers may inhibit a teen's willingness to be candid.

QUICK HIT

Abnormal menses can be a marker for numerous underlying health problems, so a thorough menstrual history should be part of adolescent female visit.

3. Ask about teen concerns related to developmental stage
   a. Younger adolescents (ages 10–13 years) will be preoccupied with ongoing physical changes
   b. Middle adolescents (ages 14–17 years) will be preoccupied with peer acceptance and parent conflict
   c. Older adolescents (ages 18–21 years) will be focused on future goals and responsibilities
4. Parental input is important for questions about past medical history, family history, and even aspects of the present illness

C. Physical exam
1. Assess growth parameters: check for short stature, obesity, or low body mass index (BMI); the latter a concern for eating disorders
2. Assess sexual maturity (Tanner stage) (Table 13-2)
   a. Used to evaluate progression of pubertal development
   b. Based on secondary sex characteristics
   c. Testicular volume can be measured with orchidometer
3. Measure blood pressure
4. Test hearing and vision
   a. Highly amplified music may result in hearing loss
   b. Pubertal growth spurt may involve optic globe, resulting in elongation and myopia

TABLE 13-2 **Sexual Maturity Ratings (Tanner Stages)**

Stage	Female Breast	Male Genitals	Pubic Hair (Male/Female)
I	Prepubertal, no glandular tissue	Testis volume <4 mL Child-like penis and scrotum	None
II	"Breast bud," breast tissue beneath areola only	Testis volume 4–6 mL Scrotum: reddened, thinner, larger	Long, downy, slightly pigmented hair at base of penis or along labia
III	Glandular tissue extends beyond areola	Testis volume 6–12 mL Scrotum: more enlargement Penis: increased length	More curly, pigmented, coarse
IV	Areola forms secondary mound projecting from breast contour	Testis volume 12–20 mL Scrotum: darker Penis: increased length and circumference	Spreads across mons pubis but not to medial thigh
V	Adult breast, areola in same plane as breast	Testis volume >20 mL Adult penis and scrotum	Extends to medial surface of thigh

5. Spine: Adam forward bend test for scoliosis (seen in 2%–4% of adolescents)
6. Skin exam: look for acne, suspicious moles, tattoos/piercings, signs of self-inflicted injuries (e.g., cutting in depressed teen)
7. Cardiovascular exam particularly important in preparticipation physical
8. In boys, check for gynecomastia and scrotal masses (tumors, varicocele, hernia); teach testicular self-exam
9. In girls, breast exam to assess Tanner stage; pelvic exam only if clinically warranted

D. Other
1. Immunizations
   a. Tdap (tetanus, diphtheria, pertussis)
   b. Human papillomavirus (HPV): 3-dose series
   c. Meningococcal vaccine
2. Fasting lipid profile if obese, hypertensive, or family history of dyslipidemia or premature cardiovascular disease
3. Screening for anemia is not recommended unless suggestive history or physical
4. Screen sexually active adolescents for sexually transmitted infections (STIs)
5. Provide anticipatory guidance on healthy habits, risk behaviors

> **QUICK HIT**
> Essential hypertension is increasingly a problem among adolescents.

> **QUICK HIT**
> Receiving the HPV vaccine does *not* increase promiscuity but *does* prevent cancer.

> **QUICK HIT**
> Both boys and girls should get the HPV vaccine.

> **QUICK HIT**
> High fasting lipids may lead to effective counseling; however, except for severe hyperlipidemia syndromes, pharmacologic treatment is controversial in adolescents.

II. Approach to Dysfunctional Uterine Bleeding (DUB)

A. Background information
1. Normal menstrual cycle
   a. Interval: 21–35 days (average 28 days)
   b. Duration: 3–7 days
   c. Average blood loss: 30–40 mL
2. DUB: abnormal changes in frequency of menses, duration of flow, or amount of blood loss
   a. Usually results in excessive, prolonged, or irregularly patterned bleeding
   b. **Menorrhagia**: prolonged or heavy uterine bleeding at regular intervals
   c. **Metrorrhagia**: uterine bleeding that occurs at irregular intervals
   d. **Menometrorrhagia**: prolonged or heavy bleeding that occurs at irregular intervals
   e. **Oligomenorrhea**: uterine bleeding at intervals >35 days
3. Most DUB (>80%) in adolescents results from anovulatory cycles secondary to immaturity of hypothalamic–pituitary–ovarian (HPO) axis
   a. Usually seen in first 2 years after menarche (~50% of cycles are ovulatory during this time)
   b. Failure to ovulate leads to absence of corpus luteum → no progesterone secretion → unopposed estrogen leads to excessive proliferation of endometrium → no cyclical hormone withdrawal → irregular, heavy bleeding
   c. Diagnosis of exclusion, so must consider other causes of abnormal uterine or vaginal bleeding (Box 13-1)

> **MNEMONIC**
> **Periods should follow the 7, 7, 21 rule:**
> **<7** pads per day
> **<7** days
> **>21** days between periods

> **QUICK HIT**
> Irregular menses occur in most girls after menarche.

BOX 13-1

Differential Diagnosis of Dysfunctional Uterine Bleeding

Anovulatory cycles (immature hypothalamic–pituitary–ovarian axis)
Pregnancy: miscarriage, ectopic, molar pregnancy
Infection: vaginitis, cervicitis, pelvic inflammatory disease
Hematologic disorders: von Willebrand disease, thrombocytopenia, platelet dysfunction, problem with coagulation factors
Endocrine disorders: hyperthyroidism, hypothyroidism, polycystic ovary syndrome, hyperprolactinemia (e.g., prolactinoma)
Trauma
Foreign body
Medications: hormonal contraception, anticoagulants, dopamine antagonists (e.g., antipsychotics), chemotherapeutic agents
Endometriosis
Structural pathology: congenital anatomic anomalies of uterus or vagina, uterine polyps, fibroids (uncommon in adolescents)

QUICK HIT

Increased time lapse between menarche and onset of DUB lessens the likelihood of anovulatory cycles as the etiology.

QUICK HIT

Postcoital bleeding is suggestive of an STI, especially *C. trachomatis* cervicitis.

QUICK HIT

Adolescents often have difficulty adhering to a daily regimen of oral contraceptive pills. Missed pills can lead to irregular breakthrough bleeding, so be sure to ask about compliance.

QUICK HIT

Dopamine regulates pituitary release of prolactin. Drugs (e.g., selective serotonin reuptake inhibitors, monoamine oxidase inhibitors, antipsychotics, atypical neuroleptics) that decrease dopamine secretion will lead to excess prolactin release, which will disrupt normal menstrual cycles.

QUICK HIT

Onset of menses for most girls occurs in Tanner stage IV and less frequently in Tanner stages III and V. If the patient is Tanner stage I or II, bleeding is most likely not menstrual in origin.

QUICK HIT

Clinical signs of androgen excess (e.g., hirsutism) are not necessary in PCOS, which can present only with irregular menses.

B. Important historical findings
   1. Age of menarche
   2. Pattern of bleeding
      a. Regular intervals with very heavy flow: consider hematologic problem
      b. Regular intervals but with bleeding in between periods: consider infection, presence of foreign body
      c. Abnormal intervals with no regularity (regardless of heaviness of flow): consider endocrinopathy or anovulatory cycles
   3. Cramping or pain
      a. Often no cramping with anovulatory cycles
      b. Pain may be consistent with structural problem
   4. History of trauma (accidental, sexual assault)
   5. Sexual activity: contraceptive use
   6. Medications that affect hemostasis (e.g., warfarin) or HPO axis
   7. Associated symptoms
      a. Dizziness, fatigue: suggests anemia secondary to menstrual blood loss
      b. Careful review of systems (ROS) may suggest underlying diagnosis (Table 13-3)
      c. Often no associated symptoms with anovulatory cycles (immature axis)
   8. Family history of menstrual or other gynecologic problems or bleeding disorders

C. Pertinent physical exam findings
   1. Exam is usually unremarkable for anovulatory cycles due to immature axis
   2. Check vital signs to assess for hemodynamic instability due to blood loss
   3. Assess Tanner stage (sexual maturity rating)
   4. Evidence of androgen excess
      a. Hirsutism, acne
      b. Clitoromegaly and deepening of voice not usually seen with polycystic ovary syndrome (PCOS) but may suggest adrenal disorder or androgen-secreting tumor
   5. Check for presence of goiter
   6. Breast exam for galactorrhea (prolactinoma) and tenderness (pregnancy)
   7. Check for signs of bleeding disorder
      a. Examine mucosal surfaces (nares, gums)
      b. Skin exam for petechiae, purpura, ecchymoses
      c. Hepatomegaly may suggest coagulopathy from liver disease
   8. If tolerated, pelvic exam can help localize source of bleeding
      a. Bleeding from cervix (e.g., uterine bleeding, cervicitis) or vagina (e.g., laceration, foreign body)
      b. Bimanual exam to assess for pelvic inflammatory disease (PID), masses, anatomic abnormalities

D. Diagnostic workup
   1. Laboratory data
      a. No significant abnormalities in anovulatory cycles due to immature axis
      b. Pregnancy test

TABLE 13-3 **Symptoms Associated with Causes of Abnormal Uterine Bleeding**

Diagnosis	Characteristic Symptoms
Hematologic disorders	History of easy bruising or bleeding, epistaxis, gingival bleeding
Sexually transmitted infection	Vaginal discharge, postcoital bleeding, pain with sex
Polycystic ovary syndrome (or other causes of hyperandrogenism)	History of hirsutism, acne, weight gain
Hyperprolactinemia	Galactorrhea, headaches, and visual deficits suggest prolactinoma
Thyroid disease	Diarrhea or constipation, heat or cold intolerance, weight changes, skin/hair changes

c. Complete blood count (CBC)
   i. Assess for thrombocytopenia as cause of heavy or prolonged bleeding
   ii. Assess degree of anemia, if any, resulting from blood loss
d. Other hematologic studies
   i. Prothrombin time (PT), partial thromboplastin time (PTT)
   ii. Testing for von Willebrand disease (not necessary if platelet count is normal because this is platelet adhesion problem)
e. Testing for STIs
f. Hormone studies: thyroid function tests, prolactin level, androgens (free and total testosterone, dehydroepiandrosterone sulfate [DHEA-S]), luteinizing hormone (LH), and follicle-stimulating hormone (FSH)

2. Radiologic imaging
   a. Ultrasound of pelvis
      i. Useful if patient cannot tolerate pelvic exam
      ii. Can identify ectopic pregnancy, assess for structural or anatomic abnormality

III. Approach to Dysmenorrhea

A. Background information
1. **Dysmenorrhea**: painful menstruation
2. Classification
   a. **Primary dysmenorrhea**: painful menses with clear physiologic etiology and no identifiable pelvic pathology
   b. **Secondary dysmenorrhea**: painful menses associated with underlying pelvic abnormality
3. Most common gynecologic complaint among female adolescents
4. Etiology
   a. Primary dysmenorrhea is due to release of prostaglandins from endometrium after progesterone withdrawal that precedes menstrual period
      i. Prostaglandins lead to potent vasoconstriction and uterine contractions, which leads to ischemia and pain
      ii. Other symptoms (e.g., bloating, diarrhea, nausea, vomiting, headaches) can result if prostaglandins are released into systemic circulation
   b. Causes of secondary dysmenorrhea are more prevalent in adulthood but should still be considered in adolescents
      i. Endometriosis
      ii. Congenital Müllerian anomaly
      iii. PID
      iv. Adhesions from prior surgery
      v. Ectopic pregnancy
      vi. Ovarian cyst
      vii. Ovarian torsion
      viii. Uterine fibroids
      ix. Intrauterine device use for contraception

B. Important historical findings
1. Interview adolescent alone and ensure confidentiality
2. Pain timing
   a. Determine whether associated only with menses
   b. Pain is usually just before or after onset of menstrual flow, usually worse in first 2 days
3. Ask patient to describe pain
   a. Often described as "cramping"
   b. Usually in lower abdomen but can radiate to lower back, buttocks, rectum, or legs
4. Determine whether symptoms have been present since menarche
5. Determine whether nonsteroidal anti-inflammatory drugs (NSAIDs) provide relief
   a. Drugs target endometrium's release of prostaglandins
   b. To be most effective, should be started before or at onset of menses, then continued for at least 24–48 hours
6. Previous abdominal or pelvic surgeries

QUICK HIT

Adolescents may be reluctant to share history of sexual activity, so do not rely on sexual history when considering pregnancy.

QUICK HIT

A pelvic exam is not necessary to test for chlamydia and gonorrhea. Nucleic acid amplification tests (e.g., polymerase chain reaction) can be sent on non–clean-catch urine specimens.

QUICK HIT

Primary dysmenorrhea is more common than secondary dysmenorrhea in adolescents (at least 90% of cases).

QUICK HIT

Primary dysmenorrhea is the leading cause of recurrent absences from school or work in young women.

QUICK HIT

Chronic pelvic pain may also be due to nongynecologic causes, especially if not only associated with menses. Consider gastrointestinal, musculoskeletal, and urinary systems as well as psychological issues and stress.

QUICK HIT

Dysmenorrhea is associated with normal ovulatory cycles, but many adolescents do not establish regular cycles in the first few years after menarche. Therefore, recurrent pain since the onset of menarche should raise suspicion for congenital malformations such as bicornuate uterus with partial obstruction.

7. Sexual activity/contraception
8. Associated symptoms
   a. Primary dysmenorrhea: nausea, vomiting, diarrhea, breast tenderness, bloating, fatigue, headache, light-headedness, and mood changes
   b. Secondary dysmenorrhea: fever, vaginal discharge, abnormal menstrual bleeding

C. Pertinent physical exam findings
1. Physical exam usually normal in primary dysmenorrhea
2. Abdominal exam
   a. Mild suprapubic tenderness possible with primary dysmenorrhea at time of menses; otherwise normal
   b. Rebound tenderness concerning for secondary causes of dysmenorrhea
3. Pelvic exam
   a. Speculum exam allows visualization of vagina and cervix but may not be necessary if history is consistent with primary dysmenorrhea and remainder of physical exam is within normal limits
   b. Inspect external genitalia to rule out imperforate hymen
   c. Bimanual exam can assess uterine size and shape; helps identify PID, ovarian mass, uterine malformation, or fibroid
   d. Rectovaginal exam can evaluate for endometriosis, which can be associated with mild posterior uterine or rectouterine pouch tenderness and uterosacral nodularity

QUICK HIT

Imperforate hymen usually presents as pain in the pelvis, abdomen, and back; difficulty with urination; and without bleeding at menarche.

D. Diagnostic workup
1. Laboratory data: done to rule out other causes of pelvic pain
   a. Pregnancy test
   b. Testing for gonorrhea and chlamydia (part of PID evaluation)
   c. If history and physical suggest nongynecologic causes of pain, consider urine culture, stool for occult blood, and erythrocyte sedimentation rate (ESR) or C-reactive protein (CRP) to assess for inflammation
2. Radiologic imaging: pelvic ultrasound
   a. Rule out anatomic abnormalities of uterus
   b. Evaluate for ovarian pathology
3. Laparoscopy
   a. Allows for direct visualization of pelvic and peritoneal cavity; can diagnose adhesions
   b. Useful for diagnosis of endometriosis
      i. Visualize ectopic nests of endometrial tissue outside of uterus
      ii. Visualize "chocolate cysts" in ovary

QUICK HIT

Primary dysmenorrhea is a clinical diagnosis. If the history and physical exam are not suggestive of a secondary etiology, further diagnostic evaluation may not be necessary.

E. Management
1. Primary dysmenorrhea: best treated by targeting endometrial prostaglandins
   a. NSAIDs: inhibit cyclooxygenase → reduction in production of prostaglandins → less vigorous uterine contractions → less pain
   b. Oral contraceptives: limit endometrial proliferation so less tissue available for prostaglandin production
   c. Others (heat, acupuncture herbs): limited data
2. Secondary dysmenorrhea: treat underlying pelvic pathology
   a. May require surgical intervention (e.g., anatomic anomalies, ovarian mass, unresolving ovarian cyst)
   b. Antibiotics for management of PID
   c. Endometriosis managed with oral contraceptive pills (OCPs) or gonadotropin-releasing hormone (GnRH) agonists

QUICK HIT

Decreasing the frequency of menstrual periods can help decrease episodes of dysmenorrhea, which can be accomplished with extended cycling of oral contraceptive pills (i.e., take placebo pills every 3 months) or with depot medroxyprogesterone acetate, which has an expected side effect of amenorrhea.

IV. Approach to Contraception

A. General considerations
1. 46% of U.S. high school students report ever having sex
2. >700,000 U.S. teen pregnancies occur annually
3. Declines in teen pregnancy rates attributed to increased use of contraception
4. Contraception options in adolescence (Table 13-4)
   a. Hormonal methods combining estrogen and progesterone
   b. Hormonal methods containing progesterone only

TABLE 13-4 **Examples of Adolescent Birth Control Methods**

Method	Hormone in Method	How Used
OCPs	Estrogen and progesterone (progesterone-only pills not discussed in this chapter)	Daily pill; 3 weeks of active hormone pills, 1 week of placebo pills (menses week)
Transdermal patch	Estrogen and progesterone	Adhesive patch worn on skin; changed weekly × 3 weeks, no patch × 1 week (menses during patch-free week)
Vaginal ring	Estrogen and progesterone	Patient inserts flexible ring into vagina; leave in place × 3 weeks, remove for 1 week (menses during ring-free week)
DMPA	Progesterone only	Intramuscular injection every 3 months; no hormone-free time
Condom	N/A	Barrier used at time of sex

DMPA, depot medroxyprogesterone acetate (Depo-Provera); N/A, not applicable; OCPs, oral contraceptive pills.

c. Barrier methods
d. Condoms are the most frequently used contraceptive method by adolescents; OCPs are most commonly used hormonal method (usually late adolescence/early adulthood)

B. Choosing a method (Table 13-5)
1. Some U.S. states allow minors to consent for health care related to sexual health and birth control
2. Selection requires consideration of several factors
a. Privacy needs
b. Challenges to adherence with regimen (e.g., daily, weekly, monthly)
c. Tolerance of method-specific side effects
d. Knowledge of contraindications to method
e. Noncontraceptive benefits (e.g., acne management, menses regulation)
3. Determine patient understanding of how various methods work

QUICK HIT

Hormonal contraception works by suppressing ovulation or by changing the cervical/uterine environment to prevent sperm from reaching the egg.

QUICK HIT

Hormonal methods are highly effective at preventing pregnancy but do not prevent STIs.

TABLE 13-5 **Advantages and Disadvantages of Birth Control Methods**

Method	Advantages	Disadvantages
OCPs	Menses shorter, lighter, predictable Decreased acne Ovarian cyst suppression	Daily adherence difficult for teens Estrogen-related side effects*
Transdermal patch	Same as OCPs Weekly dosing may improve adherence	Lacks privacy Skin irritation Estrogen-related side effects*
Vaginal ring	Same as OCPs Very private Monthly dosing may improve adherence	Requires patient comfort with idea of vaginal placement Vaginal discharge may occur Estrogen-related side effects*
DMPA	Amenorrhea, if desired Very private Infrequent dosing enhances adherence	Weight gain May see irregular periods for first few months Decreases bone mineral density
Condom	Use only when needed, rather than ongoing Minimal side effects	Interferes with spontaneity Need to remember with each sexual encounter May break or tear if used improperly Latex sensitivities or allergies

*Estrogen-related side effects include (but are not limited to) nausea, breast tenderness, headaches, possible increase in blood pressure and lipids, possible gallstones, and risk of thrombosis.

DMPA, depot medroxyprogesterone acetate (Depo-Provera); OCPs, oral contraceptive pills.

C. Clinical encounter
1. History
a. Sexual activity
b. Number of current partners; lifetime partners
c. STIs or pregnancies
d. Past forms of birth control
e. Identify medical problems that may complicate use of various methods
i. History of thrombotic disorder or migraines with aura is contraindication to estrogen-containing methods
ii. Medications that decrease effectiveness of hormones
f. Identify medical problems that may benefit from hormonal contraception (e.g., irregular menses, acne, hirsutism, menstrual migraines, catamenial seizures)
2. Physical exam
a. Pap smear is not recommended until age 21 years
b. Check weight, blood pressure
3. Laboratory findings
a. Pregnancy test should be done before starting hormonal contraceptives
b. Screening for thrombotic disorders is not necessary before starting estrogen-containing methods, unless there is a family history of thrombotic events
c. Testing for STIs can be done with urine specimen

D. Managing contraceptive use
1. Start hormonal methods in 1 of 3 ways
a. Sunday start: begin on Sunday after next menses begins
b. 1st-day start: begin on 1st day of next menses
i. Ensures patient is not pregnant
ii. Reduces chance of breakthrough bleeding during 1st cycle
c. Quick start (begin today): reduces chance of becoming pregnant before next period
2. Follow up in 3 months after starting birth control to assess compliance, tolerance of method
3. Monitor side effects, especially for symptoms concerning for thrombosis
4. Encourage use of barrier methods to prevent spread of STIs
5. Educate patients about emergency contraception in case of contraceptive failure, such as condom breaking or missed birth control pills
6. Calcium supplementation for patients on depot medroxyprogesterone acetate (DMPA)
7. Counsel about safe relationships, need for routine STI testing, and abstinence

QUICK HIT

Because adolescents rely on peers as a primary source of information, it is important to identify and correct any myths or misconceptions the teen has about birth control.

QUICK HIT

Interview the patient alone and ensure confidentiality.

QUICK HIT

Approximately 25% of 15–19-year-olds report no birth control method with their first sexual encounter.

QUICK HIT

Estrogen has procoagulant properties, so any predisposition to clotting is a contraindication to birth control containing this hormone.

QUICK HIT

Certain anticonvulsants induce cytochrome P450 activity, which decreases circulating levels of contraceptive hormones.

QUICK HIT

Although a general physical exam should be done, a pelvic exam is not necessary to initiate contraception (with the exception of intrauterine device [IUD]) and should not pose a barrier to adolescents seeking birth control.

DISEASE SPECIFIC

V. Primary Amenorrhea

A. General characteristics
1. Definition (1 of following)
a. No menarche (onset of menses) by age 14 years in absence of pubertal development (e.g., breast development)
b. No menarche by age 16 years regardless of pubertal development
2. Normal onset of menses
a. Menses is dependent on ovulation, estrogen, and progesterone (secretion and withdrawal)
b. In U.S., average age of menarche is 12.7 years
c. At least 2/3 of girls experience menarche in Tanner stage IV
3. Etiology
a. May result from genetic, endocrine, nutritional, or anatomic defects
b. Ovaries not producing sufficient estrogen to proliferate uterine lining or induce ovulation
i. Hypogonadotropic hypogonadism: inadequate release of gonadotropins (LH, FSH) from pituitary

ii. Hypergonadotropic hypogonadism: inadequate ovarian response to gonadotropins
c. Anatomic problem with reproductive tract
i. Absent uterus
ii. Genital outlet obstruction
B. Clinical features
1. Historical findings
a. Other signs of pubertal progression
i. Age of thelarche (onset of breast development)
ii. Timing of growth spurt
b. Age of menarche in mother, sisters
c. Menstrual, gynecologic, or puberty problems in family
d. Sexual activity
e. Abdominal pain or cramping
f. Diet and exercise habits
g. Careful ROS can identify underlying hormonal problems contributing to abnormal onset of menses (e.g., thyroid disease)
2. Physical exam findings
a. Assess Tanner stage
b. Check growth parameters
i. Low BMI can delay onset of menses
ii. Short stature may suggest genetic or endocrine disorder
c. Genital exam
i. Hymenal opening: obstructed by thin membrane
ii. Enlarged clitoris: suggests excess androgens
iii. Appropriate pubic hair development
iv. Vaginal exam (if tolerated)
(a) Vagina ending in "blind pouch": indicates absent uterus
d. Look for signs consistent with endocrinopathy or genetic disease
i. Acne, hirsutism, galactorrhea, brittle hair or nails, short stature
ii. See Figure 13-1 for signs consistent with Turner syndrome

QUICK HIT
Weight gain is a known side effect of the injectable progesterone-only method, but OCPs do not cause weight gain.

QUICK HIT
DMPA leads to a hypoestrogenic state, which decreases osteoblast activity and, therefore, bone mineral density.

QUICK HIT
On average, menses occur 2 years after breast bud development and 1 year after the "growth spurt."

QUICK HIT
Primary amenorrhea can occur in competitive teen athletes and those with severe anorexia.

QUICK HIT
Cyclic abdominal pain in an adolescent with primary amenorrhea should raise suspicion for an imperforate hymen or other genital outlet obstruction.

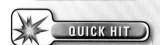

QUICK HIT
In the absence of notable history or physical findings, girls age <16 years who have initiated but not completed puberty (i.e., have not yet reached Tanner stage V) can likely be reassured about not yet reaching menarche.

QUICK HIT
Menarche requires 17% body fat; cyclic menses require 22% body fat.

FIGURE 13-1 **Clinical features of Turner syndrome.**

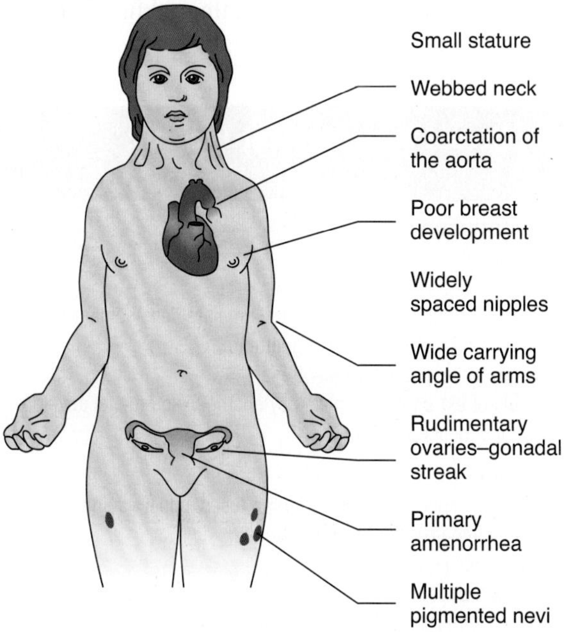

(From Rubin E, Farber JL. *Pathology.* 3rd ed. Philadelphia: Lippincott Williams & Wilkins; 1999.)

Diseases Unique to Adolescent Medicine

TABLE 13-6 **Differential Diagnosis: No Breast Development; Uterus Present**

Disorder	Defect
Problem with ovary	
Turner syndrome	Ovaries fail to develop (streak gonads)
Aromatase deficiency	Lack hormone to convert androgen to estrogen
Chemotherapy or radiation	Induces ovarian failure, follicular atresia
Autoimmune oophoritis	Autoantibodies against ovaries (e.g., Hashimoto thyroiditis)
Problem with hypothalamus or pituitary	
Kallmann syndrome	Failure of GnRH-producing cells to develop (may also see anosmia as olfactory cells develop improperly)
Tumor	Compression or infiltration of pituitary
Malnutrition	Leads to hypothalamic dysregulation, inhibits GnRH
Endocrinopathy	Disrupts hypothalamic–pituitary–ovarian axis (hyperthyroidism, elevated prolactin or androgens)

GnRH, gonadotropin-releasing hormone.

QUICK HIT

Turner syndrome is the most common cause of primary amenorrhea in adolescents, whereas Müllerian agenesis is the second most common cause.

QUICK HIT

Elevated FSH and LH levels suggest a problem with ovarian function; low levels suggest a pituitary or hypothalamus problem.

C. Diagnosis
1. Differential diagnosis
   a. Organize differential based on presence or absence of breasts and/or uterus (Tables 13-6, 13-7, and 13-8)
      i. Absent breast development indicates inadequate estrogen production (consider if problem is at level of hypothalamus, pituitary, or ovary)
      ii. Absence of uterus indicates abnormal Müllerian development or XY karyotype
      iii. Presence of uterus and breasts suggests obstruction of menstrual flow or HPO axis problems
   b. Some overlap exists with differential diagnosis for secondary amenorrhea
2. Laboratory testing
   a. Always check pregnancy test, even if patient denies sexual activity
   b. Check for abnormal hormone levels consistent with differential diagnosis (e.g., androgens [free and total testosterone, DHEA-S], thyroid function tests, prolactin)

TABLE 13-7 **Differential Diagnosis: Breast Development Present; No Uterus**

Disorder	Karyotype	Characteristics
Androgen insensitivity syndrome	Androgen receptor defect	XY karyotype Testes present but androgens cannot stimulate development of Wolffian structures or external genitalia Genetically male, phenotypically female Low levels of estrogen unopposed by androgen so breasts develop Blind vaginal pouch, no pubic hair
Müllerian agenesis (Mayer-Rokitansky-Kuster-Hauser syndrome)	Anomalous development of Müllerian system	XX karyotype Congenital absence of uterus, fallopian tubes, upper vagina Genetically female, phenotypically female Normal ovaries so breasts develop Blind vaginal pouch Associated with renal and skeletal anomalies

TABLE 13-8 **Differential Diagnosis: Breast Development and Uterus Present***

Disorder	Defect	Characteristics
Genital outlet obstruction (e.g., imperforate hymen, transverse vaginal septum)	Intact hypothalamic–pituitary–ovarian axis, normal shedding of endometrium but no outlet for menstrual flow	Leads to hematocolpos (menstrual blood trapped in vagina) Imperforate hymen seen as bulging membrane Cyclic abdominal pain at time of menses
Pregnancy	Pregnancy can occur with first ovulation	Positive pregnancy test, morning sickness, breast tenderness

*See Table 13-6 for malnutrition, endocrinopathy, effects of chemotherapy, and autoimmune oophoritis.

c. Check karyotype if
   i. Absence of uterus on exam or ultrasound
   ii. No signs of puberty by age 14 years
3. Radiology findings
   a. Pelvic ultrasound is most useful for evaluating reproductive anatomy
   b. Obtain magnetic resonance imaging (MRI) of head/pituitary if elevated prolactin level or abnormal neurologic findings

D. Treatment
1. Management strategies will depend on underlying etiology
2. Hypergonadotropic and hypogonadotropic hypogonadism necessitate estrogen and progesterone replacement (e.g., OCPs)
3. Imperforate hymen and other outlet obstructions require surgical correction
4. Refer patient to endocrinology for management of underlying endocrinopathies
5. Hypothalamic dysregulation due to malnutrition
   a. Encourage weight gain; provide nutritional supplementation
   b. Eating disorders require psychiatric and medical management
6. Look for undescended testes in patients with androgen insensitivity syndrome

QUICK HIT

Because short stature is associated with Turner syndrome, hormone replacement may also include growth hormone therapy with this disorder.

QUICK HIT

Because undescended testes have a high malignancy potential, they should be surgically removed.

VI. Secondary Amenorrhea

A. General characteristics
1. Definition: absence of menses ≥6 months in previously menstruating female (occurs anytime after menarche)
2. Pubertal development should be normal
3. Anovulatory cycles are common cause in young adolescents
4. Can result from any disruption in HPO axis (Box 13-2)
   a. Inadequate GnRH release
   b. Inadequate LH, FSH release
   c. Insufficient estrogen to stimulate LH surge and ovulation

QUICK HIT

Normal ovaries are present in patients with Müllerian agenesis, so hormone replacement is not necessary. However, body image and self-esteem issues may arise, so counseling or support groups should be offered.

BOX 13-2

Differential Diagnosis of Secondary Amenorrhea

Anovulatory cycles due to immature hypothalamic–pituitary–ovarian axis
Pregnancy
Hormonal contraception, especially Depo-Provera
Malabsorption diseases
Eating disorder
Intense or excessive exercise
Psychosocial stress
Tumor (androgen secreting, pituitary)
Endocrine disorders
  Hyperthyroidism, hypothyroidism
  Hyperprolactinemia (prolactinoma, medication induced)
  Polycystic ovary syndrome
  Late-onset congenital adrenal hyperplasia
Ovarian failure
  Autoimmune oophoritis (autoantibodies to ovary)
  Chemotherapy- or radiation-induced failure

QUICK HIT

Amenorrhea is an expected side effect of DMPA due to a thinned endometrium and suppressed estrogen levels.

QUICK HIT

A previous pregnancy complicated by Sheehan syndrome will lead to pituitary dysfunction.

QUICK HIT

Poor nutrition, weight loss, or a high level of physical activity can affect GnRH and LH pulsatile release.

QUICK HIT

The **female athlete triad** consists of disordered eating, amenorrhea, and osteoporosis.

QUICK HIT

Girls who have reached Tanner stage V are less likely to have anovulatory cycles than girls at Tanner stage III or IV.

QUICK HIT

Clitoromegaly is associated more with high androgen levels due to adrenal disorders or androgen-secreting tumors than with PCOS.

QUICK HIT

Always check a pregnancy test, even if adolescent denies sexual activity.

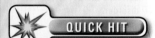

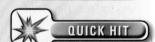

5. Excluding congenital disorders, much overlap exists between causes of primary and secondary amenorrhea

B. Clinical features
   1. Historical findings
      a. Sexual activity
         i. Pregnancy symptoms
         ii. Hormonal contraception
      b. Eating behaviors suggestive of eating disorder
      c. Competitive athlete or excessive exerciser
      d. History of chemotherapy or pelvic radiation suggests iatrogenic ovarian failure
      e. Family history of menstrual or gynecologic problems
      f. Psychotropic medications (e.g., antipsychotics) or illicit drugs
      g. Check for symptoms consistent with underlying hormonal problems (Table 13-9)
   2. Physical exam findings
      a. Assess Tanner stage
      b. Weight, height, and BMI
      c. Genital exam
         i. Clitoromegaly suggests excess androgens
         ii. Bimanual exam can assess uterus, ovaries
      d. Skin exam for hirsutism, acne, striae, acanthosis nigricans
      e. Look for signs consistent with endocrinopathy (see Table 13-9)

C. Diagnosis
   1. Differential diagnosis (see Box 13-2)
   2. Anovulatory cycles is diagnosis of exclusion
   3. Laboratory testing
      a. Pregnancy test
      b. Thyroid-stimulating hormone, free T_4 (thyroxine)
      c. Prolactin level
      d. Free and total testosterone, DHEA-S, 17-α-hydroxyprogesterone
      e. LH and FSH
      f. Elevated insulin levels in PCOS

TABLE 13-9 **Signs and Symptoms: Endocrine Causes of Secondary Amenorrhea**

Disease	Symptoms	Physical Findings
Prolactinoma	Headache Galactorrhea	Visual field deficits Galactorrhea
Hyperthyroidism	Weight loss Palpitations Heat intolerance Diarrhea	Tachycardia Tremor Warm skin, brittle nails Goiter possible
Hypothyroidism	Weight gain Constipation Fatigue Cold intolerance	Cold, dry skin Edema of face and eyelids Dry, brittle hair Goiter possible
PCOS	Acne Hirsutism Weight gain	Acne Hirsutism Obesity Acanthosis nigricans (due to insulin resistance)
Late-onset CAH or virilizing tumor	Acne Hirsutism	Acne Hirsutism Clitoromegaly

CAH, congenital adrenal hyperplasia; PCOS, polycystic ovary syndrome.

4. Radiology findings
   a. Pelvic ultrasound is most useful for evaluating reproductive anatomy
   b. Obtain MRI of head/pituitary if elevated prolactin level or abnormal neurologic findings
   c. Dual-energy x-ray absorptiometry (DEXA) scan (assesses bone mineral density [BMD]) if concerned about female athlete triad or significant hypoestrogenism
5. Other: check response to progesterone challenge test
   a. Administer oral medroxyprogesterone acetate for 5–10 days
   b. Look for withdrawal bleed after medroxyprogesterone cessation
      i. If present, endometrium has been primed by estrogen; implies ovarian function
      ii. If absent, evaluate for hypothalamic–pituitary insufficiency or ovarian failure

D. Treatment
1. Treat underlying etiology
   a. Nutritional counseling or support
   b. Refer to endocrinology or gynecology as appropriate
   c. Psychological intervention for eating disorders, significant psychosocial stressors
2. Counsel pregnant teens about pregnancy options; make appropriate referral
3. Anovulatory cycles
   a. Provide reassurance; no intervention necessary
   b. OCPs can be used to produce regular periods, if desired
4. Patients with ovarian failure will need hormone replacement
   a. Usually taken as OCP
   b. Without treatment, may experience hot flashes, other menopause-like symptoms
5. PCOS
   a. OCP (estrogen + progesterone)
      i. Restores regular menses
      ii. Decreases testosterone levels
      iii. Protects against endometrial hyperplasia from unopposed estrogen
      iv. Can use pill with drospirenone as progestin component; has antiandrogen properties
   b. Insulin-sensitizing agents (metformin)
      i. Decrease circulating androgens
      ii. Improve reproductive function
      iii. Improve metabolic complications; help with weight loss

QUICK HIT

PCOS is associated with insulin resistance, with elevated insulin playing a role in excess testosterone production.

QUICK HIT

In PCOS, the ratio of LH to FSH is often 2:1 or greater. However, diagnosis is made based on elevated free and/or total testosterone levels.

QUICK HIT

Most adolescents with PCOS do not have the classic ultrasound findings of polycystic ovaries, which are, therefore, not necessary for diagnosis.

QUICK HIT

Male levels of testosterone in a female with a normal XX karyotype necessitate imaging needed to look for an androgen-secreting tumor in the ovary or adrenal glands.

VII. Pelvic Inflammatory Disease

A. General characteristics
1. Definition: STI of upper female genital tract
   a. Complication of cervicitis
   b. Ascending spread of microorganisms from lower genital tract
   c. Spectrum of inflammatory disorders including endometritis, salpingitis, tubo-ovarian abscess (TOA), pelvic peritonitis, perihepatitis
2. Adolescent females account for 1/3 of PID cases annually in U.S.
3. Cause
   a. Common organisms are *Neisseria gonorrhoeae* and *Chlamydia trachomatis*
   b. Other organisms include *Streptococcus* species, *Escherichia coli*, *Mycoplasma hominis*, *Ureaplasma urealyticum*, *Bacteroides* species, and other anaerobes
4. Risk factors
   a. Young age at 1st sex
      i. Chlamydia and gonorrhea have predilection for columnar cells that predominate in area surrounding cervical os in adolescents (cervical ectropion); these cells transform to squamous epithelium as the adolescents enter adulthood
      ii. Higher rates of chlamydia and gonorrhea in adolescents make complication of PID more likely

QUICK HIT

Chlamydia is the most common reportable disease and has the highest rates in 15–19-year-old females in the U.S.

iii. Less likely to use barrier contraception due to cognitive stage, sense of invincibility
b. Multiple sexual partners
c. Unprotected sexual intercourse
d. Previous history of PID
e. Bacterial vaginosis (BV) associated with PID but no causal relationship established
5. Pathophysiology
a. Begins as lower genital tract infection, usually as cervicitis
b. Inflammatory disruption of cervical barrier permits ascension of inciting bacteria into uterus
c. Multiple vaginal organisms follow, creating polymicrobial upper tract infection
d. Plasma cell infiltration of endometrium
e. Decreased motility of fallopian tubes due to inflammation leads to collections of fluid (hydrosalpinx) or pus (pyosalpinx)
f. Infection may spill out end of fallopian tube, leading to complication of peritonitis, perihepatitis, TOA

QUICK HIT

Menstruation facilitates the ascension of lower tract organisms because the cervical os is open, and endometrial blood serves as a growth medium.

B. Clinical features
1. Patient may or may not have had symptoms of cervicitis prior to presentation (see Box 13-3 for clinical presentation of cervicitis)
2. Historical findings with PID
a. Lower abdominal or pelvic pain or cramping (>80% of patients)
b. Vaginal discharge (>50% of patients)
c. Dyspareunia
d. Irregular vaginal bleeding
e. Other: dysuria, fever, nausea/vomiting, difficulty ambulating secondary to pain ("PID shuffle")
3. Physical exam findings
a. Assess vital signs for fever and hemodynamic stability (patients with PID may become very ill, especially if peritonitis)
b. Abdominal tenderness (assess for peritoneal signs)
c. Pelvic exam
i. Vaginal or cervical discharge frequently seen
ii. Friable, inflamed cervix
iii. Assess for tenderness of uterus, adnexa, or with movement of cervix

QUICK HIT

A bimanual exam is essential for making the clinical diagnosis of PID.

C. Diagnosis
1. Minimum clinical criteria are used to diagnose PID, supported by additional criteria to increase specificity of diagnosis (Box 13-4)
2. Differential diagnosis includes causes of abdominal pain originating from multiple organ systems
a. Gastrointestinal (GI): appendicitis, cholecystitis, constipation, diverticulitis, hernia, inflammatory bowel disease (IBD)
b. Gynecologic: pregnancy, dysmenorrhea, endometriosis, mittelschmerz, ovarian cyst, ovarian torsion, ovarian tumor
c. Urologic: cystitis, pyelonephritis, nephrolithiasis
d. Others: musculoskeletal pain, psychosomatic pain

BOX 13-3

Clinical Features of Cervicitis

Symptoms	Physical findings
Frequently asymptomatic	Mucopurulent discharge at cervical os
Vaginal discharge	Erythema/edema of cervix
Intermenstrual vaginal spotting or bleeding	Friable cervix (bleeds when touched with swab)
Postcoital bleeding	
Dyspareunia	
Dysuria	

BOX 13-4

Criteria for Diagnosing Pelvic Inflammatory Disease

Minimum criteria

Patient should have at least one of the following:

- Cervical motion tenderness
- Uterine tenderness
- Adnexal tenderness

Additional criteria to support diagnosis (not necessary for diagnosis)

- Temperature >38.3°C (101°F)
- Abnormal cervical or vaginal mucopurulent discharge
- Presence of white blood cells on wet mount
- Elevated ESR or CRP
- Positive test for gonorrhea or chlamydia

CRP, C-reactive protein; ESR, erythrocyte sedimentation rate.

3. Laboratory findings
    a. Pregnancy test should be done on all patients suspected of PID
        i. Rule out as cause of abdominal pain
        ii. Pregnancy alters management strategy in PID
    b. Check CBC for elevated white blood cells (WBCs)
    c. ESR and CRP may be elevated
    d. Urine dip often positive for leukocyte esterase
    e. Vaginal microscopy (wet mount) shows >10 WBCs per high-power field (HPF)
    f. Testing for *N. gonorrhoeae* and *C. trachomatis* should be sent via nucleic acid amplification test (NAAT) or culture of cervical swab
    g. Test for other STIs, including HIV
4. Radiology findings
    a. Pelvic ultrasound
        i. May see fluid-filled fallopian tubes
        ii. Can use to narrow differential diagnosis (e.g., look for ovarian pathology, ectopic pregnancy)
        iii. Allows for visualization of TOA (see p. 72, Complications)
5. Other findings (rarely needed to make diagnosis in adolescents)
    a. Histopathologic evidence of endometritis on endometrial biopsy
    b. Laparoscopy can visualize swollen fallopian tubes, allow for bacterial culture of pelvic fluid or abscesses

D. Treatment
1. Antibiotics are mainstay of therapy (Box 13-5)
2. Indications for hospitalization
    a. Surgical emergencies (e.g., appendicitis) cannot be excluded
    b. Pregnancy
    c. Failed or poor response to outpatient therapy
    d. Inability to tolerate outpatient regimen
    e. Severe illness, nausea and vomiting, or high fever
    f. TOA

QUICK HIT

PID is a polymicrobial infection, so a negative test for gonorrhea or chlamydia does not rule out the diagnosis.

QUICK HIT

Unlike in adults, a speculum exam is not routinely indicated in adolescents.

QUICK HIT

Most PID can be managed on an outpatient basis. Hospitalization has not been shown to change future behavior in adolescents.

BOX 13-5

Antibiotic Regimen for Pelvic Inflammatory Disease

Outpatient management	Inpatient management
Ceftriaxone 250 mg IM × 1 dose	Cefoxitin 2 g IV every 6 hours
AND	AND
Doxycycline 100 mg PO twice daily × 14 days	Doxycycline 100 mg PO every 12 hours*
WITH OR WITHOUT	WITH OR WITHOUT
Metronidazole 500 mg PO twice daily × 14 days	Metronidazole 500 mg IV twice daily × 14 days

*Oral doxycycline is preferred because intravenous (IV) form is caustic to veins. If oral is not possible, consider alternative regimen of IV clindamycin + gentamicin.

IM, intramuscular; PO, per os.

QUICK HIT

Fitz-Hugh-Curtis syndrome is a perihepatitis, so hepatic transaminases usually are *not* elevated.

QUICK HIT

Consider Fitz-Hugh-Curtis syndrome in a sexually active adolescent who presents with right upper quadrant pain and tenderness.

QUICK HIT

Reinfection is common in adolescents treated for PID.

QUICK HIT

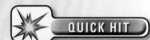

Candidiasis is a major cause of vaginitis in non–sexually active adolescents.

QUICK HIT

A retained foreign body such as a tampon or condom often leads to malodorous vaginal discharge.

3. Complications
   a. TOA
      i. Bacteria, inflammatory cells, fluid accumulate in fallopian tube, then spread beyond fimbriated end of tube to encompass adjacent ovary
      ii. Requires longer duration of antibiotic therapy (at least 21 days)
      iii. May require surgical drainage
   b. Fitz-Hugh-Curtis syndrome (perihepatitis)
      i. Infection travels up right paracolic gutter to infect liver capsule
      ii. Adhesions form between liver capsule and diaphragm ("violin strings")
      iii. Not detected on ultrasound; diagnosis made laparoscopically
4. PID leads to increased future risk of ectopic pregnancy (due to damaged fallopian tubes), infertility, and chronic pelvic pain
5. Treat sexual partners empirically for gonorrhea and chlamydia; test for other STIs
6. Prevention
   a. Educate patients on safer sexual practices (e.g., condoms), STIs
   b. Because PID is complication of untreated cervicitis, routinely screen asymptomatic adolescents for STIs

VIII. Vaginitis

A. General characteristics
1. **Vaginitis**: inflammation of squamous epithelial tissues lining vagina
   a. Most commonly leads to vaginal discharge
   b. May also see vulvar and/or labial irritation or inflammation
2. >90% of cases of vaginal discharge in adolescents are caused by 3 infections
   a. **Vulvovaginal candidiasis** (20%–25%)
   b. **BV** (40%–45%) due to overgrowth of *Gardnerella vaginalis* and other anaerobic vaginal species
   c. **Trichomoniasis** (15%–20%)
3. Risk factors
   a. Unprotected sexual intercourse
   b. Multiple sexual partners or new partner
   c. History of STIs
   d. Frequent douching or recent antibiotics
4. Pathophysiology
   a. *Lactobacillus* is predominant normal flora in vagina
   b. Normal postpubertal vagina has pH of 3.8–4.2
   c. Disruption of normal vaginal flora and/or altered pH leads to overgrowth of other flora (e.g., *Candida* species, *Gardnerella* species), leading to symptoms of vaginitis
   d. Trichomoniasis results from sexual transmission of *Trichomonas vaginalis*
      i. Anaerobic parasitic protozoan
      ii. Characteristic flagella aid in motility
      iii. Adherence to vaginal epithelial cells leads to cellular damage and mucosal inflammation

B. Clinical features (Table 13-10)
1. Historical findings
   a. Ask about onset, duration, color, odor, consistency, and quantity of vaginal discharge
   b. Ask about sexual activity, feminine hygiene habits (e.g., douching, tampon use), recent antibiotic use
2. Physical exam findings
   a. External genitalia involvement
      i. Look for vulvar erythema or edema
      ii. Genital lesions should raise suspicion for other STIs (e.g., herpes, genital warts)
   b. Palpate for inguinal lymph nodes

TABLE 13-10 **Key Clinical Features in Vaginitis**

	Trichomoniasis	Bacterial Vaginosis	Candida Vaginitis
Discharge	Greenish, frothy	Grayish white	Whitish, thick ("cottage cheese")
Pruritus	Yes	No	No
Odor	Yes	Yes	No
Dysuria	Yes	No	Yes
Bleeding	Postcoital	No	No
Edema/erythema of vulva/labia	Yes	No	Yes
"Strawberry cervix" (punctate hemorrhages seen on cervix)	Yes (although rare)	No	No

c. Speculum exam allows visualization of discharge
   i. Note color, consistency
   ii. Discharge from cervical os: more suggestive of cervicitis than vaginitis

C. Diagnosis
1. Differential diagnosis
   a. "Nonspecific" vaginitis results from poor hygiene, improper wiping, wearing tight clothes, and chemical irritation (e.g., bubble baths)
   b. Physiologic leukorrhea
      i. Normal discharge resulting from rise in estrogens during puberty
      ii. Usually precedes menarche by 3–6 months
   c. Vaginal discharge from cervicitis (e.g., chlamydia infection) may be mistaken for vaginitis
2. Laboratory findings
   a. Vaginal microscopy (i.e., wet mount) identifies most common causes of vaginitis (Table 13-11)
      i. Saline wet mount: visualization of epithelial cells, clue cells, WBCs, trichomonads
      ii. Potassium hydroxide (KOH) prep: visualization of hyphae, "whiff test"
      iii. Check pH of vaginal discharge
   b. Culture of organisms not typically needed to diagnose vaginitis in adolescents

QUICK HIT

In prepubertal children, vaginitis is often caused by respiratory organisms (e.g., group A β-hemolytic strep) and enteric organisms (e.g., *E. coli*).

QUICK HIT

A positive "whiff test" occurs when volatile amines release a fishy odor in the presence of 10% KOH.

QUICK HIT

Adolescents can self-swab and send specimens for molecular testing in lieu of speculum examination and wet-mount microscopy.

TABLE 13-11 **Findings on Vaginal Microscopy (Wet Mount)**

	Trichomoniasis	Bacterial Vaginosis	Candida Vaginitis
pH	>4.5	>4.5	<4.5
White blood cells	Yes	No	Yes
Characteristic finding	Motile organisms with flagella	Clue cells	Budding yeast, pseudohyphae
"Whiff test" with 10% potassium hydroxide (KOH)	May be positive	Positive	Negative

D. Treatment
1. Vulvovaginal candidiasis
   a. Fluconazole 150 mg per os (PO) × 1 dose
   b. Over-the-counter intravaginal antifungal creams (e.g., clotrimazole)
2. BV: metronidazole 500 mg PO twice daily × 7 days
3. Trichomoniasis: metronidazole 2 g PO × 1 dose
4. Instruct patients to abstain from sexual intercourse until completion of therapy, resolution of symptoms
5. Complications
   a. BV and trichomoniasis are associated with preterm labor, premature rupture of membranes, and low-birth-weight newborns
   b. Increased risk for acquiring STIs
6. Prevention
   a. Encourage consistent condom use
   b. Discourage douching, other intravaginal hygiene products
   c. Eating yogurt and other sources of live lactobacilli not shown to significantly prevent infections
   d. Address hygiene issues contributing to nonspecific vaginitis (e.g., wipe front to back, avoid bubble baths, wear cotton underwear)

> **QUICK HIT**
> Because adolescents may experiment with substance use, it is important to warn of the disulfiram-like effects of metronidazole when mixed with alcohol.

> **QUICK HIT**
> Recurrent vaginal yeast infections should raise concern for diabetes mellitus (DM). The higher glucose content of vaginal secretions and altered immune function permit increased proliferation of *Candida* species.

IX. Human Papillomavirus

A. General characteristics
1. Double-stranded DNA virus with >100 genotypes
2. Causes genital warts (condyloma acuminata) in sexually active adolescents
3. Although HPV (genital warts) is responsible for most cervical cancer in women, this cancer rarely manifests during adolescence
4. Epidemiology
   a. ~6 million new infections each year in U.S.
   b. At least 50% of sexually active people will acquire HPV virus
   c. "Low-risk" HPV types 6 and 11 cause 90% of genital warts in males and females
   d. "High-risk" HPV types 16 and 18 cause 70% of cervical cancer cases in females
5. Early sexual debut and history of multiple sex partners increase risk of acquiring HPV
6. Pathophysiology
   a. Transmitted through sexual contact: vaginal or anal sex, genital–genital contact, manual–genital contact
   b. Can also be transmitted to newborn during birth
   c. Virus infects basal layer of epithelial cells in skin and mucous membranes
      i. Stimulates cellular proliferation and hyperplasia, leading to wart formation
      ii. Can lead to cellular dysplasia and even anogenital and cervical carcinoma, although much less likely in adolescents

> **QUICK HIT**
> Routine Pap smear or cervical cytology is not recommended for women younger than age 21 years.

> **QUICK HIT**
> The prevalence of genital HPV infection is ~25% among 14–19-year-olds.

> **QUICK HIT**
> Condoms do not completely protect against HPV.

B. Clinical features
1. Historical findings (genital warts)
   a. Ask about sexual activity, genital–genital contact
   b. May be asymptomatic other than wart
   c. Patients may report "bumps" in genital region; may occasionally itch or bleed at site of lesion
   d. Ask if previously vaccinated with HPV vaccine
2. Physical exam findings
   a. Fleshy, exophytic, pedunculated lesions (cauliflower-like appearance)
   b. May also present as small, discrete, sessile, smooth-topped papules
   c. May appear as single lesions or in multiples
      i. Males: on penis, scrotum, inguinal, and perianal areas
      ii. Females: on vulva, cervix, vagina, urethra, and perianal area

> **QUICK HIT**
> Perinatal transmission can cause recurrent respiratory papillomatosis (RRP) in children. A serious complication of RRP is airway obstruction and respiratory distress.

> **QUICK HIT**
> In most cases, genital HPV infection is transient and has no clinical manifestations.

C. Diagnosis
  1. Primarily clinical diagnosis based on appearance of lesions
  2. Differential diagnosis
    a. Condyloma lata (due to syphilis)
    b. Molluscum contagiosum
    c. Pearly penile papules
    d. Fibromas, lipomas, adenomas
    e. Inflamed hair follicle (secondary to shaving or ingrown hair)
  3. Pap smear or liquid-based cytology is used to screen for cervical dysplasia in women age 21 years and older

D. Treatment
  1. Therapy
    a. Spontaneous regression of genital warts is seen in 70%–90% of women within 2 years if left untreated
    b. Treatments
      i. Patient applied: Imiquimod 5% cream, podofilox solution or gel
      ii. Provider administered: cryotherapy (e.g., liquid nitrogen), trichloroacetic acid, surgical or laser removal, or intralesional interferon
  2. Prognosis: recurrence of lesions is common because virus is not eliminated
  3. Prevention
    a. HPV vaccine (3-dose series) is recommended beginning at age 11 years for males and females
    b. Adolescents can receive protection against HPV types 6, 11, 16, and 18 with use of quadrivalent vaccine and against HPV types 6 and 11 with use of bivalent vaccine

X. Breast Masses

A. Background information
  1. Pubertal breast development is mainly under influence of estrogen (lactiferous ducts) and progesterone (lobular tissue and alveolar budding)
  2. Female adolescent breast tissue is very dense and very responsive to cyclic hormonal changes, especially around menses
  3. Many breast masses are found incidentally by patient

B. Cause/pathophysiology
  1. Most breast masses in adolescents are benign; fibroadenoma is most common
  2. Malignant breast lesions are very rare in adolescents (<1% of breast tumors)

C. Clinical presentation (see Table 13-12 for clinical features)
  1. Inspection: look for asymmetry, skin changes, color changes
  2. Palpation: note location, size, mobility, and consistency of any masses; note any nipple discharge

D. Testing
  1. Ultrasound is modality of choice to distinguish solid from cystic mass
  2. Mammography is not recommended in adolescents due to high density of breast tissue, low prevalence of cancer
  3. Fine-needle aspiration of breast mass can be performed to evaluate persistent (>2–3 months), nonmobile, or irregularly shaped masses

E. Therapy
  1. Most benign adolescent breast masses require only clinical follow-up to ensure resolution
  2. Surgical excision for symptomatic, rapidly growing, or persistent masses or for cosmetic reasons
  3. Breast abscesses: antibiotics, warm compresses, and surgical drainage as needed
  4. NSAIDs or OCPs may help pain associated with hormone-dependent proliferative breast changes

QUICK HIT

The HPV vaccine does not cover all HPV genotypes; therefore, a history of vaccination reduces but does not completely eliminate the possibility of acquiring HPV infection.

QUICK HIT

A diagnosis of HPV should prompt testing for other commonly acquired STIs, such as chlamydia, gonorrhea, syphilis, and HIV.

QUICK HIT

The goal of vaccination early in adolescence is to offer protection prior to the initiation of sexual activity.

QUICK HIT

Malignant breast lesions in adolescent females are more often metastases from other body sites rather than primary breast cancers.

QUICK HIT

Always perform the breast exam with the patient in upright and supine positions.

QUICK HIT

A fibroadenoma appears on ultrasound as a homogeneous, hypoechoic mass with smooth, well-demarcated borders.

QUICK HIT

Up to 50% of fibroadenomas decrease in size or resolve within 5 years.

TABLE 13-12 Common Breast Masses in Adolescents

Breast Mass	Comments	Pathophysiology	Clinical Features
Fibroadenoma	Most common adolescent breast mass (60%–80% of lesions)	Proliferating stroma around distorted ducts	Round, rubbery, firm, mobile lesion (average size 2–3 cm); nontender, well demarcated; often in upper outer quadrant
Proliferative breast changes	Also known as fibrocystic changes	Breast nodules and cord-like thickenings (connective tissue and epithelial cell proliferation); associated with fluctuations in estrogen and progesterone	Diffuse, small (<1 cm) lumps or nodules that become painful or tender around time of menstruation
Abscess or cellulitis	Introduction of bacteria from overlying skin (e.g., trauma, piercings, plucking/shaving periareolar hairs); also seen in lactating women	Most commonly *Staphylococcus aureus*; occasionally *Streptococcus pyogenes* or other streptococcal species	Swelling, erythema, warmth, induration, or fluctuance of the breast; may see purulent nipple
Cysts	Can present as single or multiple breast masses; can increase in size or tenderness in association with menstruation	Fluid accumulation in terminal duct lobar unit	Firm, well-circumscribed, freely mobile mass distinct from surrounding breast tissue
Trauma	History of trauma to anterior chest or directly to breast	Hematoma; may see accompanying fat necrosis	Tender, well-demarcated mass; skin ecchymosis

QUICK HIT

The risk of testicular cancer is increased 10–40-fold in males with a history of undescended testicles.

QUICK HIT

Torsion results from the anatomic "bell-clapper deformity," in which no gubernaculum is present to anchor the testicle in the scrotum.

XI. Scrotal Masses

A. General characteristics
1. Masses may be palpated in any scrotal structure, including testicle, epididymis, tunica vaginalis, and spermatic cord
2. Masses in scrotum may be painful or nonpainful (Box 13-6 and Figure 13-2)
   a. Painful scrotal masses may be surgical emergency (e.g., testicular torsion)
   b. Nonpainful mass arising from testicle itself (rather than other scrotal structures) is more concerning for testicular cancer
3. Most life-threatening mass is testicular cancer, which is most common solid tumor in 15–35-year-old males
   a. 95% of testicular cancers are germ cell tumors, with seminomas most common type
   b. Other testicular tumors include embryonal cell carcinoma, choriocarcinoma, Sertoli cell tumor, and Leydig cell tumor
4. Etiology of common disorders
   a. **Testicular torsion**: twisting of spermatic cord leading to obstruction of blood flow, ischemia of testis
   b. **Epididymitis**: inflammation of epididymis, usually due to STI ascending from urethra (most commonly *N. gonorrhoeae* and *C. trachomatis*)
   c. **Hydrocele**: fluid collection in tunica vaginalis surrounding testis

BOX 13-6

Painful and Nonpainful Causes of Scrotal Mass

Painful	Nonpainful
Testicular torsion	Hydrocele
Torsion of appendix testis	Spermatocele
Epididymitis	Varicocele
Orchitis	Testicular tumor
Hematoma (trauma)	Hernia (nonincarcerated)
Incarcerated hernia	

FIGURE 13-2 **Scrotal masses. A. Normal testis. B. Hydrocele. C. Spermatocele. D. Varicocele.**

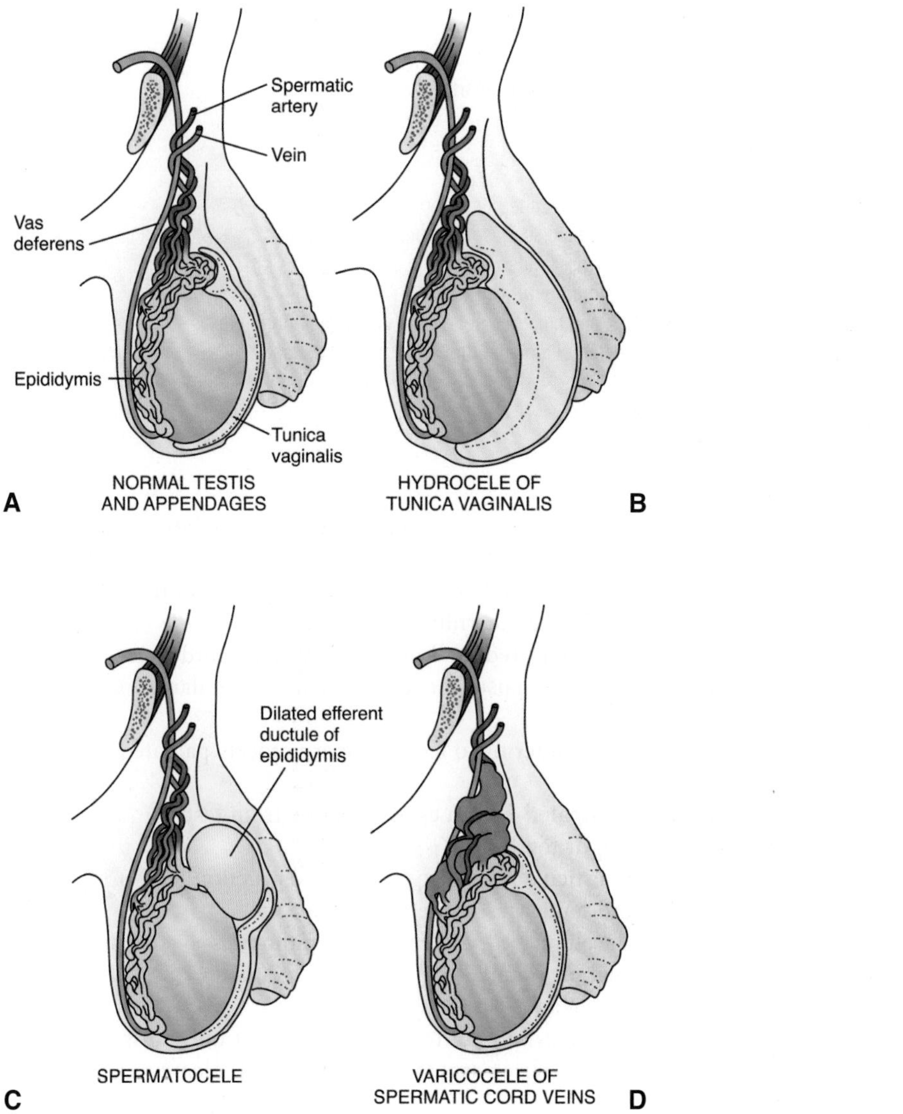

(From Rubin R, Strayer DS. *Rubin's Pathology: Clinicopathologic Foundations of Medicine*. 5th ed. Philadelphia: Lippincott Williams & Wilkins; 2008.)

QUICK HIT

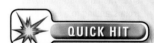

Varicoceles are usually seen on the left side due to higher pressures resulting from venous drainage into the left renal vein (versus the inferior vena cava on the right side).

QUICK HIT

Adolescents presenting with lower abdominal pain should *always* have a testicular exam, even if there are no scrotal complaints.

QUICK HIT

Urethritis is often asymptomatic prior to ascending to the epididymis, so absence of urethral symptoms does not rule out an STI.

d. **Spermatocele**: retention cyst filled with sperm located in epididymis
e. **Varicocele**: dilatation of veins in pampiniform plexus
  i. Pressure in left testicular vein > right testicular vein
  ii. Higher pressure coupled with incompetent venous valves leads to pooling of blood in plexus

B. Clinical features
  1. History
    a. Begin by establishing if painful or painless
      i. Determine onset, severity, location of pain
      ii. Scrotal pain may be referred pain to lower abdomen, lower back
    b. Trauma
    c. Sexual activity; STIs
    d. Urethral symptoms consistent with infection (e.g., discharge, burning)
    e. Mumps: can cause orchitis
    f. Undescended testis or malignancies
    g. Associated symptoms (e.g., fever, nausea/vomiting)

BOX 13-7

Components of Male Genital Exam

Examine pubic hair for Tanner stage
Examine surrounding skin for lesions (e.g., folliculitis, warts, ulcers)
Palpate for inguinal lymphadenopathy
Examine penis and scrotal skin for lesions, rash
Try to express any urethral discharge
Assess testicular volume for Tanner stage (may need orchidometer)
Check testes for masses or areas of induration, suggesting cancer
Palpate other scrotal structures for masses or tenderness
  Epididymis should be palpable on posterolateral wall
  Spermatic cord contains vas deferens and blood vessels, including pampiniform plexus
Check for presence of hernia: palpate external inguinal ring, have patient cough

QUICK HIT

Testicular cancer may present as a painless enlarged testicle rather than a palpable discrete mass.

QUICK HIT

Varicocele is often described as a "bag of worms" when palpating dilated, tortuous vessels in the pampiniform plexus.

QUICK HIT

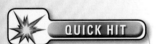

A varicocele will decrease in size when the patient moves from standing to a supine position.

QUICK HIT

An absent cremasteric reflex suggests testicular torsion when evaluating a painful scrotal mass.

QUICK HIT

Relief of pain with elevation of the scrotum is called the **Prehn sign** and supports the diagnosis of epididymitis.

QUICK HIT

Parotid gland enlargement in an unvaccinated male with testicular pain suggests mumps orchitis.

2. Physical exam
   a. Male genitourinary exam is not just examination of testis but should include all scrotal structures (Box 13-7)
   b. If mass is present, does it arise from testicle or from surrounding structures?
      i. Mass within testicle is concerning for cancer
      ii. Torsion may be appreciated as "knot" in spermatic cord
      iii. Mass palpated above or posterior to testicle may be enlarged inflamed epididymis
      iv. Hydrocele palpated anterior to testicle; spermatocele palpated within epididymis
      v. Varicoceles are palpated within cord, separate from testis
   c. Localize any swelling or tenderness
      i. Torsion leads to testicular swelling (venous obstruction leads to engorgement) and tenderness (due to ischemia)
      ii. STI will lead to swelling and tenderness of epididymis; testis usually not affected, so normal on exam
   d. Note position of testicle and epididymis
      i. Torsion will lead to elevation of testicle and bring it into horizontal lie
      ii. Epididymis not on posterior aspect of testicle may indicate twisted testicle
   e. Examine patient standing and then lying down; note changes in exam
   f. Assess cremasteric reflex
      i. Normal reflex: elevation of testis after stroking ipsilateral inner thigh
      ii. Should be normal in most cases except testicular torsion
      iii. Twisting of cord interferes with contraction of cremaster muscle along spermatic cord
   g. Transillumination of scrotum helps distinguish solid from fluid-filled mass
      i. Hold light against scrotum to see if light shines through or if blocked by mass
      ii. Illumination of mass indicates cystic structure such as hydrocele or spermatocele
      iii. Mass that does not illuminate should be further evaluated for malignancy

C. Diagnosis
1. Torsion is time-sensitive surgical emergency, so differentiate from other painful disorders as quickly as possible (Table 13-13)
2. Lab studies
   a. Suspect epididymitis if testing is consistent with urethritis (see XIII. Urethritis)
   b. NAATs to look specifically for chlamydia and gonorrhea infections
   c. If suspect cancer, check blood for tumor markers: α-fetoprotein, human chorionic gonadotropin (hCG), and lactate dehydrogenase

TABLE 13-13 **Clinical Presentation of Torsion Versus Epididymitis**

Symptoms/Exam Findings	Torsion	Epididymitis
Pain	Severe Acute onset May radiate to abdomen	Severe Gradual onset May radiate to abdomen
Fever	No	Maybe
Urethral symptoms	No	May have discharge or dysuria
Nausea/vomiting	More common	Less common
Testis position	Horizontal lie, elevated	Normal
Cremasteric reflex	Absent	Present
Swelling	Testicle may be engorged	Inflamed epididymis
Tenderness	Testis will be tender	Localized to epididymis

3. Radiologic studies
   a. Can visualize structures such as tumors, hydroceles, and dilation of pampiniform plexus vessels
   b. Doppler ultrasound can assess blood flow
      i. Decreased blood flow seen with torsion
      ii. Epididymitis is inflammatory process, so blood flow may be increased (or normal)
4. Biopsy testicular mass to confirm diagnosis of cancer

D. Treatment
1. Torsion requires surgery to untwist testicle; remove testicle if no longer viable
2. If asymptomatic, no intervention needed for hydrocele, spermatocele, or varicocele
3. Testicular cancer should be referred to oncology for further management

XII. Gynecomastia

A. Definition
1. Proliferation of glandular breast tissue in males (1 or both sides)
2. Enlargement may be localized beneath areola or extend beyond

B. Cause/pathophysiology
1. Relative excess of estrogen compared to androgens stimulates breast tissue
2. Pubertal gynecomastia is most common
   a. Transient imbalance between estrogen and testosterone occurs frequently in early puberty
   b. Spontaneous regression is seen once androgen levels rise high enough to counter stimulatory effects of estrogen
3. Pathologic causes
   a. Drug induced (e.g., anabolic steroids, antipsychotics, spironolactone, marijuana, ketoconazole)
   b. Tumors (e.g., testicular, adrenal)
   c. Endocrine causes (e.g., hyperthyroidism, primary hypogonadism such as Klinefelter syndrome)
   d. Organ dysfunction (e.g., cirrhosis, renal insufficiency)

C. Clinical presentation
1. Historical points
   a. Pubertal gynecomastia may be painful or tender
   b. Nipple discharge: suggests pathologic cause
   c. Progression of breast development
   d. Drug use
   e. Abnormalities on testicular self-exam

QUICK HIT

Ultrasound poses no radiation risk to the patient and is the best way to differentiate masses palpated in the scrotum.

QUICK HIT

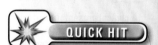

Antibiotic treatment for epididymitis is ceftriaxone (250 mg intramuscularly [IM] × 1 dose) and doxycycline (100 mg PO twice daily × 10 days).

QUICK HIT

A right-sided varicocele should prompt evaluation for a pathologic obstruction to venous flow (e.g., abdominal mass, blood clot).

QUICK HIT

At least 2/3 of males experience pubertal gynecomastia, with peak prevalence at age 14 years.

QUICK HIT

Rapid progression of breast tissue is *not* typical of physiologic gynecomastia.

QUICK HIT

Marijuana can cause gynecomastia.

2. Physical examination
   a. Firm, rubbery, mobile mass of breast tissue, often beneath areola
   b. Check for galactorrhea: suggests high prolactin, drug use
   c. Examine testes for masses; assess Tanner stage
   d. Look for signs of thyroid, liver, or renal disease

D. Testing
   1. Pubertal gynecomastia does not require any lab or radiographic evaluation
   2. Initiate workup if duration >2 years, if puberty is complete, or if abnormal findings on physical exam
   3. Consider thyroid function studies, testosterone, estradiol, LH, liver function tests (LFTs)

E. Therapy
   1. Provide reassurance for pubertal gynecomastia; reinforce transient nature
   2. Cease any contributing medications
   3. Limited data exist to support use of pharmacologic therapy
   4. Surgical intervention can be recommended if no regression and adolescent suffers significant psychological sequelae

QUICK HIT

Suspect gynecomastia if glandular tissue is >0.5 cm in diameter.

QUICK HIT

An elevated serum hCG in a male with gynecomastia indicates the presence of a germ cell tumor and necessitates an ultrasound of testes.

XIII. Urethritis

A. Definition: inflammation of urethra

B. Cause/pathophysiology
   1. Urethritis in sexually active adolescent males is usually due to STI, especially *C. trachomatis* and *N. gonorrhoeae*
      a. Other causes of urethritis
         i. *C. trachomatis*
         ii. *T. vaginalis*
         iii. *Mycoplasma* spp. (*M. hominis*, *M. genitalium*)
         iv. *Ureaplasma urealyticum*
         v. Herpes simplex virus (HSV)
   2. Infection of epithelial cells lining urethra leads to inflammation
   3. Transmission is through unprotected sexual contact

QUICK HIT

A clinical presentation of tall stature, gynecomastia, small firm testes, and elevated LH suggests Klinefelter syndrome. A karyotype should be obtained to look for XXY.

QUICK HIT

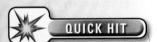

Spontaneous regression of breast tissue occurs within 6 months to 2 years for >90% of males with pubertal gynecomastia.

C. Clinical presentation
   1. Symptoms
      a. No symptoms present in most cases
      b. Symptoms may include dysuria, urinary frequency, urethral discharge, pruritus at urethral meatus, and (rarely) hematuria
   2. Signs
      a. Physical exam is often unremarkable
      b. Check for urethral discharge, inguinal lymphadenopathy
      c. Examine for skin lesions in genital area that may be indicative of other STIs (e.g., genital warts or herpes)

QUICK HIT

Clinical manifestations are absent in >90% of chlamydia and >60% of gonorrhea infections in males.

D. Testing
   1. Diagnosis suggested by any of following
      a. Positive leukocyte esterase on urine dip
      b. Microscopy of urethral swab: >10 WBCs per HPF
      c. Gram-negative intracellular diplococci on Gram stain of urethral discharge (90%–95% sensitivity for *N. gonorrhoeae* in males)
   2. NAAT to look specifically for chlamydia and gonorrhea infections

QUICK HIT

Organisms causing urethritis can ascend to the upper reproductive tract, causing epididymitis, so remember to ask about scrotal pain and examine for an enlarged, tender epididymis.

E. Therapy
   1. Treatment with antibiotics helps prevent complications (e.g., epididymitis) and reduce transmission to sexual contacts
      a. *N. gonorrhoeae*: ceftriaxone (intramuscular [IM]) or cefixime (PO) × 1 dose
      b. *C. trachomatis*, *Mycoplasma* spp., or *Ureaplasma* spp.: azithromycin (PO) × 1 dose or doxycycline (PO) × 7 days
      c. *T. vaginalis*: metronidazole (PO) × 1 dose
   2. Single-dose therapy is preferable to improve compliance with regimen
   3. Patient should notify sexual partner, encourage partner to seek treatment

4. Abstain from sex for 7–14 days after treatment and until symptoms have resolved; encourage use of barrier contraception

XIV. Genital Herpes

A. Definition
1. Recurrent viral disease leading to vesicular and ulcerative skin eruptions
2. Caused by HSV in sexually active adolescents
   a. HSV has 2 serotypes, HSV-1 and HSV-2
   b. Genital infections most commonly caused by HSV-2
   c. HSV-1 typically associated with oral ulcers (gingivostomatitis) but can cause genital lesions as well

B. Cause/pathophysiology
1. Viral shedding leads to transmission through sexual contact (genital–genital, oral–genital, anal–genital)
2. Virus replicates in epidermal and dermal cells, then spreads to sensory nerves where it remains latent after primary infection
3. Reactivation leads to asymptomatic viral shedding or recurrence of symptoms

C. Clinical presentation
1. Primary (initial) infection
   a. Vesicles on erythematous bases rupture to form painful ulcers
      i. Multiple lesions involve vulva, perineum, vagina, cervix, and penis
      ii. Episode resolves with crusting of vesicles and healing of ulcers
   b. May also see dysuria, vaginal or urethral discharge
   c. Duration of symptoms may be up to 3 weeks
   d. Constitutional symptoms occur in >50% of primary infections (e.g., fever, malaise, myalgias, headaches)
2. Recurrent infection occurs with periodic reactivation of virus
   a. Similar lesions as primary infection but usually smaller in number
   b. Prodrome of pain may precede eruption
   c. Duration of symptoms (1 week) is shorter than primary infection
   d. Constitutional symptoms are uncommon

D. Testing
1. Viral culture obtained from active lesion using culture transport swab, which has lower sensitivity but can increase yield by culturing punctured vesicles and wet ulcers rather than dry erosions or crusted lesions
2. Polymerase chain reaction (PCR) is preferred diagnostic method
   a. Higher sensitivity
   b. Detects presence of HSV DNA on swab from genital lesions
3. **Tzanck smear** shows multinucleated giant cells (rarely used because PCR is widely available and more sensitive and specific)
4. Type-specific antibody serologic tests may be helpful to identify infected partners but are not routinely used for screening in the general population

E. Therapy
1. Oral antiviral medications include acyclovir, famciclovir, and valacyclovir
   a. Decrease duration of symptoms and appearance of new lesions
   b. Shorten duration of viral shedding and, thus, transmission risk
   c. Do not eradicate latent virus
   d. Does not affect risk of future recurrences
2. Daily suppressive therapy used for frequent outbreaks (>6 per year)

XV. Syphilis

A. General characteristics
1. STI that leads to systemic disease
2. More prevalent in males than females, with highest rates in men who have sex with men
3. Caused by *Treponema pallidum*, a motile spirochete
4. Risk factors
   a. High-risk sexual behavior (e.g., multiple sex partners, unprotected sex)
   b. High rates seen in large urban areas and in southeastern U.S.

QUICK HIT

NAATs detect and amplify organism-specific DNA or RNA from *N. gonorrhoeae* and *C. trachomatis*, have high sensitivity and specificity, and can be performed on first-void urine specimens.

QUICK HIT

Multidrug-resistant gonorrhea is now reported around the globe. Know the resistance pattern of gonorrhea where you work.

QUICK HIT

Reinfection with STIs is common in adolescents.

QUICK HIT

Viral shedding of HSV can occur even in the absence of any genital lesions or other symptoms.

QUICK HIT

1 in 6 Americans have genital herpes, and most do not know they have it and are asymptomatic.

QUICK HIT

Latent HSV can be reactivated due to various stimuli including stress, fever, trauma, sunlight, and menstruation.

QUICK HIT

Epstein-Barr virus (EBV) can cause diffuse, painful vaginal ulcers in adolescent girls, which can mimic primary genital HSV.

5. Pathophysiology
   a. Transmitted through direct sexual contact with ulcerative lesions
   b. Spreads via lymph and blood vessels throughout body
   c. Also transmitted transplacentally from mother to fetus

B. Clinical features
1. Syphilis is classified in 4 stages: primary, secondary, latent, and tertiary
2. Primary syphilis
   a. Characterized by **chancre** at point of inoculation (external genitalia)
      i. Occurs 3–9 weeks after incubation
      ii. Often not recognized by patient due to asymptomatic nature
      iii. Heals spontaneously in 1–6 weeks
   b. Inguinal lymphadenopathy may be present
3. Secondary syphilis
   a. Occurs 4–10 weeks after chancre appears
   b. Characterized by rash, mucocutaneous lesions, and lymphadenopathy
   c. Condylomata lata are highly infectious hypertrophic wart-like papules seen in warm, moist areas such as vulva and anus
   d. Nonspecific findings include generalized lymphadenopathy, flu-like symptoms (sore throat, malaise, arthralgias)
4. Latent syphilis = asymptomatic phase that may last years
5. Tertiary syphilis
   a. Develops in 30% of untreated patients; usually 2–20 years later
   b. Characterized by gumma formation, cardiovascular involvement
      i. **Gummas**: granulomatous lesions with centralized tissue necrosis and rubbery texture; occur in skin, bone, or viscera
      ii. Cardiovascular involvement: aortic aneurysm
6. Neurosyphilis
   a. *T. pallidum* invades central nervous system (CNS)
   b. Can occur at any stage
   c. Findings include
      i. Acute syphilitic meningitis, often with cranial nerve palsies
      ii. Meningovascular syphilis (damage to blood vessels of meninges, brain, and spinal cord, leading to infarctions)
      iii. **Tabes dorsalis** (damage to posterior columns of spinal cord leading to impaired vibration and proprioceptive sensation, wide-based gait)

C. Diagnosis
1. Differential diagnosis
   a. Consider other causes of genital ulcers (Table 13-14)
   b. Differential diagnosis is broad for generalized rash of secondary syphilis; narrow list to disorders presenting with rash on palms/soles (Box 13-8)
2. Dark-field microscopy
   a. Examination of sample from chancre or moist lesions
   b. Can visualize corkscrew-shaped *T. pallidum*
   c. Low sensitivity; rarely used
3. Serologic tests
   a. Nontreponemal serologic tests (rapid plasma reagin [RPR], Venereal Disease Research Laboratory [VDRL] test)
      i. Quantitative tests for nonspecific anticardiolipin antibody formed in response to surface of *T. pallidum*
      ii. Used as screening test due to **high sensitivity**
      iii. Nonspecific, seen in other disease states
      iv. Titers correlate with disease activity so can follow disease progression and resolution
   b. Treponemal serologic tests (fluorescent treponemal antibody absorbed [FTA-ABS], *T. pallidum* particle agglutination [TP-PA])
      i. Measure antibody directed against specific *T. pallidum* antigens
      ii. **Highly specific tests used to confirm diagnosis following positive nontreponemal screening test**

> **QUICK HIT**
> Episodic treatment of recurrent herpes is most effective when therapy is started within 1 day of lesion onset or during the prodrome that precedes lesions.

> **QUICK HIT**
> Valacyclovir has better bioavailability than oral acyclovir but is more expensive, not covered by insurance, and is not Food and Drug Administration approved for children younger than age 2 years.

> **QUICK HIT**
> Primary syphilis presents as a nonpainful ulcer on the genitalia.

> **QUICK HIT**
> The syphilis rash is maculopapular, generalized, and may include palms and soles.

> **QUICK HIT**
> Generalized rash is the most common finding in secondary syphilis (90% of patients).

> **QUICK HIT**
> Tertiary syphilis is rarely seen in the U.S. due to widespread availability of antibiotics.

> **QUICK HIT**
> **Argyll-Robertson pupil**, seen in neurosyphilis, is a pupil that constricts during accommodation but does not react to light.

TABLE 13-14 **Differential Diagnosis of Infectious Genital Ulcers**

Disease	Painful?	Typical Lesion
Syphilis (primary)	No	Papule erodes to shallow ulcer Sharply demarcated Elevated margins Usually 1 lesion Heals in 2–3 weeks
Genital herpes (herpes simplex virus)	Yes	Vesicles on erythematous base Rupture to shallow ulcers "Punched out" border Multiple lesions Heals in 7–21 days
Chancroid	Yes	Deep ulcer Purulent base Erythematous borders 1 to few lesions Heals in 2–3 weeks
Lymphogranuloma venereum	Variable	Small nonindurated or herpetiform ulcer Often unnoticed by patient Heals within 1–2 weeks
Behçet disease	Yes	Accompanied by oral aphthous ulcers

iii. Qualitative tests; do not use to monitor disease progression or response to therapy
iv. False positives may occur with other spirochete infections (e.g., Lyme disease, leptospirosis)

4. Cerebrospinal fluid (CSF) analysis
   a. CSF VDRL test is highly specific but not sensitive
   b. CSF lymphocytic pleocytosis and elevated protein

D. Treatment
1. Penicillin is antibiotic of choice; doxycycline if allergic to penicillin
2. Dose and duration depend on stage of disease
3. Re-examine patient and repeat quantitative nontreponemal tests every 3 months
   a. Ensure titers are falling after treatment
   b. Expect 4-fold decrease in titers (e.g., 1:32 to 1:4) within 6 months in primary and secondary syphilis
4. Patients diagnosed with syphilis should be reported to public health authorities
5. Evaluate and treat sexual partners
6. Prognosis
   a. Depends on stage of disease
   b. Patients treated with primary or secondary syphilis have much better outcomes than patients with tertiary syphilis

BOX 13-8

Differential Diagnosis of Secondary Syphilis (Dermatologic Findings)

Diseases presenting with rash on palms and soles
- Syphilis (secondary)
- Enteroviral infections (e.g., coxsackievirus)
- Rocky Mountain spotted fever
- Drug eruption
- Erythema multiforme
- Psoriasis

Rash with no involvement of palms and soles
- Pityriasis rosea
- Tinea versicolor
- Systemic lupus erythematosus
- Scabies (adolescents and adults)
- Viral eruption
- Lichen planus (differential for condyloma lata)
- Condyloma acuminatum (differential for condyloma lata)

QUICK HIT

Syphilis is often called the "great imitator" because its clinical features are so diverse and can mimic other diseases.

QUICK HIT

Because of similarities in the rash, think about secondary syphilis in a sexually active adolescent with presumed pityriasis rosea and consider sending a rapid plasma reagin.

QUICK HIT

False elevation of RPR can be seen in EBV infections, pregnancy, systemic lupus erythematosus, endocarditis, and malaria.

QUICK HIT

The **Jarisch-Herxheimer reaction** (fever, chills, myalgias, nausea, vomiting) is a self-limited reaction to antitreponemal therapy that may occur 2–24 hours after therapy. It is *not* an allergic reaction to penicillin.

7. Prevention
   a. Educate patients on safer sexual practices and STIs
   b. Encourage consistent use of barrier methods during sexual activity

XVI. Depression and Suicide

A. General characteristics
1. Mood changes and emotional lability are common during adolescent years but do not necessarily fit clinical definition of depression
2. Definition: chronic and recurrent mood disorder characterized by reduced functioning in more than 1 major area of life, such as academics or familial or peer relationships
   a. Criteria for depression are detailed in *Diagnostic and Statistical Manual of Mental Disorders*, 4th Edition (*DSM-IV-TR*)
   b. **Major depressive episode**: presence of 5 or more symptoms listed in Table 13-15 during same 2-week period, representing change from previous functioning
   c. **Major depressive disorder**: 2 or more major depressive episodes
3. Epidemiology
   a. Prevalence: 1% of children and 8%–10% of adolescents
   b. Female-to-male ratio of depression is 1:1 prior to puberty but increases to 2:1 in adolescence
4. Cause
   a. Most likely caused by low brain levels of monoamines (e.g., serotonin)
   b. Complex interplay of genetic and environmental factors
5. Risk factors
   a. Parental or family history of depression, substance abuse, or suicidality
   b. Chronic illness (e.g., diabetes, asthma, IBD)
   c. Poor relationship with parents (e.g., emotionally unavailable parent)
   d. Rejection or victimization by peers (e.g., bullying)
   e. Child abuse and neglect
   f. Negative life events (e.g., death of close friend, parental divorce)
6. Comorbid mental health disorders are common: anxiety disorder, attention-deficit hyperactivity disorder (ADHD), substance abuse, eating disorders

B. Clinical features
1. Historical findings
   a. SIGECAPS (see Table 13-15)
   b. Adolescents are more likely than adults to manifest depression with irritability rather than sadness (e.g., irritability, frustration, anger)

QUICK HIT

Females are twice as likely as males to suffer from depression during adolescence.

QUICK HIT

Having a family member with depression increases a child's risk by 2–4×.

MNEMONIC

Use SIGECAPS to identify symptoms of depression:
Sleep disturbances
Interest (loss of) or anhedonia
Guilt or negative feelings about self
Energy (loss of)
Concentration/cognition (loss of)
Appetite changes
Psychomotor agitation or retardation
Suicidality

TABLE 13-15 **SIGECAPS Mnemonic for Symptoms of Depression**

	Symptom	Example
S	**Sleep** disturbances (i.e., too much or too little)	Sleeps for 12 hours now but previous norm was 8 hours
I	Loss of **Interest** or anhedonia	Quit sports teams, no longer wants to spend time with friends
G	**Guilt** or negative feelings about self	Verbal self-reproach
E	Loss of **Energy**	Feels fatigued or tired most of the time
C	Loss of **Concentration/Cognition**	School grades drop
A	**Appetite** changes	Weight loss or gain, change noted in clothing size
P	**Psychomotor** agitation or retardation	Agitated, pacing, more fretful, hair pulling, slowed speech, more sighs and pauses
S	**Suicidality**	Preoccupation with death, thoughts of death and dying

2. Physical findings
   a. Physical exam may be unremarkable
   b. Changes in weight from previous visit may be noted
   c. Look for signs of self-injurious behavior (e.g., cutting marks on wrists, rope burns on neck)

C. Diagnosis
1. Depression is clinical diagnosis made using *DSM-IV-TR* criteria
2. Differential diagnosis
   a. Differentiate depression from other mood disorders or other psychiatric diagnoses with depressive features (e.g., bipolar disorder, substance abuse)
   b. Rule out nonpsychiatric medical conditions
      i. Hypothyroidism
      ii. Anemia/nutritional deficiencies
      iii. Obstructive sleep apnea
      iv. CNS lesion (e.g., tumor, stroke)
3. Laboratory findings
   a. Lab tests do not diagnose depression but can help rule out other medical problems
   b. Evaluation should be guided by history and physical findings suggestive of particular medical conditions in the differential diagnosis (e.g., thyroid function tests, CBC, ESR, urinalysis)

D. Treatment
1. Psychotherapy
   a. Cognitive-behavioral therapy most effective form
   b. Interpersonal therapy
2. Medications
   a. Selective serotonin reuptake inhibitors (SSRIs): most effective class in adolescents
   b. Other antidepressants can be used to increase availability of monoamines (e.g., bupropion, venlafaxine, nefazodone), but SSRIs are preferred based on efficacy, side effects, and lower risks in overdose
   c. Tricyclic antidepressants: high risk of cardiotoxic side effects, including dysrhythmias in high doses and, thus, are used less often in adolescents
3. Manage comorbidities, such as substance use disorders, eating disorders, anxiety

E. Suicide
1. Suicide is 3rd leading cause of death in adolescents
2. **Females *attempt* suicide 2–4× more than males**; males *complete* suicide 3–4× more than females
3. Risk factors
   a. Previous suicide attempt (20%–50% of attempters will try again)
   b. Mood disorders
   c. Substance abuse
   d. Family history of mental illness or suicide
   e. History of sexual or physical abuse
4. Assessment for suicidality
   a. Ask about suicidal ideation, specific plans, previous attempts
   b. Ask about access (e.g., in home) to firearms and other lethal agents

XVII. Substance Abuse

A. General characteristics
1. Definitions
   a. **Substance abuse**: drug use leading to physical, psychological, financial, legal, or social distress
   b. **Substance dependence**: substance abuse accompanied by tolerance, withdrawal, unsuccessful efforts to stop, or continued abuse despite awareness of having persistent problems related to use

QUICK HIT

Several validated screening tools are available for depression in adolescents including the Beck Depression Inventory, the Mood and Feelings Questionnaire, and the Kutcher Adolescent Depression Scale.

QUICK HIT

Depression in teens is commonly unrecognized compared to adults due to differences in adolescent presentation (e.g., irritability > sadness) and reluctance to disclose depressive symptoms.

QUICK HIT

Dual treatment with medications (SSRIs) and cognitive-behavioral therapy is the most efficacious method for treating major depression.

QUICK HIT

Females are most likely to attempt suicide through ingestions, whereas males are more likely to use firearms or hanging in their attempts, which accounts for the discrepancy in completion between sexes.

QUICK HIT

Self-mutilating behaviors such as cutting may be coping mechanisms to deal with emotional stress rather than actual suicide attempts.

QUICK HIT

Suicidality is a reason to break patient confidentiality with an adolescent. Be sure patients understand the limits of confidentiality.

QUICK HIT

Drug use is frequently linked with other risk behaviors (e.g., unsafe sex, violence).

2. Epidemiology
   a. Alcohol, tobacco, and marijuana are most commonly used substances
   b. 1/3 of all 10th graders report use of illicit drug in past year
   c. Comorbid mental health conditions are common
3. Drug abuse stems from genetic, neurobiologic, and social factors
   a. Increased concordance seen with monozygotic twins compared to dizygotic twins
   b. Increased dopamine levels and stimulation of limbic system
4. Adolescent development and drug use
   a. Failure to recognize long-term consequences
   b. Primacy of peer influence, need for acceptance
   c. Struggle for autonomy leads to challenge of parental authority
   d. Underrecognition of depression, other mental health problems
   e. Experimentation and risk-taking behaviors common
5. Risk factors
   a. Parents or peers using drugs
   b. Poor parental supervision
   c. Decreased impulse control
   d. Early age of 1st exposure or intoxication
   e. Mood or anxiety disorders
   f. Conduct disorder or antisocial behaviors

QUICK HIT

When engaging an adolescent patient in a conversation about drug use, do *not* discuss your personal history, regardless of what it is; instead, redirect the conversation back to the patient (e.g., "We're here to talk about you and how I can be helpful to you").

B. Clinical features
   1. Historical findings
      a. Interview adolescent alone and ensure confidentiality
      b. Symptoms will vary, depending on substance used (Table 13-16)
      c. Ask about weight loss, mood swings, and problems with sleep
      d. Ask about drops in academic performance, school truancy, or suspensions
      e. Use CRAFFT Screening Tool to screen for adolescent substance use disorders (Box 13-9)
   2. Physical exam
      a. Findings will vary, depending on substance used (see Table 13-16)
      b. Most illicit drugs will lead to changes in vital signs

TABLE 13-16 **Common Drugs of Abuse in Adolescents**

Drug	Route of Administration	Clinical Features
Alcohol	Oral	Disinhibition, slurred speech, ataxia, emotional lability, "blackouts"
Marijuana	Smoked	Euphoria, red conjunctivae, dry mouth and throat, increased appetite, impaired reaction time, gynecomastia with chronic use
Stimulants (e.g., cocaine, amphetamines)	Oral Snorted Smoked Intravenous	Hyperalertness, restlessness, agitation, aggression, paranoia or suspicious state, tachycardia, hypertension, arrhythmias, dilated pupils, seizures
Opioids (e.g., heroin)	Oral Intravenous	Drowsiness, euphoria, flushing, floating feeling, constipation, miosis (pinpoint pupils), respiratory depression, hypotension
Hallucinogens (e.g., LSD, PCP)	Oral Smoked Snorted	Dizziness, heightened sensual awareness, nausea, hallucinations, nausea, flushing, elevated temperature, tachycardia, dilated pupils
Inhalants (e.g., organic solvents, gasoline, glue, spray paints)	Directly inhaled or inhaled from bag ("huffing")	Dizziness, headaches, slurred speech, sleepiness, lacrimation, rhinorrhea, mucous membrane irritation, ataxia, impaired memory

LSD, lysergic acid diethylamide; PCP, phencyclidine.

BOX 13-9

CRAFFT Screening Tool

- C—Have you ever ridden in a CAR driven by someone (including yourself) who was "high" or had been using alcohol or drugs?
- R—Do you ever use alcohol or drugs to RELAX, feel better about yourself, or fit in?
- A—Do you ever use alcohol or drugs while you are by yourself (ALONE)?
- F—Do you ever FORGET things you did while using alcohol or drugs?
- F—Do your family or FRIENDS ever tell you that you should cut down on your drinking or drug use?
- T—Have you gotten into TROUBLE while you were using alcohol or drugs?

NOTE: Two or more "yes" answers suggest high risk for adolescent substance abuse and require further assessment.

c. Assessment of eyes and pupils can suggest intoxication for certain drugs
   i. **Miosis** (pinpoint pupils): opiates
   ii. **Mydriasis** (enlarged pupils): stimulants
   iii. **Sluggish pupillary response**: barbiturates
   iv. **Rotary nystagmus**: phencyclidine (PCP)
d. Examine skin for track marks, cellulitis, abscesses, phlebitis
e. Examine nose for rhinitis, nasal septum damage, or perforation
f. Chronic cognitive changes or acute distortions in perceived reality may be seen on mental status exam

QUICK HIT

Patients on PCP or "bath salts" may present with excited hallucinatory delirium.

C. Diagnosis
1. See Table 13-16 for common drugs of abuse
2. Screen for other mental health problems (e.g., mood disorders, anxiety disorders, schizophrenia)
3. Laboratory findings
   a. Drug testing can be done on urine and/or blood
   b. Office-based routine urine drug screening of adolescents without suggestive history or physical is not recommended
      i. Tests are subject to limitations of lab, variable persistence in body after use
      ii. Failure to detect drug on spot test does not rule out substance use
      iii. Positive screen does not rule in habitual drug user
      iv. False positives seen with certain cough and cold medications
   c. Drug testing most helpful in following situations
      i. Assessment of medically or psychologically compromised teen suspected of drug use
      ii. Evaluation in the emergency department of patient with acute injuries possibly secondary to drug use
      iii. Monitoring abstinence in patient undergoing drug rehabilitation or in treatment program

QUICK HIT

Younger adolescents are more likely to abuse inhalants than illicit drugs due to widespread availability of substances such as organic solvents, gasoline, and paint thinners.

D. Treatment
1. Acute management of drug overdose
   a. Evaluate and manage airway, breathing, and circulation (ABCs) to ensure respiratory and hemodynamic stability
   b. Manage hypo- or hyperthermia
   c. GI decontamination (e.g., activated charcoal) if oral ingestion
   d. Naloxone for opioid overdose
   e. Pharmacologic management of aggressive or uncontrolled behavior (e.g., Benadryl, lorazepam, or Haldol)
2. Outpatient management
   a. Occasional recreational drug use may be addressed in primary care setting with counseling, setting quit dates, frequent follow-up appointments
   b. Outpatient psychological interventions
      i. Individual and/or group therapy
      ii. Family counseling

QUICK HIT

Ketamine, ecstasy, dextromethorphan, and inhalants are commonly used recreational drugs that will not show up in a routine drug screen.

iii. Structured day programs
iv. Short-term and long-term residential therapy
c. Indications for inpatient treatment
i. Detoxification
ii. Failure of sufficiently intensive outpatient therapy
iii. Danger to self or others
iv. Severe medical or psychiatric comorbidity
3. Complications
a. Drug overdose can lead to serious morbidity and mortality
b. Intravenous drug abuse is risk for endocarditis, HIV, hepatitis
c. Addiction can lead to theft, prostitution, and other criminal acts to sustain drug habit
4. Prevention
a. Begin anticipatory guidance about substance use with preadolescent patients
b. Facilitate parental awareness and monitoring of adolescent's activities
c. Help patients recognize protective factors against drug use
i. Positive self-esteem
ii. Supportive family relationships
iii. Positive role models

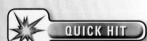

QUICK HIT
Many states allow minors to consent to their own drug and alcohol treatment without parental consent.

XVIII. Eating Disorders

A. General characteristics
1. 2 commonly described eating disorders include
a. Anorexia nervosa: prevalence ~0.5%
b. Bulimia nervosa: prevalence ~3%
2. Defined as group of conditions associated with
a. Abnormal eating habits
b. Insufficient or excessive food intake
c. Detrimental to patient's mental and physical health
3. Specific diagnostic criteria listed in *DSM-IV-TR* (Boxes 13-10 and 13-11)
a. Anorexia nervosa: characterized by intentional and extreme weight loss through restrictive eating
b. Bulimia nervosa: characterized by binge eating followed by compensatory purging or excessive exercise
4. Peak onset of symptoms and behaviors occur during puberty and late teen years
5. Etiology is multifactorial; following factors are interrelated
a. Sociocultural (media influence, cultural norms emphasizing thinness)
b. Biologic/genetic predisposition
c. Interpersonal relations with friends, family, and/or peers
d. Psychological factors (e.g., low self-esteem, perfectionism, impulsivity, obsessive-compulsive traits)

B. Clinical features
1. Historical findings
a. See Box 13-12 for questions to ask in history taking
b. Patients are often in denial, so obtain history from family members as well
c. Symptoms of inadequate caloric intake (i.e., anorexia nervosa) include amenorrhea, constipation, fainting or dizziness, cold intolerance, epigastric pain, difficulty concentrating

QUICK HIT
Purging behaviors include vomiting and laxative and diuretic use.

QUICK HIT
Girls are 2–2.5× more likely than boys to have an eating disorder.

QUICK HIT
Risk periods for developing eating disorders occur during transitions such as moving into high school or college.

QUICK HIT
Depression, anxiety, and obsessive-compulsive disorders are observed in >50% of patients with eating disorders.

BOX 13-10

DSM-IV-TR Diagnostic Criteria for Anorexia Nervosa

1. Refusal to maintain body weight at or above a minimally normal weight for age and height (<85% ideal body weight)
2. Intense fear of gaining weight
3. Disturbance in the perception of one's body weight or shape
4. Secondary amenorrhea

BOX 13-11

DSM-IV-TR Diagnostic Criteria for Bulimia Nervosa

1. Recurrent episodes of binge eating characterized by the following:
   a. Eating a larger amount of food than most people would eat
   b. A sense of lack of control over eating during the episode
2. Recurrent inappropriate compensatory behavior in order to prevent weight gain
3. Occurrence: twice a week for 3 months
4. Self-evaluation is unduly influenced by body shape or weight
5. The disturbance does not occur exclusively during episodes of anorexia nervosa

d. Bulimia nervosa symptoms can be minimal, may include bloating or abdominal fullness, lethargy, headaches, irregular menses
e. Psychological symptoms include anxiety, depression, guilt, low self-esteem, social withdrawal

2. Physical exam findings in anorexia nervosa
   a. Low BMI (often <18), cachectic appearance
   b. Hypothermia, orthostatic hypotension, bradycardia
   c. Dry skin, cold extremities, increased lanugo hair
3. Physical exam findings in bulimia nervosa
   a. Normal to increased weight
   b. Salivary gland enlargement (which correlates with elevated serum amylase concentration), dental erosion, and knuckle calluses due to self-induced vomiting

C. Diagnosis
1. Differential diagnosis
   a. Consider other causes of weight loss: hyperthyroidism, malignancy, tuberculosis, type 1 diabetes, IBD, malabsorption disorders
   b. Other causes of vomiting: GI obstruction or infection, increased intracranial pressure, pancreatitis, uremia, migraine, adrenal insufficiency
2. Laboratory findings
   a. CBC: look for anemia
   b. Serum electrolytes: may see hypokalemia with hypochloremic metabolic alkalosis with vomiting
   c. Check for disturbances in albumin, calcium, magnesium, phosphate, urinalysis, and ESR
   d. LH and FSH may be suppressed in anorexia nervosa (due to hypothalamic–pituitary dysregulation)
3. Radiology findings: DEXA scan may show decreased BMD
4. Other findings: electrocardiography can detect arrhythmias secondary to electrolytes abnormalities or decreased cardiac muscle mass

D. Treatment
1. Management of eating disorders is multifaceted and involves interdisciplinary teams (i.e., primary care physician, nutritionist, psychologist, psychiatrist)

BOX 13-12

Questions for History Taking

How do you feel about your weight?
How do you feel about your physical appearance?
Are you satisfied with your body image?
What are your eating patterns, and are you satisfied with them?
Do you ever eat in secret or eat large amounts of food in a short amount of time?
Do you feel guilty or depressed after eating?
Have you ever restricted your food intake?
Have you ever tried to lose weight? If so, how?
Have you ever tried to control your weight by vomiting, taking laxatives or diuretics, or excessively exercising?

QUICK HIT

Rigorous participation in sports increases risk of the female athlete triad: disordered eating, amenorrhea, and osteoporosis.

QUICK HIT

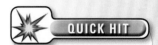

Patients with anorexia nervosa are underweight, whereas patients with bulimia nervosa are usually normal weight.

QUICK HIT

Close examination of knuckles and teeth is indicated in any patient in whom bulimia is suspected.

QUICK HIT

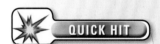

Eating disorders are diagnosed clinically, so lab studies are used to look for medical complications.

QUICK HIT

ESR should be normal in all patients with eating disorders, but an abnormal value raises suspicion for an organic pathology of weight loss.

QUICK HIT

Anorexia can lead to low estrogen levels, which will have negative consequences for bone health.

2. Treatment should focus on medical stabilization, nutritional rehabilitation, and behavioral intervention
   a. Repletion of nutritional stores
   b. Address medical complications such as hypovolemia, cardiac dysfunction, electrolyte abnormalities
   c. Psychotherapy (individual, family therapy), support groups
   d. Medications (e.g., SSRIs) can be used to treat comorbid psychiatric conditions and may have role in treating eating disorder
3. See Table 13-17 for a list of complications of eating disorders
4. Recovery rates are higher with bulimia nervosa than anorexia nervosa

TABLE 13-17 **Complications of Eating Disorders**

Related to Caloric Restriction and Weight Loss	Related to Vomiting	Related to Laxatives
Bradycardia or arrhythmias	Esophagitis	Hyperuricemia
Delayed gastric emptying	Mallory-Weiss tears	Hypocalcemia
Constipation	Gastroesophageal reflux	Fluid retention
Amenorrhea	Hypochloremic metabolic alkalosis	Hyperchloremic metabolic acidosis
Abnormal liver function	Dental erosions	
Hypercholesterolemia	Enlarged parotid glands	
Hypoglycemia		
Anemia, leukopenia, and thrombocytopenia		
Growth retardation		
Osteoporosis		

14 Diseases Unique to the Newborn

SYMPTOM SPECIFIC

I. Approach to Delivery Room

A. General characteristics
  1. >4 million infants born in U.S. every year
    a. 10% require some intervention at birth
    b. <1% require resuscitation
  2. American Academy of Pediatrics (AAP) and American Heart Association publish Neonatal Resuscitation Program guidelines
    a. Based on best available scientific recommendations
    b. Standard of care for neonatal resuscitation
  3. Normal physiology changes at birth
    a. Initial breath and cry leads to aeration and expansion of lungs
    b. Oxygenated alveoli cause pulmonary arteriole dilatation and decrease pulmonary vascular resistance
    c. Umbilical cord clamping and stimulation of sympathetic nervous system lead to increased systemic vascular resistance
    d. Pressure gradient leads to transition from fetal to adult circulation
    e. Ductus and foramen ovale close over minutes to hours after birth (Figure 14-1)
  4. Common abnormal physiology and risk factors leading to resuscitation
    a. Antepartum
      i. Multiple gestation
      ii. Maternal infection
      iii. Magnesium therapy (administered to halt preterm labor)
      iv. Maternal substance abuse
    b. Intrapartum
      i. Breech presentation
      ii. Chorioamnionitis
      iii. Meconium
      iv. Prolapsed cord
      v. Placental abruption or placenta previa

B. Preparation for resuscitation
  1. Communication between obstetricians and pediatricians is key
  2. Estimation of gestational age or weight allows preparation of endotracheal tube size, catheter sizes, and drug doses before delivery

C. Resuscitation
  1. All newborns should be assessed with following 3 questions
    a. Term gestation?
    b. Crying or breathing?
    c. Good muscle tone?
  2. Newborns who do not meet *all* of 3 should be transferred to radiant warmer and receive initial stabilization, including warmth, drying, tactile stimulation, airway suctioning (if required), and further evaluation

QUICK HIT

Hearing the infant cry during delivery is an excellent prognostic sign.

QUICK HIT

Delivery room resuscitation is focused on Ventilation! Ventilation! Ventilation! Most other problems stem from failure to adequately ventilate the newborn.

QUICK HIT

Term newborns are pink, breathing, and vigorous and do not need resuscitation. Dry the newborn, place skin-to-skin with mother, and cover with dry linen to maintain temperature.

MNEMONIC

Escalating resuscitation:
"**D**o **w**hat **p**ediatricians **s**ay **t**o, **o**r **b**e **i**nviting **c**ostly **m**alpractice!"
Drying
Warming
Positioning
Suctioning
Tactile stimulation
Oxygen
Bagging
Intubate
Chest compressions
Medications

FIGURE 14-1 Circulatory routes during gestation (A) and changes at birth (B).

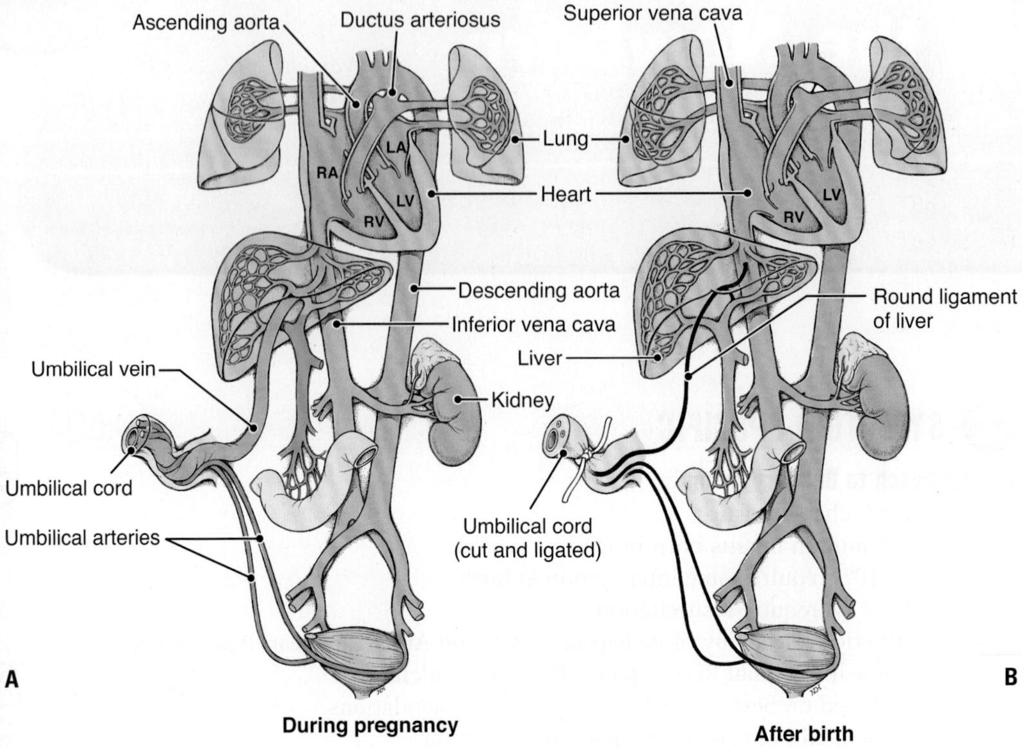

At birth, the connections between mother and fetus are severed, literally. The umbilical arteries and veins wither into ligamentous cords. By that time, the yolk sac has diminished to a trivial unit, and portions of the vitelline vessels transform into parts of other major vessels. The introduction of atmospheric oxygen to the newborn lung leads to mechanical closure of the foramen ovale and withering of the shunt between the pulmonary trunk and the aorta. LA, left atrium; LV, left ventricle; RA, right atrium; RV, right ventricle. (From Sadler TW. *Langman's Medical Embryology.* 10th ed. Baltimore: Lippincott Williams & Wilkins; 2006.)

3. Apgar scores
   a. Invented by Virginia Apgar
   b. Scores from 5 categories added up (10 is a perfect score)
   c. Measured at 1, 5, and 10 minutes
   d. Only 10-minute score is prognostically accurate
4. Ventilation
   a. Apnea or heart rate (HR) <100 beats per minute (bpm) beyond 30 seconds should prompt positive pressure ventilation with bag and mask ventilation
   b. HR <100 bpm requires ventilation initially, not chest compressions
5. Indication for endotracheal intubation
   a. Initial endotracheal tube suctioning of nonvigorous meconium-stained newborns
   b. If bag-mask ventilation is ineffective or prolonged duration
   c. When chest compressions are being performed
   d. Other circumstances: congenital diaphragmatic hernia or extremely low birth weight
6. Chest compressions
   a. Initiated if HR <60 bpm despite 30 seconds of adequate positive pressure ventilation
   b. Bag-mask ventilation provides positive pressure ventilation.
7. Oxygen therapy
   a. Blended oxygen to maintain saturation
   b. 100% oxygen reserved for bradycardia (<60 bpm) not responding to positive pressure ventilation
8. Medications (rarely required)
   a. Epinephrine and/or volume expansion considered when HR is persistently <60 bpm despite adequate ventilation and chest compressions

QUICK HIT

Note that Apgar scores are not used for resuscitation because resuscitation should be well under way before the 1-minute Apgar is assigned!

QUICK HIT

It is easiest to check the heart rate by holding the umbilicus.

b. Epinephrine: administered intravenously, via umbilical venous catheter or endotracheal tube
c. Volume expansion: for suspected blood loss
i. Isotonic crystalloid or blood recommended
ii. Higher volumes associated with intraventricular hemorrhage (IVH)
9. Continuous positive airway pressure (CPAP): used to support spontaneously breathing infants with respiratory distress
10. Temperature: steps to maintain
a. Prewarm radiant warmer; dry and wrap the baby with warm blankets
b. Additional steps for very-low-birth-weight babies include warming delivery room to 79°F, covering infant in plastic wrapping, using exothermic mattress, monitoring infant temperature in real-time with skin probes
D. Meconium-stained amniotic fluid
1. Meconium is extremely inflammatory to neonatal lung and can cause respiratory distress syndrome (RDS) and persistent pulmonary hypertension (PPHN)
2. Tracheal suctioning and meconium aspirator: beneficial, if meconium present in amniotic fluid and infant not vigorous at delivery
3. If infant is vigorous, suction mouth and nose only
E. Special scenarios: Table 14-1

QUICK HIT

Glucose, atropine, naloxone, and other therapies can have roles in postresuscitation care depending on the scenario.

QUICK HIT

In utero, an infant in distress will stool meconium; therefore, meconium may be a sign of other problems as well.

II. Approach to Newborn Examination

A. Historical findings
1. Family history: including genetic diseases, consanguinity, and health of siblings
2. Social history: maternal education, relationship with father, resources, and support at home
3. Mother's age, gravida, parity, and prior history of abortions (spontaneous and therapeutic)
4. Pregnancy history and complications
a. **Adequacy of prenatal care**
b. Maternal illness: hypertension, preeclampsia, eclampsia, diabetes, or other chronic diseases
c. **Maternal medications/drugs** used during pregnancy, including prescription, over-the-counter (OTC), or illicit drugs; tobacco; caffeine; alcohol
d. Number of fetuses
e. Prenatal ultrasound results
f. Results of prenatal genetic studies, if performed
g. **Results of syphilis**, **hepatitis**, and **HIV testing** during pregnancy and at delivery

TABLE 14-1 **Special Scenarios for Resuscitation**

Clinical Condition	Problem	Resuscitative Measures
Bilateral choanal atresia	• Obstruction of the nasal airway leads to obstructive apnea	Obtain a stable oral airway • Oral airway insertion • Endotracheal tube
Pierre-Robin sequence	• Small mandible • Posterior cleft palate • Obstruction due to posterior displacement of tongue	Open up airway and support • Prone positioning • Nasopharyngeal tube • Laryngeal mask airway insertion
Congenital diaphragmatic hernia	• Defective formation of diaphragm • Herniation of abdominal contents into chest with scaphoid abdomen	• Avoid bag-mask ventilation to prevent distension of stomach and intestines • Immediate endotracheal tube • Place large orogastric tube and suction stomach contents

QUICK HIT

Two doses of PCN administered more than 4 hours prior to delivery are needed for adequate protection against GBS in the infant.

QUICK HIT

Prolonged rupture of membranes (>18 hours) and maternal GBS status help identify risk of neonatal sepsis.

QUICK HIT

Pediatricians rely on weight of an infant to access nutrition, hydration, and growth.

QUICK HIT

The exam is not typically performed head to toe; if the infant is quiet, examine areas that require a calm infant first, such as heart sounds, prior to performing a complete physical exam.

h. **Results of group B *Streptococcus* (GBS) screening**
i. Gestational age and criteria for determination
   i. Last menstrual period most accurate
   ii. 1st-trimester ultrasound or early exam by obstetrician second most reliable

5. Labor and delivery history
   a. Medications during labor, including anesthesia, antibiotic, and opiates
   b. Indications for maternal GBS prophylaxis
      i. Preterm labor
      ii. GBS positive (any time in pregnancy)
      iii. GBS status unknown with membrane rupture >18 hours or maternal fever
   c. Duration of labor
   d. Time of rupture of membranes: prolonged (>18 hours) associated with increased risk for infection
   e. Meconium-stained fluid may be marker for stress, hypoxia
   f. Fetal HR tracing in labor may show evidence of fetal distress
6. Mode of delivery, fetal presentation, and forceps or vacuum use
7. Infant's **Apgar score** (Figure 14-2)
8. Resuscitation required by infant
   a. Most infants are vigorous at birth
   b. 10% require some type of assistance
9. Infant's birth weight
10. Mother's infant feeding preference: 1st breastfeed should occur within 1 hour of birth

B. Physical examination
   1. Vital signs and growth parameters
      a. HR: 90–160 bpm
      b. Respiratory rate (RR): 30–60/minute, infants exhibit periodic breathing, so RR should be counted for 1 entire minute to account for variation
      c. Blood pressure (BP): not typically measured, unless infant is ill
      d. Length, weight, and head circumference (HC) must be plotted for gestational age; HC is measured around largest possible fronto-occipital circumference (Figures 14-3 and 14-4)
   2. General appearance (Table 14-2)

FIGURE 14-2 **Apgar scoring data.**

Apgar Scoring Chart			
		Score	
Sign	0	1	2
Heart rate	Absent	Slow (<100)	>100
Respiratory effort	Absent	Slow, irreguar; weak cry	Good; strong cry
Muscle tone	Flaccid	Some flexion of extremities	Well flexed
Reflex irritability			
Response to catheter in nostril *or*	No response	Grimace	Cough or sneeze
Slap of sole of foot	No response	Grimace	Cry and withdrawal of foot
Color	Blue, pale	Body pink, extremities blue	Completely pink

FIGURE 14-3 **The Colorado curves give percentiles of intrauterine growth for weight, length, and head circumference.**

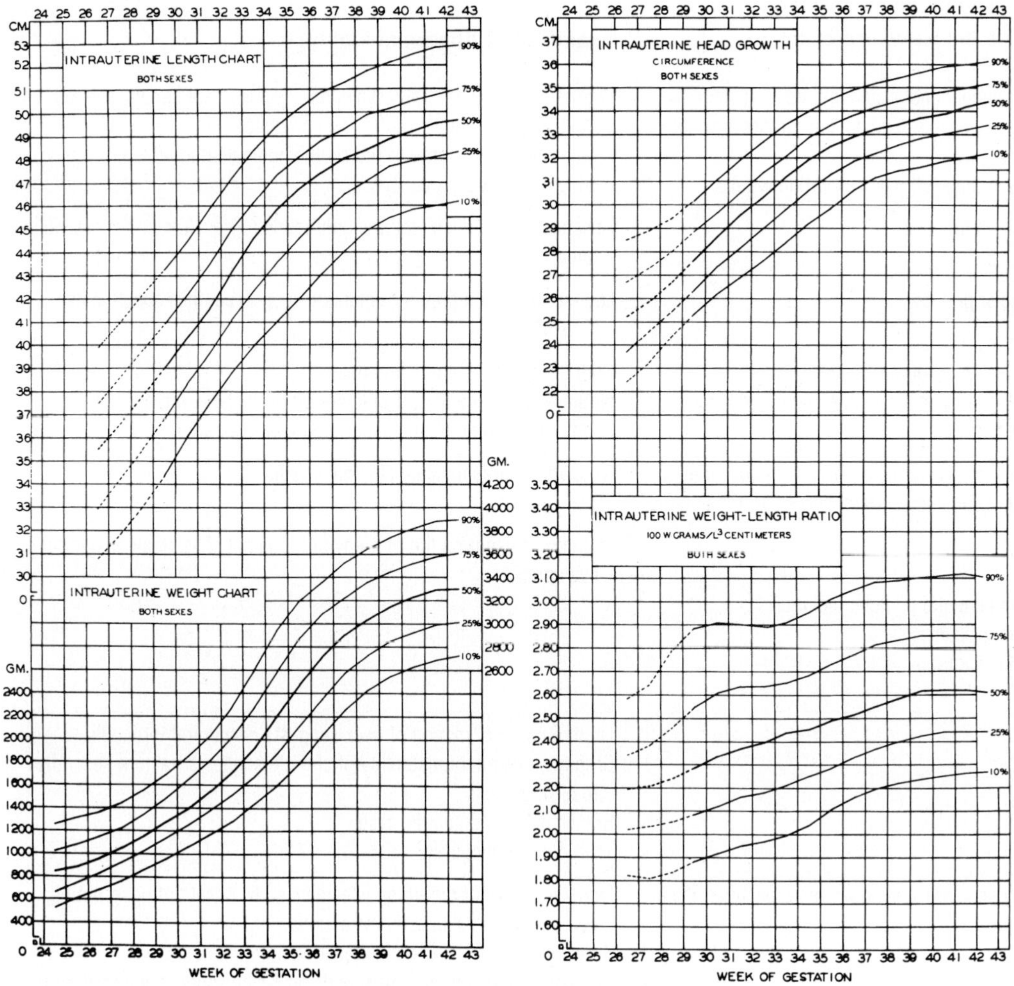

(From Lubchenco LO, Hansman C, Boyd E. Intrauterine growth in length and head circumference as estimated from live births at gestational ages from 26 to 42 weeks. *Pediatrics.* 1966;37:403. Copyright © American Academy of Pediatrics, 1966.)

FIGURE 14-4 **From left to right: Newborns are small, appropriate, and large for gestational age.**

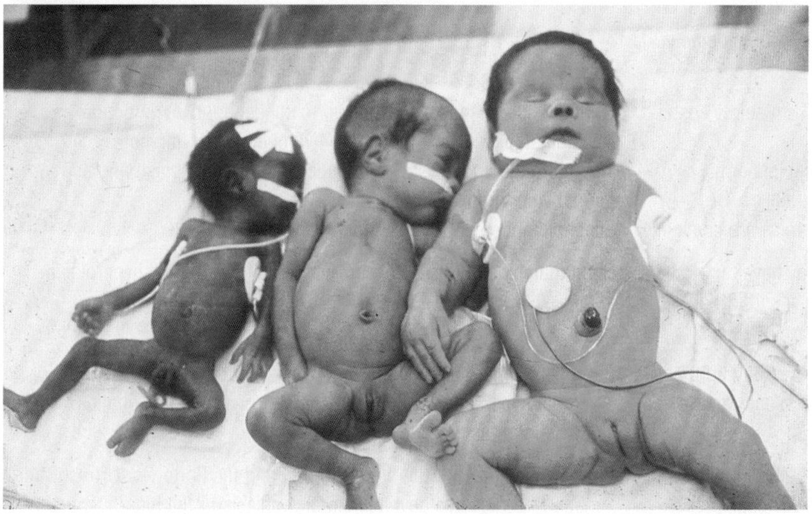

(Reprinted with permission from Korones SB. *High-Risk Newborn Infants: The Basis for Intensive Nursing Care.* 4th ed. St. Louis: CV Mosby; 1986.)

TABLE 14-2 Newborn Examination

	Normal and Common Variations Found on the Newborn Exam	Examples of Abnormal Findings
Head	Sutures, anterior and posterior fontanels (Figure 14-5) Sutures may be overlapping, but fontanels should be open Molding of the skull resolves within weeks	Premature fusion, or craniosynostosis, leads to abnormally shaped skull; sutures will be ridged and immobile. Craniotabes, a soft area of the skull when palpated feels like a ping pong ball, a benign variant
Eyes	Bilateral red reflexes	Absence of red reflex requires ophthalmology evaluation for cataracts, tumor
Ears	Preauricular pits, tags	Low-set ears: line drawn from inner to outer canthus should cross helix of ear
Mouth	Epstein pearls (retention cysts) Ankyloglossia (short lingual frenulum) rarely requires intervention	Cleft lip, palate; high arched palate Natal teeth: typically central lower incisors; these are not primary teeth and should be removed to prevent aspiration
Nose	Patency of nares can be accessed via auscultation or fogging of shiny surface held up to the nostrils	Nonpatent nares indicate choanal atresia
Skin	Vernix Milia Transient neonatal pustular melanosis Erythema toxicum Mongolian spots Lanugo	Jaundice present on the first day of life is not physiologic and requires evaluation
Neck/clavicles		Limited range of motion of neck suggests congenital torticollis Crepitus, edema, or instability of clavicle suggests fracture secondary to birth process Branchial cleft remnants, cysts Thyroglossal duct cysts
Lungs	Breath sounds are symmetric and bronchovesicular in nature	Increased work of breathing is evidenced by nasal flaring, grunting, intercostal and subcostal retractions Bowel sounds in the chest suggest diaphragmatic hernia Decreased or absent breath sounds on 1 side suggest pneumothorax
Heart	Point of maximal impulse is located just to the left of the sternum at the 4th intercostal space Many infants have transitional heart murmurs on the 1st day of life, typically soft, 1–2/6, low pitched, nonradiating, and localized to the LSB; caused by the PDA. Usually resolve within 1–2 days Brachial and femoral pulses should be palpable and equal	Point of maximal impulse on the right suggests dextrocardia Hyperactive precordium may suggest congenital heart defect Pathologic murmurs may not be present on the initial exam; they are typically coarse, louder, radiate, and persist
Abdomen	Liver is normally palpable up to 3 cm below costal margin Spleen tip is less commonly palpable; normal kidneys can be palpated in the flanks Diastasis rectus and umbilical hernias are common	Enlarged spleen may be secondary to congenital CMV infection Abdominal masses may be due to hydronephrosis, adrenal hemorrhage, multicystic-dysplastic kidneys, neuroblastoma, and renal vein thrombosis Scaphoid abdomen suggests diaphragmatic hernia
Genitalia: female	Mucoid vaginal discharge and may have pseudomenses about 5–7 days after birth due to maternal hormones	Genital ambiguity raises concern for congenital adrenal hyperplasia
Genitalia: male	Physiologic phimosis; prepuce is typically tight and adherent; hydroceles are common and resolve over 6 months	Bilateral nonpalpable testes is concerning for possible congenital adrenal hypertrophy, even in the presence of a normal phallus, unless infant is preterm
Hips	Hips should be examined using the Barlow and Ortolani maneuvers to rule out developmental dysplasia	Clunk or instability of the hip elicited during the Barlow or Ortolani maneuver indicates developmental dysplasia of the hip

TABLE 14-2 **Newborn Examination *(Continued)***

	Normal and Common Variations Found on the Newborn Exam	Examples of Abnormal Findings
Spine	Sacral pits and dimples in the natal cleft are benign	Defects such as lipomas, hemangiomas, pits, or sinuses overlying the spine may indicate underlying anomaly
Extremities	Posture and position of extremities will reflect intrauterine positioning **Acrocyanosis** (blueness of hands, feet, and perioral area): transient and normal	Remember to count the fingers and toes
Neurologic	High flexor tone present at birth in the term infant Primitive reflexes including suck, root, grasp, and Moro should be elicited DTRs including biceps, patellar, and ankle reflexes can be elicited; triceps reflex cannot be elicited secondary to high baseline flexor tone Head lag is minimal in the term infant	Asymmetry of Moro reflex may indicate brachial plexus injury

CMV, cytomegalovirus; DTRs, deep tendon reflexes; LSB, lower sternal border; PDA, patent ductus arteriosus.

III. Approach to Intrauterine Growth Restriction (IUGR)

A. Characteristics
1. Definition: fetus that fails to reach growth potential
2. Prevalence: 8% in general population; 10% perinatal mortality
3. Etiology: maternal, fetal, or placental (Table 14-3)
4. Pathophysiology: placental blood flow and insulin-like growth factor 1 receptor gene mutations may restrict intrauterine growth

B. Clinical features
1. Historical questions (see Table 14-3): detailed history to assess maternal risk factors for IUGR

QUICK HIT

Small-for-gestational age (SGA) and IUGR are *not* synonymous. SGA is defined as a birth weight below the 10th percentile for gestational age and refers to the newborn, whereas IUGR refers to the fetus.

QUICK HIT

Maternal smoking is an important cause of IUGR.

FIGURE 14-5 **Skull of a newborn, seen from above (A) and the right side (B).**

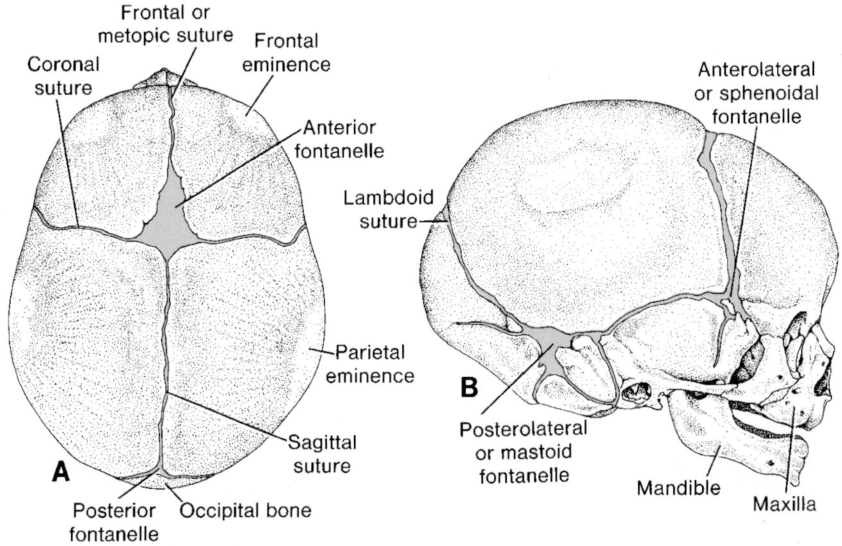

Note the anterior and posterior fontanelles and sutures. The posterior fontanelle closes about 3 months after birth; the anterior fontanelle, about the middle of the second year. Many of the sutures disappear during adult life. (From Sadler T. *Langman's Medical Embryology*. 9th ed. Image Bank. Baltimore: Lippincott Williams & Wilkins; 2003.)

TABLE 14-3 Etiology of Intrauterine Growth Restriction

Maternal	Chronic hypertension Pregestational diabetes Cardiovascular disease Autoimmune disease Renal disease Hemoglobinopathies Restrictive lung disease Substance use and abuse Malnutrition Exposure to teratogens Extremes of reproductive age (<16 years or >35 years) Low prepregnancy weight
Fetal	Infection (viral, protozoal) Malformation Chromosomal anomalies Multiple gestation
Placental	Chorioangioma Infarction Hematoma Placenta previa Circumvallate placenta Confined placental mosaicism Obliterative vasculopathy of the placental bed

QUICK HIT

Asymmetric IUGR is more common and has a much better prognosis.

2. Physical exam findings
   a. Assessment of gestation at birth (**Dubowitz chart**)
   b. Identify symmetric *versus* asymmetric IUGR
      i. **Asymmetric IUGR**
         (a) Weight affected > length
         (b) Head continues to grow; head sparing is protective mechanism to promote brain growth
         (c) Usually fetus affected in late gestation
         (d) Postnatal catch-up growth is good
      ii. **Symmetric IUGR**
         (a) Associated with genetic and metabolic conditions
         (b) Weight, height, HC equally affected
         (c) Fetus affected early in gestation: <18 weeks
         (d) Poor brain growth pre- and postnatally
         (e) High morbidity and mortality

MNEMONIC

TORCHeS infections
Toxoplasma
Other (syphilis)
Rubella
Cytomegalovirus
Herpes
Syphilis

C. Diagnosis
   1. Typically antenatal diagnosis
   2. 2 main steps to recognize IUGR in the antenatal period
      a. Clinical evaluation of uterine size in relation to gestational age
      b. Ultrasonographic evaluation of fetal size and growth
   3. Laboratory findings
      a. Maternal labs for TORCH infection and HIV screen
      b. Evaluation for gestational diabetes mellitus (DM)
      c. Fetal karyotyping, if concerns
   4. Radiology findings: done after 1st trimester and involve fetal measurements by ultrasound
   5. Monitoring: regular surveillance including umbilical artery Doppler, amniotic fluid volume, estimated fetal weights, biophysical profile, and nonstress test

QUICK HIT

Congenital infections commonly cause IUGR.

D. Treatment
1. Dependent on monitoring and gestational age
2. Normal umbilical artery Doppler and reassuring tests of fetal well-being: monitor biweekly
3. Complications of infants born after IUGR
a. Metabolic (hypoglycemia, hypothermia, dyslipidemia, acidemia)
b. Hematologic (polycythemia)
c. Cardiovascular (hypotension)
d. Stillbirth/intrapartum asphyxia
e. Meconium aspiration
f. Necrotizing enterocolitis
g. Hypoxic-ischemic encephalopathy
h. Long-term complications: neurodevelopmental outcomes

E. Prognosis: optimized by intrapartum surveillance and skilled staff at delivery
F. Prevention
1. Avoidance of smoking during pregnancy
2. Early diagnosis and treatment of infections

IV. Approach to the Floppy Infant

A. Background information and differential diagnosis
1. **Hypotonia**: reduced resistance to passive movement; it must be differentiated from *weakness*, which is decrease in muscle strength
2. Hypotonia is classified into 2 broad categories (Table 14-4)
a. **Central**: brain, brainstem, and cervicospinal junction disorders
b. **Peripheral**: anterior horn cell, peripheral nerves, neuromuscular junction, and muscle disorders

B. Historical findings
1. Family history: parental consanguinity, muscle diseases, or genetic disorders
2. Prenatal history: oligo-/polyhydramnios, poor fetal movement in utero, drug or alcohol use, exposure to infections
3. Birth history: abnormal fetal presentation, low Apgar scores, birth trauma
4. Postnatal history: weak cry, feeding difficulty, need for respiratory support

C. Physical exam findings
1. Classic "frog-like" posture with full abduction and external rotation of legs
2. Evaluate for alertness, visual tracking, dysmorphic features
3. Bell-shaped chest, hip dislocation, and joint contractures seen in severe hypotonia
4. Evaluate for abnormal movements like myotonia (congenital myotonic dystrophy [CMD]), fasciculations (Werdnig-Hoffman disease), and jitteriness (hypoxic-ischemic encephalopathy)

D. Diagnostic workup: led by history and physical
1. Systemic illness
a. Sepsis workup: complete blood count (CBC), differential count, blood culture, urine culture, cerebrospinal fluid (CSF) culture and analysis
b. Hypoxic-ischemic encephalopathy: cord arterial blood gas (ABG), liver function tests (LFTs), serum creatinine, and troponin immediately after birth
c. Metabolic abnormalities: serum electrolytes, glucose, calcium, **magnesium**, and ABG (for metabolic acidosis)

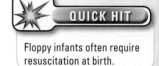

QUICK HIT
Floppy infants often require resuscitation at birth.

QUICK HIT
The floppy infant demonstrates head lag and slips through the examiner's hands when picked up under the arms.

QUICK HIT
Deep tendon reflexes differentiate between central and peripheral hypotonia.

QUICK HIT
Frog-leg posture, bell-shaped chest, feeding difficulty, and weak cry suggest severe hypotonia. Males may have undescended testes.

TABLE 14-4 **Characteristics of Neonatal Hypotonia**

Characteristics	Central Hypotonia	Peripheral Hypotonia
Deep tendon reflexes	Present (decreased or increased)	Absent
Muscle weakness	Mild to moderate	Severe
Primitive reflexes	Persistent	Absent
Pull to sit	Moderate head lag	Severe head lag

d. Evaluation for congenital infections (see Congenital TORCH Infections)
e. Evaluation for inborn errors of metabolism

2. Central hypotonia
   a. Cytogenetic studies if dysmorphic features are present (e.g., Down syndrome, Prader-Willi syndrome, fragile X)
   b. Brain magnetic resonance imaging (MRI): structural malformations
   c. Metabolic syndromes (e.g., Zellweger syndrome, carnitine deficiency)
   d. Benign congenital hypotonia is a diagnosis of exclusion
3. Peripheral hypotonia
   a. Serum creatine kinase: elevated in muscular dystrophies
   b. Specific DNA testing: for myotonic dystrophy, spinal muscular atrophy
   c. Electromyography (EMG): for myopathies and neuromuscular disorders
   d. Nerve conduction studies: to diagnose neuropathies
   e. Muscle biopsy

E. Management: once cause is identified, treatment is tailored for specific condition; supportive management includes
   1. Functional evaluation
   2. Rehabilitation program for feeding and nutrition and airway management
   3. School placement and vocational training
   4. Genetic counseling

> **QUICK HIT**
>
> If a mother received magnesium to prevent premature labor, her baby may be born hypotonic. A workup may not be indicated if the baby gradually recovers.

V. Approach to Microcephaly

A. Background information/definition
   1. **Microcephaly** ("small head"): HC measurement <3 standard deviations (SDs) below mean for age and gender
   2. Classified as **primary** *versus* **secondary** based on onset at birth or later; **congenital** *versus* **genetic** based on etiology

B. Historical questions (see Box 14-1 for differential diagnosis)
   1. Maternal history: gestational age, medications during pregnancy, infections
   2. Birth history: prolonged labor, Apgar scores, neonatal resuscitation, abnormal cord blood gas, and prolonged neonatal intensive care unit (NICU) stay

BOX 14-1

Differential Diagnosis of Microcephaly

Genetic

Isolated (microcephaly vera): familial
Autosomal recessive (1 in 40,000 births): severe mental retardation
Autosomal dominant: mild mental retardation
X-linked microcephaly
Chromosomal: due to chromosomal rearrangements and ring chromosomes

Syndromes due to chromosomal abnormalities
Trisomy 21 (Down syndrome)
Trisomy 18 (Edward syndrome)
Trisomy 13 (Patau syndrome)

Syndromes due to gene deletions
Wolf-Hirschhorn syndrome (4p deletion)
Cri-du-chat syndrome (5p deletion)
Williams syndrome (7q11.23 deletion)
Miller-Dieker (17p13.3 deletion) syndrome

Other syndromes
Cornelia de Lange syndrome
Smith-Lemli-Opitz syndrome
Rubinstein-Taybi syndrome
Miller-Dieker syndrome
Rett syndrome (postnatal onset of microcephaly)

Environmental

Congenital infections
Cytomegalovirus
Toxoplasmosis
Rubella
Herpes simplex

Maternal drugs/exposure
Fetal alcohol syndrome
Fetal hydantoin syndrome
Maternal cocaine use
Fetal radiation exposure (before 15th week of gestation)
Maternal phenylketonuria (increased phenylalanine levels)

Postnatal insults to brain
Meningitis/encephalitis
Hypoxic-ischemic encephalopathy

3. Family history: genetic disorders, microcephaly, mental retardation, seizures
4. Infant: seizures, feeding difficulty, growth and development milestones

C. Physical exam findings
1. HC measurement
a. Compare HC with length and weight
b. Measurement of parents' HC helps identify familial microcephaly
2. Dysmorphisms: may provide clues to syndromic microcephaly
3. Ophthalmic examination: evaluation with papillary dilation can help in diagnosis
a. **Chorioretinitis**: intrauterine infections (also associated with IUGR, hepatosplenomegaly, growth retardation)
b. **Optic nerve hypoplasia**: holoprosencephaly
c. **Microphthalmos**: Wolf-Hirschhorn syndrome, trisomy 13
d. **Cataracts**: Down syndrome, Rubinstein-Taybi syndrome, Smith-Lemli-Opitz syndrome
4. Skin examination for neurocutaneous markers

D. Laboratory testing and radiologic imaging
1. History and physical examination should guide appropriate evaluation
2. Laboratory data
a. Prenatal labs: TORCH and HIV screening (immunoglobulin [Ig] G by enzyme-linked immunosorbent assay [ELISA] and rapid plasma reagin [RPR] for syphilis)
b. Cytogenetic analysis
c. Karyotype, targeted fluorescence in situ hybridization (FISH), and comparative genomic hybridization microarray
d. Urine for cytomegalovirus (CMV)
e. Metabolic workup: newborn screening, serum amino acids, urine organic acids, serum ammonia
f. Electroencephalography (EEG): for seizures
g. Placenta: signs of insufficiency and infection, abruption, infarcts, calcifications, histopathology
3. Radiologic evaluation
a. Head ultrasound: diagnose IVHs, periventricular leukomalacia, porencephalic cysts, etc.
b. Computed tomography (CT) of head: synostosis, intracerebral calcifications, cortical atrophy
c. Brain MRI: preferred over CT; useful in identifying structural abnormalities (e.g., lissencephaly, holoprosencephaly, and schizencephaly)

E. Management (supportive) includes
1. Functional evaluation and rehabilitation
2. Management of seizures and other associated conditions
3. School placement and vocational training
4. Genetic and family counseling

VI. Approach to Newborn Rashes

A. Definitions and background (Table 14-5)
1. **Rash**: skin eruption that may or may not be associated with color change
a. Differential diagnosis: broad; ranges from transient and benign lesions to severe life-threatening infection
b. Always examine rash in whole patient context

B. Historical findings
1. 1st appearance of rash and evolution: some newborn rashes undergo characteristic series of changes as lesions resolve (Table 14-6)
2. Associated symptoms
a. Fever, lethargy, or other signs of systemic illness with underlying infection
b. Developmental delay, seizures, rash, and mental retardation may be secondary to neurologic condition (e.g., tuberous sclerosis)

QUICK HIT

HC soon after birth is a valuable clinical indication of the intrauterine growth of the brain and also as a baseline for future follow-up.

QUICK HIT

The best way to screen for CMV in an infant is the urine.

QUICK HIT

Early intervention is critical to maximize potential of these children.

QUICK HIT

Neonatal pustular melanosis evolves from a pustule into a hyperpigmented macule.

QUICK HIT

Hemangiomas grow in size before involution (Figure 14-6).

TABLE 14-5 Common Dermatologic Terms and Their Definitions

Term	Definition
Macule	Circumscribed flat area of discoloration of skin <1 cm
Patch	Large macule, >1 cm in diameter
Papule	Circumscribed elevated solid lesion, <1 cm
Plaque	Well-circumscribed superficial elevated solid lesion, >1 cm in diameter
Vesicle	Small superficial circumscribed elevated lesion containing serous fluid, <0.5 cm in diameter
Bulla	Raised circumscribed lesion containing serous fluid, >0.5 cm in diameter
Pustule	Small superficial circumscribed elevated lesion containing purulent fluid, <0.5 cm in diameter
Nodule	Palpable solid lesion >1 cm in diameter; sometimes in subcutaneous tissue and may be above, at the level of, or below the surface of the skin
Petechiae	1–2-mm red or purple spots on the body caused by broken capillary blood vessels that do not blanch under pressure
Purpura	Red or purple discolorations 0.3–1 cm diameter; does not blanch
Ecchymosis	Red or purple discoloration >1 cm diameter; does not blanch under pressure
Excoriated	Presence of linear abrasions produced by motion, often by scratching
Indurated	Thickening of the dermis causing it to feel firmer

TABLE 14-6 Common "Normal" Newborn Rashes

Diagnosis	Physical Exam and Histology Findings	Time to Resolution
Milia	1–2-mm papules over forehead, cheeks, nose, and in oral cavity; called **Epstein pearls** when present on palate Histologically: superficial keratin-filled cysts	Spontaneously rupture 1–2 weeks after birth
Sebaceous gland hyperplasia	1-mm yellow macules or papules over nose and cheeks found at the opening of the pilosebaceous follicle and due to maternal androgens	Resolve within 6 months
Erythema toxicum	Erythematous macules 2–3 cm in diameter with a central tiny vesicle or pustule Histologically show many **eosinophils** with Wright staining	Onset 24–48 hours of life; resolve within 1 week
Transient neonatal pustular melanosis	Vesicles, pustules, or ruptured vesicles/pustules with a collarette of scale Sites of resolving lesions develop into pigmented macules Histologically show many **neutrophils** with only occasional eosinophils	Vesicles and pustules resolve within 1 week; pigmented macules resolve within 3 months
Acne neonatorum	Multiple discrete papules that may evolve into pustules	Onset in the first 2–4 weeks of life; resolve within 6–8 months
Seborrheic dermatitis	Waxy shiny lesions to scalp and forehead due to overproduction of sebum	Onset within first 2–4 weeks of life; resolve within 3 months

FIGURE 14-6 **Hemangioma.**

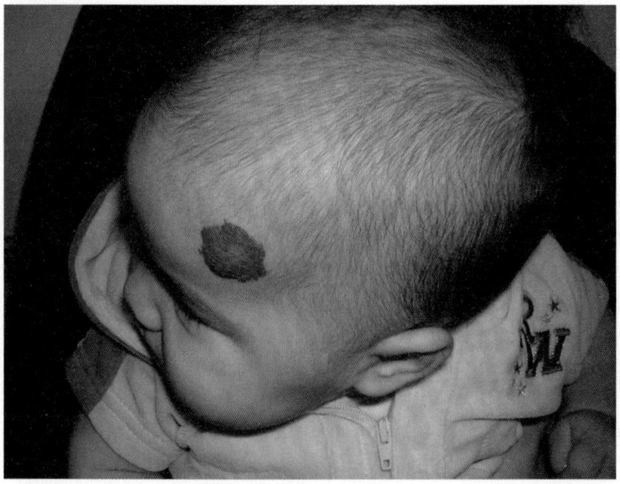

(Courtesy of Scott Van Duzer, MD.)

C. Physical exam findings
 1. Skin evaluation: identify primary lesion, secondary lesion, and configuration and distribution
  a. **Primary lesion**
   i. Predominant lesion directly associated with disease process
   ii. Terms such as **papule**, **pustule**, and **macule** may be used to describe and aid in diagnosis
  b. **Secondary lesion**
   i. Modification of primary lesion by patient or natural course
   ii. Described as **excoriated** or **indurated**
  c. **Configuration**
   i. How lesions are locally grouped
   ii. Described as **annular** (ring-like) or **targetoid**, etc.
  d. **Distribution**
   i. How lesions are localized
   ii. Described as **generalized**, **symmetric**, or **localized** to certain areas of body
  e. Skin color change should be noted
  f. Examine *all* skin, including scalp
 2. Evaluation of other systems: complete examination of all systems should be performed
  a. Hepatosplenomegaly with rash may suggest congenital infection
  b. Rashes, seizures, and abnormal neurologic exam may suggest neurocutaneous syndromes
D. Laboratory testing
 1. Newborn rashes are mostly benign
  a. Polymerase chain reaction (PCR) testing of blood, urine, and CSF samples and culture swabs indicated if suspicion for herpes simplex virus (HSV) (vesicular rash)
  b. CBC, LFT, TORCH infection screen may be indicated for newborns with petechial rash and jaundice
  c. Metabolic or genetic tests may be required for some skin condition
 2. **Skin biopsy** is rare and may be performed in consultation with dermatologist when diagnosis is unclear and rash is persistent
 3. **Treatment**: most newborn rashes are benign and do not require any treatment

QUICK HIT

Vesicular lesions of herpes simplex virus infection in a neonate may be found clustered at the site of a fetal scalp electrode used during labor.

QUICK HIT

The older term "Mongolian spot" has been replaced with the more accurate and generalizable term "dermal melanosis."

QUICK HIT

Ill-appearing newborns with a rash require a septic evaluation with blood, urine, and CSF cultures.

QUICK HIT

Capillary hemangiomas on the forehead ("angel's kisses") or the nape of the neck ("stork bites") are extremely common and benign.

QUICK HIT

"Blueberry muffin spots" are sites of dermal hematopoiesis associated with congenital rubella or CMV.

QUICK HIT

Newborn rashes are mostly benign. A complete history and physical exam including a detailed examination of the rash may help decide the need for further lab tests.

MNEMONIC

BREAST: drugs contraindicated in breastfeeding
Bromocriptine, **b**enzos
Radioactive isotopes, **r**izatriptan
Ergotamine, **e**thosuximide
Amiodarone, **a**mphetamines
Stimulant laxatives, **s**ex hormones
Tetracycline, **t**retinoin

QUICK HIT

Alcohol and caffeine in moderate amounts are okay for breastfeeding women.

QUICK HIT

Lanolin cream may be helpful for cracked nipples.

QUICK HIT

Acute fever onset without source in a breastfeeding mother is a common presentation of mastitis. Breast symptoms may be delayed by several hours.

QUICK HIT

Alcohol cleaning of the stump does not seem to reduce infection or promote detachment.

QUICK HIT

Omphalitis is a rare but life-threatening infection in children that can be caused by *Staphylococcus aureus* (including methicillin-resistant *S. aureus*), group A strep, Gram negatives, and anaerobes. Broad-spectrum antibiotics and hospitalization are indicated.

QUICK HIT

Infants should have only sponge baths before the cord falls off (at age 2–3 weeks).

VII. Approach to Anticipatory Guidance for New Parents

A. Prior to discharge, parental knowledge and ability to care safely for newborn must be assessed

B. Anticipatory guidance and parental education should include assessment of

1. Feeding
    a. Breastfeeding is recommended for nearly all infants
        i. Contraindications to breastfeeding
            (a) Maternal HIV in developed countries
            (b) Current maternal illicit drug use
            (c) Rarely, maternal medications (e.g., chemotherapy, illicit drugs)
    b. Hospital policies associated with maternal success with breastfeeding
        i. Written breastfeeding policy
        ii. Inform women of benefits of breastfeeding (see VIII. Approach to Infant Nutritional Requirements and Formulas)
        iii. Help mothers initiate breastfeeding within 30 minutes of birth
        iv. Practice rooming-in: allow mothers and infants to remain together, 24 hours/day
    c. How to know infant is getting enough milk
        i. First 2 days of life, anticipate 1–2 voids and 1–2 stools daily
        ii. Infant should lose no more than 7% of birth weight
        iii. Infant should feed 8–12 times every 24 hours and be content
        iv. By 2 weeks of age, infant should regain birth weight
    d. Problems
        i. Sore nipples: caused by poor latch, leading to cracking or soreness
        ii. Poor weight gain or excessive weight loss
        iii. Engorgement (breast is full and hard)
            (a) Caused by inadequate frequency or ineffective feeding
        iv. Plugged ducts
            (a) Massage and warm compresses before nursing and varying breastfeeding positions may resolve problem
        v. Mastitis
            (a) Typical symptoms are flu-like and nonspecific
            (b) A tender, reddened, wedge-shaped area may be noticed
            (c) May continue to breastfeed; seek medical attention for antibiotics
        vi. Jaundice (see XVII. Neonatal Hyperbilirubinemia)
    e. Formula feeding (see VIII. Approach to Infant Nutritional Requirements and Formulas)
        i. Iron-fortified cow's milk–based formula = 1st formula choice; breastfeeding still preferred
        ii. Hydrolysated formulas decrease or delay atopic disease in genetically prone infants; discuss with pediatrician
        iii. Soy formulas: appropriate for vegan families
        iv. Formula is available as concentrate, powder, and ready to feed
2. Umbilical cord care
    a. Keep cord clean and dry; fold diaper below cord
    b. If cord is dirty, wash with soap and water
    c. Cord typically falls off within 2–3 weeks of birth; if still attached at age 2 months, consider leukocyte adhesion defect
    d. If foul-smelling drainage, redness of skin around cord, or cord tenderness, consult pediatrician; infection of cord (**omphalitis**) is rare, but serious
3. Skin care
    a. Sponge baths only until cord falls off, using mild, fragrance-free soap
    b. Once cord falls off, infant may be immersed in water for bathing
    c. Change diapers frequently to avoid diaper rash
4. Genital care
    a. Vaginal drainage or pseudomenses in girls is due to hormone withdrawal at birth
    b. Circumcised boys: keep site clean and covered with Vaseline gauze until healed

5. Recognition of signs of illness; parents should seek emergency care for the following:
   a. Fever >100.5°F (38°C) measured rectally, after unwrapping infant
   b. Lethargy; sleeping through more than 1 feeding
   c. Forceful emesis occurring consecutively more than once
   d. Diarrhea, more than several episodes, large enough to leak from diaper
   e. Any cyanosis or difficulty breathing
   f. Jaundice associated with lethargy or poor feeding
6. Infant safety
   a. Car safety: all infants must be in car seat when in car
   b. Sleep safety
      i. Infants must sleep on back to decrease risk of sudden infant death syndrome (SIDS); risk of SIDS decreased by 50% in supine position
      ii. No soft bedding, baby bumpers, or toys should be in crib; they may compromise airway and lead to SIDS
   c. Immunizations
      i. Hepatitis B immunization should be given before leaving hospital
      ii. Follow immunizations schedule recommended by AAP
   d. Infant crying
      i. Infants cry for many reasons: they may be hungry, uncomfortable, tired, or wet, or it may be way to release tension
      ii. Ways to calm baby: feeding, swaddling, noise reduction
      iii. **Never shake a baby**

VIII. Approach to Infant Nutritional Requirements and Formulas

A. General considerations
1. Breastfeeding: 2/3 of U.S. mothers initiate at birth
2. Feeding: infants consume 100–110 kcal/kg/day
3. Nutrition
   a. Carbohydrates contribute ~40% total calories; lactose is main source of carbohydrates in breast milk and most formulas
   b. <10% of calories are derived from proteins: whey protein, important for immune function; casein helps increase intestinal motility and mineral absorption
   c. 50% of calories in infant diet are derived from fat
4. Growth
   a. Infants gain about 20–30 g/day
   b. Most head growth occurs in 1st year of life

B. Breast milk and breastfeeding (see VII. Approach to Anticipatory Guidance for New Parents)
1. Exclusive breastfeeding is recommended until age 4–6 months
2. Transitional/mature milk
   a. Breast milk produced from day 3–5 onward
   b. White, increased volume and calories; provides calories and satiety
3. Various oligosaccharides in breast milk serve as growth factors for intestinal microflora
4. Major whey proteins in breast milk include albumin, lactoferrin, secretory IgA, and α-lactalbumin
5. Fat is most variable nutrient in human milk
   a. Varies among women and over course of day
   b. Breast milk provides about 50% of calories from fat

C. Infant formulas (Table 14-7)
1. Used as substitute for breast milk; breast milk preferred
2. Types
   a. Cow's milk–based formulas: most commonly used; available as ready-to-feed, concentrated liquid, or powder forms
   b. Soy-based formulas: used for intolerance to cow's milk formula
   c. Hydrolyzed formulas: protein hydrolysate formulas used for cow's milk protein allergy or short-gut syndrome

QUICK HIT

Infants should sleep on a firm mattress and not sleep in the same bed with parents.

QUICK HIT

Smoking in the home and co-sleeping are associated with SIDS.

QUICK HIT

Infants should exclusively breastfeed or formula feed for the first 4–6 months.

MNEMONIC

Different forms of protein predominate in human and cow's milk: **W**omen make mostly **whey**; cows make mostly **casein**.

QUICK HIT

Babies double their birth weight by age 4–5 months and triple it by age 1 year.

QUICK HIT

Breast milk also contains nonnutritional factors, growth modulators, and enzymes.

QUICK HIT

Colostrum is calorie-dense breast milk produced from days 1–3 that is yellow in color and high in protein and maternal antibodies.

QUICK HIT

About 50% of patients with cow's milk protein allergy also have soy protein allergy and may need a protein hydrolysate formula.

QUICK HIT

IgA from breast milk coats the gut and can passively provide immunity during the time of neonatal gastrointestinal immaturity.

QUICK HIT

Major whey proteins in breast milk include albumin, lactoferrin, secretory IgA, and α-lactalbumin. The major whey protein in cow's milk is β-lactalbumin, the protein associated with cow's milk allergy.

QUICK HIT

ARA and DHA may play a role in retinal and brain development; however, supplementation in formula has no impact on development.

QUICK HIT

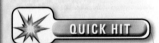

Vitamin D supplementation is required for exclusively breastfed infants.

QUICK HIT

Scurvy is extraordinarily rare. Juice can cause obesity in excess or malnourishment if substituting for formula or breastfeeding.

QUICK HIT

Emerging evidence indicates that early introduction of foods is not as allergenic as previously thought.

TABLE 14-7 Comparing Nutrition Content of Breast Milk and Formulas

	Breast Milk	Cow's Milk Formula	Soy Formula	Protein Hydrolysate Formula
Carbohydrate	Lactose	Lactose	Corn syrup/sucrose	Corn syrup/sucrose
Protein	60:40 whey:casein; lower % kcal from protein	Variable whey:casein ratios and different proteins; higher % kcal from protein than breast milk	Soy protein; higher % kcal from protein than breast milk	Casein hydrolysate; higher % kcal from protein than breast milk
Fat	Human butterfat; contains more fat content than formulas	Less fat content and cholesterol than breast milk	Less fat content than breast milk	Less fat content than breast milk

D. Breast milk *versus* formula (see Table 14-7)
  1. Breast milk protects against necrotizing enterocolitis (NEC) in infants by decreasing permeability of gut to invading bacteria
  2. Carbohydrates: lactose in both breast milk and cow's milk formulas
  3. Protein
     a. Cow's milk formula has higher protein content
     b. Whey/casein ratios vary
     c. Cow's milk formula provides slightly higher percentage of calories from protein
  4. Fat: arachidonic acid (ARA) and docosahexaenoic acid (DHA) are naturally found in breast milk but not in cow's milk; however, these fatty acids are now supplemented in most formulas
  5. Advantages of breastfeeding
     a. Psychosocial: promotes mother–infant bonding, uterine involution
     b. Nutrition: contains ideal ingredients for human body
        i. Lower rates of acute infections: infant diarrhea, otitis media, lower respiratory tract infections
        ii. Lower rates of chronic disease: Crohn disease, celiac disease, obesity, insulin-dependent diabetes, food allergies
        iii. Lower rates of SIDS
     c. Allergies rare
     d. Contains additional components that are difficult to add to formula, such as hormones, growth factors, and antibodies (i.e., secretory IgA)
  6. Vitamin and trace mineral requirements
     a. Iron: supplementation recommended for breastfed term infants after age 4–6 months
     b. Fluoride: recommended after age 6 months for exclusively breastfed infants

E. Other foods
  1. Cow's milk should not be introduced until age 1 year
  2. Fruit juices should not be introduced in 1st 6 months of life (if ever)
  3. Complementary foods are introduced around age 4–6 months
     a. New foods introduced every 3–5 days; observe for allergic reaction
     b. Good 1st foods include iron-fortified infant cereals and puréed meats

F. Prematurity and feeding
  1. Greater nutritional needs compared to full-term infants
  2. Breast milk is recommended for preterm infants, but fortification may be required; preterm infants may require 130–150 kcal/kg/day
  3. May have intolerance to enteral feedings and may need parenteral nutrition

IX. Understanding the Newborn Laboratory Screen

A. General characteristics
1. Testing of babies shortly after birth includes
   a. Blood spots on testing card
   b. Hearing screen
2. Characteristics of newborn screening test
   a. Reliable identification of healthy versus affected infants
   b. Disease course well known and treatment established, if identified early
   c. Early intervention beneficial
3. Identifying treatable conditions in healthy-appearing babies (Table 14-8)

QUICK HIT

Newborn screening is determined by *state*. Check with your department of health to see what conditions are screened for in your state.

TABLE 14-8 Clinical Disorders Detected by Newborn Screening and Their Management

Clinical Disorder	Treatment
Red cell disorders	
1. Sickle cell (SS) anemia 2. Hemoglobin SC	Prophylactic antibiotics, folic acid, monitor for crisis
3. Thalassemia	Depends on severity, may need transfusions
Fatty acid oxidation disorders	
1. Very-long-chain acyl-CoA dehydrogenase deficiency (VLCAD) 2. Long-chain acyl-CoA dehydrogenase deficiency (LCAD) 3. Medium-chain acyl-CoA dehydrogenase deficiency (MCAD) 4. Trifunctional protein deficiency	Fasting, frequent carbohydrate intake
5. Carnitine uptake deficiency	Supplement with carnitine
Amino acid metabolism disorders	
1. Phenylketonuria (PKU)	Avoid phenylalanine
2. Maple syrup urine disease (MSUD)	Limit leucine, isoleucine, valine
3. Tyrosinemia type I 4. Homocystinuria	Low-protein diet
5. Citrullinemia 6. Argininosuccinic acidemia	Low-protein diet, medication to reduce ammonia level
Organic acid metabolism disorders	
1. Methylmalonic acidemia	Low-protein diet, B_{12} supplementation
2. Multiple carboxylase deficiency	Low-protein diet, glycine and L-carnitine supplementation
3 Glutaric acidemia	Low-protein diet, riboflavin and L-carnitine supplementation
4. Propionic academia 5. β-Ketothiolase deficiency 6. Isovaleric academia 7. 3-Methylcrotonyl-CoA carboxylase deficiency	Low-protein diet, L-carnitine supplementation
8. 3-Hydroxy 3-methylglutaric aciduria	Prevent hypoglycemia, medication to reduce ammonia levels
Others	
1. Hearing loss	Speech therapy, hearing devices
2. Congenital hypothyroidism	Thyroid hormone supplementation
3. Galactosemia	Dietary changes, avoid galactose
4. Congenital adrenal hyperplasia	Mineralocorticoid and glucocorticoid
5. Biotinidase deficiency	Supplement with biotin
6. Cystic fibrosis	Fat-soluble vitamins, pulmonary regimen

CoA, coenzyme A.

4. Without early identification, these diseases can lead to morbidity or mortality

B. Clinical features
1. Most metabolic disorders are inherited (autosomal recessive pattern)
2. Infants appear healthy, and manifestations may not appear for weeks or months
3. Red blood cell (RBC) disorders: anemia; can identify carriers
4. Fatty acid oxidation defects
   a. Appear normal until body runs out of glucose
   b. Often symptomatic when ill or fasting; can lead to death
5. Amino acid metabolism disorders
   a. Inability to break down amino acids or excrete nitrogen
   b. Severity varies; buildup of toxic metabolites can cause death
6. Organic acid metabolism disorders: inability to breakdown amino acids or convert proteins or fats to sugar
7. Others
   a. Cystic fibrosis (CF): abnormal chloride channels
   b. Congenital adrenal hyperplasia (CAH) and hypothyroidism: inability to make specific hormone
   c. Galactosemia: inability to break down galactose
   d. Biotinidase deficiency: inability to reuse biotin

C. Diagnosis
1. Hearing screen is performed prior to leaving hospital by either of 2 methods
   a. Otoacoustic emissions (OAE) testing
   b. Auditory brainstem response (ABR)
2. Blood sample obtained from heel prick and placed on screening card
   a. 1st: ~24–48 hours after birth
   b. 2nd: ~1–2 weeks after birth
3. Samples analyzed at state lab and results reported to physician
4. Screening tests have higher false-positive rates and always require confirmatory testing; if confirmed by additional testing, treatment initiated

D. Treatment: depends on specific disease process

MNEMONIC

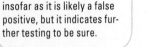

The newborn hearing test is also known as BAER:
Brainstem
Auditory
Evoked
Response

QUICK HIT

False positives are very high. A positive test should be interpreted with caution insofar as it is likely a false positive, but it indicates further testing to be sure.

DISEASE SPECIFIC

X. Complications of Extreme Prematurity

A. General considerations
1. In U.S., 10% of infants are born premature
2. Have physiologic challenges adapting to extrauterine environment
3. Extreme prematurity (<28 weeks) leads to prolonged NICU stay, high mortality (~50%) and morbidity (73%) (Box 14-2)

BOX 14-2

Classification of Prematurity Based on Birth Weight and Gestational Age

Classification	Metric
Birth weight	
Low birth weight	<2,500 g
Very low birth weight	<1,500 g
Extremely low birth weight	<1,000 g
Gestational age	
Late preterm birth	≥34 and <37 weeks
Very preterm birth	<32 weeks
Extremely preterm birth	<28 weeks

BOX 14-3

Major Problems in Extremely Low-Birth-Weight Infants

Respiratory
Respiratory distress syndrome
Apnea
Chronic lung disease

Cardiovascular
Patent ductus arteriosus

Central nervous system
Intraventricular hemorrhage
Periventricular leukomalacia
Seizures

Renal
Electrolyte imbalance
Acid–base disturbances
Renal failure

Ophthalmologic
Retinopathy of prematurity

Gastrointestinal
Necrotizing enterocolitis
Cholestasis

Immunologic
Immature immune system

4. Common complications of prematurity will be discussed in this chapter (Box 14-3)

B. IVH
1. General characteristics
   a. Bleeding occurs at subependymal germinal matrix and can spread
   b. Epidemiology: 25%–40% of all preterm infants
   c. Risk factors: extreme prematurity, hypotension, hypothermia, metabolic acidosis, thrombocytopenia, and/or coagulation disorder
   d. Physiology: variations in cerebral blood flow due to impaired autoregulation
2. Clinical features
   a. Variable; asymptomatic or seriously ill/catastrophic
   b. Dependent on degree of hemorrhage; 80% within age 72 hours
   c. Symptoms: apnea, seizures, sudden anemia, hypo-/hypertension, acidosis, and/or altered sensorium
3. Diagnosis
   a. Lab findings: low hemoglobin, elevated CSF RBCs (**xanthochromia**)
   b. Radiology findings: head ultrasound is diagnostic
      i. Grades 1–2: germinal matrix hemorrhage and IVH up to 50% of ventricular area
      ii. Grade 3: IVH >50% of ventricular area
      iii. Grade 4: parenchymal bleed
4. Treatment and prognosis
   a. Therapy: correction of hypoxia, hypotension, and bleeding diathesis
   b. Complications: posthemorrhagic hydrocephalus and periventricular leukomalacia
   c. Prognosis: correlated with grade of IVH
      i. Grades 1–2: good; neurodevelopment follow-up required
      ii. Grade 3: guarded; ~60% neurodevelopment problems
      iii. Grade 4: risk of morbidity and 90% severe sequelae

C. RDS
1. General characteristics
   a. Caused by deficiency of surfactant; affects 90% of extremely low-birth-weight infants
   b. Incidence and severity inversely related to gestational age
   c. Risk factors: prematurity, asphyxia, maternal diabetes, and cesarean section
2. Pathophysiology: high alveolar surface tension due to surfactant deficiency leads to low lung compliance and volume, causing widespread alveolar collapse

QUICK HIT

Complications from IVH increase the risk for long-term sequelae, including cerebral palsy, visual and hearing defects, and cognitive impairment.

QUICK HIT

Typically, IVH occurs within 72 hours of birth, screening is done via head sonogram at 24 hours, and serial sonograms are done thereafter depending on sonogram findings.

QUICK HIT

RDS puts infants at risk for chronic lung disease and eventually asthma.

QUICK HIT

A single dose of steroids given >24 hours but not over 7 days before premature delivery in a child <34 weeks' gestation will significantly reduce rates of RDS and improve mortality.

3. Clinical features: respiratory distress, grunting, and cyanosis
4. Diagnosis: chest x-ray (CXR)
5. Treatment and prognosis
   a. Therapy
      i. Surfactant: prophylactic therapy (intubation at birth) or rescue therapy (when symptoms develop)
      ii. CPAP: shown to improve endogenous surfactant production
      iii. Mechanical ventilation for respiratory failure
   b. Complications
      i. Barotrauma: pneumothorax or pneumomediastinum
      ii. Chronic lung disease
      iii. Retinopathy of prematurity (ROP)
   c. Prognosis: improved with surfactant and ventilator therapy
   d. Prevention: antenatal steroids

D. Apnea of prematurity
1. General characteristics
   a. Cessation of breathing >20 seconds with or without bradycardia or cyanosis
   b. Seen in 90% in infants <1,000 g
2. Risk factors: extreme prematurity
3. Pathophysiology: immaturity of respiratory regulatory function
4. Clinical features
   a. Sudden episodes of apnea
   b. May be induced by hypoxia, hypoglycemia, sepsis, seizures, IVH, or temperature instability
5. Diagnosis
   a. Cardiorespiratory monitors may identify apnea, bradycardia, or hypoxia
   b. Laboratory findings
      i. Infectious workup to rule out sepsis
      ii. Obtain glucose and serum electrolytes (abnormalities may cause apnea)
   c. Radiology findings
      i. Obtain cranial ultrasound if IVH is suspected
      ii. Chest and abdominal imaging, as needed
6. Treatment and prognosis
   a. Therapy
      i. Supportive: oxygen, metabolic balance, and hemodynamic stability
      ii. Nasal CPAP
   b. Prognosis: excellent and resolves by 42 weeks' postmenstrual age

QUICK HIT

Seizures are subtle in newborns and may result in apnea. If suspicious, an EEG may be a helpful diagnostic tool.

QUICK HIT

Oral caffeine is an effective pharmacologic treatment; it stimulates the respiratory center, increases sensitivity of chemoreceptors to carbon dioxide, and increases RR and minute ventilation.

E. Patent ductus arteriosus (PDA)
1. General characteristics
   a. Failure of ductus to close after birth
   b. Incidence: 60% of preterms
2. Physiology (normal)
   a. Placental prostaglandin E_2 (PGE_2) maintains ductal patency in utero
   b. Decreases in PGE_2 and oxygen at birth trigger ductal closure
3. Risk factors: inversely proportional to gestational age
4. Pathophysiology: congestive heart failure (CHF) due to left to right shunt
5. Clinical features
   a. Small PDAs are asymptomatic
   b. Moderate to large PDAs can present with CHF, feeding difficulty, and failure to thrive (FTT)
6. Physical exam findings
   a. Prominent left ventricular impulse and bounding peripheral pulses
   b. Heart murmur: systolic murmur and crescendo may not be present
7. Diagnosis
   a. CXR: may show increased pulmonary vascularity
   b. Echocardiography with color Doppler is diagnostic

QUICK HIT

Ironically, PDA can be lifesaving if a child has duct-dependent congenital heart disease.

8. Treatment and prognosis
   a. Therapy
      i. Medical
         (a) Fluid restriction, diuretics, indomethacin (prostaglandin inhibitor) or ibuprofen
         (b) In 20%–30% of cases, 2nd course of indomethacin needed
      ii. Surgical ligation
   b. Complications: CHF, chronic lung disease, NEC, and IVH
   c. Prognosis: excellent; most respond to medical treatment

F. Necrotizing enterocolitis (NEC)
1. General characteristics
   a. Ischemic necrosis of premature gut
   b. 1%–8% of all NICU admissions
2. Risk factors
   a. Asphyxia or ischemic insult to gut: extreme prematurity, IUGR, PDA
   b. Role of enteral feeding is controversial; breast milk protective
3. Pathophysiology: intestinal mucosal necrosis accompanied by inflammation and invasion of gas-forming organisms into muscularis and portal venous system
4. Clinical features
   a. Feeding intolerance, increased residuals, temperature instability, or lethargy
   b. Physical exam: abdominal distension, bloody stools, apnea, or hypotension
5. Diagnosis
   a. Laboratory findings
      i. CBC: anemia, thrombocytopenia, or leukocytosis
      ii. Stool occult blood is often positive
      iii. Electrolyte, glucose, blood gas: metabolic acidosis, low sodium
      iv. LFTs and coagulation studies
   b. Radiology findings
      i. Serial abdominal x-rays: dilated bowel loops, **pneumatosis intestinalis** (presence of gas within intestinal wall), and perforation
      ii. Pneumatosis is found in 70%–80% of confirmed cases
6. Treatment and prognosis
   a. Therapy
      i. Medical NEC (no perforation)
         (a) Supportive care
         (b) Nothing by mouth (NPO) and gastric decompression, total parenteral nutrition, and broad-spectrum IV antibiotics
      ii. Surgical NEC: surgical consult, resection of necrotic bowel
   b. Complications: short-gut syndrome and malabsorption (if resection)
   c. Prognosis: mortality = 10%–50%
7. Prevention
   a. Slow advancement of feedings
   b. Breast milk protective

> **QUICK HIT**
> To keep a PDA open, give prostaglandins; to close it, give indomethacin.

> **QUICK HIT**
> A complication of ligation is hurting the left recurrent laryngeal nerve, leading to vocal cord paralysis, in turn leading to stridor.

> **QUICK HIT**
> NEC will not happen until the infant is first fed. In small preemies, start feedings slowly.

> **QUICK HIT**
> Bowel perforation is a common complication of NEC.

XI. Birth Injuries

A. Characteristics
1. Definition: injuries related to birth process; may not have history of trauma
2. Risk factors
   a. Macrosomia and infant of **diabetic mother**
   b. Breech presentation/malpresentation
   c. Prolonged labor or precipitous delivery
   d. Vacuum extraction or forceps delivery

B. Musculoskeletal injuries
1. Head
   a. **Caput succedaneum** (Figure 14-7)
      i. Diffuse, edematous swelling of soft tissue of presenting part
      ii. Can cross suture lines; spontaneous resolution in days

FIGURE 14-7 **A. Caput succedaneum. From pressure of the birth canal, an edematous area is present beneath the scalp. Note how it crosses the midline of the skull. B. Cephalohematoma. A small capillary beneath the periosteum of the skull bone has ruptured, and blood has collected under the periosteum of the bone. Note how the swelling now stops at the midline. Because the blood is contained under the periosteum, it is necessarily stopped by a suture line.**

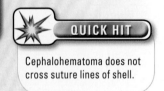

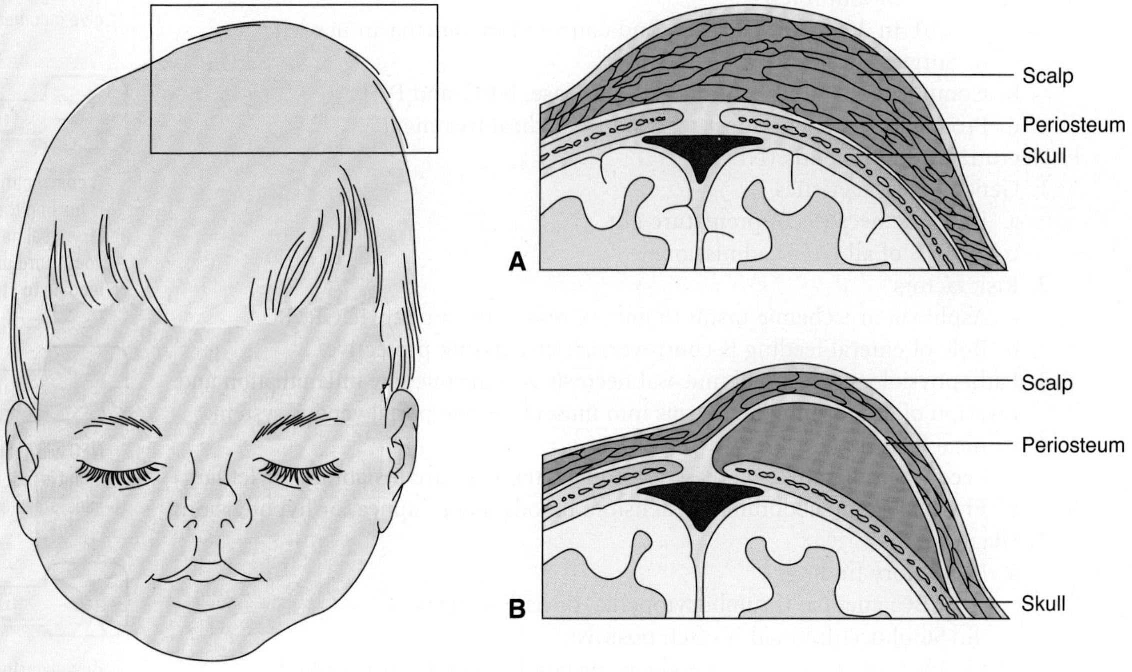

(From Pillitteri A. *Maternal and Child Nursing.* 4th ed. Philadelphia: Lippincott Williams & Wilkins; 2003.)

b. **Cephalohematoma** (Figure 14-8)
   i. May enlarge over several days; resolves in weeks to months; may lead to neonatal jaundice
   ii. No treatment; treat jaundice if indicated

c. **Subgaleal hemorrhage**
   i. Collection of blood between aponeurosis that covers scalp and periosteum
   ii. Bleeding can be extensive and lead to hemorrhagic shock; presents within hours of birth and can increase in size over 2–3 days
   iii. Mechanism of injury: linear skull fracture, suture diastasis or fragmentation of parietal bone, or rupture of emissary vein
   iv. Treatment is supportive; transfusion may be indicated

d. **Skull fracture**
   i. Compression from forceps or maternal symphysis
   ii. Linear: involve parietal bone; no treatment
   iii. Depressed fracture: surgical indications if neurologic symptoms or bone fragments

2. Clavicle fracture
   a. 40% missed at birth and present later with callus formation
   b. No treatment; heals spontaneously
3. Long bone fractures
   a. Rare
   b. Obstetrician may hear snap at delivery
   c. Treatment is pain management, splinting, and immobilization
4. Nasal septal dislocation
   a. Dislocation of triangular cartilaginous portion of septum from vomerine groove
   b. Presents with airway obstruction, deviation of nose, or asymmetrical nares
   c. Diagnosed via rhinoscopy and needs reduction by ear, nose, and throat (ENT) specialist

QUICK HIT

Cephalohematoma does not cross suture lines of shell.

QUICK HIT

Clavicles are the most frequently fractured bone in delivery.

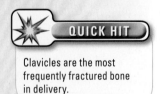

FIGURE 14-8 **Cephalohematoma.**

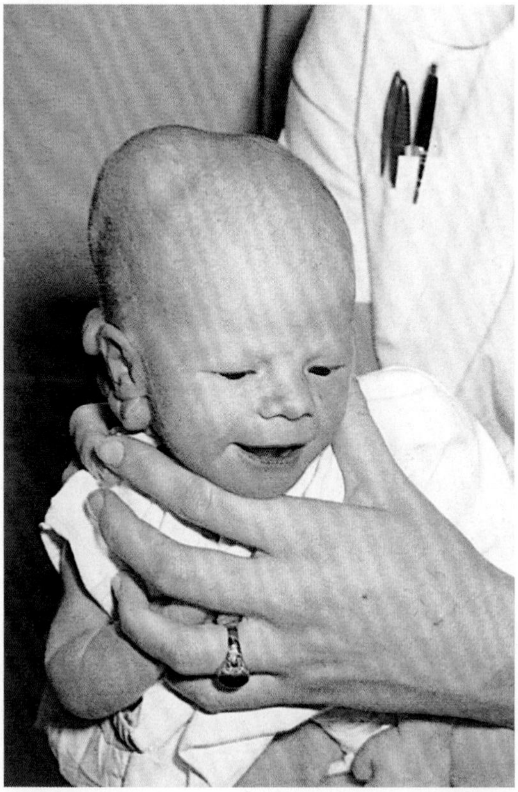

(From O'Doherty N. *Atlas of the Newborn.* Philadelphia: JB Lippincott; 1979:117, 143, with permission.)

C. Neurologic injury
   1. Facial nerve palsy
      a. Caused by compression of facial nerve as it exits the stylomastoid foramen or passes over mandibular ramus
      b. Prognosis is good: >90% complete resolution; 100% have improvement
      c. Treatment: artificial tears to prevent corneal abrasions
   2. Brachial plexus injury (Figure 14-9)
      a. Incidence ~1/1,000 (Table 14-9)
      b. Treatment: physical therapy and range-of-motion exercises
   3. Phrenic nerve palsy
      a. 75% associated with brachial plexus injury
      b. Presents late with respiratory distress; CXR shows elevation of affected hemidiaphragm in inspiration
      c. Diagnosed by fluoroscopy
      d. If supportive treatment fails, plication of diaphragm is indicated
   4. Vocal cord paralysis
      a. Recurrent laryngeal nerve injury (5%–25% of cases); increased incidence in forceps delivery
      b. Resolves spontaneously
   5. Intracranial hemorrhage
      a. Subdural hemorrhage
         i. Most frequent intracranial hemorrhage related to trauma; frequently asymptomatic
         ii. Caused by traumatic tearing of bridging veins
         iii. Presenting symptoms include apnea, dusky episodes, seizures, or neurologic deficits
         iv. Diagnosis: CT; ultrasound is usually not useful

QUICK HIT

Facial nerve palsy is more common in forceps delivery.

QUICK HIT

Vocal cord paralysis can present with stridor.

QUICK HIT

Because asymptomatic babies may have a subdural hematoma at birth, that is not necessarily a sign of child abuse if found shortly after birth.

FIGURE 14-9 **Brachial paralysis.**

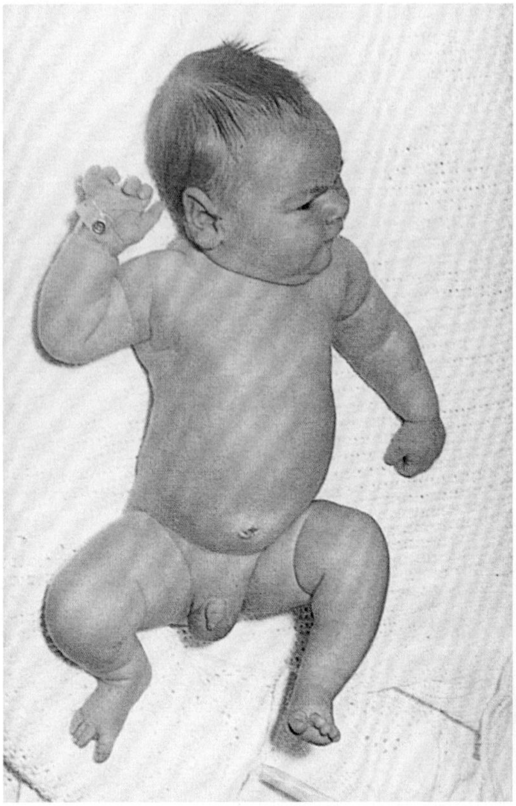

(From O'Doherty N. *Atlas of the Newborn.* Philadelphia: JB Lippincott; 1979:159, with permission.)

v. Treatment
   (a) Supportive care
   (b) Surgery if signs of compression

b. Subarachnoid hemorrhage
   i. Common in premature babies with asphyxia
   ii. Caused by rupture of bridging veins or leptomeningeal vessels
   iii. Presents with seizures on 2nd day of life
   iv. Diagnosis: CT; CSF may show large number of RBCs
   v. Treatment: supportive; resolves spontaneously in most cases

6. Spinal cord injury: rare; poor prognosis
7. Hypoxic-ischemic encephalopathy
   a. Before birth: maternal hypoxia, hypotension, uterine tetany, placental abruption, umbilical cord compression, placental insufficiency

TABLE 14-9 **Neurologic Birth Injuries**

	Location	Frequency	Clinical Findings
Erb palsy	C5–C7	90%	"Waiter's tip" posture: adduction and internal rotation at shoulder; extension of elbow, pronation of forearm, flexion at wrist and fingers, grasp is intact, Moro reflex is asymmetric, biceps reflex is absent
Klumpke paralysis	C8–T1	<1%	Absent grasp reflex, biceps reflex is present
Injury to entire plexus	C5–T1	10%	Completely flaccid arm

b. May see variable or late fetal HR decelerations or decreased beat-to-beat variability, meconium-stained amniotic fluid
c. Low cord pH: <7.0, 5-minute Apgar ≤ 3, abnormal neurologic exam, and multiorgan failure
d. Symptoms include hypotonia, respiratory failure, and seizures
e. Sarnat staging criteria
f. MRI is preferred imaging; EEG may predict outcome
g. Treatment: supportive; systemic hypothermia decreases neural injury

D. Visceral injury
1. Liver
a. Treatment is supportive
b. Surgical repair of laceration may be indicated
2. Adrenal hemorrhage
a. More common in breech delivery or large infants
b. 90% are unilateral
c. Flank mass on exam
d. If bilateral, acute adrenal failure may occur and requires hormonal treatment

XII. Infant of Diabetic Mother

A. General characteristics
1. Infant born to mother with persistently high blood sugar levels during pregnancy
2. Hypoglycemia, congenital anomalies, prematurity, macrosomia, and RDS occur with increased frequency, especially when maternal diabetes is not well controlled
3. Epidemiology
a. 3%–10% of pregnancies are complicated by DM
b. Male = female
4. Pathophysiology
a. No single mechanism clearly explains all associated problems
b. Maternal hyperglycemia causes fetal hyperglycemia, which leads to pancreatic β-cell hyperplasia and hyperinsulinemia
c. Insulin acts as growth factor and can result in fetal macrosomia, with increased fetal fat and visceromegaly, especially of heart and liver
d. Increased RBCs can lead to increased bilirubin release
e. At birth, insulin levels continue to stay elevated, but maternal supply of glucose is discontinued, resulting in hypoglycemia
f. Perinatal stress with associated catecholamine release can cause glycogen depletion, also leading to low glucose levels
g. Delay in parathyroid hormone synthesis may lead to low calcium levels

B. Clinical features (Box 14-4)
1. Physical exam findings (Figure 14-10)
2. Common findings include
a. **Large for gestational age** (LGA) (20%) or small for gestational age (SGA)
b. **Plethora** (red skin), jitteriness, jaundice, or tachypnea
c. Respiratory: tachypnea, respiratory distress

QUICK HIT

Polycythemia is common in infants of diabetic mothers (~1/3).

BOX 14-4

Common Findings in Infants of Diabetic Mothers

Metabolic: hypoglycemia, hypocalcemia, hypomagnesemia
Respiratory: respiratory distress syndrome
Cardiac: hypertrophic cardiomyopathy
Hematologic: polycythemia, hyperbilirubinemia
Central nervous system: jitteriness, caudal agenesis
Skeletal: macrosomia
Gastrointestinal: small left colon, increased frequency of duodenal atresia

FIGURE 14-10 **A macrosomic infant born to a diabetic mother (IDM).**

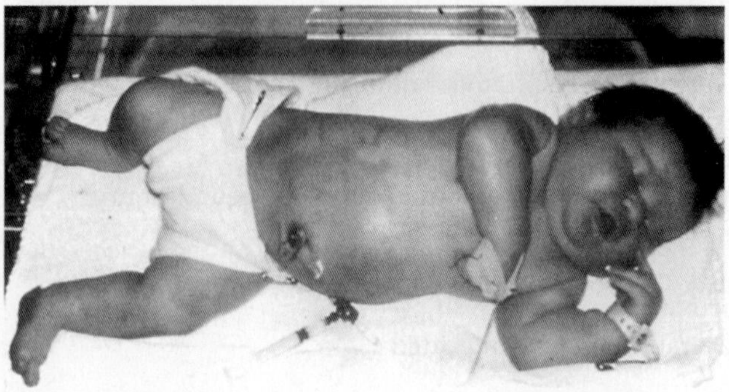

Body weight greatly exceeds the 90th percentile, and the IDM has significant fat deposition in the shoulders. Organomegaly (liver and heart) may be present as well. (From MacDonald MG, Seshia MMK, Mullett MD. *Avery's Neonatology Pathophysiology & Management of the Newborn.* 6th ed. Philadelphia: Lippincott Williams & Wilkins; 2005.)

QUICK HIT

Although infants of diabetic mothers are often LGA, with severe maternal diabetes, fetal growth may be impaired due to poor placental blood flow.

QUICK HIT

In the newborn period, consider maternal diabetes for any LGA infant presenting with hypoglycemia.

QUICK HIT

Untreated hypoglycemia can have long-term psychomotor complications; therefore, prompt recognition and treatment of hypoglycemia are essential.

d. Cardiac: tachypnea, murmur, cyanosis
e. Gastrointestinal (GI): poor feeding, vomiting, **inability to pass meconium**
f. Neurologic: sacral dimple, tuft of hair, poor tone in lower limbs
g. Skin and skull: signs of birth trauma

C. Diagnosis
1. Differential diagnosis for LGA: Beckwith-Wiedemann syndrome including macroglossia, abdominal wall defects, hemihypertrophy, and/or genitourinary abnormalities
2. Laboratory findings: as per symptoms
   a. Dextrose sticks or blood glucose
   b. Calcium and magnesium levels
   c. Hematocrit and bilirubin levels
3. Radiology
   a. CXR
   b. If respiratory distress: echocardiogram
   c. Spine sonogram: if concern for caudal regression
   d. Barium enema: if symptomatic for small left colon syndrome

D. Treatment
1. Identification and treatment of associated metabolic conditions
   a. Hypoglycemia
      i. Preventable by early and frequent feedings; gavage feedings may be tried initially, persistently low glucose (<40 mg/dL) and/or symptomatic hypoglycemia (not responding to oral/gavage feeds) should be treated promptly with IV glucose
      ii. Bolus of dextrose followed by constant infusion of 6–8 mg dextrose/kg/min may be required
   b. Hypocalcemia and hypomagnesemia require replacement
2. Identification of associated systemic conditions and anomalies
   a. Polycythemia may require partial exchange transfusion
   b. RDS may require surfactant, oxygen, or ventilation
   c. Cardiology evaluation for abnormal echocardiogram
   d. Prompt evaluation of small left colon or caudal regression

E. Duration and prognosis
1. Early recognition and treatment have reduced number and severity of associated problems
2. Overall prognosis is good
3. Hypertrophic cardiomyopathy may take months to resolve

XIII. Transient Tachypnea of Newborn (TTN)

A. General characteristics: benign parenchymal lung disorder of immediate newborn period

B. Pathophysiology
   1. Failure of fetal alveolar fluid clearance leads to poor compliance and tachypnea
   2. Risk factors include cesarean section, male gender, and maternal diabetes

C. Clinical features
   1. Respiratory distress: tachypnea, grunting, hypoxia, and increased work of breathing
   2. Symptoms may begin at birth and last up to 24 hours

D. Diagnosis
   1. Clinical diagnosis and diagnosis of exclusion
   2. Differential diagnosis: sepsis; pneumonia; pneumothorax; structural/anatomic causes;RDS; and cardiac, metabolic, and hypoxic brain injury CXR findings

E. Treatment: supportive; oxygen or CPAP may be required

> **QUICK HIT**
> Babies delivered by cesarean section have a higher risk for TTN.

XIV. Laryngomalacia

A. Background information: common and benign congenital laryngeal anomaly

B. Pathophysiology
   1. Potential genetic basis but unclear pathogenesis
   2. Due to collapse of supraglottic structures during inspiration

C. Clinical presentation
   1. Presents as "noisy breathing" or stridor in early infancy and resolves by ages 1–2 years
   2. Physical examination: stridor with mild to moderate respiratory distress

D. Diagnostic workup
   1. Clinical diagnosis; reassure parents if mild stridor
   2. Moderate to severe stridor: CXR and airway assessment by ENT to evaluate for other causes of stridor
      a. Supraglottic web
      b. Hemangioma
      c. Vascular ring
      d. Lingual thyroid or thyroglossal duct cyst
      e. Subglottic stenosis
      f. Laryngeal papilloma (rare)

> **QUICK HIT**
> Stridor worsens with agitation or sleeping on the back due to decreased muscular tone.

> **QUICK HIT**
> Placing the child in the prone position often diminishes stridor.

XV. Tracheoesophageal Fistula (TEF)

A. General characteristics
   1. Abnormal connection between trachea and esophagus (Figure 14-11)
   2. Disruption of tracheoesophageal septum in utero prevents separation of trachea from esophagus, preserving abnormal connection

> **QUICK HIT**
> Proximal atresia with distal TEF is the most common form of TEF.

FIGURE 14-11 **Esophageal atresia and tracheoesophageal fistula.**

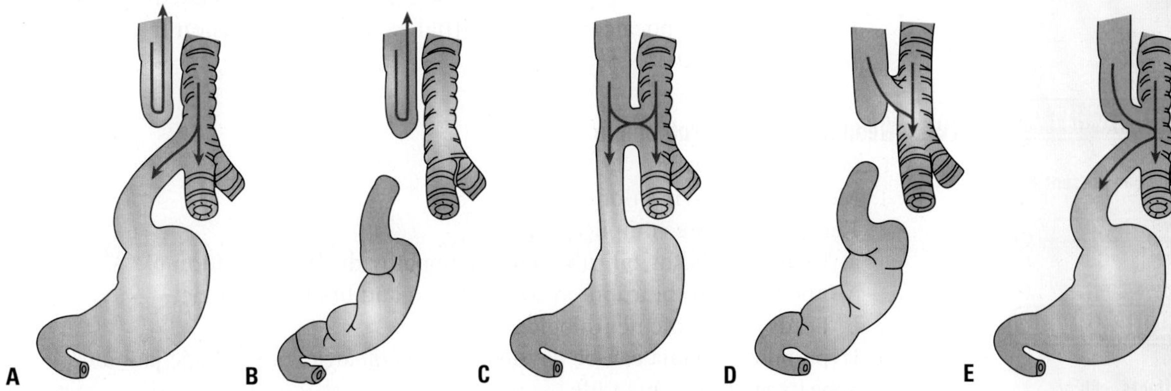

A. In the most frequent type of esophageal atresia, the esophagus ends in a blind pouch. The trachea communicates by a fistula with the lower esophagus and stomach (approximately 90% of infants with the defect have this type). **B.** Both upper and lower segments end in blind pouches (5%–8% of infants with the defect have this type). **C.** Both upper and lower segments communicate with the trachea (2%–3% of infants with the defect have this type). **D.** Very rarely, the upper segment ends in a blind pouch and communicates by a fistula to the trachea, or **(E)** a fistula connects to both upper and lower segments of the esophagus. (From Pillitteri A. *Maternal and Child Nursing*. 4th ed. Philadelphia: Lippincott Williams & Wilkins; 2003.)

MNEMONIC

VACTERL
Vertebral
Anorectal
Cardiac
Tracheal
Esophageal
Renal
Limb

MNEMONIC

CHARGE
Coloboma of the eye
Heart defects
Atresia of the nasal choanae
Retardation of growth and/or development
Genital and/or urinary abnormalities
Ear abnormalities and deafness

QUICK HIT

Polycythemia in an infant can cause a stroke.

QUICK HIT

The H-type TEF can present in infancy with chronic choking/coughing with feedings.

QUICK HIT

Maternal polyhydramnios suggests intestinal obstruction.

QUICK HIT

Polycythemia can present as priapism.

QUICK HIT

Jaundice affects ~60% of term infants and 80% of preterm infants.

3. 50% have associated anomalies; most common: VACTERL and CHARGE
4. Without intact esophagus, liquid either cannot reach stomach or is diverted to lungs, causing aspiration pneumonia

B. Clinical features
1. Feeding problem: vomiting or frothing at mouth
2. Respiratory distress

C. Diagnosis
1. Inability to pass nasogastric (NG) or orogastric (OG) tube at birth
2. Chest radiograph: coiled NG in esophagus suggests proximal atresia
3. Esophagogram or bronchoscopy (direct visualization of connection)

D. Treatment
1. Initial supportive: maintain airway, suction secretions, and avoid feedings
2. Surgical correction: ligation of TEF with end-to-end anastomosis
3. Prognosis: excellent in isolated TEF

XVI. Polycythemia

A. Definition
1. **Polycythemia (hyperviscosity)**: central venous hematocrit >65% in symptomatic infant and >70% in asymptomatic infant
2. Primary concern is hyperviscosity and its related complications

B. Pathophysiology
1. Maternal factors
   a. Preeclampsia
   b. DM or gestational diabetes
   c. Smoking
   d. Medications (e.g., propranolol)
2. Infant factors
   a. IUGR
   b. Twin pregnancy
   c. Cyanotic congenital heart disease
   d. Chromosomal abnormalities (e.g., Down syndrome)
   e. Hypothyroidism

C. Clinical features
1. Most newborns are asymptomatic
2. Common symptoms: jitteriness, tachypnea, irritability, lethargy, poor suck, vomiting, jaundice, plethora (red skin), and apnea
3. Other findings: hypoglycemia, hypocalcemia, respiratory distress, hypotonia, oliguria, seizures, priapism, coagulation disorders, and focal neurologic deficits

D. Testing: CBC with hematocrit, blood glucose, and calcium

E. Treatment
1. Asymptomatic (hematocrit <70%): IV hydration and close monitoring
2. Symptomatic (hematocrit >65%): IV hydration, treat associated hypoglycemia/hypocalcemia, and partial exchange transfusion to reduce hematocrit to 50%–55%

XVII. Neonatal Hyperbilirubinemia

A. General characteristics
1. Mostly benign condition
2. **Kernicterus**: rare complication
   a. Characterized by bilirubin encephalopathy due to deposition of unconjugated bilirubin in basal ganglia and brainstem nuclei
   b. Leads to chronic neurologic sequelae
3. Hyperbilirubinemia can be *physiologic* or *pathologic*; physiologic jaundice appears after 1st day of life
4. Pathologic hyperbilirubinemias
   a. Unconjugated hyperbilirubinemia
      i. Occurs due to increased bilirubin load, or
      ii. Decreased ability of liver to metabolize bilirubin

FIGURE 14-12 **Neonatal bile pigment metabolism.**

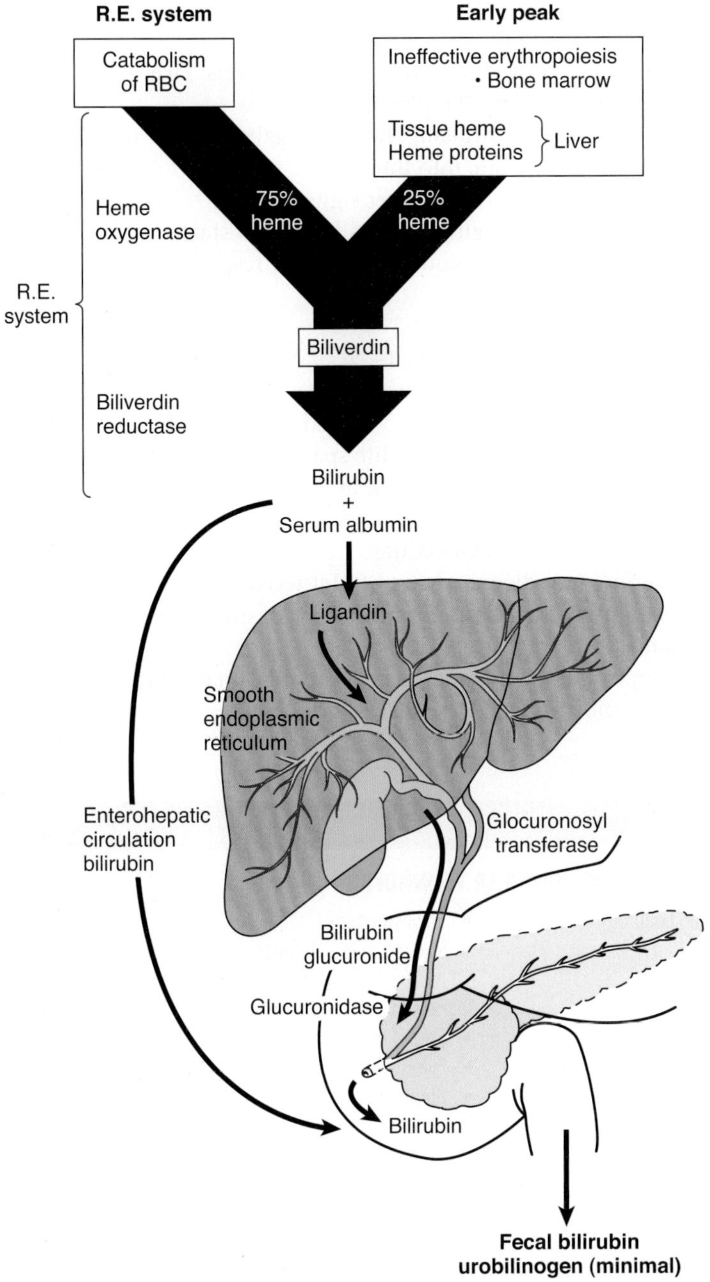

RBC, erythrocytes (red blood cells); R.E., reticuloendothelial. (Modified from Maisels MJ. Jaundice. In: MacDonald MG, Seshia MMK, Mullett MD, eds. *Neonatology: Pathophysiology and Management of the Newborn.* Philadelphia: Lippincott Williams & Wilkins; 2005:768–846.)

b. Conjugated hyperbilirubinemia (**cholestasis**)
   i. Failure of bile excretion secondary to obstruction
   ii. Potentially serious disorder; never physiologic

5. Pathophysiology (Figure 14-12)

B. Clinical features
1. Historical findings
   a. Time of onset and duration of jaundice
   b. Presence of sepsis-like symptoms
   c. Feeding history/hydration status
   d. Past medical history
      i. Estimated gestational age (preemies can have prolonged jaundice)
      ii. Birth complications (caput, cephalohematoma)

QUICK HIT

Jaundice that occurs on the first day of life is *not* physiologic.

QUICK HIT

Always check conjugated *and* unconjugated bilirubin in the first blood sample when investigating newborn jaundice.

QUICK HIT

Unconjugated bilirubin is water soluble and can cross the blood–brain barrier, whereas conjugated bilirubin cannot.

QUICK HIT

Although the cephalocaudal progression is taught (and tested!), in reality, it is an inaccurate estimation.

iii. Maternal blood type and Rh group (infant's if known)
iv. Maternal prenatal infectious workup (GBS and TORCH)
v. Family history of hyperbilirubinemia (metabolic conditions)

2. Physical exam findings: depend on etiology of jaundice
   a. Jaundice: **cephalocaudal progression** (approximate levels: face = 5 mg/dL, abdomen = 15 mg/dL, soles = 20 mg/dL)
   b. Cephalohematomas, excessive bruising, hepatomegaly, rash, or petechiae
   c. Stool color (indicates flow of bile into intestine)
   d. Lethargy, dehydration, poor suck, or other signs of sepsis
   e. Current weight versus birth weight to assess hydration status
   f. Others: dysmorphic features, abdominal distension, respiratory distress

C. Diagnosis
1. Differential diagnosis
   a. Unconjugated hyperbilirubinemia (Box 14-5)
      i. Physiologic jaundice: benign form of jaundice
         (a) Starts after day 1, peaks at days 3–4, and disappears by days 7–10
         (b) Develops due to short fetal RBC life span, immature liver enzymes, and poor enterohepatic circulation in newborns
         (c) Clinical diagnosis
      ii. Jaundice associated with breastfeeding
         (a) **Breastfeeding jaundice**: early onset (1st week of life)
            (i) Bilirubin >12 mg/dL occurs in <13% of exclusively breastfed infants
            (ii) Pathophysiology includes decreased milk intake with dehydration and/or decreased caloric intake

BOX 14-5

Causes of Indirect Hyperbilirubinemia in Newborns

Increased Production or Bilirubin Load on the Liver

Hemolytic Disease
- Immune-mediated
  - Rh alloimmunization, ABO and other blood group incompatibilities
- Heritable
  - Red cell membrane defects: Hereditary spherocytosis, elliptocytosis, pyropoikilocytosis, stomatocytosis
  - Red cell enzyme deficiencies: Glucose-6-phosphate dehydrogenase deficiency,[a] pyruvate kinase deficiency, and other erythrocyte enzyme deficiencies
  - Hemoglobinopathies: Alpha thalassemia, beta thalassemia
  - Unstable hemoglobins: Congenital Heinz body hemolytic anemia

Other Causes of Increased Production
- Sepsis[a, b]
- Disseminated intravascular coagulation
- Extravasation of blood: Hematomas; pulmonary, abdominal, cerebral, or other occult hemorrhage
- Polycythemia
- Macrosomia in infants of diabetic mothers

Increased Enterohepatic Circulation of Bilirubin
- Breast milk jaundice
- Pyloric stenosis[a]
- Small or large bowel obstruction or ileus

Decreased Clearance
- Prematurity
- Glucose-6-phosphate dehydrogenase deficiency

Inborn Errors of Metabolism
- Crigler-Najjar syndrome, types I and II
- Gilbert syndrome
- Galactosemia[b]
- Tyrosinemia[b]
- Hypermethioninemia[b]

Metabolic
- Hypothyroidism
- Hypopituitarism[b]

[a] Decreased clearance also part of pathogenesis.

[b] Elevation of direct-reading bilirubin also occurs.

Reprinted with permission from Maisels MJ. Jaundice. In: MacDonald MG, Seshia MMK, Mullett MD, eds. *Neonatology: Pathophysiology and Management of the Newborn.* Philadelphia: Lippincott Williams & Wilkins; 2005:768–846.

(b) **Breast milk jaundice**: late onset (2nd–3rd week of life)
  (i) Bilirubin 10–30 mg/dL by 2nd–3rd week of life
  (ii) Clear etiology unknown; possibly secondary to unidentified product in maternal milk

iii. Hemolytic diseases (see XVIII. Hemolytic Disorders of Newborn)

iv. Inborn errors of metabolism

(a) **Gilbert syndrome**: autosomal recessive variation of uridine diphosphate glucuronyltransferase (UDPGT) deficiency
  (i) Mild, fluctuating, nonhemolytic jaundice
  (ii) Can be exacerbated by certain drugs or fasting
  (iii) Benign prognosis

(b) **Crigler-Najjar syndrome**
  (i) Absence (type I) or nearly complete absence (type II) of UDPGT
  (ii) Type I is fatal due to inability to eliminate bilirubin by glucuronidation

b. Conjugated hyperbilirubinemia (Table 14-10)

i. Biliary atresia: most common surgical cause of neonatal cholestasis
  (a) Incidence 6.5/100,000
  (b) Jaundice develops around 3–6 weeks of age
  (c) Pale or clay-colored stools
  (d) Unknown etiology

ii. α_1-Antitrypsin deficiency: affects 1:2,000–4,000 newborns
  (a) Homozygous for Z allele (PiZZ) have clinical deficiency
  (b) Variable prognosis depending on degree of liver injury

iii. Alagille syndrome: familial intrahepatic cholestasis; autosomal dominant
  (a) Associated with dysmorphic facies (broad forehead, widely spaced eyes), peripheral pulmonic stenosis, vertebral anomalies (butterfly or fused vertebrae), and tubulointerstitial nephropathy
  (b) Secondary to "paucity" of bile ducts

iv. Choledochal cyst: congenital dilatation in common bile duct; if untreated, can lead to progressive biliary obstruction and cirrhosis

2. Laboratory findings (Box 14-6)

QUICK HIT

Commonly tested! Breastfeeding jaundice is *early*, whereas breast milk jaundice is *late*.

QUICK HIT

Gilbert syndrome is a lifelong condition. Some patients use tanning to control the yellow color of jaundice.

QUICK HIT

Patients with α_1-antitrypsin deficiency may also have pulmonary symptoms.

TABLE 14-10 **Most Frequent Causes of Neonatal Cholestasis**

Obstructive Cholestasis	Intrahepatic Cholestasis
Biliary atresia Choledochal cysts Bile duct paucity Neonatal sclerosing cholangitis Inspissated bile syndrome Gallstones/biliary sludge Cystic fibrosis	Viral infection • Herpes, CMV, HIV, Epstein-Barr virus • Parvovirus B19, others Bacterial infection • Sepsis, urinary tract infection, syphilis Genetic/metabolic disorders • α_1-Antitrypsin deficiency • Tyrosinemia • Galactosemia • Progressive familial intrahepatic cholestasis • Alagille syndrome • Other Endocrine disorders • Hypothyroidism • Hypopituitarism Toxic • Drugs, parenteral nutrition Systemic • Shock, heart failure, neonatal lupus

From Suchy FJ. Neonatal cholestasis. *Pediatr Rev.* 2004;25(11):388–396.

BOX 14-6

Evaluation of the Infant Who Has Cholestasis

Initial Investigations

(Establish the presence of cholestasis, define severity of liver dysfunction, and detect readily treatable disorders)

- Fractionated serum bilirubin concentration
- Serum liver chemistries: AST, ALT, alkaline phosphatase, γ-glutamyl transferase
- Tests of liver function: serum glucose, albumin, cholesterol, ammonia, and coagulation studies (prothrombin time, partial thromboplastin time, coagulation factor levels)
- Complete blood count
- Bacterial cultures of blood, urine, other as indicated
- Paracentesis if ascites (examine for bile and infection)

Investigations to Establish a Specific Diagnosis

- Ultrasonography of liver and biliary system (magnetic resonance cholangiography in selected cases)
- Serum α_1-antitrypsin level and phenotype
- Serologies and cultures for viruses (TORCH agents, parvovirus B19, human herpesvirus type 6, HIV, other)
- Sweat chloride analysis
- Metabolic screen (urine and serum amino and organic acids)
- Endocrine studies (thyroxine, thyroid-stimulating hormone, evaluation for hypopituitarism as indicated)
- Urine and serum bile acid analysis
- Specific enzyme assays on liver tissue, fibroblasts, others such as red blood cells (e.g., red cell galactose-1-phosphate uridylyl transferase activity)
- Hepatobiliary scintigraphy (HIDA) in selected cases (e.g., assess for bile flow and duct obstruction or perforation)
- Percutaneous liver biopsy (routine histology, immunohistochemistry, viral culture and nucleic acid assays, electron microscopy, enzymology as required)
- Genetic testing as indicated
  - Cystic fibrosis, Alagille syndrome
  - 3 forms of progressive familial intrahepatic cholestasis
- Exploratory laparotomy and intraoperative cholangiography if biliary obstruction not excluded

ALT, alanine aminotransferase; AST, aspartate aminotransferase.

Modified from Suchy FJ. Approach to the infant with cholestasis. In: Suchy FJ, Sokol RJ, Balistreri WF, eds. *Liver Disease in Children.* Philadelphia: Lippincott Williams & Wilkins; 2001:191.

QUICK HIT

A choledochal cyst is found by ultrasound.

QUICK HIT

The rules about when to light a hyperbilirubinemic baby are complicated. Online calculators exist that can help figure out when to use phototherapy (bilitool.org).

QUICK HIT

Accidental phototherapy of conjugated hyperbilirubinemia causes a baby to turn bronze in color.

QUICK HIT

Unconjugated bilirubin is stooled out. The more a baby eats, the better.

QUICK HIT

Maternal IgG causes hemolytic disease of the newborn. IgM does not cross the placenta.

D. Treatment
   1. Dependent on etiology and type of hyperbilirubinemia
      a. Unconjugated hyperbilirubinemia
         i. Phototherapy to prevent neurotoxicity
         ii. Exchange transfusion (rare), when intensive phototherapy fails
      b. Pharmacotherapy (rare)
         i. IV immunoglobulin (IVIG) for isoimmune hemolytic disease
         ii. **Phenobarbital** and ursodeoxycholic acid: improve bile flow
      c. Conjugated hyperbilirubinemia: to relieve obstruction
         i. Biliary atresia: portoenterostomy or **Kasai procedure**
         ii. Surgical resection followed by creation of new biliary drainage tract
         iii. Survival >90%, if done before age 8 weeks
      d. α_1-Antitrypsin deficiency and Alagille syndrome
         i. Symptomatic support
         ii. Liver transplant used for patients progressing to cirrhosis
      e. Choledochal cyst: complete surgical removal and biliary drainage
   2. Prevention
      a. Regular nursing: 8–12 times per day for first several days
      b. Screening for ABO and Rh(D) blood types
      c. Possible cause of jaundice should be sought in every child

XVIII. Hemolytic Disorders of Newborn

A. Characteristics
   1. Immune-mediated hemolysis results from maternal antibodies directed against surface antigens on newborn's RBCs

2. Alloimmune hemolytic disease typically involves major blood groups of Rh (Rhesus), A, B, AB, and O; occasionally, minor blood group incompatibilities (i.e., Kell, Duffy, MNS system, P system) may be involved
3. Infants make antibodies to unexposed antigens (found in food and bacteria)
4. Epidemiology
   a. ABO incompatibility is found in 15% of pregnancies; only 4% associated with neonatal hemolytic disease
   b. Rh(D) immunoglobulin prophylaxis has reduced incidence of Rh incompatibility
5. Pathophysiology
   a. ABO incompatibility
      i. Group O mother produces IgG anti-A or anti-B alloantibodies that cross placenta and bind to infant's type A or B erythrocytes
      ii. Groups A or B mother produces anti-A or anti-B alloantibodies (also called **isohemagglutinins**); they are IgM class and do not cross placenta
6. Rh incompatibility
   a. In Rh disease, sensitization of Rh− mother occurs when small amount of Rh+ blood enters maternal circulation, leading to IgG antibody formation (usually occurs at delivery but may also occur from blood transfusions or miscarriages)
   b. With future pregnancy, maternal antibodies cross placenta and bind to Rh+ fetal RBCs, leading to hemolysis

B. Clinical features
1. Historical findings
   a. Range from mild hemolytic disease and jaundice to complications of severe anemia
   b. Jaundice: typically, appears within 1st 24 hours of life; secondary to increased hemolysis and poor hepatic conjugation
   c. Pallor
2. Physical exam findings
   a. Newborns with hemolytic disease present with pallor, jaundice, tachycardia, and lethargy
   b. **Hydrops fetalis**
      i. Results from massive RBC destruction
      ii. Characterized by severe anemia, CHF, generalized edema, pleural effusion, ascites, hepatosplenomegaly, and extramedullary erythropoiesis

C. Diagnosis
1. Differential diagnosis of hemolytic anemia (see XVII. Neonatal Hyperbilirubinemia)
2. Laboratory findings
   a. Evidence of blood group incompatibility (e.g., ABO or Rh set-up)
   b. Rapid progressive anemia and indirect hyperbilirubinemia
   c. Cord blood bilirubin level >4 mg/dL, cord hemoglobin <12 g/dL, or both suggests moderate to severe disease
   d. Positive direct antiglobulin test (DAT)
   e. Peripheral smear
      i. Hemolysis, including reticulocytosis (usually 5%–15%) and polychromasia
      ii. Microspherocytes may be seen in ABO incompatibility cases resulting from partial membrane loss
3. Prevention and treatment: prophylaxis has reduced risk of sensitization to <1%
   a. Antepartum management
      i. Potential ABO incompatibility: invasive intervention (e.g., amniocentesis) not indicated due to low prevalence of severe hemolytic disease

> **QUICK HIT**
> Check the blood type of a jaundiced infant's mother. If she is O−, that is a "set up" for immune-mediated hemolysis. If she is AB+, that is much less likely.

> **QUICK HIT**
> ABO incompatibility can occur with the first pregnancy (A and B antigens are ubiquitous in food) in contrast to Rh disease, in which the mother needs prior sensitization.

> **QUICK HIT**
> The direct or indirect antiglobulin (Coombs) test is crucial to help diagnose an immune-mediated hemolytic disease and to differentiate it from other disorders.

> **MNEMONIC**
> The **direct** Coombs looks for antibodies that are bound **directly** on the patient's cells. The **indirect** Coombs looks **indirectly** at the patient's serum for what kind of antibody is there.

> **QUICK HIT**
> Rh(D) immunoglobulin prophylaxis, given at 28 weeks' gestation and/or within 72 hours of suspected Rh antigen exposure (postpartum), prevents Rh sensitization.

ii. Potential Rh incompatibility: if mother is sensitized, serial antibody titer determinations are mandated during pregnancy
   (a) If maternal antibody titers indicate risk of fetal death (1:16–1:32), amniocentesis performed for fetal Rh genotype and amniotic fluid bilirubin level
   (b) Depending on level of amniotic fluid bilirubin: fetuses may be followed by serial amniocentesis or may require intrauterine transfusion or delivery
   (c) Combined maternal plasmapheresis and high-dose IVIG can decrease circulating maternal antibodies levels in severe cases

b. Postpartum management
   i. Hyperbilirubinemia: phototherapy; in severe cases, exchange transfusion
   ii. IVIG: for severe hemolysis; may reduce need for exchange transfusion
   iii. Transfusion may be required for severe anemia

c. Complications
   i. Hydrops fetalis
   ii. Complications related to elevated bilirubin, including kernicterus

QUICK HIT

Gastroschisis is a full-thickness defect with no sac and is not in the midline.

XIX. Gastroschisis and Omphalocele

A. Background information/definition
   1. **Gastroschisis**: full-thickness defect in abdominal wall with evisceration of bowel without covering membrane or sac; seen in 1:10,000 live births
   2. **Omphalocele (exomphalos)**: midline abdominal wall defect with herniation of viscera contained within peritoneal sac; seen in 1:4,000–7,000 live births

B. Pathophysiology (Table 14-11)

C. Clinical presentation (see Table 14-11)
   1. Evaluate for location and extent of defect, presence of sac, and complications
   2. Presence of other associated congenital anomalies

D. Testing
   1. Prenatal diagnosis: elevated serum α-fetoprotein, ultrasound, karyotype
   2. Evaluation after birth: echocardiogram, renal and spinal ultrasound for other anomalies; blood for chromosomal analysis

TABLE 14-11 **Differences between Gastroschisis and Omphalocele**

Clinical Attribute	Gastroschisis	Omphalocele
Maternal age	Younger	Older
Location of defect	Usually to right of the umbilical cord	Midline
Covering membrane	Absent. Fetal abdominal contents exposed to amniotic fluid	Membrane consists of peritoneum on the inner surface, amnion on the outer surface
Embryologic defect	Premature involution of the right umbilical vein or the left omphalomesenteric arteries	Arrest of normal involution of the physiologic bowel herniation through the umbilical ring
Associated anomalies	Usually low (10%–20%) Intestinal atresias, undescended testes, and intestinal duplications	Usually high (50%–70%) Cardiac, renal, skeletal, and neural tube defects
Association syndromes	Usually none	Trisomy 13, 18, and 21 and Beckwith-Wiedemann syndrome
Complications	Poor gut motility; intestinal malrotation and volvulus Necrotizing enterocolitis	Depends on associated anomalies
Prognosis	Excellent for small defect	Depends on associated anomalies

E. Therapy/management
   1. Surgical
      a. Small gastroschisis and omphaloceles: reduction and primary closure
      b. Large gastroschisis: silastic silo to reduce over 3–10-day period

XX. Ophthalmia Neonatorum

A. General characteristics
   1. Conjunctivitis occurring within 1st 4 weeks of life
   2. Commonly caused by bacteria, usually transmitted during vaginal delivery
      a. Bacterial causes: *Chlamydia trachomatis*; *Neisseria gonorrhoeae*; and *Staphylococcus*, *Streptococcus*, *Haemophilus*, and *Pseudomonas* species
      b. Other etiologies are viral (HSV) and chemical irritation
B. Clinical features: inflammation of conjunctiva, eyelid swelling, and purulent eye discharge
   1. *N. gonorrhoeae*: occurs early, and is most severe.
   2. *C. trachomatis*: occurs late, may be mild or severe conjunctivitis
C. Diagnosis: Gram stain, bacterial eye culture, scrape epithelial cells for chlamydia testing
D. Treatment
   1. Irrigation of eye with saline and oral or IV antibiotics
      a. Ceftriaxone or cefotaxime for gonorrhea
      b. Erythromycin or azithromycin for chlamydia
   2. Prevention
      a. Ocular prophylaxis for all newborns shortly after birth: wipe eyelid with sterile cotton and apply 1 cm ribbon of erythromycin
      b. Prenatal screening and appropriate treatment of pregnant women

> **QUICK HIT**
> Ophthalmia neonatorum is a clinical diagnosis. Gram stain, eye culture, or scrapings from the epithelial cells of the eyelid may help identify a common infectious etiology.

> **QUICK HIT**
> Neonatal chlamydia of the eye, called **trachoma**, is responsible for 3% of worldwide blindness.

XXI. Neonatal Abstinence Syndrome

A. Definition
   1. Nonspecific central and autonomic nervous system regulatory dysfunction seen when exposure to drugs used by mother in pregnancy ceases after delivery of infant
   2. Caused primarily by opiates
      a. Opiate agonists: heroin, methadone, morphine, oxycodone, codeine
      b. Opiate mixed agonists/antagonists: nalbuphine, buprenorphine
B. Cause/pathophysiology
   1. Abrupt cessation of opiates at delivery
   2. Symptoms typically occur within 24–48 hours of birth
C. Clinical presentation
   1. Multiple organ systems affected
      a. GI: vomiting, diarrhea, poor feeding, poor weight gain
      b. Neurologic: irritability, jittery/tremulous, shrill cry, hypertonia, myoclonic jerks, seizures
      c. Autonomic: fever, sweating, tachypnea
   2. Testing
      a. Abstinence scoring scales like Finnegan, Lipsitz, Neonatal Withdrawal Index: infants scored serially to assess for treatment and response
      b. Urine toxicology screen: can be performed within 24–48 hours of birth
      c. Meconium toxicology screen: reflects prior drug use (days to months before); rarely sent
D. Therapy
   1. Supportive measures: low lights, swaddle, and minimal stimulation
   2. Pharmacologic therapy: once symptoms are controlled, opiates are weaned by 10% of dose daily
   3. Treatment of mother

> **QUICK HIT**
> Neonatal abstinence syndrome generally presents as a jittery, irritable baby with diarrhea.

XXII. Congenital Myotonic Dystrophy

A. Background information/definition: most common heritable (autosomal dominant) neuromuscular disease

QUICK HIT

CMD is not the same as congenital muscular dystrophy.

QUICK HIT

Mild CMD can be undiagnosed in women until they have an affected child.

QUICK HIT

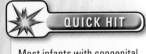

Most infants with congenital CMV are asymptomatic.

B. Pathophysiology; CTG triplet repeat expansion in the noncoding region of *DMPK* gene (DM1) on chromosome 19q13.3, encoding myotonin
C. Clinical presentation
  1. At birth: hypotonia and respiratory and feeding difficulty; has high mortality
  2. Infancy: hypotonia and respiratory difficulty improve in childhood
  3. Maternal history of myotonic dystrophy may help with diagnosis
  4. Physical exam findings
    a. Facial features: tenting of upper lip or inverted V-shape often referred to as "fish-shaped" or "carp mouth"; bitemporal flattening
    b. Others: respiratory distress, poor suck or swallow, hypotonia, arthrogryposis (multiple joint contractures), and developmental delay
D. Testing
  1. EMG, molecular DNA analyses
  2. Prenatal diagnosis available
E. Therapy
  1. Supportive care
  2. Prognosis variable

XXIII. Congenital TORCH Infections

A. General characteristics
  1. Infections that can be transmitted in utero via placenta
  2. TORCH: **T**oxoplasmosis; "**O**ther" (including syphilis, parvovirus, HIV, varicella-zoster virus [VZV]); **R**ubella; **C**MV; and **H**SV
  3. Term coined in 1974; less useful as "other" category grows
  4. Many congenital infections share common phenotype because fetal pathophysiology is similar (Table 14-12)
  5. Clinical signs can be apparent at birth or may manifest months to years later
B. Clinical features
  1. Historical features
    a. Depend on suspected agent (see below)
    b. Mothers should be interviewed regarding
      i. Past medical history (HSV, syphilis, VZV)
      ii. Results of maternal screening (HIV, syphilis, rubella)
      iii. Any febrile illnesses during pregnancy

TABLE 14-12 **Shared and Agent-Specific Signs of Congenital Infection**

Cytomegalovirus	Syphilis	Toxoplasmosis	Rubella	Herpes Simplex Virus
Growth restriction	Growth restriction	Growth restriction	Growth restriction	Growth restriction
Hepatosplenomegaly	Hepatosplenomegaly	Hepatosplenomegaly	Hepatosplenomegaly	Hepatosplenomegaly
Petechiae	Petechiae	Petechiae	Petechiae	Petechiae
Jaundice	Jaundice	Jaundice	Jaundice	Jaundice
Thrombocytopenia	Thrombocytopenia	Thrombocytopenia	Thrombocytopenia	Thrombocytopenia
Anemia	Anemia	Anemia	Anemia	Anemia
Rash	**Rash (bullous/peeling)**	Rash	**Blueberry muffin spots**	**Rash (vesicular/scarring)**
Periventricular calcifications	**Metaphyseal lucencies**	**Calcifications throughout cortex**	**Cardiac lesions**	**Calcifications throughout cortex**
Sensorineural hearing loss	**Rhinitis**	**Hydrocephalus**	**Sensorineural hearing loss**	**Brain destruction**
Microcephaly	Pneumonia	**Chorioretinitis**	**Cataracts**	**Chorioretinitis**
Blueberry muffin spots	Blueberry muffin spots	Blueberry muffin spots		

Bold shows "classic" findings.

iv. Common exposures (children in day care, CMV, cat exposure [toxoplasmosis])

2. Clinical presentation
   a. Symptomatic infants may present with similar physical exam and laboratory findings, regardless of pathogen (see Table 14-12)
   b. IUGR, SGA, hepatosplenomegaly, early jaundice, thrombocytopenia, and anemia are nonspecific manifestations of congenital infection (Figure 14-13)

C. Diagnosis
1. Laboratory findings: common labs that may be abnormal include
   a. CBC: anemia, thrombocytopenia
   b. LFTs: hyperbilirubinemia, elevated alanine aminotransferase (ALT), aspartate aminotransferase (AST)
   c. Bacterial cultures for blood, urine, and CSF are not positive in congenital infection but should be obtained if perinatal infection is suspected
2. Radiology findings
   a. Head sonogram or other cranial imaging to assess for calcifications
   b. Long-bone roentgenograms (syphilis)

D. Treatment
1. Treatment dependent on identification of causative organism
2. Supportive care for liver disease, thrombocytopenia or anemia, and jaundice
3. Screening for hearing loss, visual impairment, and neurodevelopmental outcome

E. Prevention
1. Active screening of mothers and counseling regarding preventative behaviors
2. Treatment of mothers
3. Vaccines are available for some pathogens and have resulted in near-elimination of congenital infection in developed world, as in congenital rubella

F. Specific agents
1. CMV
   a. Most common cause of congenital infection (U.S.: ~1/1,000 live births)
   b. Virus is shed in secretions, including saliva and urine
   c. ~90% of infants asymptomatic at birth
   d. Urine or saliva CMV PCR before 21 days (otherwise, cannot differentiate congenital versus postpartum CMV acquisition)
   e. IV ganciclovir, for 6 weeks, decreases hearing loss in infants with congenital CMV involving CNS
2. *Treponema pallidum* (syphilis)
   a. Rising incidence in U.S. since 2006
   b. Pathophysiology
      i. Spirochetes can cross placenta as early as 1st trimester
      ii. Highest transmission during secondary syphilis (**spirochetemia**)

QUICK HIT

It is difficult to differentiate the agents of congenital infection in an infant with these signs without more specific examination and testing; congenital infections cannot be diagnosed "from the doorway!"

QUICK HIT

Microcephaly, with or without cortical dysplasia or periventricular calcifications, is classically associated with congenital CMV (Figure 14-14).

QUICK HIT

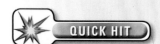

Hearing loss is the most common sequela of congenital CMV.

FIGURE 14-13 Congenital rubella infection at birth.

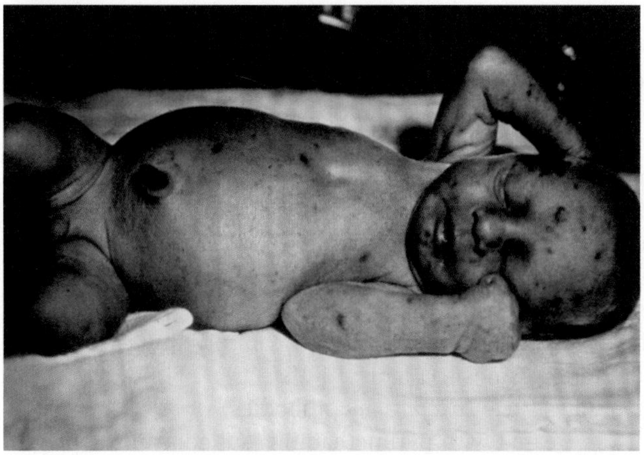

(From Sweet RL, Gibbs RS. *Atlas of Infectious Diseases of the Female Genital Tract.* Philadelphia: Lippincott Williams & Wilkins; 2005.)

FIGURE 14-14 **Computerized axial tomogram of a microcephalic 3-month-old boy with symptomatic congenital CMV following primary maternal gestational CMV infection. Shown are subependymal periventricular calcifications, enlarged ventricles and CSF spaces, and loss of periventricular and subcortical white matter volume.**

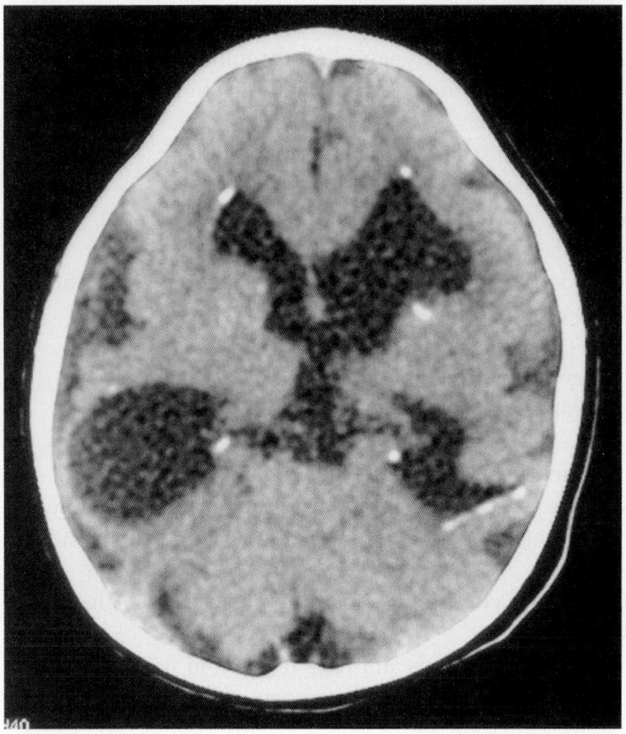

CMV, cytomegalovirus; CSF, cerebrospinal fluid. (From MacDonald MG, Seshia MMK, Mullett MD. *Avery's Neonatology Pathophysiology & Management of the Newborn.* 6th ed. Philadelphia: Lippincott Williams & Wilkins; 2005.)

c. Fetal infection can lead to stillbirth, preterm birth, and congenital infection
d. 60%–70% of infected infants are asymptomatic at birth
e. Symptomatic infants can present with hepatosplenomegaly, adenopathy, rash, jaundice, rhinitis, metaphyseal lucencies (periostitis) on radiography
f. Late findings include notched teeth (**Hutchinson teeth**), sensorineural hearing loss, **snuffles**, saddle nose, **saber shins**, and neurodevelopmental delay
g. Diagnosis
   i. All mothers to be screened with RPR and confirmatory treponemal-specific immunoassay, if RPR reactive
   ii. Symptomatic infants or those born to inadequately treated mothers should be evaluated by CBC, x-rays of long bones (periostitis), and lumbar puncture (for reactive Venereal Disease Research Laboratory [VDRL] test)
h. Treatment
   i. IV penicillin
   ii. Duration depends on extent of maternal treatment and the presence or absence of abnormalities on infant's exam or labs

3. *Toxoplasma gondii*
   a. Parasite with cats as definitive host
   b. Human infection can occur by direct contact with cat stool or ingestion of encysted muscle in raw or undercooked meat
   c. Immunocompromised mothers can have reactivation of prior toxoplasmosis that leads to congenital infection
   d. Hydrocephalus, diffuse cerebral calcifications, and chorioretinitis are classic findings of congenital toxoplasmosis (Figure 14-15)
   e. Diagnosis: serologic studies (i.e., *Toxoplasma* antibodies)
   f. Symptomatic infants are treated with pyrimethamine, sulfadiazine, and leucovorin for 12 months

QUICK HIT

T. gondii spores have not been found in U.S. beef, but they are somewhat common in pork.

FIGURE 14-15 **Computerized axial head tomogram of a 5-month-old girl with congenital toxoplasmosis. Notice the diffuse parenchymal calcifications and the prominent subarachnoid space bilaterally.**

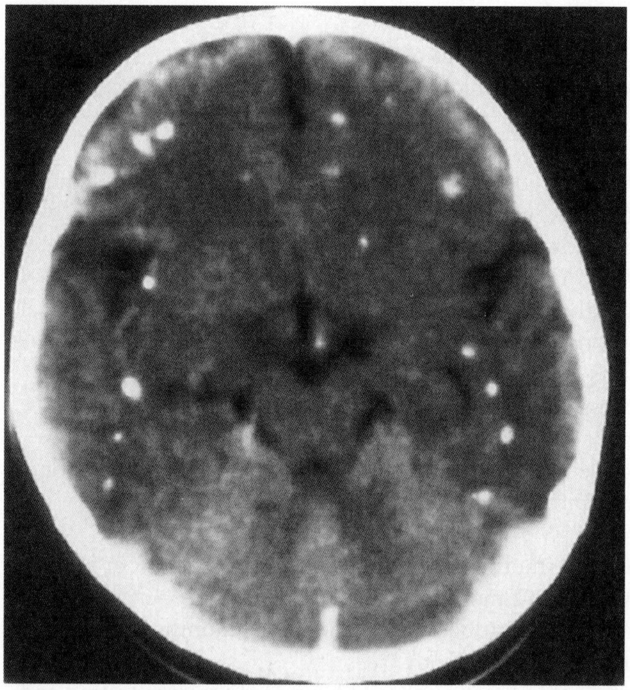

(From MacDonald MG, Seshia MMK, Mullett MD. *Avery's Neonatology Pathophysiology & Management of the Newborn.* 6th ed. Philadelphia: Lippincott Williams & Wilkins; 2005.)

g. Prevention: pregnant mothers should avoid litter boxes and raw or undercooked meat and use good hand hygiene

4. Rubella
   a. Rare in developed world following development of live vaccine in 1969
   b. RNA virus that can penetrate placenta at all stages of pregnancy
      i. Can lead to abortion, stillbirth
   c. **Classic triad** includes cataracts, sensorineural hearing loss, and cardiac defects
   d. Diagnosis
      i. Serologic studies traditionally used for diagnosis
      ii. Virus culture or PCR detection from nasopharynx, conjunctiva, urine, and CSF are gold standard for diagnosis
   e. Treatment
      i. No specific antiviral treatment
      ii. Prevention by universal vaccination
5. HSV
   a. Epidemiology
      i. HSV-2 more common but HSV-1 can also cause congenital and perinatal infection
      ii. Perinatal infection (e.g., skin lesions, sepsis, meningitis) more common than congenital infection
   b. Pathophysiology
      i. Maternal viremia leads to transplacental passage of virus and fetal viremia
      ii. HSV is tropic for brain, liver, and eyes; all organs can be affected
      iii. Can lead to stillbirth, anencephaly, or severe congenital infection
   c. **Classic triad** for HSV is severe brain destruction, eye involvement (generally chorioretinitis), and skin lesions or scarring
   d. Hepatitis, coagulopathy, pneumonitis, and NEC can also be present
   e. Diagnosis
      i. Detected by culture or PCR; PCR is preferred for CSF and blood and is commonly being used for surface sites

QUICK HIT

Vaccination of a pregnant woman with rubella vaccine has not been associated with congenital rubella or pregnancy loss but is not recommended.

QUICK HIT

Most infants with HSV get it if the mother is having her first outbreak during birth. A history of previous HSV *reduces* the likelihood of infantile disease.

QUICK HIT

Unlike other congenital infection, congenital HSV is *not* asymptomatic.

QUICK HIT

There are 3 types of neonatal HSV: (1) skin-eye-mouth, (2) meningitis, and (3) disseminated.

ii. HSV samples should be taken from surface (eyes, nasopharynx, axilla, rectum), CSF, and blood
iii. Cranial imaging and eye exam may help quantify extent of disease

f. Treatment
i. High-dose acyclovir for minimum of 21 days
ii. Severe disease with high morbidity and mortality

6. HIV

a. Epidemiology
i. 400,000 children acquired HIV in 2009; >85% were perinatally acquired
ii. Transmission decreased with access to highly active antiretroviral therapy (HAART); slower decreases in developing world

b. Pathophysiology
i. Transmission directly associated with maternal viral load and is inversely proportional to mother's immune status
ii. ~2%–5% of infants are infected congenitally via placenta; 85%–90% during birth process, and ~10% postnatally via breastfeeding

c. Clinical manifestations
i. Most common presentation of perinatal HIV is *Pneumocystis* pneumonia
ii. **FTT** and/or recurrent bacterial infections are also common

d. Diagnosis
i. Infants born to HIV+ mothers should be screened with PCR at regular intervals (1–2 weeks, 1–2 months, 4 months)
ii. Infants should have HIV antibody test after age 18 months to ensure disappearance of maternal antibody
iii. Infants with positive viral testing should have confirmatory testing and CD4 count and baseline blood and chemistry studies

e. Treatment
i. Confirmed HIV infant should be started on HAART
ii. Infants should be treated with azidothymidine (AZT) for 6 weeks, then with trimethoprim-sulfamethoxazole prophylaxis until they are known to be HIV-negative
iii. Prevention of mother-to-child transmission
(a) Optimizing maternal status with HAART therapy (or AZT during 3rd trimester if HAART not available)
(b) IV AZT during delivery
(c) AZT orally for infant for 6 weeks after delivery
(d) Cesarean section
(i) If mother's viral load is >1,000 copies/cc to decrease exposure to virus
(ii) Not beneficial if viral load <1,000 copies/cc
iv. Vertical transmission decreased to <1% with this regimen

QUICK HIT

Rates of pediatric HIV are related to maternal testing rates, *not* rates of disease in adults.

QUICK HIT

Likelihood of vertical transmission relates to mother's viral load during delivery. Knowing the mother's status can reduce transmission to <2%. Without treatment, transmission rate is 25%.

QUICK HIT

If mother's HIV status is not known prior to delivery, postnatal AZT for the infant is still beneficial even if mother did not receive AZT.

15 Developmental and Behavioral Disorders

SYMPTOM SPECIFIC

I. Health Supervision/Anticipatory Guidance

A. Regularly scheduled visits to optimize child's growth and development
   1. Listening to parents' or child's concerns
   2. Charting of weight, length (up to age 2 years), height, and head circumference (up to age 5 years) to monitor child's growth trajectory
   3. Documenting patterns of feeding, elimination, sleep, adjustment to school, family stressors
   4. Guidance for care of routine childhood illnesses including identifying when medical attention is required
   5. Immunizations at recommended schedules
   6. Supervision for injury prevention
   7. Routine use of screening tools to identify early medical, developmental, or behavioral problems

B. Well-child visits: newborn to age 6 months
   1. Growth/nutrition
      a. Exclusive breastfeeding is recommended until age 6 months; if breastfeeding is not chosen, then recommend iron-fortified infant formula
      b. Elimination
         i. Newborns should urinate at least 3–4 times/day
         ii. Bowel movement frequency is variable; stools should be soft, not firm or watery
      c. Introduce solid foods when infant has good head and trunk control and is able to feed from spoon, usually ~age 6 months
         i. Separate new food introduction by 1-week intervals
         ii. Monitor for signs of allergy
   2. Health supervision
      a. Discuss developmental milestones and screen for atypical development with referral to early intervention as needed
      b. Discuss appropriate use of over-the-counter medications and homeopathics
         i. Do *not* administer *any* medication or substance to infant age <6 months without supervision of physician
         ii. Ibuprofen is not recommended in infants age <6 months
      c. Water is not recommended in infants age <6 months
      d. All infants should receive vitamin D supplementation: American Academy of Pediatrics (AAP) recommends 400 International Units/day
   3. Anticipatory guidance
      a. Sleep
         i. AAP "Back to Sleep" campaign
         ii. Pacifier may be used for self-calming
         iii. Newborns sleep at least 20 hours/day

> **QUICK HIT**
> Full-term infants should be gaining ~1 ounce/day in the first 3 months, 1/2 ounce/day from ages 3 to 6 months, and 1/4 ounce/day from ages 6 to 12 months.

> **QUICK HIT**
> Birth weight should double by age 5 months and triple by age 12 months.

MNEMONIC

Age	Weight
Newborn	3 kg
5 months	6 kg (2× birth weight at 5 months)
1 year	10 kg (3× birth weight at 1 year)
3 years	15 kg (+ 5 kg every other year until 11 years old)
5 years	20 kg
7 years	25 kg
9 years	30 kg
11 years	35 kg

> **QUICK HIT**
> Breastfed babies stool more often.

> **QUICK HIT**
> Do not give honey to children age <1 year due to the risk of infant botulism.

QUICK HIT

Any infant age <2 months with a rectal temperature of 100.4°F (38°C) or greater should be evaluated for serious bacterial infections as soon as possible.

MNEMONIC

Safe Sleeping ABCs
Infants should sleep **A**lone
On their **B**acks
In their own **C**ribs

QUICK HIT

Do recommend supervised "tummy time" daily to improve head and trunk control.

QUICK HIT

Risk factors for sudden infant death syndrome include sleeping on the side or stomach, co-sleeping, maternal age <20 years, household smoking, parental substance abuse, and overheating.

QUICK HIT

AAP recommends no television or videos for children age <2 years and <1–2 hours/day after age 2 years.

QUICK HIT

Parasomnias, such as night terrors and sleepwalking, although frightening to the parents, are generally benign and are occur in 1%–3% of children ages 2–12 years.

QUICK HIT

Hypertrophy of the tonsils and/or adenoids is the primary cause of OSA in children age <7 years.

b. Household safety
   i. Inquire about **smoke exposure**; offer counseling for smoking cessation
   ii. Ask about presence of guns in house, smoke detectors, fire evacuation plans
   iii. Reduce water heater temperature to <120°F to prevent scalding
c. Car safety: current recommendations include using approved **rear-facing** car seat in middle back seat of car until child is age 24 months or until maximum height and weight for car seat is reached

4. Screening
   a. Obtain results of state newborn metabolic screen and hearing screen
   b. Refer for hip ultrasound at age 4–6 weeks if breech presentation

C. Well-child visits: late infancy, toddler, and preschool

1. Growth/nutrition
   a. At age 12 months, transition from infant formula to whole cow's milk and continue until age 24 months
   b. Avoid **choking hazards** such as peanuts, popcorn, hot dogs, carrots, grapes
2. Elimination: children are generally ready to begin potty training by age 2 years
3. Sleep
   a. By age 12 months, most children sleep 12 hours/night and take 1–2 naps/day
   b. Persistent snoring is never "normal"; sleep evaluation for obstructive sleep apnea (OSA) may be indicated
4. Health supervision
   a. Discuss developmental milestones and screen for atypical development with referral to early intervention as needed
   b. Dental hygiene
      i. Develop brushing habits early
      ii. Supplement with **fluoride drops** if community water supply is not fluoridated
      iii. Begin regular dentist visits at age 1 year
5. Risk reduction
   a. Car safety
      i. All children age <13 years should ride in back seat
         (a) <40 pounds: front-facing car seat in back seat
         (b) >40 pounds: booster seat in back seat
         (c) Belt positioning: booster seat should be continued until 4 feet 9 inches tall and ages 8–12 years
   b. Household safety: locks and gates to prevent access to dangerous areas such as stairs, cabinets, sharp objects, electronic appliances, outlets, swimming pools
6. Screening
   a. Purified protein derivative test for at-risk children: urban, immigrant from endemic area, or other known tuberculosis exposure
   b. Anemia: at ages 9–12 months
   c. **Lead level** at ages 9–12 months and repeat at 24 months if increased risk
      i. Spends time in home built <1970
      ii. History of immigration from developing country
   d. Formal visual screening at age 3 years
   e. Blood pressure: beginning at age 3 years

D. Well-child visits: school-age and adolescence

1. Growth/nutrition
   a. Encourage appropriate exercise and balanced diet
   b. Avoid sugary drinks
2. Elimination: ask about bowel habits, enuresis, and **encopresis**
3. Health supervision
   a. Sleep hygiene
      i. Adolescents need ~9 hours of sleep/night
      ii. Snoring/sleep apnea may need further evaluation
   b. Puberty: educate about expected physical and emotional changes

4. Risk reduction
   a. Encourage use of proper protective gear for sports and recreational activities and educate about concussion symptoms and treatment
   b. Personal risk behaviors: Counsel adolescents about safe sex, smoking, alcohol and drug avoidance, and safe driving practices
5. Screening tests
   a. Vision/hearing
   b. Anemia in menstruating girls
   c. Body mass index **(BMI)**
   d. Blood pressure
   e. Hyperlipidemia if risk factors
   f. Immunizations (see Chapter 10)

II. Approach to Developmental Milestones and Developmental Delay

A. Principles of child development
   1. Most children develop motor, language, and adaptive (cognitive and social) skills in predictable sequence, for example, roll → sit → pull up → stand → walk
   2. Development proceeds in **head-to-toe** (cephalocaudal) and proximal–distal sequences
      a. Baby learns to push up on arms before legs
      b. 1st vocalizations are grunts (from chest) and progress to pharyngeal vowel sounds ("ah," "oh") to consonants ("ba," "ma") with lips
   3. Developmental milestone charts are meant to guide health care providers' and parents' understanding of expected progression of skills

B. Motor development
   1. Early motor development influenced by presence of primitive reflexes
      a. Newborns' behavior is largely driven by innate physiologic reflexes
      b. Extinguish over time as brain matures and cortical control emerges
   2. **Moro**: extension of head elicits symmetric outward abduction and extension of extremities followed by flexion of arms and legs (Figure 15-1)
   3. **Sucking**: reflex present at birth, mature sucking by age 3 months
   4. **Rooting**: stimulus to side of infant's mouth causes infant to turn mouth toward source
   5. **Stepping**: placing upright infant's foot on firm surface elicits alternating steps (Figure 15-2)

QUICK HIT

Premature infants should develop milestones in an appropriate sequence but should have their age "corrected" to their gestational ages when assessing milestones. For example, a 28-week premature infant who crawls at 12 months chronologic age is developing typically.

QUICK HIT

Using consonants is "babbling" and happens at ~age 4 months.

QUICK HIT

The persistence of primitive reflexes beyond the expected stage of development is a signal of abnormal upper motor neuron function.

QUICK HIT

The degree to which an infant displays the Moro reflex varies; however, **asymmetric** response is concerning.

FIGURE 15-1 Reflexes and behaviors of the neonate. Moro reflex.

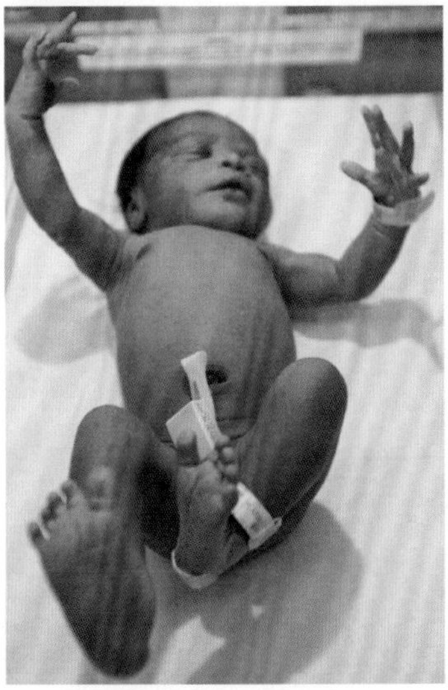

(Photo by Joe Mitchell.)

FIGURE 15-2 **Normal newborn reflexes. The nurse elicits the stepping reflex.**

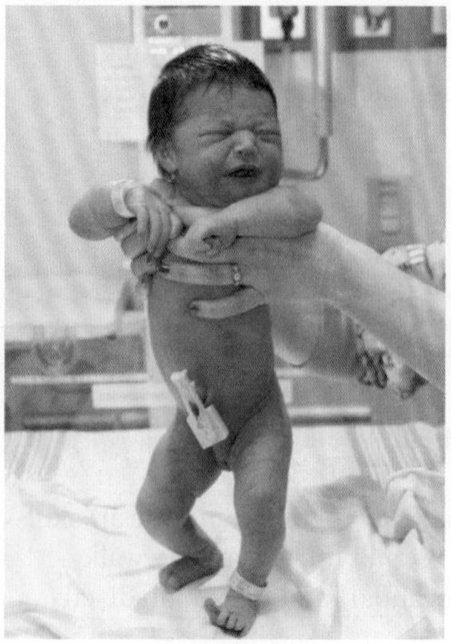

6. **Babinski**: stroking lateral foot in heel-to-toe direction elicits extension of great toe and fanning of toes
7. **Plantar/palmar grasp**: touching center of palm or sole elicits flexion of fingers/toes
8. **Galant**: stroking infant's back upward produces ipsilateral flexion of trunk
9. **Asymmetric tonic neck** (fencer's pose): turning head to side elicits extension of limbs on same side, flexion of limbs on opposite side (Figure 15-3)
10. **Parachute**: when baby is turned upside down, arms reach above head to protect from fall

FIGURE 15-3 **Asymmetrical tonic reflex (ATNR) A sleeping infant demonstrates the typical posture assumed by a healthy child exhibiting an ATNR.**

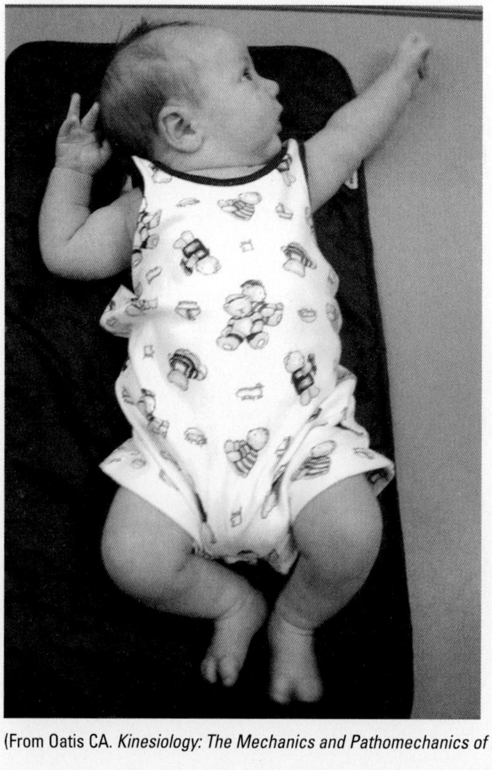

(From Oatis CA. *Kinesiology: The Mechanics and Pathomechanics of Human Movement.* Baltimore: Lippincott Williams & Wilkins; 2004.)

C. Developmental surveillance and screening
  1. Surveillance should occur at every office visit
    a. All 4 areas of development: gross motor, fine motor, cognitive/adaptive/social, and language
    b. Review risk factors for developmental delays
      i. Psychosocial: parental stress/impairment, food and shelter insecurity, neglect, abuse
      ii. Medical: illnesses/infections, trauma, seizures, visual or hearing impairments, genetic factors
      iii. Environmental: lead exposure
  2. AAP recommends formal screening with standardized tools at 9, 18, and 24/30 months, and additional autism-specific screening at 18 and 24/30 months
  3. Screening for school-aged children should focus on school-related skills
    a. Attention-deficit hyperactivity disorder (ADHD)
    b. Achievement IQ and behavior

D. Developmental delays
  1. Language and/or speech delays most common, either in isolation or with delays in other areas of development
  2. Intellectual disability ([ID] formerly called *mental retardation*)
    a. Diagnosed by trained mental health professional/psychologist: *Diagnostic and Statistical Manual of Mental Disorders* (*DSM-IV-TR*) diagnostic criteria
      i. IQ score ≤70 *and*
      ii. Impairment in at least 2 of these areas of function: communication, self-care, home living, social and interpersonal skills, use of community resources, functional academic skills, work and leisure, health and safety
    b. Affects 2.5% of population
    c. Boys > girls
      i. 2:1 in mild category
      ii. 1.5:1 in severe category
    d. Prevalence of mild ID is decreasing, whereas prevalence of severe ID is stable
    e. Mild ID: IQ >50–70
      i. Children with mild ID may be incorporated into other diagnostic categories, such as autism spectrum disorders (ASDs)
      ii. Most correlated with environmental factors: maternal education, poverty, neglect, and malnutrition
    f. Severe ID: full-scale IQ <35
      i. More likely due to biologic or genetic etiology
      ii. Some examples include trisomy 21 and fragile X, Angelman, Prader-Willi, and Rett syndromes
  3. Medical evaluation of developmental delays
    a. Start with comprehensive history and physical exam
      i. Review detailed family history and newborn screen
      ii. Hearing and vision screening
    b. Consider chromosomal studies and **fragile X** testing if positive family history
    c. Positive exam or history: further workup may include brain magnetic resonance imaging, thyroid function tests, complete blood count, lead levels, electroencephalography (EEG), metabolic testing (serum amino acids, urine organic acids, lactate/pyruvate, acylcarnitine)

III. Approach to Child Temperament

A. Characteristics
  1. Definition: behavioral style with which a person experiences and responds to environment
  2. Separate from behavioral adjustment, physical and neurologic status, and cognitive skills

QUICK HIT

Prevalence of all developmental delays is 10%.

QUICK HIT

Early identification and referral to early intervention services can significantly improve outcomes for children with developmental delays.

QUICK HIT

The Individuals with Disabilities Act (IDEA) mandates providers to refer children with suspected delays to early intervention services (ages 0–3 years) or early childhood services (ages 3–5 years).

QUICK HIT

Language is most closely correlated with intellectual potential.

QUICK HIT

Global developmental delay is significant delay in 2 or more areas of development.

QUICK HIT

The most common cause of motor impairment/delays is **cerebral palsy**.

QUICK HIT

Remember—many patients with cerebral palsy do *not* have ID.

QUICK HIT

Even very mild lead poisoning causes cognitive impairment.

QUICK HIT

Temperament is somewhat stable over place and time but never completely fixed or completely changeable. By ages 5–6 years, children can often learn to suppress expression of some challenging traits such as shyness.

QUICK HIT

More incidents of child abuse occur with challenging children.

QUICK HIT

AAP recommends alternative disciplinary techniques due to the limited effectiveness of corporal punishment and the risk for physical and emotional injury.

3. Certain individual traits can lead to stressful relationships with caregivers in certain situations (e.g., low adaptability or negative mood)
4. Origins: predominantly inborn; ~50% genetic

B. Clinical importance
1. Appropriate management is different from that of reactive behavior problems, being more directed at caregiver accommodation of young child's style rather than attempts at eradication of it
2. Goodness or poorness of fit between values and expectations of parents, teachers, or other caregivers and child
3. Impact of poor fit
   a. On parents: may influence how they feel about themselves as parents
   b. On children
      i. May impact prevalent mood/level of contentment or adjustment
      ii. Difficulties with impulse control
      iii. Physical problems: increased incidence of some conditions and problems in feeding, sleep, elimination
      iv. Development may be influenced by temperament and ability to adapt to environmental stimuli like social skills or language

C. Diagnosis
1. Requires skillful interviewing of caregiver
2. Differential diagnosis: temperament must be distinguished from
   a. Behavioral adjustment problems (content)
   b. Parental misperceptions of abnormal behavior
3. Clinical management of aversive temperaments
   a. Recognition of temperament by clinician or teacher
   b. Revising caregiver's understanding and handling of it, whether associated behavior problem exists or not
   c. Emphasis on improving goodness of fit (e.g., giving advance notice to children who are slow to adapt)
   d. Respite and support for caregivers

IV. Approach to Discipline

A. General principles
1. Way for parents/caregivers to teach children responsibility, self-reliance, and social skills
2. Successful discipline
   a. Developmentally appropriate and has reasonable expectations
   b. Used in context of supportive environment and loving relationship between caregiver and child
   c. Uses **positive reinforcement** and **modeling** of desired behaviors
   d. Consistency between caregivers and across situations is critical
   e. Uses removal of reinforcement to reduce undesired behaviors

B. Parenting styles: continuum from highly controlling to highly permissive, often influenced by cultural or religious beliefs
1. Authoritarian
   a. Parental authority valued over independent behavior of child
   b. Highly controlling, restrictive, and/or punitive
      i. Limited or no discussion about rules
      ii. "You will do this because I said so"
      iii. May use corporal punishment (i.e., spanking)
   c. Children can become rebellious/aggressive *or* submissive and dependent on parents as adolescents or adults
2. Permissive
   a. Child's independence valued over parental authority
   b. Undemanding, passive, allows children to stretch or break rules
   c. Belief that adult's role is to provide love and warmth and to allow child to make his or her own decisions
   d. Children may have difficulty with self-control and poor social skills as adolescents and adults

3. **Authoritative**
   a. Values parental authority to guide child's development
   b. Keeps consistent and firm limits and rules but listen to child's views
   c. Children more likely to be more socially competent, responsible, and independent as adolescents and adults

C. Developmental approach to effective discipline
1. Model appropriate behavior and be consistent with rules/expectations
2. Ages 0–24 months
   a. Say "no" calmly but firmly
   b. Provide distraction with different activity or object if child does not relinquish object or stop behavior
3. Beginning at age ~24 months, children learn rules and understand consequences of behavior
   a. "**Time-out**" is effective
      i. Verbally explain how behavior has broken rules
      ii. Place child in a consistent, safe, quiet but boring place
      iii. Caregiver should be removed from but aware of child and should not interact with child verbally until time-out is over
   b. Positive reinforcement
      i. Discuss expected behaviors with child and reward desired behaviors
      ii. Use sticker chart or other tokens for young child or obtaining privileges to reinforce desired behaviors
4. School-aged and adolescent children
   a. Continue to use positive reinforcement
   b. Natural consequences of behaviors can be instructive
   c. Remove privileges if rules are disobeyed

> **QUICK HIT**
> The authoritative parenting style is most effective.

> **QUICK HIT**
> Brief interventions on parenting early in childhood may have significant long-term impact on health.

> **QUICK HIT**
> A "time-out" should last 1 minute per year of age.

> **QUICK HIT**
> Spanking is used by >90% of U.S. families at some time.

DISEASE SPECIFIC

V. Attention-Deficit Hyperactivity Disorder

A. General characteristics
1. Significant impairment in functioning in at least 2 settings due to impulsivity, inattention, and/or hyperactivity
2. Classes of ADHD
   a. **Combined type**: most common; children have difficulty with attention/focus and some hyperactive/impulsive behaviors
   b. **Inattentive type**: 2nd most common; children do not have significant hyperactive or impulsive behaviors
   c. **Hyperactive-impulsive type**: more common in preschool age
3. Epidemiology
   a. Boys are affected 3:1 over girls
   b. U.S. rates are 5–10× greater than in other developed countries
4. Risk factors/causes: likely multifactorial
   a. Genetic
      i. Child of parent with ADHD has 25% chance of having ADHD
      ii. 55%–90% monozygotic twin concordance
      iii. Chromosomal abnormalities: Klinefelter, Turner syndrome, fragile X, neurofibromatosis type I, Williams, 22q11 deletion
   b. Environmental
      i. Low socioeconomic status
      ii. Parental mental disorder
      iii. Foster care
   c. Other
      i. Prematurity/low birth weight
      ii. Acquired traumatic brain injury
5. Pathophysiology: neural
   a. Neurotransmitters dopamine and norepinephrine modulate attention to and responses to environment

> **QUICK HIT**
> ADHD is one of the most prevalent neurodevelopmental conditions in childhood, affecting 7%–10% of school-aged children in the United States.

b. Putative defect in dopamine receptor D4 (*DRD4*) receptor gene and overexpression of dopamine transporter-1 (*DAT1*)
c. Imaging studies suggest anatomic differences
   i. Smaller right prefrontal cortex, caudate nucleus, and globus pallidus than age-matched controls
   ii. May suggest lack of connectivity of key brain regions that modulate attention, stimulus processing, and impulsivity

B. Clinical features
1. Preschool age
   a. Hyperactive or impulsive
   b. Not flexible
   c. May be aggressive toward peers
2. Elementary age
   a. Struggles with listening and compliance
   b. Difficulty completing tasks and poor organization skills
   c. Struggles with social interaction
   d. Not able to function independently
3. Adolescence
   a. Often able to cope early on in academic career, but history of some struggles with attention and focus
   b. Increased academic demands along with need for organization and independence become overwhelming
   c. Struggles with attention, learning, and executive functions

C. Diagnosis
1. Perform complete history to assess for symptoms of ADHD
2. Complete medical evaluation to evaluate growth and look for neurologic and genetic differences
   a. Rule out conditions with similar symptoms
      i. Anxiety disorders, depression
      ii. Auditory processing difficulty
      iii. Social difficulty
      iv. Sleep disturbance
      v. Substance abuse
      vi. Motor coordination: handwriting difficulty, problems with athletics
   b. Look for coexisting conditions: up to 2/3 of children with ADHD have coexisting disorder
      i. Anxiety, depression, or bipolar illness
      ii. Oppositional-defiant (50% concordance) (ODD) or conduct disorder (see Disruptive Behavioral Disorders)
      iii. Learning disorder
3. Review *DSM-IV* criteria (Table 15-1)
4. Recommend educational testing to look for learning disability

D. Treatment
1. Behavioral and family counseling
   a. Avoid distractions
   b. Family to increase praise and positive reinforcement
   c. Establish consistency
2. Social skills support to model, practice, and reinforce appropriate behavior
3. Educational interventions
   a. Modify class environment and class work
   b. Help with organization
   c. May require testing modifications
   d. Allow use of technology including tape recorder, laptop, and calculator to assist in meeting learning goals
4. Medication
   a. Stimulants (short- and long-acting options): 1st-line therapy
      i. Methylphenidate and mixed amphetamine salts

QUICK HIT

Use parent and teacher rating scales such as the Vanderbilt, ADHD 4, and Connors scales to evaluate for ADHD.

QUICK HIT

Consider getting a hearing test because it is common for children with a hearing deficit to be mislabeled as having an attention problem.

QUICK HIT

Implement a 504 plan and/or an individualized educational plan, if needed, for a child with ADHD.

QUICK HIT

Monitor growth and blood pressure while on stimulants; consider getting a baseline electrocardiogram prior to starting stimulants.

TABLE 15-1 ***DSM-IV* Criteria for Attention-Deficit Hyperactivity Disorder**

Inattention/distractibility
Often fails to give close attention to details or makes careless mistakes in schoolwork, work, or other activities
Often has difficulty sustaining attentions in tasks or play activities
Often does not seem to listen when spoken to directly
Often does not follow through on instructions and fails to finish schoolwork, chores, or duties in the workplace (not due to oppositional behavior or failure to understand instructions)
Often has difficulty organizing tasks and activities
Often avoids, dislikes, or is reluctant to engage in tasks that require sustained mental effort (such as schoolwork or homework)
Often loses things necessary for tasks or activities (e.g., toys, school assignments, pencils, books, or tools)
Often easily distracted by extraneous stimuli
Often forgetful in daily activities
Hyperactivity
Often fidgets with hands or feet or squirms in seat
Often leaves seat in classroom or in other situations in which remaining seated is expected
Often runs about or climbs excessively in situations in which it is inappropriate (in adolescents or adults, may be limited to subjective feelings of restlessness)
Often has difficulty playing or engaging in leisure activities quietly
Often "on the go" or acts as if "driven by a motor"
Often talks excessively
Impulsivity
Often blurts out answers before the questions have been completed
Often has difficulty waiting turn
Often interrupts or intrudes on others (e.g., butts into conversations or games)
To make a diagnosis
At least 6 symptoms from just Category A (ADHD, inattentive subtype), or just Category B (ADHD, hyperactive-impulsive subtype), or at least 6 symptoms from both categories (ADHD, combined subtype)
Symptoms are chronic (some symptoms were functionally impairing from before the age of 7), are clearly significantly impairing (in social, academic, or occupational functioning), ***are present across settings***
Symptoms do not occur exclusively during the course of a pervasive developmental disorder, schizophrenia, or other psychotic disorder and are not better accounted for by another mental disorder (e.g., mood, anxiety, dissociative, or personality disorder).

From American Psychiatric Association. *Diagnostic and Statistical Manual of Mental Disorders*. 4th ed. Arlington, VA: American Psychiatric Association; 1994.

ii. Side effects: **decreased appetite**, headache, stomachache, sleep difficulty, moodiness, tics, social withdrawal, elevated blood pressure, activation of mania or psychosis (very rare)

iii. **Rebound effects** (temporary worsening of symptoms when medication wears off)

b. Nonstimulants: norepinephrine reuptake inhibitor (atomoxetine)

i. Food and Drug Administration–approved for ADHD (age 6 years and older)

ii. Less effective than stimulants; may take several weeks to see benefit

iii. Can be used if coexisting conditions exist, including tics and anxiety, which may worsen with stimulants

iv. Side effects: **fatigue**, abdominal upset (decreases if given with food), dizziness, irritability, somnolence (but not as likely to cause sleep disturbance as stimulants are)

QUICK HIT

Atomoxetine includes a black box warning about suicidal ideation. Monitor the child for depression, mood instability, and activation.

c. α_2-Adrenergic agonists: clonidine and guanfacine
   i. Do not exacerbate tics
   ii. Can be helpful for sleep disturbance
   iii. Side effects: **sedation** (most common and may decrease over time), dry mouth, decreased compliance due to need for frequent dosing, decrease in blood pressure
   iv. Must be taken every day and cannot stop abruptly

VI. Autism Spectrum Disorders

A. Characteristics
   1. Definition: neurodevelopmental disorders categorized in *DSM-IV* under Pervasive Developmental Disorders
   2. Characterized by pervasive difficulties in
      a. Reciprocal social interaction
      b. Communication
      c. Repetitive or restricted behaviors, interests, or activities
   3. Categories (Table 15-2)
      a. Autism
      b. Asperger syndrome (AS)
      c. Pervasive developmental disorder not otherwise specified (PDD-NOS)

B. Epidemiology
   1. Prevalence estimated rate 1:110 children
   2. Boys > girls (4:1), ratio is closer to 2:1 with severe autism
   3. Risk for siblings is 5%–19%; if 2 siblings, recurrence risk = 8%–35%

TABLE 15-2 *DSM-IV* Diagnostic Criteria for Autistic Disorder

Six (or more) items from (1), (2), and (3), with at least 2 from (1), and 1 each from (2) and (3)
1. Qualitative impairment in social interaction, as manifested by at least 2 of the following: (a) Marked impairment in the use of multiple nonverbal behaviors such as eye-to-eye gaze, facial expression, body postures, and gestures to regulate social interaction (b) Failure to develop peer relationships appropriate to developmental level (c) Lack of spontaneous seeking to share enjoyment, interests, or achievements with other people (e.g., by a lack of showing, bringing, or pointing out objects of interest) (d) Lack of social or emotional reciprocity
2. Qualitative impairments in communication as manifested by at least 1 of the following: (a) Delay in, or total lack of, the development of spoken language (not accompanied by an attempt to compensate through alternative modes of communication such as gesture or mime) (b) In individuals with adequate speech, marked impairment in the ability to initiate or sustain a conversation with others (c) Stereotyped and repetitive use of language or idiosyncratic language (d) Lack of varied, spontaneous make-believe play or social imitative play appropriate to developmental level
3. Restricted repetitive and stereotyped patterns of behavior, interests, and activities, as manifested by at least 1 of the following: (a) Encompassing preoccupation with 1 or more stereotyped and restricted patterns of interest that is abnormal either in intensity or focus (b) Apparently inflexible adherence to specific, nonfunctional routines or rituals (c) Stereotyped and repetitive motor mannerisms (e.g., hand or finger flapping or twisting, or complex whole-body movements) (d) Persistent preoccupation with parts of objects
Delays or abnormal functioning in at least 1 of the following areas, with onset prior to age 3 years: (1) social interaction, (2) language as used in social communication, or (3) symbolic or imaginative play
The disturbance is not better accounted for by Rett disorder or childhood disintegrative disorder

C. Causes
  1. Idiopathic: most common
  2. Genetics: association with known genetic conditions = <10% of cases
  3. Risk factors
    a. Prenatal risk factors
      i. Teratogens (e.g., valproic acid, thalidomide)
      ii. Maternal infections
      iii. Advanced maternal and paternal age
    b. Perinatal factors
      i. Term newborn encephalopathy
      ii. Prematurity (age <35 weeks) and small for gestational age

D. Clinical presentation
  1. Pertinent clinical history signs and symptoms
    a. Social
      i. Lack of coordination of nonverbal communication, including gaze, facial expression, gesture, and sound
      ii. Lack of appropriate gaze
      iii. Lack of response to own name even while being aware of environmental sounds
    b. Language/communication
      i. No single word by age 16 months
      ii. No 2-word spontaneous language (nonechoed) phrases by age 24 months
      iii. Loss of language or speech at any age
      iv. No response to name after several attempts
      v. **Echolalia**: child repeats examiner's or parent's words
    c. Atypical behaviors
      i. **Stereotypies**: repetitive nonpurposeful movements such as flapping hands
      ii. Self-injurious behavior
      iii. Atypical play
        (a) Spinning wheels
        (b) Peering: examining toys/objects from odd angles
        (c) Lining objects up
        (d) Collecting objects but not using them
  2. Pertinent physical exam findings: may be found in some, but not all, children with an ASD
    a. Dysmorphic features: suggestive of genetic disorder (<10%)
    b. Macrocephaly (20%–30%): generally seen during 1st 2 years of life
    c. Hypotonia, motor delays (gross and/or fine motor), postural instability, motor incoordination, toe walking, and other gait abnormalities
  3. Common comorbidities and symptoms
    a. ID (30%–60%)
    b. Language disorders (5%–63%)
    c. Anxiety, depression, and/or obsessive-compulsive disorder (OCD) (25%–84%)
    d. Symptoms of ADHD (25%–60%)
    e. Self-injurious behaviors (up to 50%)
    f. Aggressive, irritable, or disruptive behavior (3%–32%)
    g. Hypo- or hypersensitivity to environmental stimuli (80%–90%)
    h. Seizures or tics (11%–49%)
    i. Gastrointestinal (GI) problems: food selectivity, gastroesophageal reflux (GER), constipation, and diarrhea (up to 70%)
    j. Sleep difficulties (44%–84%)

E. Testing
  1. Diagnosis: based on observed behaviors, and educational, developmental, and psychological evaluations
  2. Differential diagnosis
    a. Global developmental delay
    b. Speech and language disorder
    c. ADHD with associated social difficulties

QUICK HIT

There are *no* known causal links between vaccines (including measles-mumps-rubella and thimerosal-containing vaccines) and autism.

QUICK HIT

Children with ASDs typically present when socialization begins at daycare or at the start of schooling.

QUICK HIT

Children with ASDs do not show objects of interest to others.

QUICK HIT

Children with ASDs do not point or otherwise gesture by age 12 months.

QUICK HIT

ASD-specific screening should be done at the 18- and 24/30-month well-child visits.

QUICK HIT

There are *no* medical tests to confirm a diagnosis of an ASD.

QUICK HIT

For patients with ASD, early detection and treatment are critically important for improved outcomes.

QUICK HIT

Every child with a suspected ASD should be referred for an education assessment. Referral should not wait for an official diagnosis.

QUICK HIT

There are no confirmatory laboratory tests for ASDs, but consider supplemental testing.

QUICK HIT

Comprehensive individualized treatment programs are necessary for children with ASDs.

QUICK HIT

Out of desperation, some parents may turn to ineffective and even harmful so-called cures for ASD such as chelation therapy.

QUICK HIT

Separation anxiety from caregivers is a *normal* developmental milestone in infancy seen at ages 10–18 months.

- d. Anxiety and other affective disorders
- e. Hearing impairment
- f. Seizure disorder
- g. Rett syndrome
- h. Neurodegenerative disorders

3. Educational evaluation with a comprehensive, multidisciplinary ASD team
4. Audiologic evaluation
5. Supplemental laboratory testing
   - a. If estimated IQ or developmental quotient (DQ) = 50–75: consider sending genome-wide array, fragile X testing
   - b. In females with estimated IQ or DQ <50: send above and add MECP2 to test for **Rett syndrome**
   - c. If macrocephaly present, consider genome-wide array and fragile X testing
   - d. If dysmorphic features seen, refer to genetics and send genome-wide array
   - e. For children with history of substantial regression or lethargy, consider metabolic workup and EEG in addition to the previously mentioned tests
   - f. Radiologic imaging: *not* routinely recommended unless neurologic abnormalities present (e.g., microcephaly, new-onset or rapidly progressing macrocephaly, or focal neurologic signs)
   - g. EEG
     - i. *Not* routinely recommended
     - ii. If history concerning for seizures or significant regression, consider obtaining EEG and/or neurology evaluation

F. Treatment

1. Provide parent education/parent training and family support
2. Educational interventions
   - a. Behavioral, communication, and socialization interventions should be incorporated into **educational program**
   - b. Adjunctive therapies: speech, occupational and physical therapy
3. Pharmacotherapy: medications for associated symptoms
   - a. Irritability including aggression, tantrums, self-injurious behaviors: may improve with atypical antipsychotics and anticonvulsants
   - b. ADHD symptoms: stimulants, α_2-agonists
   - c. Anxiety: selective serotonin reuptake inhibitors (SSRIs)
   - d. Repetitive behaviors: SSRIs, risperidone
4. Complementary and alternative medications and treatments (CAMs): common in families of children with an ASD (52%–95%); providers should ask about and inform families of risks and benefits of CAM therapies
5. Prognosis: most children (at least 81%) continue to be on spectrum throughout their lives

VII. Anxiety Disorders

A. Definition

1. Functional impairment due to inappropriate worries, ruminations, and/or fears inconsistent with child's developmental stage and situation
2. Symptoms are persistent and cause significant distress and dysfunction

B. Causes

1. 36%–65% with family history of anxiety disorder
2. Environmental risk factors
   - a. Insecure parent–child attachment
   - b. Anxious/controlling parenting styles
   - c. Food/shelter insecurity
   - d. Exposure to violence or traumatic events
   - e. Parental substance abuse

C. Clinical presentation

1. **Generalized anxiety disorder**
   - a. Excessive worry/anxiety on most days, which is *not* situation or object specific and is *not* triggered by recent stressful events

b. Difficulty concentrating and feelings of restlessness
c. Sleep disturbances
2. **Separation disorder**
a. Persistent/excessive **fear** of being alone or separated from parent/caregiver/attachment figure
b. Distress with anticipated or actual separation
c. Persistent school refusal
d. Worry about harm/death to attachment figure
3. OCD
a. Persistent, recurrent, or intrusive thoughts or behaviors that cause significant distress
b. **Repetitive behaviors** or mental processes that child feels compelled to perform (e.g., handwashing, ritualistic cleaning)

D. Treatment: multimodal approach
1. Parent–child and family behavioral strategies and psychotherapy
2. Cognitive-behavioral therapy
3. Medication: should be used cautiously
a. SSRIs: some short-term efficacy in pediatric anxiety disorders (especially OCD), but long-term efficacy/risks have not been evaluated
b. Benzodiazepines: limited efficacy; can develop dependency

QUICK HIT

Anxiety disorders are due to multifactorial causes.

QUICK HIT

Separation disorder interferes with daily life. Separation anxiety does not interfere with daily life and occurs in younger children.

VIII. Disruptive Behavioral Disorders

A. Definition: mental health disorders with features of disobedience, anger, explosiveness, and defiance of authority figures causing significant impairment in social and school functioning

B. Causes/risk factors
1. Biologic: often family history of DBD, ADHD, mood or personality disorders
2. Environmental/social
a. **Authoritarian** or coercive parenting
b. Poverty and food/shelter insecurity
c. Exposure to violence and traumatic events

C. Clinical presentation
1. **ODD**
a. Persistent anger, argumentativeness, and resistant behaviors directed especially toward **authority** figures
b. Usually presents in *preschool* years
2. **Conduct disorder**
a. Persistent, serious, and potentially destructive behaviors that violate societal or legal rules
b. Characterized by **physical aggression** resulting in destruction to persons, animals, or property

D. Testing
1. Screening tools
a. Connors Rating Scales
b. Buss-Perry Aggression Questionnaire
c. Anger, Irritability, and Aggression Questionnaire
2. Referral to mental health professional for *DSM-IV-TR* diagnosis

E. Treatment: multimodal
1. Parent management training aimed at redirecting parent–child interactions
2. Social skills training with child
3. Medication
a. Atypical antipsychotics are most commonly prescribed medications
b. Divalproex sodium and lithium carbonate are used as mood stabilizers

QUICK HIT

Boys are more prone to DBDs than girls by a ratio of 3:1.

IX. Mood Disorders

A. Definition: mental health disorders characterized by depressed, elevated, or mixed moods, resulting in significant functional impairment in school or social environment

QUICK HIT

Mood disorders have a high comorbidity rate with other psychiatric disorders.

QUICK HIT

Depressive disorder is equally common in young boys and girls, but, by adolescence, it is more common in girls.

QUICK HIT

Suicide is the 3rd leading cause of death of all 15–18-year-olds, after accidents and homicide.

B. Causes/risk factors
  1. 4–6× increase in risk if mood disorder in 1st-degree family member
  2. Psychosocial deprivation
  3. Exposure to violence and trauma
C. Clinical presentation
  1. **Depressive disorder**
    a. Depressed mood
    b. Decreased interest in activities
    c. Disturbances of sleep and appetite
    d. Fatigue
    e. Feelings of worthlessness or inappropriate guilt
    f. Difficulty concentrating or making decisions
    g. Thoughts of death/suicidal ideation without plan
    h. Suicide attempt with plan
  2. **Bipolar 1 disorder (BPD)**
    a. Exaggerated self-esteem/grandiosity
    b. Limited need for sleep (*less common in children than adults*)
    c. Pressured speech
    d. Flight of ideas/racing thoughts
    e. Psychomotor agitation or obsession with completing tasks
    f. Engaging in high-risk behaviors
    g. Irritability, rage, and explosive behaviors may be phenotype of "mania" in children
D. Treatment
  1. Depressive disorders: best response with combination of medication and supportive therapy
    a. Family/individual psychotherapy
    b. Cognitive-behavioral therapy
    c. Medications: SSRIs (1st line), tricyclic antidepressants (TCAs)
  2. Bipolar disorders: medication is primary treatment
    a. "Mood stabilizers": lithium, valproate
    b. Atypical antipsychotics: aripiprazole, olanzapine, risperidone, quetiapine, ziprasidone

X. Hearing Impairment

QUICK HIT

In the U.S., 1–3 per 1,000 infants have some form of hearing loss.

QUICK HIT

Signs of potential hearing loss include not turning the head to sound by age 6 months and delayed language development.

A. General characteristics: types of hearing loss
  1. **Conductive**: mechanical problem of conduction of air from middle/outer ear to inner ear
  2. **Sensorineural**: caused by damage to inner ear and/or cranial nerve VIII
  3. **Mixed**: both conductive and sensorineural components
B. Causes
  1. Conductive hearing loss
    a. Otitis externa, otitis media, eustachian tube dysfunction
    b. Genetic craniofacial syndromes such as **Treacher-Collins**, Apert
  2. Sensorineural hearing loss
    a. Neonatal intensive care unit stay >5 days
    b. Family history of permanent hearing loss
    c. Genetic syndromes: CHARGE, Cornelia de Lange, **neurofibromatosis type II**, trisomy 21
    d. Congenital infections: cytomegalovirus, rubella
    e. Sequelae of meningitis
    f. Exposure to ototoxic medications
    g. Very high neonatal bilirubin levels
C. Testing
  1. Physical exam
    a. Examine outer ear for any anomalies
    b. Look at patency of external auditory meatus and for obstruction in external auditory canal

c. Evaluate tympanic membrane for mobility, signs of infection, and effusion
2. Audiometry
a. **Tympanograph**: physiologic exam of tympanic membrane mobility
b. Otoacoustic emissions: measures acoustic transduction from external auditory meatus to cochlear outer hair cells
c. **Auditory brainstem response**: measures auditory stimulus transduction to brainstem

D. Treatment
1. Hearing aids
a. Electronic amplification of sounds
b. Bone conduction hearing aides
c. Cochlear implants: for severe to profound sensorineural hearing loss
2. Early intervention referral for appropriate speech therapy

XI. Colic

A. Definition
1. Intense crying in infants ages 1–6 months who are not consoled with common calming techniques such as feeding, changing diaper, rocking, burping, holding
2. Crying tends to happen at same time every day, often in early evening
3. Usually starting at ages 2–6 weeks; symptoms often start/stop quickly
4. Not attributed to medical causes (Box 15-1)

B. Causes
1. No clear single etiology; likely a combination of GI discomfort, nervous system immaturity, and psychosocial influences
a. GI causes including milk protein intolerance, GER, gassiness
b. Psychosocial
i. Temperament: "goodness of fit" of child's temperament and parent's coping skills (see III. Approach to Child Temperament)
ii. Parental anxiety about caring for infant
c. Neurologic: immature self-regulation/self-calming ability
d. Environmental: overstimulation with noise, light, handling

C. Testing: thorough history and physical exam including appropriate growth
1. Look for signs of musculoskeletal, neurologic injury
2. Laboratory investigation is rarely indicated

D. Treatment
1. Acknowledge parent's stress and emphasize that colic is a common phenomenon and is not due to poor parenting
2. Trial of antacids or simethicone is commonly used, but there is little evidence of efficacy
3. Feed baby in upright position with frequent burping
4. Reduce extra stimulation
5. Try soothing music, **swaddling**, massaging
6. Babies may calm while sucking on pacifier with gentle swaying on their side

BOX 15-1

Differential Diagnosis of Crying Infant: IT CRIESS

I: Infections (urinary tract infection, meningitis, osteomyelitis)
T: Trauma (nonaccidental and accidental), testicular torsion
C: Cardiac problems
R: Reflux, reactions to formula, reactions to medications
I: Immunizations, insect bites
E: Eye, corneal abrasions
S: Surgical issues: volvulus, intussusception, inguinal hernia
S: Strangulation from hair tourniquet

QUICK HIT

All infants should receive a newborn hearing screen by age 1 month and then be informally screened in the office regularly. Formal hearing testing should be performed at ages 4, 5, 6, 8, 10, 12, 15, and 18 years.

QUICK HIT

Cochlear implants are controversial in the deaf community.

MNEMONIC

"Rule of 3s" can help identify colic:
Crying lasts at least **3** hours/day
Occurs on >**3** days/week
Present for at least **3** weeks

QUICK HIT

Although changing formula is commonly done, true milk protein intolerance is a very rare cause of colic.

QUICK HIT

Colic is a diagnosis of exclusion for the fussy baby.

QUICK HIT

For acute-onset fussiness, do a fluorescein exam of the eyes and inspect the digits and genitals for a hair tourniquet.

QUICK HIT

Up to 40% of infants experience colic.

TABLE 15-3 Comparison of Nightmares and Night Terrors

Nightmares	Night Terrors
Any age	Ages 3–8 years
Boys = girls	More common in boys
Occur in REM sleep	Occur in non-REM sleep
Occur in last 1/3 of sleep	Occur in first 1/3 of sleep
Child awakens	Child *appears* awake
Child can be consoled	Child is inconsolable
Child remembers episode	Child does not remember episode

non-REM, non-rapid eye movement; REM, rapid eye movement.

XII. Sleep and Sleep Disorders

A. Normal sleep
  1. Normal circadian sleep with true rapid eye movement (REM; dreaming), non-REM (deep sleep) cycles becomes established ~age 3 months
  2. Most infants sleep through night by age 3 months

B. Clinical presentation
  1. Night terrors (Table 15-3)
    a. Caused by immaturity of nervous system
    b. Often associated with stress, illness, overtiredness
    c. History alone is usually sufficient for diagnosis
    d. Treatment includes reassurance of parents of benign nature of events and that child will eventually outgrow
  2. Nightmares (Table 15-3)
  3. Obstructive sleep apnea (see Chapter 19)

XIII. Breath-Holding Spells

A. Definition
  1. Paroxysmal events resulting in apnea, **color change**, change in muscle tone, and brief **loss of consciousness** in young child
  2. Typically seen at ages 6–18 months

B. Causes and clinical presentation (Table 15-4)
  1. Immature brain regulation of autonomic nervous system
  2. Possible genetic link: family history is positive in 25%–35% cases

> **QUICK HIT**
> With night terrors, emphasize the importance of a calm bedtime routine and avoiding scary television or movies.

> **QUICK HIT**
> "Breath holding" is a misnomer: the event is triggered by exhalation not inhalation.

> **QUICK HIT**
> A breath-holding spell is *not* a seizure, but anoxia can induce seizures and cardiac arrhythmias in 15% of cases.

> **QUICK HIT**
> Breath-holding spells are often mistaken for seizures by parents.

TABLE 15-4 Clinical Presentation of Breath-Holding Spells

Cyanotic Breath-Holding (most common)	Pallid Breath-Holding
Forced expiration or Valsalva increases intrathoracic pressure ↓ decreases cardiac output ↓ decreases flow of blood to the brain ↓ loss of consciousness	Vagally mediated *cardiac* inhibition ↓ bradycardia or asystole ↓ decreases cerebral blood flow ↓ loss of consciousness
Triggered by temper tantrum, crying, anger, frustration, hyperventilation	Triggered by sudden stimulus (acute pain, fright) Generally no or very little crying preceding event
Child holds breath on exhalation, turns blue (cyanotic), becomes limp or stiff, and may lose consciousness (generally <1 minute)	Child becomes pale, apneic with rapid loss of consciousness

Developmental and Behavioral Disorders

C. Testing, primarily a clinical diagnosis with no workup necessary
D. Treatment
1. Largely supportive; provide reassurance to frightened caregivers
2. Emphasize benign nature of event
3. Educate parents to management of temper tantrums
4. Emphasize avoidance of precipitating events
5. Iron supplementation (even in absence of anemia) has been shown to reduce frequency of episodes

XIV. Toilet Training

A. Definition
1. Training young child to control his or her bladder and bowels
2. Bladder control usually precedes bowel control beginning around 2 years
3. Girls usually achieve continence before boys
4. Generally, continence is achieved by ages 3–4 years
B. Treatment
1. Child-oriented approach is recommended
2. Start when child is emotionally and developmentally ready
a. Has ability to sense urge to urinate or defecate
b. Has ability to tighten external sphincters
c. Has ability to follow simple directions and communicate simple desire
3. Emphasize and praise success
4. Avoid punishment and showing signs of disappointment; *never* punish child for soiling
5. Toilet-training technique
a. Start by letting child sit on "potty seat" while clothed, then sit on potty with diaper off
b. Show child that stool from diaper goes into toilet; let child flush toilet
c. Put child on toilet when he or she signals urge to go and/or at frequent intervals

XV. Enuresis

A. Definition
1. Voluntary or involuntary release of urinary bladder contents after developmental age when bladder control should be achieved
2. Occurring at least twice weekly for at least 3 consecutive months
3. **Primary enuresis** if continence has never been achieved
4. **Secondary enuresis** if child had achieved at least 6 months of dryness before developing enuresis
5. Daytime continence usually achieved between ages 2 and 4 years
6. Nighttime continence usually achieved by ages 4–5 years
B. Causes/pathophysiology
1. **Nocturnal enuresis**
a. Immaturity of cortical control of bladder
b. Genetic: strong family history
c. Decreased functional bladder capacity
d. Alteration in circadian vasopressin
2. **Daytime incontinence**: more common in girls; most commonly caused by waiting too long to void
3. Children with both forms at age 5 years are more likely to have anatomic abnormalities
C. Testing: rule out organic etiology if suspected from history or exam, especially in cases of secondary enuresis
1. Urinary tract infection
2. Diabetes mellitus
3. Spinal cord lesion/anomaly, compression, or mass
4. Overactive bladder
5. Chemical urethritis irritation from bubble baths or soap

QUICK HIT

75% of children with enuresis wet only at night.

QUICK HIT

Giggle (or **stress**) **incontinence** is seen most commonly in girls between ages 7 and 15 years and is due to sudden relaxation of the urinary sphincter during giggling or the Valsalva maneuver, resulting in loss of total urinary volume in the bladder.

QUICK HIT

Treatment for enuresis needs to focus on positive reinforcement, not punishment.

QUICK HIT

A monitor will wake the child the instant moistness is detected.

QUICK HIT

Boys are more commonly affected than girls, by about 6:1!

QUICK HIT

The child experiences "leakage" around the mass that is difficult to expel.

QUICK HIT

Parents can mistake encopresis for diarrhea.

QUICK HIT

Consider referral to a mental health provider if tantrums are disrupting the ability of the child, class, or family to function, *or* if behavior includes significant aggression or a self-injurious component.

QUICK HIT

Approximately 6% of school-aged children in the United States receive special educational services.

6. Physical trauma
7. Sexual abuse

D. Treatment
1. Behavior modification
   a. Waking child up during night to void
   b. Use buzzer or other aides to wake child when wet
2. Medication
   a. **Antidiuretic hormone**: immediate effect, for episodic use
   b. TCAs (e.g., imipramine)
3. Reassurance: many outgrow symptoms

XVI. Encopresis

A. Definition: daytime or nighttime stool soiling beyond stage of typical toilet training, usually ~age 4 years

B. Causes
1. Chronic constipation
   a. Causes rectal distension
   b. Larger volumes of stool are required to produce sensation to defecate
2. Emotional stressors can cause temporary regression in child's ability to control bowels

C. Clinical presentation
1. "Streaking" of stool in underwear
2. Large stools, which can clog toilet
3. Abdominal pain, loss of appetite

D. Testing
1. Digital rectal exam to assess tone and presence of hard stool in rectal vault
2. Abdominal x-ray may reveal large amount of stool in large intestine

E. Treatment
1. Complete evacuation of bowels with **polyethylene glycol**, stool softeners, enemas
2. Next establish good bowel habits with frequent trips to bathroom
3. **High-fiber diet**; increase fluids and limit consumption of milk
4. If constipation is not cause, consider psychological counseling

XVII. Temper Tantrums

A. Definition
1. Episodes of crying, yelling, screaming, falling to floor, flailing arms/legs, throwing objects often in response to being told "no"
2. Typical of children ages 1–4 years

B. Causes
1. Immature ability to communicate wants, needs, feelings, or frustrations
2. Inflexible or explosive temperament
3. Inconsistent parental expectations

C. Clinical presentation
1. Physical examination to ensure no other underlying pathologic process or illness can explain child's behavior
2. History of any delays or atypical qualities in development
3. Review triggers that can contribute to worsening tantrum behaviors

D. Treatment
1. Ignore behaviors
2. Respond calmly without raising voice
3. State limits and expectations for child's behaviors
4. Use **time-out** technique
5. Praise child when expectations for behavior are met
6. **Consistency** of rules between caregivers is critical

XVIII. Learning Disorders

A. Definition: difficulty mastering age-expected academic material including oral and written expression, reading skills, and math skills *despite normal IQ*

B. Causes
   1. Children with neurogenetic syndromes have higher risk
   2. Often strong family history of learning disorders, ADHD, or special education
   3. Prematurity: 50%–70% of low-birth-weight infants (<1,500 g) have learning disorders
C. Clinical presentation
   1. History of developmental delays, especially in speech and language
   2. Academic problems, incomplete homework, failing grades
   3. Behavioral and emotional problems
D. Testing/screening
   1. Psychoeducational testing by qualified school psychologist
   2. Medical workup rarely indicated unless suggested by history or exam
E. Treatment
   1. Modified classroom instruction
   2. **Individualized educational plan (IEP)**/special education
   3. Grade retention *not* generally recommended

QUICK HIT

The cause of most learning disorders is unknown.

16 Dysmorphology and Genetic Disorders

QUICK HIT

Taking a family history can be life changing for a patient. For example, identification of a strong family history of breast cancer may trigger *BRCA* testing and result in prophylactic mastectomy.

QUICK HIT

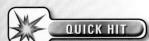

Mitochondrial inheritance refers to inheritance from the mitochondrial DNA, which is only passed on through the maternal oocyte. The nuclear genome also codes for many components of the mitochondria. Therefore, mitochondrial disease can have classic mitochondrial inheritance or can be autosomal dominant, autosomal recessive, or X-linked.

QUICK HIT

Some diseases have variable penetrance, which can make the inheritance pattern challenging on family history.

QUICK HIT

Recognition of dysmorphology aids in diagnosis. Once a genetic diagnosis is suspected, genetic testing may be offered.

SYMPTOM SPECIFIC

I. Approach to Taking a Family History and Genetic Counseling

A. Standard family history questions include
  1. Ethnic background
  2. Presence/absence of consanguinity
  3. Family members' ages, health problems, and causes of death
  4. Issues with pregnancy for patient and other relatives
  5. History of unintentional spontaneous abortion in family
  6. Degree of relationship (Table 16-1)

B. Pedigree symbols (Figure 16-1)

C. Diagnosis: analyze pedigree for pattern of inheritance (Table 16-2)

D. Genetic counseling provides information regarding disease presentation, management, inheritance, and future prenatal counseling

II. Approach to Child with Unusual Physical Findings and Clinical Malformations

A. General characteristics
  1. History
    a. Details of pregnancy, delivery, and neonatal course
    b. Medical and developmental history
    c. Family history
  2. Complete physical examination looking for signs of dysmorphology

B. Clinical presentation
  1. **Major congenital anomalies**: abnormalities of major surgical or cosmetic significance, such as congenital heart defects and diaphragmatic hernia
  2. **Minor congenital anomalies**: unusual morphologic features not of serious consequence, such as transverse palmar creases or preauricular ear pits; ~15% may be present in otherwise normal infants

C. Pathophysiology: important definitions
  1. **Malformation**: morphologic defect of organ, part of organ, or larger region that results from intrinsically abnormal developmental process (Tables 16-3 and 16-4)

TABLE 16-1 **Degree of Relationship**

Degree of Relationship	Example
First degree	Parents, children, brothers, sisters
Second degree	Grandparents, aunts and uncles, nieces and nephews, grandchildren
Third degree	First cousin

FIGURE 16-1 **Pedigrees.**

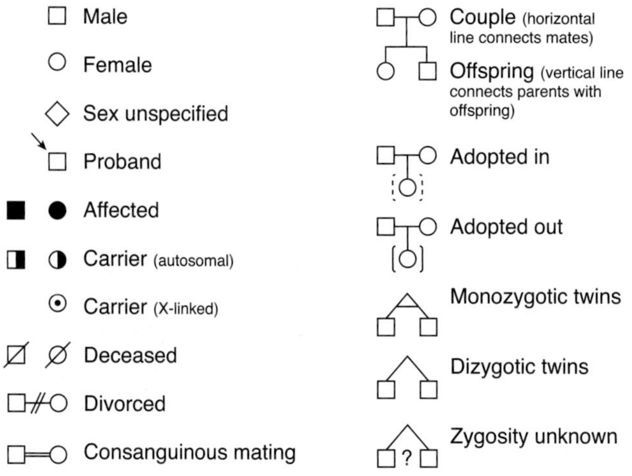

QUICK HIT

Dysmorphology is the study of abnormal development of tissue.

QUICK HIT

Major congenital anomalies are present in ~3%–5% of the general population.

QUICK HIT

When 3 or more minor anomalies are present, examine carefully to look for a more serious defect.

TABLE 16-2 Patterns of Inheritance

Pattern of Inheritance	Description	Characteristics in a Pedigree	Example(s)
Autosomal dominant	1 mutated copy of a gene in each cell is sufficient to cause a problem	Often an affected parent; often seen in every generation; males = females	Huntington disease, neurofibromatosis type I
Autosomal recessive	2 mutated copies of the gene necessary to cause disease	Look for sibships; consanguinity increases risk; some disorders have an increased carrier frequency in certain ethnic groups	Cystic fibrosis, sickle cell anemia, Tay-Sachs disease, spinal muscular atrophy
X-linked	Females often asymptomatic or less severely affected than males	Males cannot pass on to sons but can pass on to daughters; females may have multiple affected sons	Hemophilia; Duchenne muscular dystrophy
X-linked commonly lethal in males	Manifests very severely in males, and if lethal in utero, the disease may paradoxically only manifest in girls	Male miscarriages may be present	Incontinentia pigmenti; Rett syndrome
Mitochondrial	Refers to inheritance of genes in mitochondrial DNA	Males do not pass on to children; mothers pass on to all children (although some signs may be subtle or manifest later in life)	Leigh syndrome (LS), mitochondrial encephalomyopathy with lactic acidosis and stroke-like episodes (MELAS)
Multifactorial	Combination of multiple genes and interactions between genes and environment	Familial clustering sometimes seen; often shows predilection for one gender (pyloric stenosis more common in males)	Normal traits: height, intelligence Diseases: type 2 diabetes, hypertension, obesity, isolated cleft lip and palate, isolated clubfoot

TABLE 16-3 Patterns of Malformation

Type	Definition	Example(s)
Syndrome	A pattern of anomalies due to or thought to be due to a single specific cause	Down syndrome, Marfan syndrome, fetal alcohol syndrome
Sequence	An underlying anomaly giving rise to a cascade of secondary problems	Pierre-Robin sequence: micrognathia, leading to posterior displacement of the tongue → failure of the palatine shelves to fuse → cleft palate
Association	A nonrandom combination of anomalies that occur together more frequently than expected by chance	VACTERL (vertebral, anal, cardiac, tracheo-esophageal, renal, limb anomalies)

2. **Deformation**
   a. Abnormal shape or position caused by mechanical forces
   b. Many deformations are produced by intrauterine constraint, but some are associated with underlying abnormality that causes susceptibility to mechanical forces
   c. Example: spina bifida → poor motor innovation of leg in utero → leg more likely to incur mechanical forces → clubfoot

TABLE 16-4 Genetic Causes of Malformations

Etiology	Definition	Example	Common Testing Strategy
Chromosomal	An extra chromosome is present, or a chromosome is absent	Trisomy 21, trisomy 18, trisomy 13, Turner syndrome (XO), Klinefelter syndrome (XXY)	Karyotype or array comparative genomic hybridization (aCGH), a test that looks across all of the chromosomes for deletions or duplications
Microdeletion/ microduplication syndrome	A piece of a chromosome, sometimes too small to see on a conventional karyotype, is either missing or doubled	Williams syndrome (7q11.2), 22q11 deletion syndrome, 1p36 deletion syndrome	Fluorescent in situ hybridization (FISH) or aCGH
Trinucleotide repeat syndromes	Caused by expansion of certain nucleotide triplets, which leads to instability of the DNA or abnormal expression of the involved genes	Fragile X syndrome, Huntington disease, myotonic dystrophy	DNA with polymerase chain reaction and Southern blot to count repeat number
Epigenetic changes	A change not in the sequence or amount of DNA, but rather gene expression, such as methylation (turning off a gene) or hypomethylation (turning on a gene)	Beckwith-Wiedemann syndrome, some cases of Prader-Willi or Angelman syndrome	DNA methylation studies

3. **Disruption**
   a. Morphologic defect of organ or larger region resulting from extrinsic breakdown of, or interference with, originally normal developmental process
   b. Example: amniotic band syndrome
4. **Dysplasia**
   a. Abnormal development at macroscopic level
   b. Example: ectodermal dysplasia (abnormal development of sweat glands, skin, teeth, nails)

DISEASE SPECIFIC

III. Trisomy 21/Down Syndrome (DS)

A. General characteristics
1. Due to 3 copies of chromosome 21, associated with characteristic facial features, hypotonia, intellectual disability, and congenital malformations
2. Genetics
   a. 94% of DS cases occur de novo due to meiotic nondisjunction
   b. 6% of DS cases are due to **Robertsonian translocations**
      i. Common form of chromosomal rearrangement occurring in acrocentric chromosome pairs (those with short arm)
      ii. Typically, between 2 of these chromosomes, p-arms will form own very small chromosome, called a "**satellite**," and q-arms will form new, larger chromosome
      iii. Satellite may be lost, but contains very little important genetic information, so carrier is usually phenotypically normal because there are 2 copies of all essential genes
      iv. However, offspring of carrier may inherit extra 21, causing DS
   c. Rarely, **mosaicism** (some cells contain trisomy 21, some do not); does not guarantee that child will be less affected (Figure 16-2)
3. Risk factors
   a. Risk in general population is 1:800
   b. Risk increases with advanced maternal age: at age 35 years, risk is ~1:270 at time of delivery

FIGURE 16-2 Typical features of a child with Down syndrome: (A) facial features and (B) horizontal palm crease (simian line).

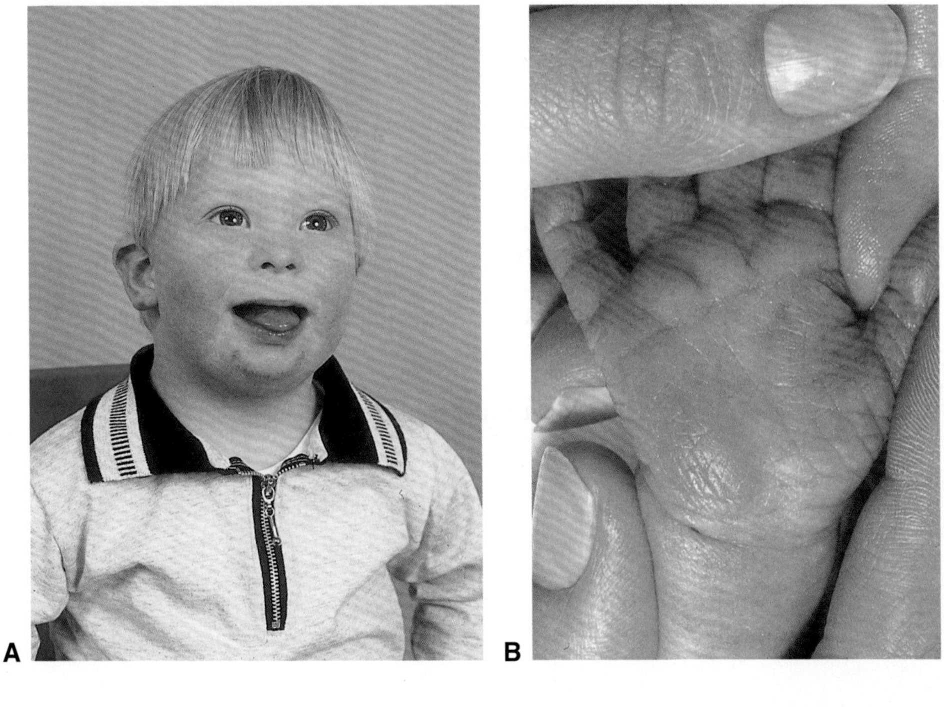

Dysmorphology and Genetic Disorders

QUICK HIT

Hypotonia is the most common presenting sign of DS.

B. Clinical presentation
   1. Historical findings at birth include hypotonia and feeding difficulties
   2. Physical exam findings
      a. Dysmorphic features
         i. Epicanthal folds and upslanting palpebral fissures
         ii. Midface hypoplasia
         iii. Brachycephaly
         iv. Excessive skin behind neck
         v. Transverse palmar creases
         vi. "Sandal gap" (large space between 1st and 2nd toes)
         vii. Brushfield spots (common; white/gray/brown spots in iris)
      b. Systemic features
         i. Congenital heart disease (CHD) (50%); most common is endocardial cushion defect
         ii. Duodenal atresia (~12%)
         iii. Congenital hypothyroidism (1%) and acquired thyroid disease
         iv. Hearing loss and otitis media
         v. Eye disease such as cataracts and refractive errors
         vi. Poor growth (use special growth charts for DS patients)
         vii. Hematologic problems and increased risk for childhood leukemia
         viii. Increase risk for celiac disease
         ix. Atlantoaxial instability

C. Testing
   1. Diagnostic screening tests
      a. Maternal serum screening
         i. 1st-trimester screening (performed between 11 and 14 weeks of pregnancy)
         ii. 2nd-trimester triple or quad screen (performed between 15 and 17 weeks of pregnancy)
      b. Level II fetal ultrasound scan may show abnormalities
   2. Diagnostic tests
      a. Chorionic villus sampling ([CVS] performed between 10 and 12 weeks' gestation)
      b. Amniocentesis (between 16 and 20 weeks' gestation)
      c. Rapid fluorescence in situ hybridization (FISH) for trisomy 18 followed by karyotype or array comparative genomic hybridization (aCGH)
      d. Karyotype after birth on baby's blood confirms diagnosis and determines whether de novo or associated with translocation

QUICK HIT

Routine neck x-rays to rule out atlantoaxial instability were previously recommended, but in 2011, that recommendation changed to verbal screening for signs/symptoms of neck instability because x-rays do not predict severity of symptoms or future instability.

IV. Trisomy 18 (Edwards Syndrome)

A. General characteristics
   1. Due to 3 copies of chromosome 18 and associated with characteristic dysmorphic features, severe intellectual disability, congenital malformations, and greatly reduced life expectancy
   2. Epidemiology
      a. Incidence ~1/8,000 live births
      b. Females > males
      c. 95% of trisomy 18 conceptions are spontaneously aborted (Figure 16-3)
   3. Genetics: >90% caused by meiotic nondisjunction of maternal chromosomes
   4. Risk factors: increased risk with advanced maternal age

B. Clinical presentation
   1. Low birth weight
   2. CHD (90%), most commonly ventricular septal defect
   3. Dysmorphic features
      a. **Micrognathia** (small jaw)
      b. Microcephaly
      c. Prominent occiput

QUICK HIT

Of babies born with trisomy 18, 50% die within the 1st week, and most babies die within the 1st year. However, there are some long-term survivors who may live until late childhood.

FIGURE 16-3 **Infant with trisomy 18. A. Note the low-set ears and micrognathia. B. Note clenched hands.**

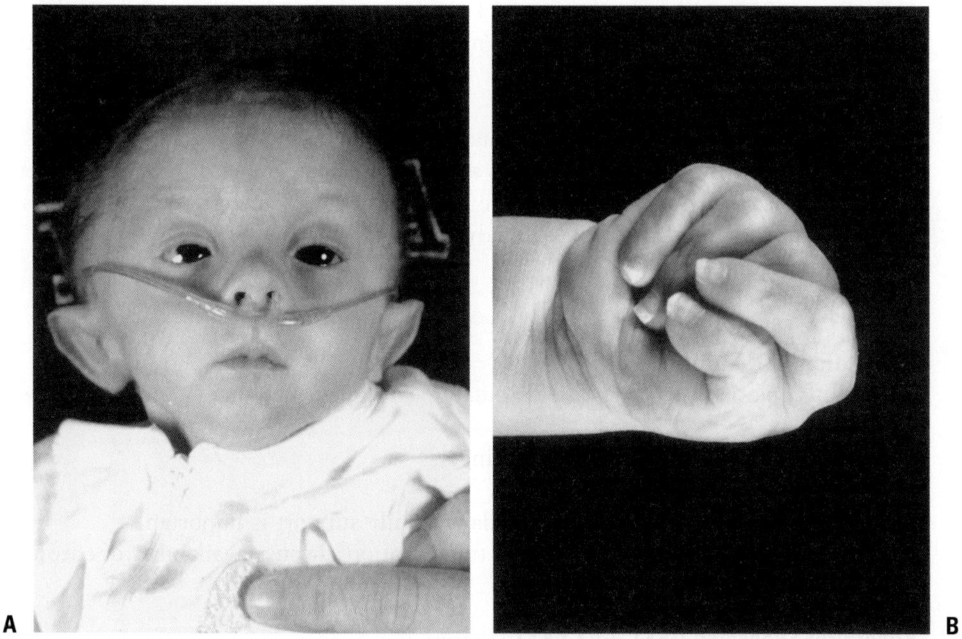

(From MacDonald MG, Seshia MMK, Mullett MD. *Avery's Neonatology Pathophysiology & Management of the Newborn.* 6th ed. Philadelphia: Lippincott Williams & Wilkins; 2005.)

d. Low-set ears
e. Clenched hands
f. "Rocker-bottom" feet (prominent calcaneus and inverted, round arch) (Figure 16-4)

4. Severe intellectual disability
5. Kidney defects: horseshoe kidney, hydronephrosis, polycystic kidney
6. Digestive tract abnormalities: esophageal atresia, omphalocele

C. Therapy varies according to anomalies
1. Cardiopulmonary arrest is most common cause of death
2. Hospice, grief counseling, and support group services
3. Parental chromosomal studies if baby's karyotype was due to a Robertsonian translocation

QUICK HIT

"Rocker-bottom feet" and characteristically clenched hands with overlapping digits are the most distinct clinical feature of trisomy 18.

FIGURE 16-4 **Rocker-bottom feet.**

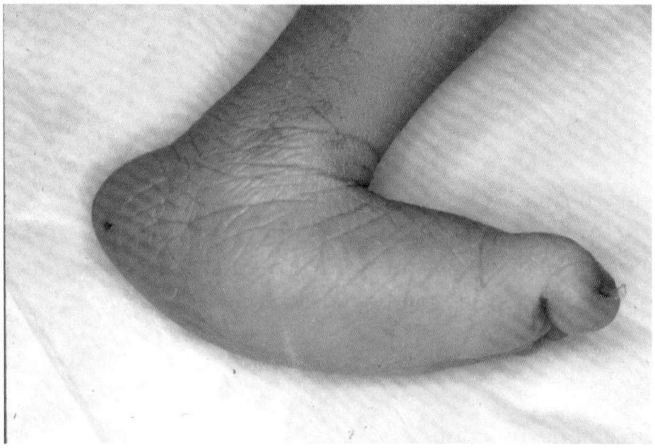

(Courtesy of Gerardo Cabrera-Meza, MD.)

QUICK HIT

Many of the congenital abnormalities of trisomy 13 are not compatible with life; 80% of newborns do not survive past their first month. However, if babies survive past the first year, they may live until early childhood.

QUICK HIT

Postaxial polydactyly (pinky side) or ulnar polydactyly can be familial and isolated or part of a syndrome, so it is important to always ask whether other family members have polydactyly.

QUICK HIT

Most chromosomal abnormalities are the result of maternal nondisjunction, but TS is an exception and can be due to paternal nondisjunction.

QUICK HIT

Of TS pregnancies, 99% miscarry by the 2nd trimester due to lymphedema. When a female is born with swollen hands and feet, TS should be considered.

V. Trisomy 13 (Patau Syndrome)

A. General characteristics
1. Due to 3 copies of chromosome 13 and associated with severe intellectual disability and multiple congenital malformations, resulting in greatly reduced life expectancy
2. Epidemiology
    a. 1/9,500 live births; females > males
    b. 60% of trisomy 13 conceptions are spontaneously aborted in 2nd trimester
3. Genetics: >90% caused by meiotic nondisjunction of maternal chromosomes
4. Risk factors: increased risk with advanced maternal age

B. Clinical presentation
1. **Holoprosencephaly**
2. Cleft palate
3. **Microphthalmia**
4. Cutis aplasia of scalp (punched out–appearing lesions)
5. CHD
6. Postaxial **polydactyly** (extra 5th fingers)

C. Therapy
1. Median age of survival is 7 to 10 days; family support is important
2. If karyotype reveals Robertsonian translocation, discuss availability of chromosome studies for parents

VI. Klinefelter Syndrome ([KS] +47,XXY) *(Figure 16-5)*

A. General characteristics
1. Due to additional copy of X chromosome and associated with tall stature, gynecomastia, and small testes with reduced germ cell counts and progressive failure of Sertoli cells
2. Epidemiology: 1/650 live births
3. Genetics
    a. Occurs due to maternal or paternal nondisjunction during meiosis
    b. Slightly increased risk with advanced maternal age
    c. Fertile KS patients have low recurrence risk (<1%) of KS but slightly increased risk of offspring with chromosomal abnormalities

B. Clinical presentation (see Figure 16-5)

C. Testing
1. Diagnosis is based on karyotype or aCGH
2. Screening indicated for infertility in adult males
3. May show decreased sperm count, decreased testosterone, hypogonadotropic hypogonadism, with increased luteinizing and follicle-stimulating hormone levels

D. Therapy
1. Testosterone therapy thought to improve facial/body hair, strength/muscle size, energy level, libido, self-confidence, and concentration
2. Reproductive options for infertility specialist

VII. Turner Syndrome ([TS] 45,X) *(Figure 16-6)*

A. General characteristics
1. Definition: chromosomal abnormality in which all or part of X chromosome is absent
2. Epidemiology: 1/2,000 live births
3. Genetics
    a. >60% caused by de novo meiotic nondisjunction of paternal sex chromosomes
    b. TS occurs in females; however, males can be mosaic for TS (45,X; 46,XY)

B. Clinical presentation
1. Symptoms
    a. Delayed puberty
    b. Amenorrhea from gonadal dysfunction
    c. Premature ovarian failure (POF)

FIGURE **16-5** **Clinical features of Klinefelter syndrome (47,XXY).**

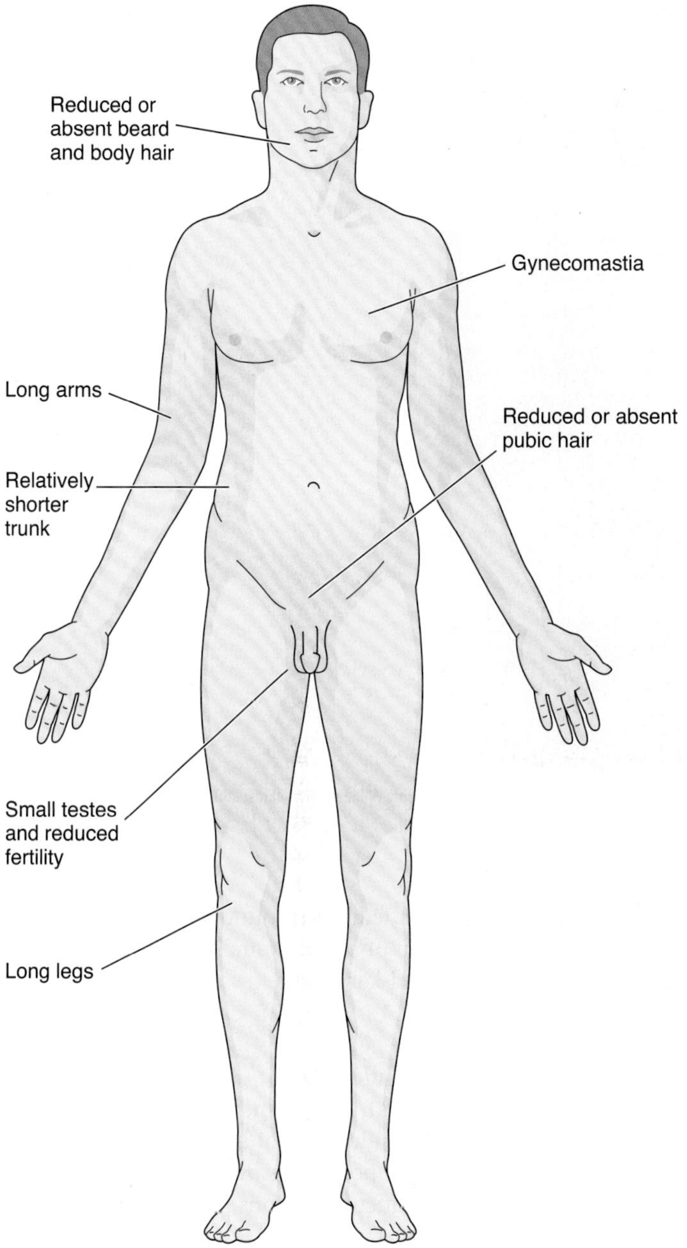

(From McConnell TH. *The Nature of Disease Pathology for the Health Professions.* Philadelphia: Lippincott Williams & Wilkins; 2007.)

QUICK HIT

Some patients with Klinefelter syndrome have learning problems, but many have normal intelligence, and we have patients who are artists, chess champions, and business leaders. Some men do not find out that they have Klinefelter syndrome until an infertility work-up reveals the diagnosis.

d. Infertility
e. Some patients with a learning disability, especially in math

2. Physical exam findings
   a. Short stature
   b. Low-set ears
   c. Low hairline
   d. Webbed neck
   e. Small jaw
   f. "Shield" chest
   g. Cubitus valgus (outward-turned elbows)
   h. Shortened 4th metatarsal
   i. Horseshoe kidney
   j. CHD including coarctation of aorta, bicuspid aorta, and aortic stenosis

QUICK HIT

Coarctation of the aorta is the most common CHD in patients with TS; 20%–40% of patients have some type of CHD.

FIGURE 16-6 A 3-year-old with Turner syndrome. Note the webbed neck.

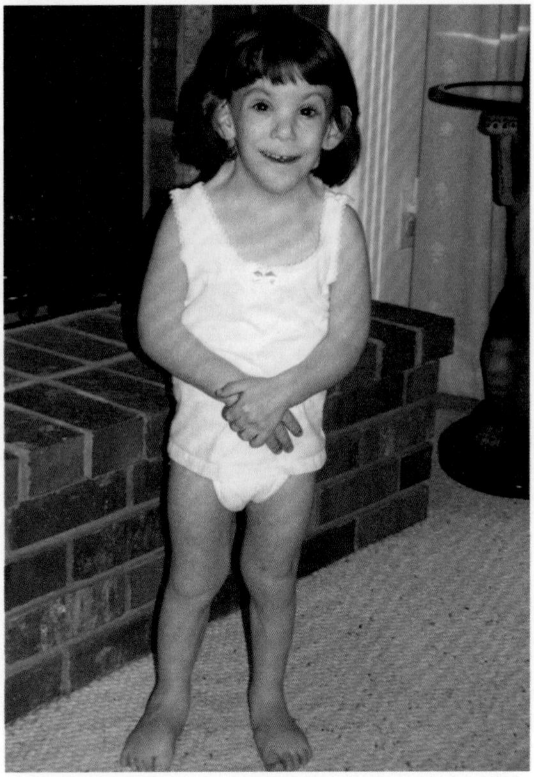

(From Nettina SM. *The Lippincott Manual of Nursing Practice*. 7th ed. Lippincott Williams & Wilkins; 2001.)

C. Testing
   1. Prenatal diagnosis can be considered when fetal ultrasound shows intrauterine growth restriction, fetal edema, coarctation of aorta, cystic hygroma
   2. CVS or amniocentesis, with rapid FISH and karyotype
   3. Postnatal diagnosis: karyotype or aCGH

D. Therapy
   1. Initial screening: echocardiogram and renal ultrasound
   2. Follow-up care: thyroid function tests (TFTs), eye exam, check for scoliosis
   3. Referral to pediatric endocrinologist for consideration of hormonal replacement therapies, including estrogen, progestin, and possibly growth hormone (GH)
   4. Refer to fertility specialist to discuss reproductive options

VIII. 22q11 Deletion Syndrome

A. General characteristics
   1. Epidemiology: 1 in 4,000–1 in 6,000 live births
   2. Genetics
      a. Microdeletion of 22q11.2 (missing small piece of chromosome)
      b. Most cases are de novo mutations
      c. 7% inherited in autosomal dominant manner from affected parent

B. Clinical presentation: physical examination and laboratory findings (Table 16-5): in general, affects central head, neck, and chest structures

C. Testing
   1. Definitive
      a. aCGH or FISH testing
      b. Prenatal diagnosis is available
      c. Deletion may not be seen by karyotype
   2. Associated labs to check for involved structures
      a. Electrocardiogram (ECG) and cardiac echocardiography (echo)
      b. Serum calcium, phosphorus

QUICK HIT

Each of the anomalies seen in 22q11 deletion syndrome can be found as an isolated anomaly.

Dysmorphology and Genetic Disorders

TABLE 16-5 **Clinical Features of 22q11 Deletion Syndrome**

Finding	Description of Finding	Frequency
Congenital heart disease	Most commonly tetralogy of Fallot and aortic arch anomalies, but many structural problems are possible.	>50%
Palatal abnormalities	Most common is velopharyngeal insufficiency (VPI), a term used when the palate does not close the nose off from the back of the mouth completely when speaking, which can cause regurgitation through the nose when swallowing and hypernasal speech. Also: cleft palate, cleft palate alone, and cleft lip and palate. May result in severe feeding problems.	
Developmental problems	Hypotonia, global developmental delays, intellectual disability, and autistic spectrum disorder.	
Immunodeficiency	Immunodeficiency occurs as a result of thymus hypoplasia with impaired T-cell function.	
Hypocalcemia	A result of hypoparathyroidism.	5%–50%
Growth deficiency	Younger children may fall below the 5th percentile in height, and endocrine referral could be considered.	
Renal anomalies	Includes single kidney, multicystic dysplastic kidney/small kidneys, horseshoe kidney, and duplicated collecting system.	
Craniofacial findings	Include auricular abnormalities, nasal abnormalities, hooded eyelids, ocular hypertelorism, and a long face and malar flatness.	Variable
Psychiatric illness	Impulsiveness, attention-deficit disorder, and anxiety. Acute psychosis and schizophrenia in adolescence have been described.	
Other	Ectopic internal carotid arteries can pose risk during pharyngeal surgery.	

c. Immune function evaluation
   i. Complete blood count (CBC): look for lymphopenia from absence of thymus
   ii. T- and B-cell subsets
   iii. Immunoglobulin levels
   iv. Posteroanterior and lateral chest x-ray (CXR) to check for physical presence of thymus

d. Renal ultrasound for anomalies

D. Treatment
1. Therapy
   a. If immune workup shows T-cell abnormalities, avoid live vaccines
   b. Treat structural abnormalities as needed
   c. Early intervention and developmental evaluations; psychiatric evaluation as needed
2. Prognosis
   a. Highly variable (some patients have normal facies and only minor cardiac abnormality; others severely affected)
   b. Many individuals hold jobs and have families

IX. Williams Syndrome (WS)

A. General characteristics
1. Epidemiology: 1/10,000 live births
2. Genetics
   a. Microdeletion of chromosome 7q11.23, which contains Williams-Beuren syndrome critical region (WBSCR)
   b. WBSCR contains many critical genes responsible for aspects of syndrome, including *ELN* (codes for elastin), *LIMK1* (cognitive defects), *GTF2* (personality)
   c. Autosomal dominant inheritance pattern, but mostly de novo; rarely transmitted from parent to child

B. Clinical presentation
1. Distinctive facial features
2. Cocktail type personality
3. Cardiovascular disease including supravalvular aortic stenosis

4. Developmental delay and/or intellectual disability
5. Failure to thrive (FTT)
6. Connective tissue abnormalities

C. Testing
1. Diagnosis based on aCGH or FISH
2. Screen with echo, renal ultrasound, ophthalmology and audiology examinations, calcium, TFTs

X. Fragile X Syndrome

A. General characteristics
1. Trinucleotide repeat disorder characterized by intellectual disability, characteristics physical features, and connective tissue abnormalities (Figure 16-7)
2. Epidemiology: prevalence of 1 in 3,600–4,000 in males, 1 in 4,000–6,000 in females
3. Genetics: usually caused by CGG repeat expansions in promoter region of *FMR1* gene
   a. CGG expansion → abnormal methylation (attachment of methyl groups to DNA) → silencing of *FMR1* gene transcription → loss of FMRP protein, which is critical in brain and testicular development
   b. Repeats tend to expand more in female premutation carriers than in male premutation carriers
   c. More repeats in subsequent generations, resulting in worsened symptoms

B. Clinical presentation (see Figure 16-7)
1. Females with >200 repeats on at least 1 allele have fragile X syndrome
2. Females are usually less severely affected, often presenting with mild intellectual disability
   a. Difference in severity between males and females due to X inactivation: men have 1 X chromosome; women have 2
   b. Result: female cells randomly turn off 1 X chromosome by **methylation**
   c. If female has most fragile X cells in her body turned off, she is considered "favorably skewed"

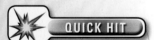

QUICK HIT

Idiopathic hypercalcemia is a common finding in WS. Children diagnosed with WS should not be given multivitamins with calcium or vitamin D. Children with diagnosed hypercalcemia often respond to diet modification with calcium-restricted formula and require close follow-up.

QUICK HIT

Sedate with great caution and expertise only! Sedated procedures in children with WS have an increased risk of sudden death.

QUICK HIT

Fragile X syndrome is the most common cause of X-linked intellectual disability.

QUICK HIT

Facial features include a long face with a prominent chin and ears.

QUICK HIT

Macro-orchidism (large testes) is a common feature of fragile X syndrome that only presents at puberty.

FIGURE 16-7 **A. Fragile X syndrome in a 2.5-year-old boy. Note the long, hypotonic face; high forehead; epicanthal folds; and prominent ears. B. Five-year-old fragile X–positive girl, referred because of behavior problems and autism.**

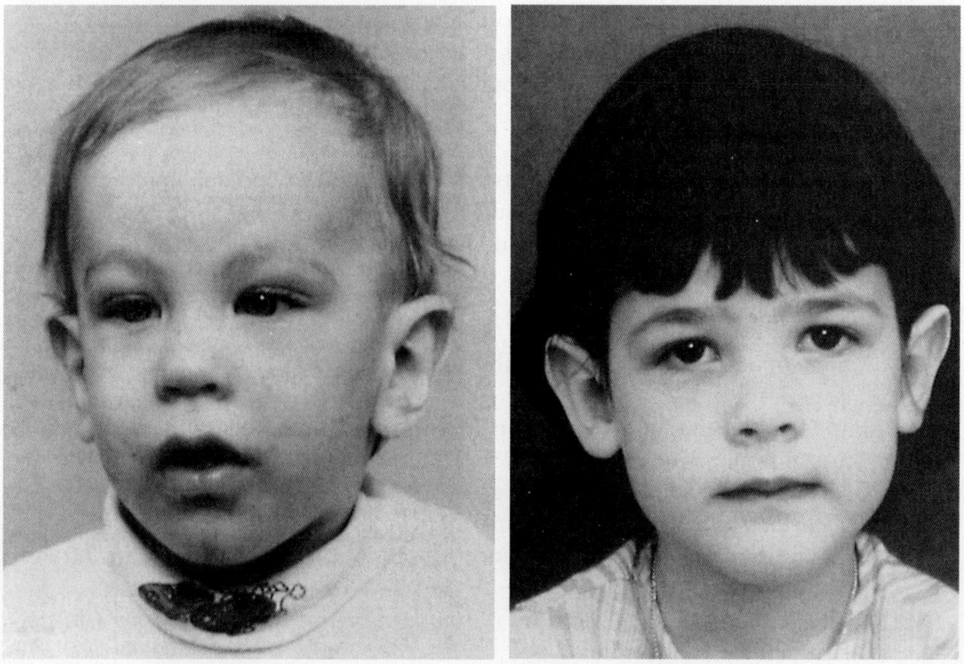

A B

(From Chudley AE, Hagerman RJ. Fragile X syndrome. *J Pediatr.* 1987;110:821–831. With permission.)

C. Testing
   1. Molecular genetic testing to count CGG repeats and analysis of *FMR1* gene's methylation status are often done for confirmation in affected patients
   2. Echo: to rule out cardiac anomalies
D. Therapy
   1. Early intervention; special education; speech, language, occupational, and physical therapy; and vocational training
   2. Developmental and psychiatric assessment, evaluate for possible autism spectrum disorder

XI. Prader-Willi Syndrome (PWS) and Angelman Syndrome (AS)

A. General characteristics
   1. Definition of genomic imprinting
      a. **Imprinted genes**: genes whose expression is determined by contributing parent
         i. For most genes, we inherit 2 expressed copies: 1 from mother + 1 from father
         ii. With imprinted genes, we inherit only 1 expressed copy
      b. In cases of imprinted genes, either mother's or father's copy is epigenetically silenced through **methylation** (the addition of methyl groups during egg or sperm formation)
   2. Cause/pathophysiology
      a. On chromosome 15, *SNRPN* is expressed only on paternally inherited copy
      b. *E6-AP ubiquitin protein ligase* (*UBE3A*) is expressed only on maternally inherited chromosome 15
         i. Paternal *SNRPN* deleted or methylated (silenced) = PWS
         ii. Maternal *UBE3A* deleted or methylated = AS
B. Clinical presentation
   1. PWS characteristics
      a. Early infancy: hypotonia, global delay, and feeding difficulties
      b. Small palpebral fissures
      c. Genitourinary (GU) abnormalities (>90% of males will have undescended testicle or other GU abnormality)
      d. Small hands and feet
      e. Short stature
      f. Adolescence and adulthood: excessive eating, obesity, compulsive behaviors, hypertension, diabetes
   2. AS characteristics
      a. Severe intellectual disability (most patients are nonverbal)
      b. Paroxysms of laughter
      c. Feeding difficulties
      d. Seizures common
      e. Exam findings include protruding jaw and small head size, scoliosis, short stature, stiff ataxic gait
C. Testing: DNA methylation analysis
D. Treatment
   1. PWS
      a. Rigid diet modification and behavior therapy
      b. GH therapy may have some possible benefits
         i. Controversial because of early reports of death due to tonsillar hypertrophy
         ii. Before starting GH, get sleep study to rule out obstructive sleep apnea (OSA)
      c. Selective serotonin reuptake inhibitors may be indicated for obsessive-compulsive behaviors
   2. AS
      a. Baseline electroencephalogram and treatment of seizures
      b. Special education plus physical and speech therapy

QUICK HIT

Mothers of patients with fragile X should be tested to determine if they are premutation carriers and counseled regarding increased risk for POF.

QUICK HIT

Maternal grandfathers should consider testing and receive counseling regarding fragile X–associated tremor/ataxia syndrome.

QUICK HIT

Prader-Willi and Angelman syndromes serve as classic examples of the role of genomic imprinting in human disease.

MNEMONIC

For deletion cases, remember the parental chromosome of origin:
"**P** = paternal" for **PWS**
"**ANGEL**ic mother" (maternal) for **AS**

QUICK HIT

In PWS, as infants, patients have hypotonia, often requiring nasogastric (NG) feeding tubes. In childhood, they develop **hyperphagia** and weight gain.

QUICK HIT

When patients with AS walk, ataxia and a wide-based gait with uplifted flexed arms are often noted; excessive laughter is also a well-known feature.

FIGURE 16-8 Patient with Beckwith-Wiedemann syndrome.

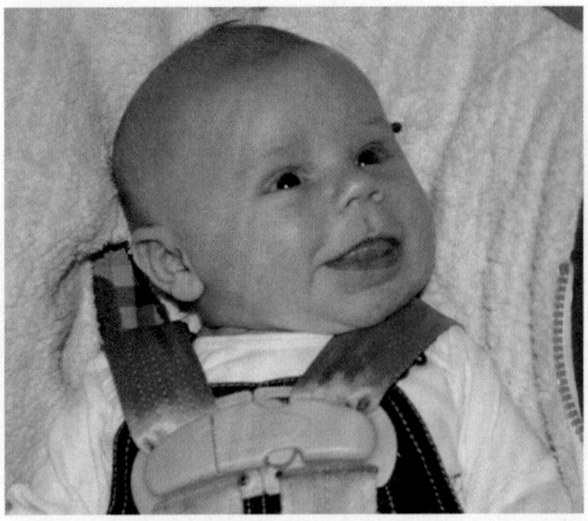

(Courtesy of Natasha Shur, MD, Hasbro Children's Hospital.)

QUICK HIT

Patients present at birth with severe **macroglossia**, which may impede with breathing.

QUICK HIT

BWS is most commonly caused by methylation errors in imprinted genes at 11p15.5, where there are 2 main imprinting centers that contain important genes that regulate growth, *IC1* and *IC2*.

QUICK HIT

Most patients with BWS have normal intelligence; however, if hypoglycemia is undiagnosed and untreated, intellectual disability can be a dire consequence.

XII. Beckwith-Wiedemann Syndrome (BWS) *(Figure 16-8)*

A. General characteristics
   1. Epidemiology: 1/13,700 live births
   2. Genetics: usually sporadic but may rarely be autosomal dominant
   3. Cause/pathophysiology
      1. Genetic error in certain growth regulators resulting in overgrowth disorder
      2. **Methylation**: addition of methyl groups to DNA, which silences gene to which it attaches

B. Clinical presentation
   1. Large birth weight and neonatal hypoglycemia
   2. Omphalocele
   3. Macroglossia
   4. **Hemihyperplasia** (one arm, leg, or side of the body is larger than the other)
   5. Embryonal tumors
   6. Renal abnormalities

C. Testing: methylation study for chromosome 11 and chromosome analysis

D. Therapy
   1. Increased risk of embryonal tumors including Wilms tumor, hepatoblastoma, neuroblastoma, and rhabdomyosarcoma
      a. Close surveillance for tumors with routine ultrasound and α-fetoprotein throughout early childhood
      b. After age 8 years, tumor risk becomes much lower (close to general population's risk)
   2. Treat hypoglycemia
   3. Special feeding techniques for macroglossia
   4. Cardiac evaluation including ECG and echo prior to any surgical procedures or when cardiac abnormality is suspected

XIII. Achondroplasia

A. General characteristics
   1. Epidemiology: ~1/25,000 live births
   2. Genetics
      a. Autosomal dominant inheritance, 80% de novo gene mutations
      b. >99% of cases caused by point mutation, resulting in glycine-to-arginine amino acid substitution
      c. Increasing risk with advanced paternal age
   3. Cause/pathophysiology
      a. Skeletal dysplasia characterized by disproportionately short limbs, normal-sized trunk, and large head
      b. Mutation in *FGFR3* gene, which encodes for fibroblast growth factor receptor
      c. Mutation leads to gain of function → overinhibition of chondrocytes in cartilage → decreased long bone growth

Dysmorphology and Genetic Disorders

B. Clinical presentation
  1. Short stature with large-appearing head with frontal bossing
  2. **Rhizomelia** (proximal limbs are disproportionately short)
  3. Tibial bowing
  4. **Trident hand** configuration
  5. Thoracolumbar kyphosis or **gibbus** (a small hump) often present in infancy; when babies start walking, gibbus usually replaced by **lordosis**

C. Therapy
  1. Monitor head circumference to screen for hydrocephalus
  2. Monitor for secretory otitis media ("glue ear")
  3. Monitor and counsel regarding obesity
  4. Monitor and treat OSA
  5. **Thoracolumbar kyphosis (gibbus)** improves with age, sitting modifications, and, in some cases, braces; spinal fusion may be done in severe cases

QUICK HIT

If a child with achondroplasia presents with vomiting or headaches, he or she may have **cervicomedullary junction myelopathy**, or compression at the foramen magnum, which can lead to sudden death. Urgent computed tomography/magnetic resonance imaging and neurosurgical decompression are indicated.

XIV. Marfan Syndrome (MFS)

A. General characteristics
  1. Connective tissue disorder that affects multiple systems; in particular, cardiovascular, skeletal, and ocular systems
  2. Epidemiology: ~1/5,000 live births
  3. Cause/pathophysiology: most cases are caused by mutation in *FBN1* gene on chromosome 15, which encodes for fibrillin-1
  4. Genetics: autosomal dominant inheritance
     a. 75% of patients with MFS have affected parent
     b. 25% have de novo gene mutation

B. Clinical presentation (Table 16-6 and Figure 16-9)

C. Diagnosis
  1. **Revised Ghent criteria**
     a. Standardized systemic score considers many clinical findings
     b. Score ≧6, combined with aortic dilatation, family history, and slipped lens of eye
  2. Diagnostic testing: sequencing of *FBN1* to look for mutation

QUICK HIT

Babies with achondroplasia should not be forcibly propped up, which can worsen their gibbus.

QUICK HIT

In MFS, cardiovascular symptoms are the main causes of morbidity and mortality.

TABLE 16-6 **Clinical Findings of Marfan Syndrome**

Aorta	Root dilatation* Aneurysm* Regurgitation
Cardiac (other)	Mitral valve prolapse*
Skeletal	Arachnodactyly* Tall stature* Arm span > height* Pectus deformity Hindfoot valgus Long legs (decreased upper:lower body ratio) Scoliosis/kyphosis Protrusion of hip acetabulum on x-ray
Face	Dolichocephaly (thin, long head) Enophthalmos (sunken eyes) Retrognathia (small chin)
Eyes	Ectopia lentis (upward dislocated lens)*
Spine	Dural ectasia (enlarged spinal canal)
Pulmonary	Spontaneous pneumothorax
Skin	Striae

*Common/important findings.

FIGURE 16-9 **The wrist sign in a patient with Marfan syndrome. In a positive test, the first phalanges of the thumb and fifth digit substantially overlap when wrapped around the opposite wrist.**

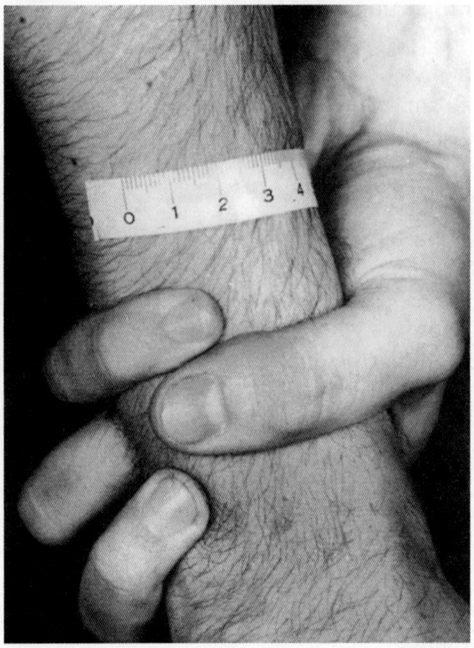

(From Koopman WJ, Moreland LW. *Arthritis and Allied Conditions: A Textbook of Rheumatology.* 15th ed. Philadelphia: Lippincott Williams & Wilkins; 2005.)

D. Therapy
1. Multidisciplinary approach necessary: cardiology, genetics, ophthalmology, orthopedics, and cardiothoracic surgery
2. Follow with echo
3. β-Blockers (reduce hemodynamic stress)
4. Angiotensin II inhibitors/transforming growth factor-β inhibitors
5. Strict blood pressure control
6. Aortic graft for aortic dilation >5 cm (or rapidly progressing dilation)
7. Avoid caffeine and stimulants and heavy exercise/contact sports
8. Treat scoliosis as indicated

XV. Ehlers-Danlos Syndrome (EDS)

A. General characteristics
1. Connective tissue disorder characterized by hyperextensibility, connective tissue fragility, and delayed wound healing
2. Many types of disorders all due to collagen mutations
   a. **Collagen**: triple helical protein widely distributed throughout body and responsible for structural integrity
   b. Collagen is expressed through multiple genes on many chromosomes
   c. Type of EDS depends on location/nature of mutation
3. Epidemiology: incidence: 1/5,000–1/10,000

B. Clinical presentation
1. Historical findings
   a. Parent with known diagnosis: 50% recurrence risk
   b. Many, especially those with benign hypermobile type, are unaware of their diagnosis even well into adulthood
2. Physical exam findings vary based on type, but some findings may include
   a. Hypermobile joints with increased risk of dislocations and subluxations
   b. Stretchy, fragile skin
   c. Increased skin, tissue, and vascular fragility

C. Diagnosis
1. For common types, diagnosis is based on clinical examination and Beighton Scale
2. Baseline echo to rule out aortic dilatation in patients with classical type

QUICK HIT

A score of 5 or more on the Beighton Scale is clinically significant

Dysmorphology and Genetic Disorders

D. Treatment
   1. Therapies
      a. Prevention of complications: frequent low resistance and small weight-bearing exercise to improve tone and bone strength and density, calcium and vitamin D supplementation, avoiding high impact and contact sports
      b. For classical type
         i. Perform clotting studies and check bleeding time
         ii. Avoid aspirin; pain management with experienced team
         iii. Referral to EDS support group
         iv. For deep cuts: try glue when possible instead of or in association with sutures; keep sutures in place for longer; inform emergency room and surgeons of diagnosis

QUICK HIT

EDS patients should be told to avoid "party tricks." Laxity demonstrations of affected joints lead to chronic osteoarthritis.

XVI. Stickler Syndrome

A. General characteristics
   1. Epidemiology: ~1/10,000 births
   2. Genetics: autosomal dominant inheritance for most cases
   3. Cause: mutations in several collagen genes
   4. Risk factors: affected parent has 50% chance of having affected child with each pregnancy; low de novo mutation rate
B. Clinical presentation
   1. Ocular findings: myopia, cataract, and retinal detachment
   2. Hearing loss: both conductive and sensorineural
   3. Midfacial underdevelopment
   4. Cleft palate (either alone or as part of Pierre-Robin sequence)
   5. Precocious osteoarthritis

QUICK HIT

Children with Stickler syndrome have characteristic facial features including prominent eyes; a small, upturned nose; and a small jaw.

XVII. Pierre-Robin Sequence

A. General characteristics
   1. **Micrognathia** and **glossoptosis** (retrodisplacement of tongue in pharynx) causing upper airway obstruction
   2. Incidence: ~1/8,500 live births
   3. Cause/pathophysiology
      a. At 9–11 weeks of embryonic development, mandibular hypoplasia leads to posterior displacement of tongue
      b. In turn, prevents palatine shelves from growing together horizontally and fusing, causing U-shaped cleft palate
B. Clinical presentation: small chin and posteriorly displaced tongue on exam
C. Diagnosis
   1. Based on clinical findings
   2. In ~50% of cases, syndromic cause is found (most frequently, Stickler syndrome, connective tissue disorder, or 22q11 deletion syndrome)
D. Therapy
   1. Airway options include
      a. Repositioning
         i. Prone position and specialized feeding techniques
         ii. Nasopharyngeal airway
         iii. In severe cases: tracheostomy
      b. Lip–tongue adhesion
         i. Surgical attachment of front tip of tongue to inside of lower lip to keep tongue from falling back and blocking airway
         ii. Reversible, typically detached when cleft palate is repaired at age 9 months
      c. Jaw distraction (alternative to tracheotomy tube): jaw bone is lengthened by turning screw daily and allowing gap between bones to be filled in by new bone
   2. Overcoming feeding difficulties
      a. Use special cleft palate nursing bottle
      b. Manage gastroesophageal reflux
      c. Gastrostomy tube in severe cases

QUICK HIT

In Pierre Robin sequence, untreated airway obstruction may lead to apnea; feeding difficulties; hypoxia; and, in the worst case, sudden death.

QUICK HIT

If a baby has Pierre-Robin sequence and trouble breathing, putting the baby in the prone position allows the tongue to fall forward and may be a temporary alleviating measure.

XVIII. Noonan Syndrome (NS)

A. General characteristics
1. Definition: disorder characterized by short stature, CHDs, webbed neck, chest wall deformities, and variable degrees of developmental delay
2. Incidence: 1:1,000–1:2,500 live births
3. Genetics: autosomal dominant inheritance either occurring de novo or from affected parent

B. Clinical presentation
1. Typical facial features
   a. Hypertelorism, low-set/posteriorly rotated ears with thickened helices, short upturned nose
   b. Patients often have excess nuchal skin with low posterior hairline
2. Cardiovascular defects
   a. Pulmonary valve stenosis is most common finding
   b. Hypertrophic cardiomyopathy present in 20%–30%
3. Unusual shaped chest with superior pectus carinatum and inferior pectus
4. Cryptorchidism
5. Developmental delay and hypotonia; attention problems in school
6. Bleeding abnormalities

C. Testing
1. Diagnosis made clinically by observation of key features
2. "**Noonan chip**": sequences most common genes
3. Screen for bleeding diathesis
4. Imaging: echo, renal ultrasound, and (if neurologic symptoms present) brain and cervical spine magnetic resonance imaging

D. Therapy: typically focused on symptoms
1. Cardiac: treat depending on echo result
2. Developmental: individualized educational plan strategies
3. Hematologic: check for bleeding disorders
4. Growth: GH is approved for short stature and should be considered

QUICK HIT

NS and TS share many physical features; however, in NS, females and males are equally affected.

QUICK HIT

Prenatal ultrasound may show cystic hygroma; polyhydramnios; and, rarely, fetal hydrops in NS.

QUICK HIT

Because of variability in expression, a parent with NS may not be diagnosed until after a child.

QUICK HIT

The most common cardiac anomaly in NS is pulmonic stenosis, whereas the most common anomalies in TS involve the aortic valve.

QUICK HIT

Hypertrophic cardiomyopathy is a major cause of morbidity and mortality. Otherwise, the prognosis is excellent with NS.

XIX. CHARGE Syndrome

A. General characteristics
1. "CHARGE" acronym: coloboma, heart defects, choanal atresia, retardation of growth and development, genital abnormalities, and ear abnormalities/deafness
2. Epidemiology: occurs in 1/10,000 births
3. Genetics
   a. *CHD7* is only gene known to be associated with CHARGE
   b. Typically sporadic; rare familial cases have been reported and inherited in autosomal dominant manner
   c. If neither parent is affected, risk to siblings of affected child = 1%–2% (due to possibility of germline mosaicism)

B. Clinical presentation (Table 16-7)

C. Diagnosis: based on clinical findings (see Table 16-7)
1. Definite CHARGE syndrome: all 4 major or 3 major plus 3 minor characteristics
2. Possible CHARGE syndrome: 1–2 major and several minor characteristics

D. Testing: sequence analysis of *CH7* coding region detects 60%–70% of cases

E. Therapy
1. Neonates: immediate evaluation of airway, heart, and feeding
2. Neurologic: low muscle tone predisposes children to rapid exhaustion, so frequent rest may be needed; assess cranial nerve function
3. Growth/development: psychological and school evaluations
4. Surveillance: echo, renal sonogram, dilated eye exam, audiology evaluation

QUICK HIT

Patients with CHARGE syndrome often have very distinctive-appearing ears that are square shaped, asymmetrical, and have helices and small lobules.

QUICK HIT

Bilateral choanal atresia causes respiratory distress in newborns, requiring immediate resuscitation. Unilateral choanal atresia may go undiagnosed until the child presents with persistent unilateral rhinorrhea.

TABLE 16-7 **Clinical Features of CHARGE Syndrome**

Clinical Finding	Description of Finding
Major characteristics	
Ocular coloboma	Unilateral or bilateral coloboma
Choanal atresia/stenosis	Unilateral/bilateral, bony or membranous choanal atresia or stenosis (usually, a suction catheter cannot be passed through the nasopharynx)
Cranial nerve abnormality	Facial palsy, hypoplasia of auditory nerve
Ear anomalies	Ossicular malformation, cochlear defects, temporal bone abnormalities
Minor characteristics	
Genital hypoplasia	Males: micropenis, cryptorchidism; females: hypoplastic labia
Development	Most commonly intellectual disability
Cardiovascular	Tetralogy of Fallot, atrioventricular canal defects, aortic arch anomalies
Growth	Short stature with occasional growth hormone deficiency
Facial features	Square face with broad prominent forehead, prominent nasal bridge, flat midface
Other	Tracheoesophageal fistula, cleft palate

XX. Treacher-Collins Syndrome (TCS)

A. General characteristics
1. Disorder characterized by hypoplasia of zygomatic bone and mandible, external ear abnormalities, conductive hearing loss, and coloboma of lower eyelid
2. Epidemiology: 1/10,000–1/50,000 live births
3. Genetics
   a. Autosomal dominant inheritance; *TCOF1* is main gene associated with TCS
   b. 40% of individuals with TCS have affected parent
   c. 60% from de novo mutations

B. Clinical presentation
1. Major
   a. Hypoplasia of zygomatic bones and mandible
   b. Small malformed ears (**microtia**)
   c. Coloboma of eyelid; sparse or absent eyelashes
2. Minor
   a. External ear abnormalities such as atresia
   b. Conductive hearing loss
   c. Cleft lip with or without cleft palate
   d. Preauricular hair displacement with hair growth extending in front of ears to lateral cheekbones

C. Testing: diagnosis is clinical, but genetic testing for mutations in *TCOF* and newly discovered rarer genes is available

QUICK HIT

In TCS, intelligence is usually normal.

QUICK HIT

TCS shows variable expression even within the same family. Some patients have subtle findings and require little to no intervention at birth, whereas other patients have severe feeding difficulties, requiring gastrostomy, and life-threatening airway compromise, requiring tracheostomy.

XXI. VACTERL Association

A. General characteristics
1. Definition: nonrandom association of three or more of the following
   a. Vertebral defects
   b. Imperforate anus
   c. Cardiac malformations
   d. Tracheoesophageal fistula (TEF)
   e. Renal anomalies
   f. Limb anomalies
2. Incidence: 1–2/10,000 births

QUICK HIT

VACTERL is a diagnosis of exclusion: syndromes such as trisomy 18 should be ruled out before making the diagnosis.

3. Genetics
   a. Empiric recurrence risk after 1 affected child = 0.5%–2%
   b. Rises to 20% if more than 1 sibling affected
4. Risk factors
   a. Most commonly sporadic
   b. More commonly found in white males
   c. More frequently in infants of type 1 diabetic mothers or with intrauterine thalidomide exposure

B. Clinical presentation

C. Testing
1. Spinal ultrasound and spinal x-ray to rule out vertebral anomalies
2. Echo
3. Renal ultrasound
4. Observation for respiratory distress or feeding problems (concerning for TEF)

QUICK HIT

An NG tube shows coiling in the mediastinum on CXR if a TEF is present.

XXII. Klippel-Feil Sequence

A. General characteristics: congenital fusion of at least 2 of 7 cervical vertebrae

B. Clinical presentation
1. Short neck, decreased cervical range of motion, and low hairline
2. Some present with torticollis or facial asymmetry
3. Additional abnormalities may include Sprengel deformity (25% of cases): shoulder muscle hypoplasia or atrophy resulting from scapula malformation

C. Testing: diagnosis is based on plain radiograph

QUICK HIT

Patients with Klippel-Feil syndrome generally have normal intelligence.

XXIII. Fetal Alcohol Syndrome (FAS) *(Figure 16-10)*

A. General characteristics
1. Epidemiology: as high as 1% of all live births
2. Risk factors
   a. Increases with high-dose exposure (blood alcohol level ≥150 mg/dL), chronic ingestion of 2 g/kg/day of alcohol, or binge drinking
   b. Alcoholics have 30%–50% risk of having child born with multiple problems

QUICK HIT

Klippel-Feil sequence can be seen in both fetal alcohol syndrome and oculoauricular vertebral dysplasia, which are associated with other congenital anomalies.

FIGURE 16-10 **An 8-year-old boy with facial features typical of fetal alcohol syndrome: short palpebral fissures, short nose with flat nasal bridge, and thin lips with a smooth philtrum.**

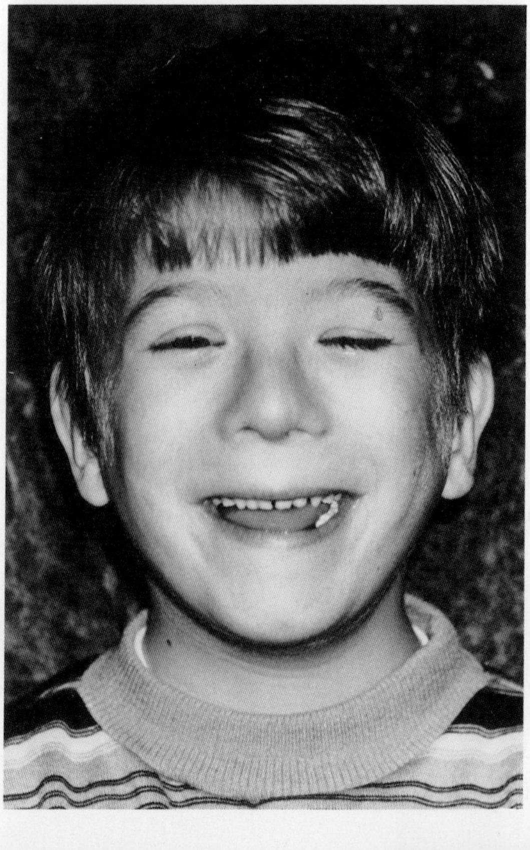

Dysmorphology and Genetic Disorders

3. Pathophysiology
    a. Alcohol crosses placenta and rapidly reaches fetus
    b. Fetus depends on maternal hepatic detoxification because activity of alcohol dehydrogenase in fetal liver is much less than that in adult liver
    c. Amniotic fluid acts as reservoir for alcohol, prolonging fetal exposure; ethanol and its metabolite acetaldehyde can alter fetal development

B. Clinical presentation
1. Facial features: short palpebral fissures, flat midface, long and flat philtrum, thin vermillion border of upper lip
2. Growth retardation: birth weight <2.5 percentile for gestational age; decelerating weight over time not due to malnutrition; thin body habitus
3. Central nervous system anomalies: microcephaly; structural brain anomalies such as partial or complete agenesis of the corpus callosum, cerebellar hypoplasia
4. Cognitive abnormalities: poor impulse control, attention-deficit hyperactivity disorder, language deficits, mathematical deficits
5. Birth defects: CHD (ventricular septal defect most common), urinary tract anomalies
6. Extremities: abnormal palmar crease pattern ("**hockey stick crease**" that runs between 2nd and 3rd fingers), small distal phalanges, small 5th fingernails

C. Testing: clinical diagnosis

D. Therapy includes early intervention and good school placement

QUICK HIT

Children with FAS tend to be thin with decreased body fat and hyperkinetic with poor attention.

QUICK HIT

A diagnosis of FAS with known alcohol exposure requires the presence of 4 major exam findings. If a child has not had a known exposure, then genetic syndromes should certainly be considered. If a patient meets some but not all criteria, fetal alcohol effects is a possible description.

17 Diseases of the Eye

QUICK HIT

A newborn's eye is 2/3 the size of an adult eye and grows fast in the first 2 years.

QUICK HIT

The uvea is the iris, the ciliary body, and the choroid.

QUICK HIT

Most newborn irises appear blue due to lack of pigment.

QUICK HIT

A **cataract** is any opacity in the normally clear lens.

QUICK HIT

You do not see with your eyes; you see with your brain!

QUICK HIT

Anything that interferes with visual stimulation while an infant is 1–3 months old (e.g., a cataract) can result in irreversible **amblyopia** (brain maldevelopment causing poor vision).

SYMPTOM SPECIFIC

I. Approach to Eye Anatomy and Visual Development

A. Normal eye anatomy
1. Eyelids (also called palpebrae)
2. Conjunctiva (transparent membrane that covers inside of eyelids [palpebral] and sclera [bulbar])
3. Cornea (transparent structure on anterior surface of globe)
4. Sclera (white fibrous layer forming primary structure of globe)
5. Anterior chamber (space posterior to cornea, anterior to iris): filled with aqueous humor, which is produced by ciliary body and drains through canal of Schlemm
6. Iris
7. Lens (provides 1/3 of focusing power; 2/3 is from cornea)
8. Ciliary body (produces aqueous humor)
9. Vitreous (gel that fills posterior 2/3 of globe)
10. Retina
    a. Neurosensory organ of eye, containing cone and rod photoreceptors
    b. **Macula**: central posterior area responsible for central vision
    c. **Fovea**: small pit in macula with densest concentration of cone cells giving highest resolution vision
11. Choroid (vascular structure between retina and sclera)
12. Optic nerve (ends in **optic disc**, which is visible on exam)

B. Visual pathway
1. Retina → optic nerve → optic tract → optic chiasm → optic radiations → lateral geniculate nucleus → primary visual cortex
2. At optic chiasm, nasal fibers (responsible for temporal visual fields) decussate (cross)
3. Behind chiasm
    i. **Right brain** is responsible for **left visual field**
    ii. **Left brain** is responsible for **right visual field**

C. Normal visual development
1. Vision during 1st 2–3 months of life critical for cortical development
2. Vision is very poor at birth (20/200) and gradually improves through age 7 or 8 years

II. Approach to Eye and Vision Assessment

A. Historical information
1. Important symptoms: vision loss, diplopia, eyes crossing or drifting, eye or eyelid redness, eye pain, photophobia
2. Past ocular history: eye disease, injury, surgery, eye drops, eyeglasses, contact lenses
3. Past medical history: other medical issues, prematurity, allergies, medications
4. Family history: strabismus, cataract, glaucoma, retinal dystrophy

B. Physical examination
  1. Extent of exam depends on patient's age and degree of cooperation
  2. Visual acuity
    a. Check each eye separately with glasses on
    b. Verbal children
      i. Optotypes: Snellen letters, tumbling Es, or symbols to check visual acuity
      ii. If patient cannot see largest letter on chart, see if he or she can count fingers, detect hand motion, and perceive light
    c. Preverbal children
      i. **Fixation**: check ability to follow colorful toys or even your face
      ii. Light aversion tells you child sees light (normal): check response to bright light, even with closed lids
      iii. Grating acuity: tests preferential gaze to progressively smaller line gratings on cards
  3. Pupil exam
    a. Check each pupil's response to light separately
    b. Check for **afferent pupillary defect (APD)**
  4. Visual fields: response to toys presented in fields of peripheral vision
  5. Ocular alignment and motility
  6. Ocular exam
    a. Use systematic approach from anterior to posterior
    b. Eyelids, conjunctiva, sclera: check for redness, lesions, tumors, discharge, ptosis (Figure 17-1)
    c. Cornea: look for opacifications, check for abrasions with fluorescein
    d. Anterior chamber: check for white cells, red cells (hyphema), depth
    e. Iris: check for pupil irregularities, heterochromia
    f. **Red reflex**: can pick up abnormalities in lens, vitreous, retina (Figure 17-2)
    g. Optic nerve: use ophthalmoscope to rule out optic disc edema
    h. Retina: direct ophthalmoscope is only a partial exam; consider referral
  7. Radiology tests
    a. Plain films of orbits
      i. Orbital/ocular metallic foreign bodies
      ii. *Not* sufficient for orbital fracture evaluation
    b. Computed tomography (CT) of brain and orbits
      i. Need fine cuts (1 mm) in axial and coronal planes
      ii. Good for evaluation of bone, fractures, trauma, proptosis, cellulitis
    c. Magnetic resonance imaging (MRI) of brain and orbits: good for evaluation of soft tissues, optic nerves
    d. Ocular ultrasound: used to evaluate posterior segment of globe when media opacity (cataract, hemorrhage, etc.) prevents direct view

QUICK HIT

Squinting is an important symptom in children and can signify strabismus, eye pain, photophobia, or vision loss.

QUICK HIT

Delay in meeting developmental milestones can sometimes be related to visual impairment, and, once treated, patients may resume normal developmental growth.

QUICK HIT

Visual acuity is the "vital sign of the eye."

QUICK HIT

A flat or shallow anterior chamber in the presence of trauma is an **open globe** until proven otherwise.

QUICK HIT

Red reflex testing is a very important screening tool for serious eye diseases and should be done in every infant and young child even if there are no eye complaints.

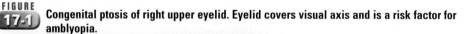

FIGURE 17-1 **Congenital ptosis of right upper eyelid. Eyelid covers visual axis and is a risk factor for amblyopia.**

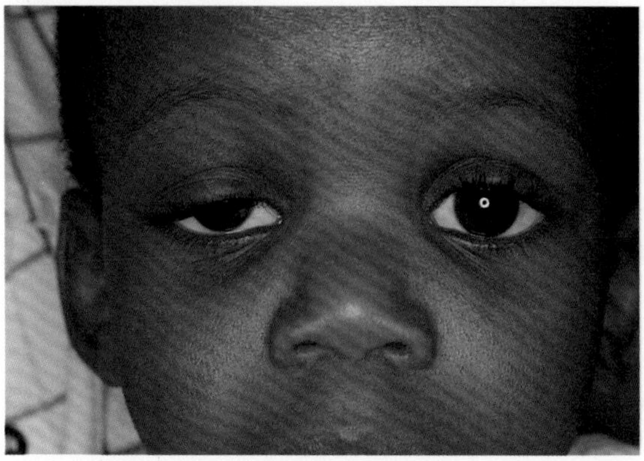

(From Tasman W, Jaeger E. *The Wills Eye Hospital Atlas of Clinical Ophthalmology.* 2nd ed. Philadelphia: Lippincott Williams & Wilkins; 2001.)

QUICK HIT

ERG and VEP are often ordered together when an infant is not developing normal visual behavior and the eyes look normal.

QUICK HIT

Optic disc swelling from other causes is *not* papilledema.

QUICK HIT

Headache is a cardinal symptom of elevated ICP. It worsens with recumbence and is worst when awakening from sleep.

QUICK HIT

Early morning emesis is a sign of raised ICP.

QUICK HIT

Idiopathic intracranial hypertension should be suspected in overweight females with papilledema.

QUICK HIT

The **Cushing triad** is hypertension, widened pulse pressure, and bradycardia.

FIGURE 17-2 **Leukocoria in patient with retinoblastoma. Patient requires immediate ophthalmology referral for life-threatening condition.**

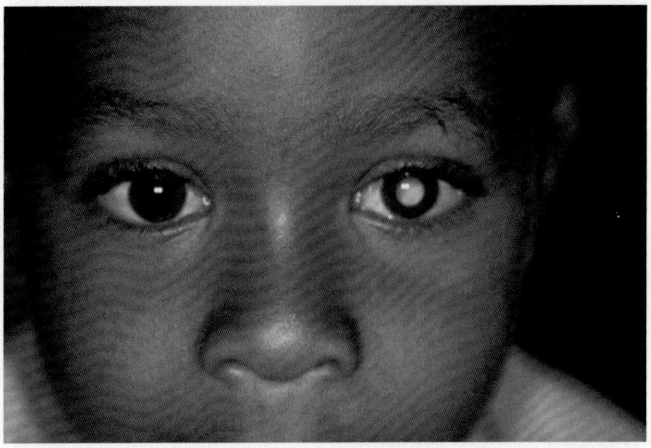

(From Rubin E, Farber JL. *Pathology.* 3rd ed. Philadelphia: Lippincott Williams & Wilkins; 1999.)

8. Electrophysiologic tests
   1. Electroretinogram (ERG)
      i. Evaluates retinal photoreceptor function
      ii. Helpful in diagnosis of retinal dystrophies
   2. Visual evoked potential (VEP): evaluates neurologic and electrophysiologic response to visual stimuli (useful in infants)

III. Approach to Optic Disc Swelling/Papilledema

A. Differential diagnosis
   1. **Papilledema** is due to raised intracranial pressure (ICP)
      a. Caused by increase in volume of any intracranial component
         i. Brain tissue (tumor, encephalitis)
         ii. Blood (hemorrhage, venous sinus thrombosis), brain
         iii. Cerebrospinal fluid (CSF) (hydrocephalus)
         iv. Idiopathic (pseudotumor cerebri)
   2. Bilateral disc swelling: usually from **papilledema**, malignant hypertension, optic neuritis
   3. Unilateral disc swelling: may be from papilledema, optic neuritis, uveitis, neuroretinitis, orbital tumor, anterior ischemic optic neuropathy

B. Historical findings
   1. **Headache, nausea, vomiting**
   2. Change in vision
      a. **Horizontal diplopia** from sixth nerve palsy may be caused by high ICP
      b. **Transient visual obscuration** that clears completely in few seconds
         i. May occur spontaneously or commonly with changes in position
         ii. Occurs in 2/3 of patients with papilledema
      c. **Visual field loss** prior to **visual acuity loss**, often late in course
      d. **Photopsias**: brief flashes provoked by positional changes or Valsalva
   3. Changes in hearing
   4. Medications or exposures
      a. Toxin-induced disc swelling: ethambutol, methanol, ethylene glycol
      b. Increased ICP: steroids, retinoids, tetracyclines
   5. Eye pain or redness may indicate intraocular inflammation or infection
   6. Obesity associated with idiopathic intracranial hypertension

C. Physical examination findings
   1. Signs of increased ICP
      a. Bulging fontanelles in infants whose cranial sutures have not yet closed
      b. **Esotropia** (crossed eyes) and poor abduction of eyes from cranial nerve (CN) VI palsy
      c. Pupillary dilatation (compression of CN III)

2. Fundus exam key findings: blurred optic disc margins, elevated optic disc, obscured retinal vessels passing out of disc
3. Visual acuity
   a. May be normal with papilledema unless severe
   b. May be decreased with optic neuritis, orbital tumor
4. Visual field testing usually normal with mild disease

D. Laboratory testing and radiologic imaging
1. Disc swelling requires an emergent workup for raised ICP
2. CT best for suspected bleeding/emergency, otherwise MRI ± magnetic resonance venography (MRV)
3. Lumbar puncture (LP)
   a. Done if neuroimaging has ruled out space-occupying lesion
   b. Manometry to determine high opening pressure (pseudotumor cerebri)
   c. CSF cell count for suspected infection

IV. Approach to Red Eye

A. Differential diagnosis
1. **Blepharitis** (inflammation of eyelid margin) can lead to "styes," which are **hordeola** (acute) and **chalazia** (chronic) (Figure 17-3A)
2. **Dacryocystitis**: inflammation of lacrimal sac; pain, tearing, redness, and discharge common (Figure 17-3B)
3. **Periorbital ("preseptal") cellulitis**
4. **Orbital cellulitis**
5. **Bacterial conjunctivitis**: frequently (but not always) unilateral, discharge often purulent, conjunctival papillae, typically *no* preauricular adenopathy
6. **Viral conjunctivitis**: 2nd-eye involvement few days after 1st; watery, mucus discharge; preauricular lymphadenopathy, conjunctival follicles
7. **Herpes simplex virus (HSV) conjunctivitis**: unilateral, occasionally recurrent, follicular conjunctivitis; may see herpetic vesicles on eyelid
8. **Allergic conjunctivitis**: characterized by itching, watery discharge, history of allergies, conjunctival papillae
9. **Subconjunctival hemorrhage**: blood under conjunctiva from trauma, Valsalva, hypertension, bleeding disorder, idiopathic; resolves spontaneously
10. **Corneal abrasions**: history of trauma, contact lens wear; often have strong foreign body (FB) sensation and photophobia; redness may not be prominent
11. **Corneal ulcer and keratitis**: trauma, contact lens wear, herpetic; pain, decrease in vision, cloudy cornea, white spot on cornea, vision- and eye-threatening condition

QUICK HIT

MRI is preferable to CT insofar as it provides more detail, avoids radiation for the child, and permits simultaneous MRV.

QUICK HIT

Nasolacrimal duct obstruction may cause the eyelid skin to be red, but the eye itself is still white.

QUICK HIT

Signs of *orbital* cellulitis (rather than *preseptal* cellulitis) include proptosis, conjunctival injection, motility limitation, decreased vision, and afferent pupillary defect.

QUICK HIT

Suspected cases of Stevens-Johnson syndrome need emergent ophthalmologic evaluation and treatment to prevent complications that can lead to blindness.

FIGURE 17-3 **A. Chalazion of right upper eyelid. B. Infantile acute dacryocystitis. Note the erythema and edema overlying the lacrimal sac.**

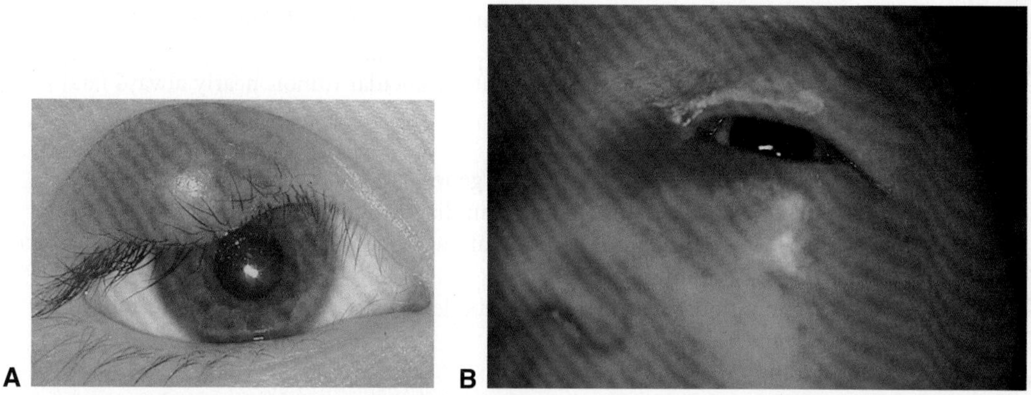

(**A:** From Berg D, Worzala K. *Atlas of Adult Physical Diagnosis*. Philadelphia: Lippincott Williams & Wilkins; 2006. **B:** From Tasman W, Jaeger E. *The Wills Eye Hospital Atlas of Clinical Ophthalmology*. 2nd ed. Philadelphia: Lippincott Williams & Wilkins; 2001.)

> **QUICK HIT**
> The classic triad of congenital glaucoma is blepharospasm, epiphora, and photophobia.

> **QUICK HIT**
> **"Red eye red flags"** for urgent ophthalmology consult include vision loss, pain, contact lens use, status as neonate, chronic red eye not responding to treatment, and severe discharge.

12. **Pterygium**: wing-shaped fibrovascular growth on conjunctiva and cornea, related to sun (ultraviolet [UV] light) and wind; can become acutely inflamed
13. **Acute glaucoma**
    a. Angle closure glaucoma: painful red eye, mid-dilated pupil, hazy cornea, nausea; can be precipitated by certain medications (topiramate, some antipsychotics)
    b. Congenital glaucoma: epiphora (tearing), cloudy cornea, enlarged globe and corneal diameter
14. **Dry-eye syndrome**: redness, irritation; often exacerbated during activities of infrequent blinking (reading, watching television, computer games)
15. **Pharmacologic**: allergic or toxic reaction to topical eye drops (especially "get the red out" medications)

B. Historical findings
1. Duration of redness: acute versus chronic
2. Associated symptoms: photophobia, eye pain, FB sensation, discharge, vision loss, trauma

C. Common physical examination findings
1. Papillae: look at inside of upper eyelid for **cobblestone appearance**; present in bacterial and allergic conjunctivitis, contact lens irritation
2. Follicles: look at inside of lower eyelid for elevated pink follicles; present in viral conjunctivitis, topical medication toxicity
3. Membranes/pseudomembranes: gray-white fibrinous sheets often found on inside of eyelids in moderate-to-severe conjunctivitis, Stevens-Johnson syndrome
4. Discharge: extreme purulence points to bacterial etiology; however, viral disease has some discharge
5. Fluorescein staining essential in evaluation to rule out abrasion, keratitis
6. Intraocular pressure (IOP): difficult to check in children
7. "**Red flags**" for ophthalmology consult: vision loss, cornea or intraocular structure involved, irregular pupil, poor red reflex, vesicles on lids

D. Ancillary testing
1. Cultures: bacterial cultures if copious or purulent discharge; viral culture for HSV if presence of eyelid vesicles
2. Inflammatory processes (scleritis, uveitis): consider workup for rheumatologic disease

V. Approach to Abnormal Red Reflex and Leukocoria

> **QUICK HIT**
> Abnormal red reflex or leukocoria in young children requires immediate ophthalmologist evaluation to rule out a life- or vision-threatening condition!

> **QUICK HIT**
> Retinoblastoma is the most common primary intraocular malignancy in children.

A. Definitions
1. Red reflex test
    a. Very important screening tool for detecting opacity or abnormality in visual axis (cornea, anterior chamber, pupil, lens, vitreous, retina)
    b. Abnormal when reflexes in either or both eyes are dim, absent, or asymmetric in color, intensity, or clarity
2. **Leukocoria** (see Figure 17-2)
    a. "White pupil"
    b. White spot or opacity in pupillary space or on red reflex testing

B. Differential diagnosis
1. **Retinoblastoma**: primary malignant intraocular tumor, nearly always fatal if untreated
    a. Pathophysiology
        i. Mutation tumor suppressor gene (*RB1*) on chromosome 13q14
        ii. 2/3 sporadic; unilateral; mean diagnosis 18–24 months
        iii. 1/3 germline mutation; unilateral or bilateral; diagnosis typically earlier (<12 months)
    b. Presentation: abnormal red reflux, leukocoria, strabismus (esotropia), or chronic red eye
    c. Testing
        i. Dilated fundus exam in clinic and under anesthesia reveals tumor
        ii. Ocular ultrasound: heterogeneous mass, calcifications

iii. MRI of brain and orbits: brain metastases, eye calcifications
iv. Examine parents and siblings
d. Therapy
i. Goals are 1st to preserve life, then eye, then vision
ii. >90% survival in developed countries
iii. Discrete unilateral tumor: focal treatment
iv. Large, advanced tumor: enucleation
v. Chemotherapy and orbital radiation
vi. Genetic testing/counseling for parents
vii. Long-term follow-up: new ocular tumors; bilateral has increased risk of other tumors (pinealoblastoma, osteogenic sarcoma, others)

2. **Congenital cataract**
   a. Opacity of lens present at birth
   b. Requires cataract surgery within 4–6 weeks of life to prevent irreversible vision deficit from amblyopia
3. **Corneal opacity**
   a. Corneal ulcer
   b. Cloudy cornea from congenital glaucoma
4. **Strabismus**: eyes are not straight; light reflects off different parts of retina; bright red reflex in deviated eye
5. **High refractive errors** (high myopia or hyperopia): dim red reflex
6. **Retinal detachment**
7. **Uveitis**, **endophthalmitis**: intraocular inflammation/infection

C. Historical questions
1. Onset, visual behavior, eye crossing or drifting, red eye, pain
2. History of prematurity; maternal infection or rash; pre- or perinatal exposure to toxins, drugs, alcohol; trauma; steroid use
3. Family history of retinoblastoma/eye cancer, congenital eye disorder

D. Physical examination findings
1. To best examine for red reflex
   a. Darken room to maximize pupil dilation
   b. Examine both pupils simultaneously looking through direct ophthalmoscope about arm's length away
2. Normal results
   a. Symmetric reflexes; equal in size, color, intensity
   b. Bright reflexes; reddish, or lightly gray in dark-eyed patients
3. Abnormal results
   a. Dim, absent, white, or asymmetric reflexes in 1 or both eyes
   b. Requires immediate referral to ophthalmologist for full dilated exam and management
4. Remainder of eye exam
   a. Vision: poor tracking
   b. Other abnormalities to look for
      i. Strabismus
      ii. Nystagmus
      iii. Small abnormal eye (microphthalmos)
      iv. **Conjunctival injection**

VI. Approach to Vision Loss and Visual Impairment

A. Differential diagnosis
1. Distinguish chronic/congenital *versus* acute/acquired
2. **Media opacities**: corneal opacities, cataracts, hyphema, vitreous hemorrhage
3. **Inflammatory diseases**: keratitis, uveitis, endophthalmitis, scleritis, retinitis
4. **Retinal abnormalities**: retinopathy of prematurity (ROP), retinal detachment
5. **Optic nerve abnormalities**: coloboma, hypoplasia, glaucoma
6. **Refractive errors**
7. **Amblyopia**: can occur in conjunction with other ocular abnormalities
8. **Visual pathway lesions**: tumor, ischemic injury, neurologic abnormalities

QUICK HIT

Persistent flashes of light, new large floaters, and "curtain" pulled down over vision are symptoms of retinal tear or detachment and require immediate evaluation.

9. **Delayed visual maturation**: infants with poor vision/fixation but normal ocular/neurologic exam may still develop normal vision

B. Important historical characteristics
1. Timing: vision impairment present since birth or recently acquired
2. Unilateral or bilateral
3. Central or peripheral vision
4. Other visual/ocular symptoms: pain, flashing lights, red eye
5. Developmental milestones: poor vision can cause developmental delay or be part of an underlying syndrome
6. Family history: refractive error, retinal dystrophies, cataracts
7. Birth history: prematurity, birth trauma, perinatal apneic events

C. Physical examination findings
1. Poor visual acuity or fixation behavior
   a. Infants should fix and follow by age 2–3 months
   b. Premature infants develop by corrected age (6-month-old, former 28-week premature infant has vision like 3-month-old full-term infant)
2. Pupils: APD with retinal, optic nerve, or brain lesion
3. Color vision abnormalities: with optic neuropathy and neuritis
4. Visual field deficit
   a. **Congruous visual field deficits**: lesion posterior to chiasm
   b. **Incongruous visual field deficits**: anterior visual pathway issues
5. Nystagmus: can be sign of poor vision early in life, often from ocular etiology
6. Strabismus: can be cause or a sign of visual impairment
7. Complete ocular exam: corneal opacities, inflammation, leukocoria, cataract
8. Fundus exam: optic nerve edema or abnormalities, retinal abnormalities
   a. "**Cherry red spot**": central retinal artery occlusion
   b. Retinal detachment: painless, associated with flashes, floaters
9. Neurologic exam: abnormalities may point to central visual processing defect, tumor, infection, demyelination

QUICK HIT

The "cherry red spot" can also be seen in patients with Tay-Sachs disease.

D. Laboratory testing and radiologic imaging
1. Brain and orbits MRI: rule out cortical and optic nerve tumors, abnormalities
2. Inflammatory and infectious workup as indicated by exam
3. ERG: evaluates photoreceptor function of retina
4. VEP: measures cortical electrical activity in response to visual stimuli

DISEASE SPECIFIC

VII. Ocular and Orbital Trauma

QUICK HIT

Do not delay irrigation! Forgo history and exam until irrigation has been done.

QUICK HIT

Alkali burns to the eye tend to be worse than acidic burns.

A. Chemical exposure
1. Characteristics
   a. True ocular emergency; every second counts; immediate copious irrigation is paramount
   b. Ocular surface damage from chemical exposure can result in permanent loss of vision from corneal, conjunctival, and eyelid scarring, destruction
2. Clinical features
   a. Identify chemical substance
   b. Determine extent of irrigation performed thus far
   c. Check pH other than neutral (base is worse than acid)
   d. Examine eye for injection or opacification
   e. Test for corneal abrasion with fluorescein exam
3. Treatment
   a. Apply proparacaine if immediately available
   b. Copious irrigation; if acid/base, continue irrigation until pH neutral

B. Open globe injury
1. Characteristics
   a. Definition: full-thickness wound in eye wall including cornea, sclera
   b. Vision- and eye-threatening condition, emergent ophthalmology consult

2. Clinical features
    a. Consider open globe injury if
        i. Obvious wound: corneal laceration, uvea (brown tissue) visible
        ii. Collapsed/shallow anterior chamber
        iii. Hyphema
        iv. Newly irregular or peaked pupil
3. Diagnosis: based on clinic exam and index of suspicion
4. Treatment
    a. Once open globe is suspected, stop exam
    b. Cover eye with shield (*not* patch) to prevent further trauma; avoid painful procedures; strict bed rest; pain control; antiemetic
    c. Emergent ophthalmology consult
    d. **Sympathetic ophthalmia**: uveitis induced in uninjured *other* eye from bad open globe injury

C. **Hyphema**
1. Characteristics
    a. Definition: blood in anterior chamber
    b. Cause: typically blunt trauma, but occasionally penetrating trauma
    c. Spontaneous hyphema: retinoblastoma, juvenile xanthogranuloma
2. Exam: layered blood in anterior chamber (Figure 17-4)
3. Treatment
    a. Main concern is acute glaucoma (rise in IOP), causing permanent optic nerve damage and vision loss; red blood cells (RBCs) clog drainage in anterior chamber
    b. Emergent ophthalmology consult
    c. Risk factors for IOP spike
        i. "Re-bleed": risk highest in 1st 5 days
        ii. Sickle cell disease or trait: RBCs sickle in anterior chamber
    d. Prevention of IOP spike
        i. Daily exams
        ii. Strict bed rest for 5 days; shield (not patch) over eye
        iii. Topical prednisolone and homatropine; no nonsteroidal anti-inflammatory drugs (NSAIDs)
        iv. Sickle cell testing for all African Americans
    e. Management of IOP spike
        i. Topical glaucoma agents; systemic acetazolamide
        ii. Surgical "wash out" of anterior chamber clot for refractory IOP

D. **Corneal abrasion**
1. Characteristics
    a. Causes
        i. Direct trauma
        ii. Contact lens abuse

QUICK HIT

Have a high index of suspicion for open globe injury; consider timing and mechanism of trauma, projectile injury, pain, vision loss, and recent ocular surgery.

QUICK HIT

Once an open globe injury is identified, *stop* the exam and contact ophthalmology!

QUICK HIT

In children, examination under anesthesia is sometimes necessary to know the full extent of injuries.

QUICK HIT

An **eye shield** *does not* touch the eye, whereas an **eye patch** *does* touch the eye.

FIGURE 17-4 **Hyphema, or blood in the anterior chamber.**

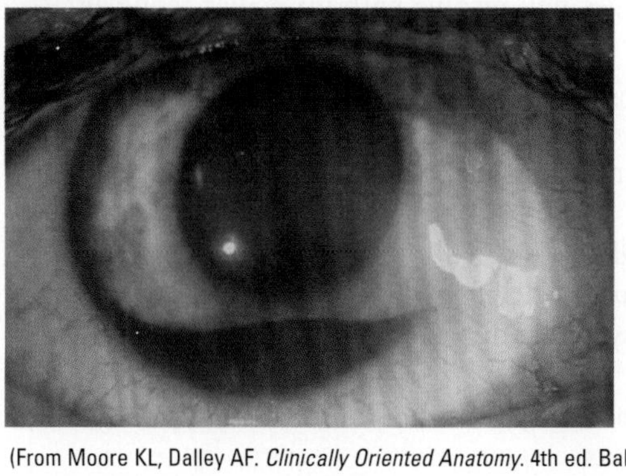

(From Moore KL, Dalley AF. *Clinically Oriented Anatomy*. 4th ed. Baltimore: Lippincott Williams & Wilkins; 1999.)

QUICK HIT

Topical proparacaine completely relieves pain and allows exam, but it is toxic if used chronically, so never prescribe it!

QUICK HIT

Extraocular muscle entrapment can be a surgical emergency in children if the oculocardiac reflex causes a vagal response or bradycardia.

QUICK HIT

Get an ophthalmology consultation for corneal abrasion with concerning signs including a large or central abrasion, contact lens wearer, and poor eyelid closure.

QUICK HIT

Retinal hemorrhages are "present" in about 85% of cases of abusive head trauma, but the severity of retinal hemorrhage is important for diagnostic implications.

QUICK HIT

The **conjunctiva** is the membrane covering the sclera and inside of the eyelid.

QUICK HIT

Neonatal conjunctivitis, or **ophthalmia neonatorum**, is a condition that occurs in the 1st month of life.

QUICK HIT

Gonococcal conjunctivitis can cause rapid (<24 hours) corneal perforation and blindness if not recognized and treated promptly!

iii. Exposure from poor eyelid closure (i.e., from CN VII palsy, sedation in intensive care unit [ICU])
b. If infected, becomes **corneal ulcer**
2. Clinical features
a. Symptoms include pain, tearing, photophobia, FB sensation
b. Physical exam: fluorescein staining with blue light or Wood's lamp
3. Treatment
a. Most abrasions heal quickly, within 24–72 hours
b. Antibiotic ophthalmic ointment to prevent infection and reduce pain (coats exposed nerve endings)
c. Close follow-up (1–2 days) to ensure healing

E. Orbital fracture
1. Characteristics
a. Orbital fracture from blunt trauma
b. "Trap door" fracture: more common in children; orbital floor fracture pieces "snap back" up into place, trapping extraocular muscle
2. Clinical features
a. History: mechanism, pain with eye movements, double vision
b. Physical exam
i. Eyelid bruising or swelling (may be absent in children)
ii. Motility restriction
iii. **Enophthalmos** (eye displaced backward into orbit)
iv. Infraorbital nerve hypoesthesia (numbness of cheek)
3. Diagnosis: CT orbits, fine cuts, axial and coronal (plain films not sufficient)
4. Treatment: surgical repair of fracture

F. Retinal hemorrhage in abusive head trauma
1. Characteristics
a. Abusive head trauma (**shaken baby syndrome**): repetitive acceleration–deceleration injury with or without impact
b. Intracranial hemorrhage, retinal hemorrhage, and ischemic brain injury, with or without bony (e.g., rib) fractures or other systemic injuries
2. Clinical features
a. History: injury inconsistent with alleged accident, changing stories, repeated hospital admissions (see Chapter 18, Child Physical Abuse and Neglect)
b. Exam: requires dilated fundus exam by an ophthalmologist
3. Differential diagnosis for retinal hemorrhage in this age group
a. Abusive head trauma
b. Accidental head trauma: uncommonly (<10%) causes retinal hemorrhages, which when present are few and limited to posterior pole
c. Birth trauma: common (35%) but resolves in 2–4 weeks
4. Diagnosis
a. Multidisciplinary team offers best approach, led by suspected child abuse and neglect team in hospital
b. Radiology findings
i. Head CT: may show subdural hemorrhage
ii. Skeletal survey: to identify occult fractures
5. Treatment: most retinal hemorrhages will resolve without ocular sequelae

VIII. Conjunctivitis

A. General characteristics
1. Conjunctival inflammation due to infection, allergy, toxin, rheumatologic, dryness
a. Neonatal conjunctivitis
i. Acquired from vaginal canal
ii. Bacterial: *Neisseria gonorrhoeae* or *Chlamydia trachomatis*
iii. HSV: may involve cornea; systemic disease often fatal
b. Older infants and children
i. **Viral**: most commonly adenovirus, but numerous others; typically self-limited; highly contagious

ii. **Herpetic**: HSV, varicella-zoster virus (VZV)
iii. **Bacterial**: staphylococci, streptococci, *Haemophilus influenzae*, *C. trachomatis*, *Pseudomonas aeruginosa* (with contact lens wear), *N. gonorrhoeae*; produces "hyperacute" copious purulent conjunctivitis
iv. **Allergic**: mast cell release of histamine; common triggers include pollen, perfumes, smoke, dust mites
v. **Toxic**: chemical exposure

B. Clinical features
1. Historical findings (Box 17-1)
a. **Viral**: clear, watery discharge; "cold" symptoms, family or classmates with red eyes; often begins unilaterally but most spread to become bilateral
b. **Bacterial**: overdiagnosed; mucopurulent discharge; commonly but not always unilateral; contact lens wearers especially susceptible
c. **Allergic**: bilateral itching and tearing; may be seasonal
d. Toxic exposure, eye drops ("get the red out" drops with vasoconstrictors like tetrahydrozoline hydrochloride)
2. Physical exam findings
a. **Conjunctival injection**: hallmark finding
b. **Discharge**
c. **Chemosis** (conjunctival edema): allergic
d. **Fluorescein staining**: "dendrite" HSV keratitis, corneal ulcer
3. Laboratory findings
a. **Neonatal conjunctivitis**: appearance and timing do not give diagnosis
i. **Gram stain**: sight threatening gonococcal infection (gram-negative intracellular diplococci); chlamydia shows intracytoplasmic inclusion bodies
ii. Culture: do *not* wait to start treatment
b. Any age: if suspicion for HSV in absence of dermatitis: direct fluorescent antibody staining; polymerase chain reaction/culture

C. Treatment
1. Neonatal conjunctivitis
a. Admission, culture, Gram stain, ophthalmology consult
b. Check closely for corneal involvement
c. Topical antibiotic drops (polymyxin, moxifloxacin)
d. Intravenous (IV) agent (ceftriaxone) and irrigation of discharge if *N. gonorrhoeae* suspected
e. IV acyclovir if HSV suspected
f. Oral and topical erythromycin for *C. trachomatis*, high risk for treatment failure
2. Children
a. Infectious in general
i. Topical antibiotics (Polytrim [polymyxin and trimethoprim] first, quinolone for severe cases)
ii. No contact lenses
b. HSV: acyclovir, ophthalmologist consult
c. Allergic: avoid triggers, antihistamines, artificial tears
d. Toxic: immediate irrigation, artificial tears

BOX 17-1

Conjunctivitis Red Flags for Urgent Ophthalmology Referral

History	Physical Exam
1. Vision loss	**1.** Corneal involvement
2. Pain	**2.** Irregular pupil
3. Severe photophobia or discharge	**3.** Abnormal red reflex
4. Chronic not responding to treatment	**4.** Vesicles on lids
5. Neonate	**5.** Motility deficit
6. Contact lens use or eye surgery	

QUICK HIT

With any red eye, contact lens wearers should remove contacts immediately! They can be infected, causing repeated trauma and preventing oxygenation.

QUICK HIT

Itch = allergy.

QUICK HIT

The presence of pus indicates a bacterial infection, whereas no pus only means that a bacterial cause cannot be ruled out—pus = bacterial; no pus = no pus.

QUICK HIT

Corneal involvement is *not* simple conjunctivitis and may be an abrasion or ulcer.

QUICK HIT

Congenital glaucoma presents with tearing, **hyperemia**, a cloudy cornea, and an enlarged eye.

QUICK HIT

Crusting or discharge does *not* mean conjunctivitis if the conjunctiva itself is not red!

QUICK HIT

Do not send discharge for culture if the eye is not red; it is a tear duct obstruction!

QUICK HIT

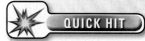

Chronic conjunctivitis not responding to treatment requires urgent referral!

> **QUICK HIT**
> With an irregular pupil in a red eye, think scarring from uveitis.

> **QUICK HIT**
> The cornea should *always* be clear with iris details clearly visible.

> **QUICK HIT**
> Conjunctivitis, with few exceptions, is a clinical diagnosis.

> **QUICK HIT**
> Cultures are not routinely sent for conjunctivitis.

> **QUICK HIT**
> Oral macrolide therapy in neonatal conjunctivitis due to chlamydia prevents the development of pneumonia.

> **QUICK HIT**
> About 10% of normal full-term newborns have congenital nasolacrimal duct obstruction, due to incomplete canalization of the duct, typically at the distal end.

> **QUICK HIT**
> Nasolacrimal duct obstruction causes discharge and tearing, but the eye is *not* red.

> **QUICK HIT**
> Tearing in a newborn is not necessarily a nasolacrimal duct obstruction; check for signs of congenital glaucoma.

IX. Dacryostenosis and Dacryocystitis

A. Definitions
   1. **Dacryostenosis**: nasolacrimal duct obstruction; most common cause of persistent tearing and ocular discharge in infants
   2. **Dacryocystitis**: infection of lacrimal sac (see Figure 17-3B)

B. Clinical features
   1. History: tearing, crusting on lashes, mucoid discharge
   2. Exam findings
      a. Nasolacrimal duct obstruction
         i. **Epiphora**: overflow of tears down cheeks
         ii. **Crusting** of eyelids/eyelashes
         iii. **Mucoid discharge**
      b. Acute dacryocystitis (see Figure 17-3B): erythema, warmth, swelling, tenderness over lacrimal sac (medial and inferior to corner of eye near nose)

C. Treatment
   1. Congenital nasolacrimal duct obstruction
      a. Massage: pressure "milking" duct from lacrimal sac downward alongside the nose for 30 seconds, 2–3 times/day
      b. 90% resolve spontaneously within 1st year of life
      c. Nasolacrimal duct probing by ophthalmologist for persistent obstruction or excessive crusting not responsive to antibiotic ointment
   2. Acute dacryocystitis
      a. IV antibiotics (group A *Streptococcus* or *Staphylococcus aureus*)
      b. Probing required (in contrast to isolated cellulitis)

X. Hordeolum and Chalazion

A. Definitions
   1. **Hordeolum**: acute purulent inflammation of glands at edge of eyelid
   2. **Chalazion** (see Figure 17-3A): focal, subacute, noninfectious chronic inflammation of eyelid glands

B. Cause: gland ducts blocked with sebum and cell debris

C. Clinical presentation
   1. Eyelid bump: edge of eyelid = hordeolum; distal from lid margin = chalazion
   2. Swelling, redness, and tenderness around bump

D. Treatment
   1. **Warm/hot compresses** for 10 minutes, 4 times/day
   2. Most lesions resolve spontaneously within 1 month

XI. Pterygium

A. Definition: growth of fibrovascular tissue within conjunctiva; may grow onto cornea

B. Related to repeated wind, sun, sand, or dust exposure (e.g., American southwest)

C. Clinical presentation
   1. Symptoms
      a. Painless wedge of red/tan tissue; can become inflamed and irritating
      b. Growth onto cornea may affect vision by causing **astigmatism** or obstruction
   2. Grows over months or years, although may be stable for years

D. Therapy
   1. Redness and irritation: topical lubricants, mild steroid drops
   2. **Surgical excision**: for lesions affecting vision or chronic inflammation

XII. Keratitis and Corneal Ulcer

A. Definition
   1. **Keratitis**: inflammation or infection of cornea
   2. **Corneal ulcer**: is focus of keratitis with overlying corneal defect

B. Causes
   1. Predisposing factors
      a. Contact lens wear, particularly soft contact lenses worn overnight or during swimming

b. Trauma
c. Chronic incomplete lid closure
d. HSV, VZV infection
2. Pathophysiology
a. Predominantly bacterial: *S. aureus, P. aeruginosa*
b. HSV keratitis: look for eyelid vesicles, history of oculofacial herpes
c. Fungal keratitis after trauma with vegetative matter (e.g., tree branch)
d. *Acanthamoeba*: swimming in fresh water with contact lenses

C. Clinical presentation
1. Symptoms: FB sensation, photophobia, blurred vision, pain, discharge, edema
2. Signs: conjunctival injection, focal or diffuse corneal whitening

D. Testing: fluorescein staining to look for corneal epithelial defect or abrasion

E. Therapy
1. Sight-threatening and even eye-threatening conditions; requires immediate ophthalmology consultation and management
2. Frequent (every hour) use of topical broad-spectrum antibiotic eye drops
3. Cycloplegic ("dilating") eye drops: for comfort if photophobia present
4. Cease contact lens use; discard contacts, lens case, lens solution

XIII. Uveitis

A. Definition: inflammation of uveal tract (iris, ciliary body, choroid)

B. Causes
1. Infections: HSV, cytomegalovirus, toxoplasmosis, syphilis
2. Rheumatologic disorders: sarcoidosis, Behçet syndrome, juvenile idiopathic arthritis (JIA), others
3. Trauma (traumatic iritis, sympathetic ophthalmia)

C. Clinical presentation
1. Symptoms: pain, photophobia, blurred vision, floaters
2. Signs
a. Conjunctival injection, particularly ciliary flush
b. Posterior synechiae: adhesions from iris to lens; causes pupil irregularities
c. Cataract
d. Retinal changes (hemorrhages, inflammatory lesions, vasculitis)

D. Workup of uveitis requires evaluation and management by ophthalmologist and possibly rheumatologist

E. Therapy: topical steroids, cycloplegic drops, treat underlying rheumatologic disease

XIV. Nystagmus

A. Characteristics
1. **Nystagmus**: involuntary, often rhythmic, oscillation of 1 or both eyes
2. **Jerk nystagmus**: slow-drift phase, then corrective quick phase (**saccade**)
3. **Pendular nystagmus**: just back and forth motion, no corrective saccade
4. **Opsoclonus**: just multidirectional quick movements ("saccade-o-mania")

B. Causes
1. Infantile (congenital) nystagmus
a. *With* vision loss: aniridia, albinism, retinal dystrophy, optic nerve hypoplasia, congenital cataracts, high refractive errors
b. *Without* vision loss: idiopathic ocular motor disorder
2. Acquired nystagmus: onset age >3 months
a. Central nervous system (CNS) lesions
b. **Opsoclonus/myoclonus syndrome** (paraneoplastic syndrome from neuroblastoma) is also called "dancing eyes, dancing feet"
c. Vestibular system disease (peripheral or central)
d. Drugs: anticonvulsants, sedatives, others
3. Spasmus nutans: onset age 4–12 months; pendular
a. **Torticollis**, head nodding, asymmetric shimmering nystagmus
b. Spontaneously resolves by age 5 years, but rule out chiasmal tumor

QUICK HIT

Hordeolum and chalazion are commonly referred to as "styes."

QUICK HIT

Heat helps melt secretions and promotes spontaneous drainage of a stye.

QUICK HIT

Epithelial defects occur commonly in contact lens wearers, predisposing them to bacterial keratitis. Corneal ulcer should always be considered in any contact lens user with a painful red eye.

QUICK HIT

Use lubricating ophthalmic ointment to prevent keratitis in patients with incomplete lid closure.

QUICK HIT

JIA-associated uveitis commonly produces no symptoms or redness in children; therefore, children with JIA require regular screening for uveitis regardless of symptoms.

QUICK HIT

With uveitis, ask historical questions to recognize risk factors for inflammatory conditions, such as about the presence of arthritis, rashes, oral/genital ulcers, or fever; inquire about recent travel and any family history of inflammatory disease.

QUICK HIT

Lymphoma and leukemia can cause masquerade syndromes mimicking uveitis and should be considered in atypical uveitis presentations.

QUICK HIT

JIA-associated uveitis is most common in pauciarticular, antinuclear antibody–positive, rheumatoid factor–negative disease.

QUICK HIT

50% of children with opsoclonus have neuroblastoma.

QUICK HIT

The classic triad of symptoms for congenital glaucoma is **epiphora** (tearing), **photophobia**, and **blepharospasm** (lid squeezing).

QUICK HIT

In babies, glaucoma typically causes eye enlargement; in adults, there may be no external signs of glaucoma.

QUICK HIT

Congenital glaucoma is a surgical disease; medical treatment is only temporizing.

QUICK HIT

Early intervention for congenital cataracts is critical to prevent long-term visual impairment!

C. Testing
   1. Complete ocular exam for structural abnormalities
   2. Consider ERG, VEP, MRI
   3. Opsoclonus: neuroblastoma workup (urine testing, body imaging)

XV. Glaucoma

A. Definitions
   1. Elevated IOP resulting in optic nerve damage and vision loss
   2. Congenital glaucoma is present at birth or within 1st year of life
   3. Juvenile glaucoma presents later, often secondary to other conditions
   4. **Open angle**: drainage angle between cornea and iris is open
   5. **Closed angle**: drainage angle is closed off; typically much higher IOP

B. Causes/pathophysiology
   1. Primary congenital glaucoma: caused by structural abnormalities of aqueous outflow tract (trabecular meshwork, iris, cornea)
   2. Secondary acquired glaucoma from trauma, uveitis, surgery, cataract

C. Clinical presentation
   1. Congenital glaucoma usually presents early in infancy with parent noticing clouding or eye enlargement; most are bilateral
   2. Symptoms
      a. Glaucoma is often painless, unless IOP is very high (IOP >30 mm Hg), in which case can have eye pain, headache, nausea/vomiting
      b. Peripheral vision affected first, so may be asymptomatic, then central vision loss later
   3. Key signs
      a. External: large eye (**buphthalmos**), enlarged cornea (>12 mm), cloudy cornea (corneal edema), dull red reflex
      b. Raised IOP (>21 mm Hg)

D. Testing
   a. IOP measurement (**tonometry**)
   b. Visual field testing in older children and adults
   c. Ophthalmology exam (sedated if necessary)

E. Therapy
   1. Medical treatment
      a. Topical eye drops (β-blocker, carbonic anhydrase inhibitor, prostaglandin analogue, and adrenergic agent)
      b. Systemic acetazolamide, mannitol
   2. Surgical treatment: goniotomy and trabeculotomy to open outflow tract, shunt placement

XVI. Cataract

A. General characteristics
   1. Definition: opacity in lens of eye; may be congenital or acquired
   2. Opacities blocking vision can impair development; early diagnosis is critical

B. Etiology
   1. Congenital cataracts are 1/3 idiopathic, 1/3 inherited, 1/3 systemic association
   2. Systemic conditions: intrauterine TORCH infections, galactosemia, hypoparathyroidism, JIA, neurofibromatosis type II diabetes, steroid use
   3. Chromosomal abnormalities: Turner syndrome (XO), trisomy 13 or 21

C. Clinical presentation
   1. Physical exam
      a. Red reflex testing is key screening tool
      b. Diagnosis based on direct physical exam through dilated pupils
      c. Inability to fix and follow by age 3 months: concerning for cataract
      d. Strabismus and nystagmus: worrisome for loss of vision

D. Testing: Consider TORCH infection, galactosemia (in newborn screening), karyotype

E. Treatment
1. Urgent ophthalmology evaluation
2. Visually significant cataracts (block visual axis) must be removed surgically
3. Aggressive amblyopia treatment (patching and glasses)

XVII. Optic Neuritis

A. **Optic neuritis**: optic nerve inflammation, associated with myelin sheath destruction
B. Causes
1. Demyelinating disorders: multiple sclerosis (MS), acute disseminated encephalomyelitis
2. Infectious or postinfectious: meningitis, encephalitis, Lyme disease, postviral (VZV, Epstein-Barr virus, influenza)
C. Clinical presentation
1. Symptoms: decreased/altered vision, decreased color vision, pain with eye movements
2. Signs
a. Disc swelling or optic nerve pallor/atrophy
b. **Dyschromatopsia**: decreased color vision (hallmark)
c. Abnormal visual fields, with reduced visual acuity
D. Diagnosis
1. Brain and orbits MRI: optic nerve inflammation, other CNS signs
2. LP: to rule out CNS infection if suspected (fever, meningismus)

XVIII. Strabismus

A. General characteristics
1. Definition: eye misalignment
a. "Phoria" versus "tropia": **hetero*phoria*** = tendency to deviate; **hetero*tropia*** = deviated
b. Prefixes
i. *Ortho-*: aligned
ii. *Eso-*: inward; *exo-*: outward (e.g., **exophoria** = tendency for eyes to drift apart; **esotropia** = eyes are crossed now)
iii. *Hyper-*: upward; *hypo-*: downward
c. **Comitant** versus **incomitant**: comitant = amount of deviation same in different gaze directions; incomitant = deviation amount changes with gaze direction
2. Epidemiology: 4% of children age <6 years; 30%–50% children with strabismus develop amblyopia
3. Common causes of strabismus
a. **Infantile (congenital) esotropia**: comitant; large-angle esotropia; presents age <6 months; surgical treatment
b. **Accommodative esotropia**: comitant esotropia associated with farsightedness; average age 2.5 years; treatment = glasses
c. **Intermittent exotropia**: comitant; varying control of exotropia; onset = infancy to age 5 years
d. **Convergence insufficiency**: comitant; exotropia at near fixation; blurred vision and headaches with reading; typically age >10 years
e. **Sensory-deprivation esotropia** or **exotropia**: comitant; horizontal deviation in patients with monocular or binocular poor vision; any age
f. **CN III palsy**: incomitant; eye down and out; ptosis and dilated pupil seen in complete CN III palsy
g. **CN IV palsy**: incomitant; often congenital
h. **CN VI palsy**: incomitant; esotropia and limited abduction; postviral; increased ICP
i. **Myasthenia gravis**: incomitant; ptosis; variable limitation of motility
j. **Thyroid eye disease**: incomitant; restricted motility and proptosis
k. **Orbital tumors**, **abscesses**: incomitant; inflammatory signs, proptosis

QUICK HIT

Treatment does not end with cataract surgery; amblyopia therapy is critical to visual outcome!

QUICK HIT

An initial episode of CNS demyelination is called a **clinically isolated syndrome (CIS)**. Children are less likely than adults to progress from CIS to clinically definite MS.

QUICK HIT

In patients without disc swelling, consider retrobulbar optic neuritis (behind the globe).

QUICK HIT

With **tropia**, the eyes are *not* straight; with **phoria**, the eyes *are* straight right now.

QUICK HIT

Incomitant strabismus is concerning for a focal neurologic cause (CN palsy, myasthenia) or restrictive process (thyroid, tumor).

QUICK HIT

Congenital CN IV palsy often presents with a head tilt/torticollis and causes asymmetric facial growth if not treated.

QUICK HIT

Blunt head trauma is commonly a cause of CN IV palsy given that nerve's long intracranial course.

B. **Clinical features**
 1. History: diplopia, onset and duration of strabismus, recent trauma, other neurologic symptoms, family history, eyeglasses
 2. Physical exam
  a. Visual acuity; look for nystagmus, ptosis, facial asymmetry, head tilt
  b. Check pupillary, slit-lamp, and fundus examinations
  c. Assess alignment
   i. With patient looking at flashlight, light reflection should be symmetric
   ii. Red reflexes
   iii. Cover–uncover test: with child fixating on object, cover 1 eye and look for movement of uncovered eye, which signifies tropia
   iv. Alternate cover test: rapidly shift cover from 1 eye to other to see both tropia and phoria
  d. Ocular motility: look for restricted or limited movements

C. Treatment
 1. Tailored to cause of strabismus
  a. Eyeglasses, sometimes with added prism
  b. Chemodenervation with botulinum toxin injections
  c. Eye muscle surgery: muscles are moved or shortened
 2. Early recognition and treatment required to prevent amblyopia

QUICK HIT

The hallmark of myasthenia gravis is variability; it can cause any strabismus pattern.

QUICK HIT

Most pediatric strabismus does not cause persistent diplopia insofar as children learn to suppress the second conflicting image. The presence of diplopia signals an acute onset of strabismus.

QUICK HIT

The light reflex test is helpful to differentiate true strabismus from **pseudostrabismus**, the appearance of esotropia from broad, flat nasal bridges or prominent epicanthal skin folds.

QUICK HIT

Suspected CN III palsy requires emergent imaging with magnetic resonance angiography or CT angiography.

QUICK HIT

Botox was first invented to treat strabismus.

QUICK HIT

In nonverbal children, look for fixation preference and visual attention to objects with each eye.

XIX. Amblyopia

A. General characteristics
 1. Definition: decrease of visual acuity caused by developmental defect in central visual processing
 2. Prevalence: 2%–4% in children and adults
 3. Causes
  a. **Strabismus**: suppression of deviating eye
  b. **Anisometropia**: difference in refractive errors between eyes; suppression of eye with higher refractive error
  c. **Stimulus deprivation**: visual deprivation (unilateral or bilateral) early in life
 4. Pathophysiology
  a. Visual cortex develops in response to receiving clear images from each eye
  b. Early critical period during 1st 3 months of life; visual deprivation can result in dense, irreversible amblyopia
  c. "Amblyogenic period": visual pathways and cortex develop through age 8 years; require clear images from eyes for normal development
  d. Blurred images from refractive error (anisometropia and high refractive error), lack of transmitted images (deprivation), and selective suppression of image from deviated eye (strabismic amblyopia) cause impaired development of visual system

B. Clinical features
 1. History
  a. Child's ability to fixate on objects and faces
  b. Strabismus or other risk factors
  c. Family history of ocular disease
 2. Physical exam findings
  a. Visual acuity: difference between eyes (unilateral amblyopia) or bilateral poor acuity that does not improve even with eyeglasses
  b. Look for risk factors: strabismus, nystagmus, leukocoria, ptosis, facial hemangioma or other lesion

C. Treatment
 1. Therapy
  a. Correct underlying causes
  b. Occlusion of normal eye: patching used to encourage use of amblyopic eye, used part time to avoid inducing "reverse amblyopia" of normal eye

2. Prognosis
   a. Younger treatment age = better treatment response
   b. Sensitive period for amblyopia reversal: best before age 7 years; can see response up to 14 years

XX. Retinal Detachment

A. Definition: detachment of neurosensory retina from underlying pigment epithelium (RPE)
B. Pathophysiology
   1. Fluid in potential space between neurosensory retina and RPE
   2. Types
      a. Rhegmatogenous: tear or break in retina, caused by trauma, Stickler syndrome, coloboma
      b. Tractional: abnormal neovascularization pulls on retina, caused by ROP, sickle cell
C. Clinical presentation: flashes, floaters, decreased vision
D. Testing: emergent ophthalmologist referral for dilated fundus exam, ocular ultrasound
E. Therapy
   1. Surgical intervention
   2. Prophylactic laser retinopexy for diseases with high rate of retinal detachment

> **QUICK HIT**
> Retinal detachment is *painless.*

XXI. Retinopathy of Prematurity

A. General characteristics
   1. Definition: potentially blinding disease of developing retinal vasculature in premature infants
   2. Epidemiology
      a. Incidence is inversely related to birth weight
         i. Birth weight <750 g: 90% infants
         ii. Birth weight 1,000–1,250 g: 50% infants
   3. Risk factors
      a. Degree of prematurity: birth weight and gestational age at birth
      b. **High supplemental oxygen**, poor postnatal growth, sepsis, necrotizing enterocolitis, respiratory distress syndrome
   4. Pathophysiology
      a. Retinal vessels normally grow on surface of retina from optic disc forward to periphery, finishing at full-term age
      b. In ROP, vessels stop and grow into vitreous instead, causing retinal detachment and blindness if severe
      c. Results from hyperoxia (early) and alterations in local retinal vascular endothelial growth factor (VEGF) and systemic insulin-like growth factor-1 (IGF-1)
B. Classification
   1. Severity
      a. **Stages 1 to 5**: in peripheral retina, stages 4 and 5 are retinal detachment
      b. **Plus disease**: dilation and tortuosity of vessels near optic disc
   2. Location: zone I (posterior) to III (anterior/peripheral)
C. Diagnosis
   1. U.S. screening criteria: birth weight <1,501 g or gestational age <30 weeks
   2. Infants receive repeated dilated fundus exams to identify treatment-requiring disease; continue in neonatal ICU or clinic until no longer at risk
   3. 85% of ROP resolves spontaneously; <5% of screened infants require treatment
D. Treatment
   1. Indications
      a. Zone I, plus disease, *or* stage 3
      b. Zone II, stage 2 or 3, *and* plus disease
   2. Modalities: **laser photocoagulation** (current standard) or **cryotherapy**

> **QUICK HIT**
> Degree of prematurity is the greatest risk factor for ROP, with low birth weight as the predominant factor.

> **QUICK HIT**
> **Plus disease** is a key driver of treatment for ROP.

3. Prognosis
   a. 90% success with laser; retreatment sometimes necessary
   b. Visual outcome poor once retinal detachment develops
   c. Risk of retinal hemorrhage or detachment later in life
   d. Increased risk of high myopia, strabismus, nystagmus
4. Prevention
   a. Ensure infants at risk receive eye exams
   b. Titrate supplemental oxygen only high enough to meet recommended saturation levels

18

Emergency Medicine, Critical Care, Toxicology, and Child Abuse

SYMPTOM SPECIFIC

I. Shock

A. Definitions: failure to deliver adequate oxygen (O_2) and substrate to meet metabolic demand; circulatory dysfunction, with impaired perfusion to tissues, end organs
   1. **Compensated** (early): blood pressure (BP) is normal; compensate with increased heart rate (HR)
   2. **Decompensated** (late): hypotension and end-organ damage are present

B. Classification of shock by cause (Table 18-1)
   1. **Hypovolemic**: ↓ circulating blood volume (dehydration, fluid loss, bleeding, third spacing)
   2. **Distributive**: vasodilation causes ↓ blood volume to organs (sepsis, neurogenic from spinal injury, anaphylactic)
   3. **Cardiogenic**: ↓ cardiac output (cardiomyopathy, arrhythmia)
   4. **Obstructive**: impediment to blood flow (tamponade, pulmonary embolism [PE], tension pneumothorax)

C. Clinical presentation
   1. Vital signs
      a. Temperature: elevated (or depressed in neonates) in septic shock
      b. HR: tachycardia; bradycardia particularly in neonates
      c. BP: hypotension, seen in decompensated shock
      d. Respiratory rate (RR): increases in response to metabolic acidosis
   2. Altered mental status (confusion, lethargy, irritability)
   3. Alterations in peripheral perfusion

D. Testing
   1. Tests that elucidate etiology of shock will depend on presentation (chest x-ray [CXR], electrocardiogram [ECG], cardiac echocardiography [echo] for presence/severity of cardiogenic shock)
   2. Electrolytes, blood gas, complete blood count (CBC), liver function tests (LFTs) may be useful
   3. Invasive monitoring may be required in decompensated shock

E. Treatment
   1. Stabilize airway, breathing, and circulation (**ABCs**)
      a. Give 100% O_2 via facemask, assist with ventilation
      b. Immediate correction of mechanism of shock if possible
         i. Needle decompression of pneumothorax; pericardiocentesis of tamponade
         ii. Epinephrine for anaphylaxis
         iii. Direct pressure to site of blood loss
      c. Fluid bolus: give rapidly
         i. 20 cc/kg of 0.9% saline, lactated Ringer's
         ii. Multiple boluses until perfusion restored or fluid overload
         iii. Give blood transfusion early if hemorrhagic shock

> **QUICK HIT**
> Untreated shock will progress to organ injury and cardiac arrest.

> **QUICK HIT**
> Fluid loss from diarrhea is the leading cause of shock in children worldwide.

> **QUICK HIT**
> Loss of sympathetic tone in neurogenic shock leads to hypotension without compensatory tachycardia or vasoconstriction.

> **QUICK HIT**
> Cases of shock may cross classifications; for instance, cardiogenic shock and distributive shock are often seen in septic shock, and an infant with ductal-dependent congenital heart disease may have both obstructive and cardiogenic features. Therapies must be adjusted accordingly.

QUICK HIT

Although symptoms of shock may overlap with dehydration and benign febrile illness, altered mental status is an ominous predictor of more severe illness.

MNEMONIC

Differential diagnosis of the septic-appearing infant: THE MISFITS
T: Trauma
H: Heart disease
E: Endocrine
M: Metabolic
I: Inborn errors of metabolism
S: Sepsis
F: Formula mishaps
I: Intestinal catastrophes and dehydration
T: Toxins
S: Seizures

Used with permission from Brousseau T, Sharieff GQ. Newborn emergencies: the first 30 days of life. *Pediatr Clin North Am.* 2006 Feb;53(1):69–84.

QUICK HIT

If shock is suspected based on clinical examination, treatment should begin immediately. Laboratory testing is useful in refining treatment, and testing should be tailored to the type of shock suspected.

QUICK HIT

A large base deficit or high lactate level indicates tissue hypoxia.

QUICK HIT

Fluid should be given quickly via a "push-pull" in-line syringe or pressure bag. In cases of suspected cardiogenic shock, fluid should be given in small amounts with close monitoring to avoid precipitating congestive heart failure.

TABLE 18-1 Pathophysiology, Compensation, Clinical Features, and Treatment for Different Classes of Shock

Type of Shock	Compensatory Mechanisms	Specific Clinical Features	Treatment
Hypovolemic	Increased SVR Increased cardiac contractility	Delayed capillary refill Cool/mottled extremities Weak peripheral pulses Skin tenting Pallor Traumatic injuries may be visible in hemorrhagic shock.	Fluid boluses Blood transfusion
Distributive	SVR high in cold shock SVR low in warm shock Cardiac output normal or increased	"Cold shock" - Narrow pulse pressure - Delayed capillary refill - Cool/mottled extremities - Weak peripheral pulses "Warm shock" - Widened pulse pressure - Brisk capillary refill - Warm extremities - Bounding peripheral pulses	Fluid boluses Dopamine Epinephrine for cold shock, anaphylaxis Norepinephrine for warm shock
Cardiogenic	Increased heart rate Increased SVR	Congestive heart failure: rales, hepatomegaly, jugular venous distension	Dopamine Dobutamine
Obstructive	Increased heart rate Increased SVR	Weak pulses Jugular venous distension Muffled heart sounds with pericardial effusion Tracheal deviation/decreased breath sounds with hemo-/pneumothorax	Physical relief of obstruction Pericardiocentesis Needle decompression Prostaglandin E_1 in cases of ductal-dependent lesions, thrombolysis in pulmonary embolism

SVR, systemic vascular resistance.

d. Vasoactive agents (most commonly used for pediatric shock)
   i. **Dopamine** (β_1, β_2, dopamine stimulation)
      (a) 1st-line agent in pediatrics
      (b) Increases cardiac output, systemic vascular resistance (SVR)
   ii. Others: norepinephrine, dobutamine; epinephrine for anaphylaxis

II. Initial Approach to Trauma

A. Historical findings
   1. Mechanism of injury to assess severity, likelihood/location of injuries: assess if consistent with injury and developmentally appropriate
   2. Preceding events to assess for precipitating etiologies: syncope, seizure, cardiac arrhythmias
B. Physical examination findings
   1. **Primary survey: ABCDEFG**
      a. Components
         i. **A**irway and cervical spine control; interventions may include suctioning of secretions, repositioning airway, or placement of advanced airway (Tables 18-2 and 18-3)
            (a) Cervical spine immobilization manually/with collar
         ii. **B**reathing and ventilation: assess for adequate ventilation, oxygenation; interventions may include supplemental O_2, pneumothorax decompression, chin lift, or intubation

TABLE 18-2 **Indications for Endotracheal Intubation in Children with Trauma**

Inability to ventilate by bag-mask ventilation
Glasgow Coma Scale score ≤8
Concern for impending brain herniation
Respiratory failure from hypoxemia/hypoventilation
Decompensated shock resistant to initial fluid resuscitation
Loss of laryngeal reflexes

TABLE 18-3 **Some Primary Survey Findings and Life-Threatening Conditions**

	Abnormal Findings	Life-Threatening Conditions
Airway	Hoarseness, stridor, subcutaneous emphysema, airway foreign body or secretions	Obstruction by blood, secretions, laryngeal fracture/tear
Breathing	Decreased, asymmetric breath sounds, flail chest, tracheal deviation, hypoxia	Tension pneumothorax, hemopneumothorax, flail chest, pulmonary contusion
Circulation	Tachycardia, abnormal pulses or perfusion	Hemorrhagic shock, pneumothorax, pericardial tamponade
Disability	Abnormal Glasgow Coma Scale score, mental status, pupillary response	Intracranial injury, increased intracranial pressure, brain herniation

iii. Circulation and hemorrhage control
   (a) Assess pulses, perfusion, HR, BP; interventions may include external bleeding injury pressure, fluid resuscitation, transfusion
iv. Disability, decontamination, dextrose
   (a) **Disability** (assess mental status): **Glasgow Coma Scale** (GCS) (Table 18-4) and pupillary response to light
   (b) **Decontamination**: remove toxin-covered clothing
   (c) **Dextrose**: bedside glucose level
v. Exposure: undress patient and log roll to find injuries, then cover
vi. Fasting: when was the last time the patient ate and/or drank
vii. General health

TABLE 18-4 **Glasgow Coma Scale (GCS) and Modified Infant GCS**

Action	GCS	Infant GCS	Score
Eye opening	Spontaneous	Spontaneous	4
	To voice	To voice	3
	To pain	To pain	2
	None	None	1
Verbal response	Oriented	Coos, babbles, smiles	5
	Confused	Irritable cry, consolable	4
	Inappropriate	Cries to pain	3
	Incomprehensible	Moans to pain	2
	None	None	1
Motor response	Obeys commands	Spontaneous movements	6
	Localizes pain	Withdraws to touch	5
	Withdraws to pain	Withdraws to pain	4
	Flexion (decorticate)	Flexion (decorticate)	3
	Extension (decerebrate)	Extension (decerebrate)	2
	Flaccid	Flaccid	1

QUICK HIT

Vasoactive agents should be considered when perfusion does not improve after 60 mL/kg of intravenous fluid boluses.

QUICK HIT

The primary survey is the organized, rapid assessment of the patient with the goal of immediately identifying and treating the life-threatening condition(s). Ideally, it should be performed by a single team member not directly involved in patient care or decision making. It should be done loudly, accurately, and efficiently. It is performed on patient's initial arrival, after any intervention and when the patient's status worsens.

QUICK HIT

Hemorrhagic shock is the most common life-threatening circulatory condition and often due to intra-abdominal, intrathoracic, or pelvic injury.

QUICK HIT

Asymmetric pupillary response, especially with contralateral weakness, is concerning for cerebral herniation and requires immediate treatment to decrease intracranial pressure.

QUICK HIT

The goals of the secondary survey are to stabilize the patient, perform laboratory and radiologic exams, refine the differential diagnosis, identify less threatening injuries, and determine patient disposition.

MNEMONIC

AMPLE history
Allergies
Medications
Past medical history
Last meal
Events surrounding injury

QUICK HIT

Always ensure that the mechanism of injury is consistent with the injury and developmental age of the child.

QUICK HIT

Inconsistencies in history obtained from caregivers individually is another warning sign for potential child abuse.

2. **Secondary survey**: head-to-toe examination and focused history
   a. Inspect entire body
   b. Head/face: intraoral trauma, cerebrospinal fluid (CSF), rhinorrhea
   c. Eyes: pupil size and reactivity, eye movements, **raccoon eyes**
   d. Ears: hemotympanum, CSF otorrhea, **Battle sign**
   e. Neck: deformity, tenderness, tracheal deviation
   f. Chest: accessory muscle use; breath and heart sounds
   g. Abdomen/pelvis: tenderness, guarding; compress pelvis for integrity
   h. Urogenital: urethral and vaginal bleeding
   i. Rectal: exam if concerned for spinal cord injury, trauma
   j. Musculoskeletal: examine all joints and limbs; assess pulses
   k. Neurologic: level of consciousness (LOC), cranial nerves, strength, sensation, deep tendon reflexes
3. **Tertiary survey**: identify potentially missed injuries, consider comorbidities

C. Laboratory testing and radiologic imaging
1. Laboratory testing
   a. Routine serum laboratory screening testing may not be useful
   b. Type and screen, CBC, hepatic enzymes, pancreatic enzymes, and electrolytes
   c. Urine pregnancy, toxicology screen for appropriate patients
2. Radiologic evaluation guided by mechanisms and physical exam findings

III. Approach to Head Trauma

A. Background information
1. Categorized based on mechanism, anatomic involvement, symptoms
2. Mild traumatic brain injury and concussion
   a. May be subtle: physical, cognitive, and emotional symptoms
   b. Cognitive and physical rest necessary while symptomatic

B. Historical findings
1. Mechanism of injury to determine severity, likelihood of additional injuries
2. Events around injury, timing of injury
3. Symptoms following event: LOC, vomiting, headache, amnesia
4. Past medical history for comorbid conditions

C. Physical examination findings
1. **ABCDEFG** (see Initial Approach to Trauma)
2. GCS (see Table 18-4)
3. External signs of head trauma (include hemotympanum, CSF from nose/ears)
4. Full-body exam to assess for other injuries

D. Radiologic imaging
1. Skull radiographs: screen for skull fracture in children age <2 years old
2. Computed tomography (CT)
   a. Severe injuries: altered mental status, focal neurologic deficits
   b. Nonsevere injuries: head trauma prediction rule (Table 18-5) to determine very low risk for intracranial injury and no need for head CT

IV. Approach to Burns

A. Pathophysiology
1. Burn severity related to type of burn, location, duration of exposure, timing
2. Loss of skin integrity alters vital functions
   a. Epidermis: prevents water loss and has antimicrobial properties
   b. Dermis: contains blood vessels that regulate heat loss
3. Systemic effects associated with burned body surface area (BSA) >20% and can lead to shock

B. Historical findings
1. Circumstances of injury
2. Associated symptoms: respiratory distress, vomiting, pain
3. Home treatment (e.g., analgesia, wound cleansing/debridement)

C. Physical examination and initial stabilization
1. General examination: assess for systemic injury
   a. Altered mental status: smoke inhalation, burn shock
   b. Vital signs: tachycardia, tachypnea, hypoxia, hypotension

TABLE 18-5 **Head Trauma Prediction Rules to Determine Patients at Very Low Risk of Intracranial Injury Who Do Not Need Head Computed Tomography (CT)***

Head Trauma Decision Rules for <2 Years Old	Head Trauma Decision Rules for ≥2 Years Old
• Normal mental status	• Normal mental status
• No hematoma or isolated frontal hematoma	• No loss of consciousness
• No loss of consciousness or loss of consciousness for <5 seconds	• No vomiting
• Nonsevere injury mechanism Severe defined as any of the following: motor vehicle crash with patient ejection, death of another passenger, or rollover; pedestrian or bicyclist without helmet struck by a motorized vehicle; falls of >3 feet; or head struck by a high-impact object	• Nonsevere injury mechanism Severe defined as any of the following: motor vehicle crash with patient ejection, death of another passenger, or rollover; pedestrian or bicyclist without helmet struck by a motorized vehicle; falls of >5 feet; or head struck by a high-impact object
• No palpable skull fracture	• No signs of basilar skull fracture
• Acting normally according to caretaker	• No severe headache

*This rule does not predict who does need to undergo a CT.
Adapted from Kuppermann N, Holmes JF, Dayan PS, et al. Identification of children at very low risk of clinically-important brain injuries after head trauma: a prospective cohort study. *Lancet.* 2009;374:1160–1170.

c. Stridor, wheezes, retractions: smoke inhalation
d. Traumatic injuries from escaping fire

2. Burn examination
   a. **Superficial**: involves only epidermis; red, painful
   b. **Superficial partial-thickness**: into dermis; blisters, red, moist, and edematous, painful
   c. **Deep partial-thickness**: involves most of dermis; pale and dry, white/red, minimal pain
   d. **Full-thickness**: involves all of epidermis and dermis; leathery/charred, not painful
3. Estimating BSA: "Rule of 9's" does not apply to small children; use pediatric estimation guide; do not count superficial areas

D. Laboratory testing and radiologic imaging
   1. Fire: carboxyhemoglobin; consider cyanide poisoning in house fires
   2. Electrical injury: urinalysis, serum creatine kinase, ECG
   3. Imaging studies: chest radiograph if injury from fire, respiratory symptoms

E. Management: moderate to severe burns
   1. Trauma evaluation if indicated; stabilize **ABCs**
      a. Red flags: facial burns, nasal soot, respiratory distress
      b. Give O_2: pulse oximetry may be normal in carbon monoxide poisoning
      c. Rapid fluid resuscitation with isotonic fluids
   2. Secondary survey: compartment syndrome in circumferential burns
   3. Prophylactic antibiotics not indicated
   4. Tetanus prophylaxis if not up-to-date or vaccine status unknown
   5. Consider transfer to burn center if extensive or high-risk burns

F. Management: minor burns
   1. Superficial burns typically require only supportive care
   2. Partial-thickness burns
      a. Clean and dress burns
      b. Topical antibiotics, pain medications

QUICK HIT

Estimating burned BSA is used to assess injury severity and calculate fluid replacement volumes.

QUICK HIT

A child's palm (including fingers) = ~1% BSA.

QUICK HIT

Half calculated fluid requirements should be given over the first 8 hours and the remainder over the next 16 hours.

QUICK HIT

Children who get an electrical mouth burn from sucking on plugs at the labial commissure are at risk of delayed hemorrhage when the eschar sloughs (usually 1–2 weeks after injury).

QUICK HIT

Patients with a higher Mallampati grade tend to have poorer visualization during direct laryngoscopy and are, therefore, more difficult to intubate.

QUICK HIT

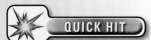

Patient anxiety and perception of pain may be reduced by nonpharmacologic developmentally appropriate distraction techniques, such as singing, reading, watching a video, or blowing bubbles.

QUICK HIT

LET is used for cuts prior to suturing. EMLA is used over intact skin prior to phlebotomy or lumbar puncture.

MNEMONIC

SOAP ME: ensure proper preparation for procedural sedation
Suction
Oxygen
Airway equipment
Pharmacy and personnel
Monitoring **e**quipment

QUICK HIT

The normal exploratory behavior of toddlers partly explains the high rate of toxin exposure for this age group. But, because the toxin usually does not taste good, they rarely ingest a large amount, which accounts for the low mortality.

QUICK HIT

Remember to protect yourself! Wear protective gear if the patient is externally contaminated.

V. Approach to Sedation and Analgesia

A. Background
  1. Definitions
    a. Minimal sedation (**anxiolysis**): responds normally to verbal commands
    b. Moderate sedation: responds purposefully to verbal commands
    c. Deep sedation: patient is difficult to arouse
    d. **Analgesia**: relief of pain without LOC
  2. Sedation-related adverse events (↑ risk with ↑ degree of sedation)
    a. Hypoventilation, apnea, O_2 desaturation
    b. Hypotension
    c. Increased secretions, vomiting, paradoxically increased agitation
B. Important historical findings
  1. Level of pain and/or anxiety
  2. Global assessment of patient factors: ABCDEFG
C. Pertinent physical exam findings
  1. **Mallampati score**: classification system for describing tongue size relative to size of oral cavity
  2. Risky if significant underlying findings affecting airway or cardiovascular status
D. Agents: depends on type of procedure and needs of patient
  1. Anxiolysis: medications (e.g., benzodiazepines such as midazolam)
  2. Sedation: may use combination of anxiolytics, analgesics, and dissociative agents
  3. Analgesia (medications)
    a. Topical (LET = lidocaine, epinephrine, tetracaine; EMLA = lidocaine, prilocaine)
    b. Local/regional (infiltration of lidocaine)
    c. Systemic: nonsteroidal anti-inflammatory drugs, opiates
  4. Safe discharge: upon recovery, patient must meet specific criteria to be eligible for discharge such as awake, alert, tolerating liquids

VI. Approach to Poisonings

A. Background
  1. Epidemiology: common reasons for ingestions
    a. Children <5 years old: unintentional (accidental ingestion, dosing error)
    b. Teens: intentional (suicide attempt, recreational substance abuse)
    c. Any age: forced (child abuse)
B. Historical findings
  1. History may not be accurate or available if intentional, unwitnessed, unknown
  2. Drug(s) or chemical(s), concentration and dose, type (sustained release, enteric coated), time of ingestion
C. Physical exam findings
  1. Vary; provide clues to diagnosis, severity, and progression of illness
  2. **Toxidrome**: set of clinical signs and symptoms that suggest specific class of poisoning (Table 18-6)
  3. Vital signs, mental status, and pupillary size and response especially important
    a. Sympathomimetics/stimulants: tachycardia, hypertension, hyperthermia, agitation, tachycardia, mydriasis (normal light response)
    b. Anticholinergics: tachycardia, hypertension, hyperthermia, agitation, **mydriasis** (relatively sluggish light response)
    c. Opioids and barbiturates: lethargy, bradycardia, hypotension, and decrease in RR, **miosis**
D. Laboratory testing and radiologic imaging
  1. Depends on suspected toxin, clinical status; may include
    a. Urine toxicology screen: mostly illicit drugs
    b. Serum toxicology screen: acetaminophen, salicylate, ethanol, other drugs
    c. Other tests depending on situation (pregnant?) or toxidrome (LFTs?)
E. Management
  1 Supportive care is mainstay of therapy
  2. Specific therapy will depend on toxin, clinical status, and time since exposure

TABLE 18-6 Toxidromes: Constellations of Symptoms and Signs Expected for Major Classes of Toxins

Toxidrome	Temperature	HR	RR	BP	O_2 Saturation	Mental Status	Pupils	Skin	Other
Salicylates (aspirin)	↑	NL (↑)*	↑	—	—	Agitated, delirium to coma	—	Pale diaphoretic	Vomiting, hypoglycemic, acidotic
Calcium channel blockers (verapamil)	—	↓ (NL)	—	↓↓	—	NL to coma	—	—	Heart block; hyperglycemia
β-Blockers (propranolol)	—	↓	—	↓ (NL)	—	Coma	—	—	Heart block; hypoglycemia
Oral hypoglycemics (sulfonylureas)	↓	NL to ↑	—	—	—	Agitated, delirium to coma	— (↑)	May be cool, diaphoretic	Seizures possible; hypoglycemia
Ethanol	↓	—	↓	—	NL (↓)	Agitated, depressed to coma	↓ (in large OD)		Nystagmus; hypoglycemia in toddlers
Sedative hypnotics (benzodiazepine)	↓	NL or ↓	↓	↓	↓	Depressed to coma	—	—	
Tricyclic antidepressants (amitriptyline)	— or ↑	↑	NL (↓)	NL (↓)	—	Confusion, agitation, coma	NL (↑)	Dry	Dysrhythmias, seizures
Sympathomimetics (Cocaine)	↑	↑	NL or ↑	NL or ↑	NL	Agitated, hallucinations	Dilate	Cool, pale, diaphoretic	Seizures possible

BP, blood pressure; HR, heart rate; NL, normal or at baseline; OD, overdose; RR, respiratory rate.

*Effects in parentheses indicate less commoNLy seen or secondary effects.

QUICK HIT

Acetaminophen for infants and children comes in 2 different concentrations, which often leads to dosing errors.

QUICK HIT

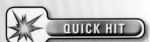

Single doses of acetaminophen <150 mg/kg in children are likely to be harmless.

QUICK HIT

The Rumack-Matthew nomogram plots the serum acetaminophen level versus time of ingestion to help predict risk of liver injury and the need for antidotal therapy with NAC. The nomogram starts at 4 hours after ingestion, when the level is expected to peak in an acute ingestion.

QUICK HIT

Liver transplantation may be indicated in fulminant hepatic failure with severe acetaminophen ingestion.

QUICK HIT

Besides aspirin, salicylates are found in bismuth salicylate (Pepto-Bismol®), salicylic acid (wart remover), and methyl salicylate (oil of wintergreen) and some herbal remedies.

QUICK HIT

The classic triad in salicylate poisoning is hyperpnea, metabolic acidosis, and tachycardia.

3. Decontamination
   a. Activated charcoal
      i. Works best if given within 1 hour of ingestion
      ii. Does not absorb heavy metals, corrosives, alcohols, hydrocarbons, inorganic ions
   b. Whole bowel irrigation: large-volume balanced electrolyte solution usually given by nasogastric (NG) tube; for sustained-release drug, concretions
   c. Syrup of ipecac, gastric lavage: *no longer recommended*
4. Antidotes
   a. Reverse or reduce effects of poisoning
   b. Use depends on clinical status, risk/benefit ratio, contraindications
   c. Examples: naloxone for opioids, atropine for organophosphates
5. Resources: American Association of Poison Control Centers (1-800-222-1222; no charge to callers)
   a. Toxicology consultation available 24 hours/day nationwide
   b. Contact Poison Control *first* for any serious or puzzling poisoning cases
6. Prevention is key
   a. Family anticipatory guidance
   b. Medication child safety devices
   c. Teen screening for depression, psychiatric issues

DISEASE SPECIFIC

VII. Acetaminophen Poisoning

A. Epidemiology
   1. Most commonly used analgesic and antipyretic in U.S.
   2. More overdoses and deaths in U.S. than any other drug
   3. Outcome usually good if antidote (**N-acetylcysteine** [**NAC**]) given quickly

B. Pharmacokinetics
   1. Metabolized in liver, excreted in urine
   2. Toxic dose (after liver stores of conjugating agent **glutathione** are used up)
      a. Peak serum concentration: 4 hours after ingestion
      b. Minimum single toxic dose: 150 mg/kg
      c. Chronic toxic ingestion (usually worse): 150 mg/kg over 2–4 days

C. Clinical features
   1. **Stage 1** (30 minutes–24 hours after ingestion): nausea, sweating, lethargy, or asymptomatic; normal labs
   2. **Stage 2** (24–72 hours): hepatotoxicity, nephrotoxicity
   3. **Stage 3** (72–96 hours): peak of LFT levels, hepatic encephalopathy, hyperammonemia, bleeding, hypoglycemia, lactic acidosis, death
   4. **Stage 4** (4–14 days): recovery, improved symptoms, LFTs recover

D. Laboratory evaluation
   1. Acetaminophen level drawn 4–24 hours after dose: plot value on **nomogram**
   2. Toxicology screens for co-ingestants
   3. Additional tests: serial LFTs, blood urea nitrogen (BUN)/creatinine (Cr) ratio, arterial blood gas (ABG) if ingestion is severe

E. Management
   1. Stabilize ABCs
   2. Activated charcoal indicated if within 4 hours of ingestion
   3. NAC antidote
      a. NAC functions as glutathione precursor
      b. Indications
         i. Level above "possible hepatic toxicity" line on nomogram
         ii. Single ingestion of >150 mg/kg when level not obtainable
         iii. Unknown ingestion time and acetaminophen level >10 mcg/mL
         iv. Hepatotoxicity and history of acetaminophen ingestion

VIII. Salicylate Poisoning

A. Epidemiology
1. Declined use of aspirin in children due to association with Reye syndrome
2. Most pediatric exposures are intentional ingestions in adolescents

B. Mechanism of action
1. Activates respiratory center of medulla causing tachypnea, respiratory alkalosis
2. Uncouples oxidative phosphorylation and inhibits Krebs cycle (metabolic acidosis and hyperpyrexia)
3. Significant coagulopathy through ↓ platelet function and clotting factors
4. Mild overdose: ↑ RR, ↑ HR, tinnitus, vertigo, nausea, diarrhea
5. Later findings: noncardiogenic pulmonary edema, altered mental status, death

C. Management
1. Stabilize ABCs
   a. Beware of endotracheal intubation: must maintain very high minute ventilation to avoid acidosis
   b. Careful fluid resuscitation with alkalinized fluids
2. Correct hypokalemia, hypoglycemia
3. Gastrointestinal (GI) decontamination
4. Urine alkalinization to improve salicylate removal: goal = urine pH 7.5–7.6
5. Hemodialysis in severe cases
6. Consider early consultation with Poison Control Center, toxicologist

IX. Calcium Channel Blocker (CCB) and β-Blocker (BB) Poisoning

A. Physical exam
1. CCBs: abnormal atrioventricular (AV) node conduction or AV block
2. Lipophilic BBs: changes in mental status

B. Laboratory evaluation
1. Glucose
   a. BB: ↓ glucose, especially in younger patients

C. ECG
1. Prolonged PR interval
2. Bradyarrhythmias
3. Can see prolonged QRS in BB with membrane-stabilizing properties

D. Differential diagnosis
1. CCB versus BB: history, glucose level (high in CCB, low in BB)
2. Specific therapies
   a. Aggressive fluid resuscitation for hypotension
   b. Atropine for bradycardia, vasopressors (norepinephrine) for ↓ BP
   c. Vasopressors for hypotension: norepinephrine
   d. Intravenous (IV) calcium for CCBs
   e. Glucagon for BBs
3. GI decontamination

X. Oral Hypoglycemic Poisoning

A. Epidemiology: sulfonylureas, metformin most common agents

B. Pharmacokinetics
1. Sulfonylureas: cause **hypoglycemia**, generally 8–12 hours after ingestion
2. Metformin: **metabolic acidosis** (normal glucose), peak 4–6 hours after ingestion

C. Clinical features
1. Sulfonylureas: lethargy or seizure from lack of brain glucose
2. Metformin: nausea, abdominal pain, ↑ HR, ↑ RR, ↓ BP from metabolic acidosis

D. Laboratory evaluation: fingerstick glucose, electrolytes, ABG, toxicology screen for co-ingestions

QUICK HIT

Be careful to note the units the lab uses to report salicylate levels when comparing to the Done nomogram. Most U.S. toxicology literature uses mg/dL.

QUICK HIT

Declining salicylate levels may be associated with a worsening clinical picture as the toxin redistributes into the central nervous system with the onset or worsening of acidemia.

QUICK HIT

CCBs are highly lethal ingestions. Although CCBs are involved in only 16% of cardiac medication overdoses, they cause ~50% of the cardiac medication–related deaths!

QUICK HIT

Vital sign changes in CCB ingestion are bradycardia and hypotension.

QUICK HIT

Glucose is elevated in CCB ingestion and decreased in BB ingestion.

QUICK HIT

In toddlers, CCBs and BBs can be fatal after the ingestion of only 1 pill.

QUICK HIT

Single-tablet ingestions of sulfonylureas can be toxic in children.

E. Management
1. Stabilize ABCs, consider activated charcoal
2. Sulfonylureas with hypoglycemia
   a. IV dextrose
   b. Octreotide: inhibits insulin release from pancreas (consider if unable to maintain blood glucose despite dextrose)
   c. Observe for at least for 12–24 hours
3. Metformin
   a. Bicarbonate and/or dialysis only if severe acidosis
   b. Observe at least 6–8 hours after ingestion to monitor for symptoms

QUICK HIT

Consider sulfonylurea exposure in a child with hypoglycemia and recent contact with diabetic adults (e.g., baby-sitting grandparent, family holiday gatherings).

XI. Anticholinergic Ingestions

A. Pathophysiology
1. Acetylcholine actions
   a. **Muscarinic receptors**: sweating, salivation, intestinal and urinary motility, pupil constriction; decrease HR via AV node
   b. **Nicotinic receptors**: sympathetic ganglia, neuromuscular junctions
   c. **Central receptors**: memory, cognition, motor coordination

B. Clinical presentation (severe): extreme hyperthermia, myoclonus (can lead to rhabdomyolysis), seizure, coma

C. Evaluation: ECG (arrhythmia, ↑ QT and ↑ QRS intervals), drug screen

D. Management
1. Stabilize ABCs, activated charcoal if alert, benzodiazepines for agitation, bicarbonate IV for ECG abnormalities
2. Physostigmine (anticholinesterase inhibitor) in severe cases

QUICK HIT

Anticholinergic ingestions can include tricyclic antidepressants (TCAs), atropine, antihistamines, over-the-counter diphenhydramine-containing products, scopolamine, and tainted illicit drugs, as well as plants (e.g., deadly nightshade and Jimson weed).

MNEMONIC

Classic anticholinergic toxidrome
Mad as a hatter—agitated to delirious mental status
Hot as Hades—anhydrotic hyperthermia
Red as a beet—cutaneous vasodilation
Blind as a bat—mydriasis, loss of accommodation
Dry as a bone—anhydrosis
Full as a flask—urinary retention
Heart runs alone—tachycardia

XII. Organophosphate Poisoning

A. Mechanism of action: irreversible acetylcholinesterase (AChE) inhibitors

B. Clinical features of toxidrome
1. Muscarinic: often improve with atropine challenge
2. Nicotinic: muscle fasciculations, weakness, paralysis
3. Central nervous system (CNS): coma, seizures, apnea
4. Cardiovascular collapse: unknown etiology
5. Intermediate syndrome: delayed onset, improves in 2–3 weeks
6. Delayed neurotoxicity: occurs 1–3 weeks after ingestion of some agents

C. Management
1. Stabilize ABCs, activated charcoal as indicated, benzodiazepines for seizure
2. Atropine IV/intramuscular (IM): improves muscarinic activity, repeat until findings relieved
3. Pralidoxime: treats muscarinic and nicotinic blockade

QUICK HIT

TCA ingestions are associated with many arrhythmias including premature ventricular contractions, ventricular tachycardia, and a prolonged QRS interval, which may progress to heart block.

XIII. Caustic Ingestions

A. Epidemiology
1. Most common in children ages 1–3 years
2. Most common agents: cosmetics, cleaning agents, button batteries

B. Mechanism of injury
1. **Alkalis**: usually cause more injury than acids
   a. Esophagus usually most severely affected
      i. Cause liquefaction necrosis, resultant burn, perforation
      ii. Delayed injury from scar and stricture formation
2. **Acids**: penetrate less deeply, mostly cause gastric or upper airway injury
3. **Button battery injuries**: electrical discharge in esophagus and rapid corrosive injury to esophagus

C. Physical exam
1. Signs of upper airway injury: stridor, hoarseness, respiratory distress
2. Oral injury: oral lesions do not predict esophageal lesions
3. Abdominal pain

D. Diagnostic evaluation
1. Abdominal radiographs for esophageal or gastric perforation
2. Chest/abdominal radiograph for button battery ingestion (Figure 18-1)

QUICK HIT

Organophosphates include insecticides (organophosphates and carbamates) and are the basis of nerve gases (e.g., Tokyo sarin exposure, 1995). They are also used medically to reverse the neuromuscular blockade in myasthenia gravis, glaucoma, and anesthesia.

FIGURE 18-1 Radiographic identification of an esophageal button battery. On this anterior-posterior view, the double ring of the battery can be seen. A coin would look like a single ring. On a lateral x-ray, the battery has a stacked or step-off appearance.

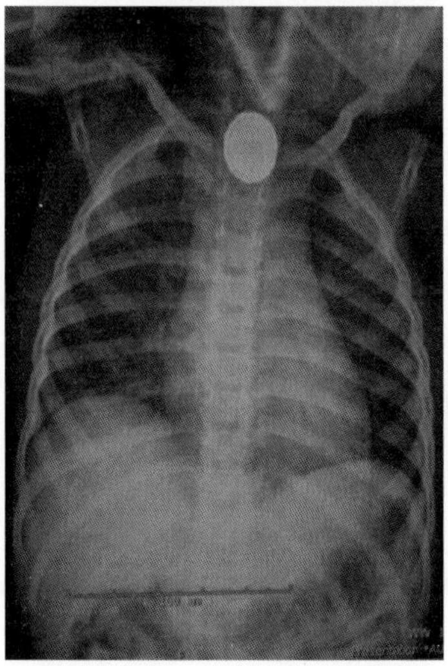

E. Management
  1. Stabilize ABCs
  2. *Emergent* operating room removal of esophageal button battery
  3. Immediate consultation with surgical and GI subspecialists
    a. Upper airway laryngoscopy or upper GI endoscopy
  4. Questionable history of ingestion: observation; assess drinking

XIV. Hydrocarbon Poisoning

A. Pathophysiology
  1. Due to low viscosity, often inhaled: pulmonary toxicity
    a. Destruction of surfactant, alveoli collapse, pneumonitis
  2. Systemic toxicity with only some compounds: most poorly absorbed from GI tract
B. Clinical presentation
  1. Aspiration: immediate or delayed coughing, wheezing, respiratory distress, fever common with pneumonitis
  2. Large ingestions: emesis, CNS symptoms, arrhythmias, hepatic/renal injury possible with some compounds
C. Laboratory evaluation: chest radiograph is initially normal, progresses to diffuse pneumonitis
D. Management is supportive; admission for respiratory symptoms/abnormal CXR

XV. Opioid Ingestion

A. Clinical presentation: CNS depression, respiratory depression, ↓ BP, ↓ HR, ↓ temperature, flushing, pinpoint pupils
B. Management
  1. Stabilize ABCs
  2. Naloxone trial
    a. Repeat dose: half-life of reversal agent is shorter than some opiates

XVI. Ethanol Poisoning

A. Specific historical findings: occurrence of any witnessed trauma, suspected sexual assault in teens
B. Clinical presentation
  1. Altered mental status, slurred speech, ataxia, agitation, lethargy, seizure, coma
  2. Signs of trauma: abrasions, hematomas, fractures
C. Laboratory evaluation
  1. Bedside blood glucose (associated with hypoglycemia), serum alcohol level
  2. Head CT if abnormal mental status and concern for head trauma
D. Management: stabilize ABCs; GI decontamination usually not indicated

MNEMONIC

Cholinergic excess muscarinic effects: DUMBeLS
Defecation
Urination
Miosis
Bronchorrhea/**b**ronchospasm/**b**radycardia
Lacrimation
Salivation

QUICK HIT

Avoid depolarizing paralytics like succinylcholine for rapid-sequence intubation.

QUICK HIT

During decontamination of organophosphates, health care providers should don protective gear.

QUICK HIT

Although children commonly ingest household bleach, mucosal injury is rare because of the typically neutral pH. However, industrial-strength formulations can cause significant injuries.

QUICK HIT

Toilet bowl and drain cleaners contain acid corrosives. Lye, oven and drainpipe cleaners, and powdered laundry and dishwasher detergents are examples of alkali caustics.

QUICK HIT

Common sources of hydrocarbons are household cleaners, solvents, gasoline, mineral spirits, pine oil, lamp oil, and lighter fluids.

QUICK HIT

Hydrocarbons, such as gasoline and kerosene, have a low viscosity, high volatility, and low surface tension; therefore, even small aspirated amounts can cause significant respiratory symptoms.

QUICK HIT

Extracorporeal membrane oxygenation and exogenous surfactant administration have been successfully used in children with severe pneumonitis after a massive hydrocarbon poisoning.

QUICK HIT

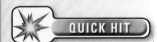

In the early course after toxin exposure, avoid catecholamines (e.g., epinephrine) and bronchodilators (e.g., albuterol) after a halogenated hydrocarbon exposure because they may lead to ventricular arrhythmias.

QUICK HIT

Opioids include natural products such as morphine, heroin, codeine, and paregoric (tincture of opium) as well as synthetic and semisynthetic products such as fentanyl, methadone, meperidine, nalbuphine, hydrocodone, and oxycodone.

QUICK HIT

Methadone is particularly toxic in that it may be deadly in small doses to children, intoxication may last 1–2 days, it may not be detected by routine drug screens, and it prolongs the QT interval.

XVII. Methemoglobinemia

A. Definitions
  1. **Congenital:** ↓ reduction of methemoglobin (metHg) back to hemoglobin reductase
  2. **Acquired**
    a. Ingestion: agents that cause metHg (nitrites, lidocaine, dapsone)
    b. Infectious: diarrhea in young children with nitrite-forming bacteria

B. Historical elements
  1. Congenital: usually asymptomatic or "cyanotic"
  2. Acquired
    a. Low levels (<20%): usually asymptomatic
    b. Moderate levels (20%–40%): headache, lethargy, fatigue, dyspnea
    c. High levels (>40%): altered mental status, shock, seizure, death

C. Physical exam
  1. Cyanosis ("slate gray" in severe cases) in presence of normal FiO_2
  2. Pulse oximeters often inaccurate

D. Laboratory evaluation: serum testing for metHg presence and level

E. Management
  1. Hereditary: avoid exposure to aniline derivatives and nitrates
  2. Acquired, if symptomatic: **methylene blue**

XVIII. Acute Iron Poisoning

A. Epidemiology
  1. Most ingestions in children are unintentional and cause little to no harm
  2. Intentional ingestions are associated with high mortality
  3. Highest risk: prenatal vitamins; children's vitamins less likely to cause harm

B. Clinical features of toxidrome
  1. GI phase: 30 minutes–6 hours
    a. Abdominal pain, vomiting, diarrhea, hematemesis, melena, shock
    b. Vomiting most sensitive sign of severe toxicity
  2. Latent phase: 6–24 hours; usually asymptomatic
  3. Shock/metabolic acidosis/hepatotoxicity: 6–96 hours
  4. Bowel obstruction: 2–8 weeks later from scarring

C. Laboratory evaluation
  1. Serum iron level within 4–6 hours of ingestion (8 hours if slow release)
  2. Electrolytes, glucose (↑ if severe), LFTs and coagulation studies, CBC, ABG for metabolic acidosis

D. Radiographic studies (abdominal x-ray): radiopaque densities in large overdoses

E. Management
  1. Stabilize ABCs, GI decontamination through NG lavage/bowel irrigation (*not* charcoal)
  2. Chelating agent: deferoxamine; if severe, dialysis/exchange transfusion (adverse reactions of chelation: hypotension, acute respiratory distress syndrome)

XIX. Lead Poisoning

A. Epidemiology
  1. Toxic level threshold: 10 mcg/dL
  2. Children age <6 years more susceptible due to immature blood–brain barrier
  3. More common in urban than rural children

B. Pharmacokinetics: route of absorption
  1. Inhaled (dust): almost complete absorption from lower respiratory tract
  2. Ingested (paint chips): children absorb more than adults
  3. Absorbed lead then is distributed in blood, soft tissue, bones, and teeth

C. Historical elements
  1. Often asymptomatic and identified through lab screening
  2. Low levels: vomiting, cognitive delay, behavior problems
  3. High levels: colicky abdominal pain, anemia, developmental delay, seizures, encephalopathy
  4. Nutritional history: worse if low iron/calcium in diet

5. History of **pica** (eating nonfood materials such as dirt)
6. Exposure source: parents' occupation, industrial sites nearby, age of home

D. Clinical features of toxidrome
1. Neurologic
   a. Range from **developmental delay** to encephalopathy
   b. Neurodevelopmental effects may persist despite treatment
   c. Hearing loss, **peripheral neuropathy**, slowed nerve conduction
   d. Altered mental status, ataxia, seizures, coma, cerebral edema
2. Hematologic
   a. **Anemia** may be microcytic or normocytic
   b. Microcytic anemia more common if in conjunction with iron deficiency

E. Laboratory evaluation
1. Blood lead levels (if capillary sample elevated, confirm with venous sample)
2. Erythrocyte protoporphyrin (increased if lead level >30 mcg/dL)
3. CBC with reticulocyte count
4. Iron testing: iron, ferritin, iron-binding capacity

F. Radiologic studies
1. Abdominal x-rays for flecks of lead in acute ingestion and pica
2. Long bone radiographs: **lead lines** if chronic high lead levels (>45 mcg/dL)

G. Management
1. Cognitive-behavioral effects irreversible: prevention critical
2. **Mild** (<44 mcg/dL) level
   a. Confirmatory venous sample within 1 month, repeat testing in 2 months
   b. Consider chelation if level 20–44 mg/dL
3. **Moderate** (45–60 mcg/dL *and* asymptomatic): chelation therapy in consultation with toxicologist
   a. Edetate disodium calcium (CaNa2EDTA) IV
   b. Succimer (dimercaptosuccinic acid [DMSA]) oral
4. **Severe** (>70 mcg/dL *or* encephalopathy)
   a. Immediate hospitalization
   b. Control seizures with diazepam infusion
   c. Chelation therapy
      i. Dimercaprol, may cause hemolysis in glucose-6-phosphate dehydrogenase deficiency
      ii. CaNa2EDTA 4 hours after dimercaprol
5. Monitoring postchelation for rebound levels and long-term development

XX. Apparent Life-Threatening Event (ALTE)

A. Characteristics
1. Definition: event in which infant has episode frightening to observer; may include combination of apnea, color change (cyanotic/pallid, erythematous), change in muscle tone (usually limpness), choking, gagging, or breath holding
2. Cause
   a. ALTE is not a diagnosis but a grouping of symptoms
   b. ~50% ALTE cases: no etiology is found
   c. Most common identified causes related to GI, neurologic, and respiratory systems (Box 18-1)
3. Risk factors
   a. Premature infants
   b. Age <1 month and history of previous ALTE predictive of need for subsequent resuscitation or significant underlying pathology
   c. Viral upper respiratory infections (URIs)

B. Clinical features
1. Historical findings
   a. Antecedent events: awake, asleep, or crying; relationship to last meal; child's location (e.g., crib, car seat, being held); caretaker
   b. Description of event: duration, central cyanosis, eye rolling, choking or gagging, vomiting, respiratory effort, muscle tone

QUICK HIT

Body packing refers to the practice of intentionally swallowing large amounts of packaged drugs for the purpose of smuggling; the packets may rupture internally. **Body stuffers** swallow smaller amounts of drugs as a means of quick concealment.

QUICK HIT

Apneic newborn infants of opioid-addicted mothers may have life-threatening withdrawal seizures when treated with the usual dosing of naloxone. This antidote should be used with extreme caution; immediate airway stabilization and ventilation may be preferred.

QUICK HIT

Ethanol can be found in alcoholic beverages, solvents, beverages, perfumes, and mouthwash.

QUICK HIT

Infants with ethanol ingestion may present with the triad of coma, hypothermia, and hypoglycemia.

QUICK HIT

Inebriated teenagers with an abnormal mental status may have co-ingested other drugs or have associated head trauma.

QUICK HIT

To estimate peak blood alcohol level = volume ingested × (% alcohol × 0.8)/weight (kg) × 0.6.

QUICK HIT

Younger children's immature hepatocyte alcohol dehydrogenase function may prolong the elimination of alcohol.

QUICK HIT

In methemoglobinemia, the blood will look darker, even chocolate colored in severe cases. When exposed to air or O_2, it will remain dark, unlike normal blood, which will become redder.

QUICK HIT

Patients with glucose-6-phosphate dehydrogenase deficiency should not be treated with methylene blue insofar as not only will it be ineffective, but it can also be dangerous because its oxidant potential may induce hemolysis.

QUICK HIT

If no GI symptoms have developed within 6 hours of iron ingestion, toxicity is unlikely. However, if the iron was an enteric-coated formulation, symptoms may be delayed.

QUICK HIT

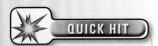

Common sources of lead are paint (especially during home renovations), imported food cans, lead plumbing, automobile emissions, and lead-using industries.

QUICK HIT

Cognitive deficits may be present even at low lead levels.

BOX 18-1

Causes of Apparent Life-Threatening Events

Idiopathic: 25%–50%

Gastrointestinal: 25%–33%
- Gastroesophageal reflux disease
- Gastroenteritis
- Gastric volvulus
- Intussusception
- Swallowing problems

Neurologic: 15%
- Seizure
- Structural malformations
- Trauma (accidental or nonaccidental)/head bleed
- Central nervous system infection
- Malignancy
- Increased intracranial pressure

Respiratory: ~10%
- Respiratory syncytial virus
- Pertussis
- Pneumonia
- Upper respiratory tract infection
- Bronchiolitis/reactive airway disease
- Foreign body

Otolaryngologic: 4%
- Laryngomalacia
- Subglottic or laryngeal stenosis
- Obstructive sleep apnea

Cardiovascular: 1%–2%
- Arrhythmias
  - Long QT syndrome
  - Wolff-Parkinson-White syndrome
- Congenital heart disease
- Myocarditis
- Cardiomyopathy

Metabolic abnormalities: <2%
- Inborn errors of metabolism
- Electrolyte disorders
- Endocrinopathies

Other infections
- Sepsis
- Urinary tract infection

Child maltreatment
- Shaken baby
- Intentional suffocation/Munchausen by proxy

Other diagnoses
- Physiologic event
- Breath-holding spell
- Choking
- Drug or toxin reaction
- Anemia
- Congenital anomalies

c. Interventions required: self-resolution, gentle stimulation, cardiopulmonary resuscitation (CPR)
d. Intercurrent illnesses: lethargy, **URI**
e. Past medical history: prematurity, previous events, birth history, **gastroesophageal reflux** (GER)
f. **History of trauma**: accidental or inflicted
g. Family history: sudden death, arrhythmias

2. Physical exam findings
   a. Vital signs including pulse oximetry
   b. General appearance: presence of dysmorphology, head circumference
   c. Respiratory: wheezing, rhonchi, crackles, stridor
   d. Cardiac exam: rate and rhythm, murmurs, femoral pulses
   e. Abdominal distension or tenderness
   f. Neurologic: tone, reflexes, mental status
   g. Evidence of trauma: bruises, hemotympanum, **retinal hemorrhages**

C. Diagnosis
1. Laboratory and radiology evaluation
   a. Routine lab and radiology workup is rarely contributory (<6%); many admit for a 24-hour observation period, pursue workup depending on concerns in history, physical exam
   b. High clinical suspicion for nonaccidental trauma; abusive head injury in about 2% of infants with ALTE

D. Treatment
1. Hospitalization for patients with unexplained ALTE
   a. Patients placed on cardiorespiratory monitor/pulse oximetry
   b. CPR teaching for caregivers
   c. Discharge typically after 24 hours if event free
2. Home apnea monitoring: does not reduce mortality, no specific indication

E. Duration/prognosis
   1. Infants with ALTE as herald for significant underlying diagnosis have higher mortality and less optimum outcomes
   2. Most infants never experience another event
   3. *Not* a predictor of sudden infant death syndrome (SIDS)

XXI. Sudden Infant Death Syndrome

A. Definition: sudden death of infant age <1 year, which remains unexplained after thorough case investigation (history, death scene exam, history review)
B. Epidemiology
   1. Leading cause of infant mortality ages 1–12 months in United States
   2. Median age = 11 weeks; peak incidence 2–4 months; 90% age <6 months
C. Risk factors
   1. Maternal: prenatal and postnatal **smoking**, young age, nutritional deficiency, **bed sharing** with infant
   2. Infant: male, minority, premature, **prone sleep position**, use of pillows and soft bumpers in cribs
D. Important historical questions
   1. Assess for other etiology, especially child abuse, metabolic disorder
      a. Previous death in siblings, cousins
      b. Previous events of cyanosis, apnea
      c. Who was the caretaker during previous and current events?
   2. Assess risk factors for SIDS: smoking, cosleeping, bedding environment
E. Emergency department (ED) management
   1. Attempt CPR, confirm asystole/pulselessness, do not call a code unless family present (if possible), then let them hold the baby once death is pronounced
   2. Postmortem skeletal survey, contact medical examiner
   3. Remind family death is likely SIDS but search for other causes will occur
   4. Nonaccusatory compassion, provide religious support/grief counseling
F. Reducing risk: safe sleeping ("Back to Sleep," no cosleeping), smoking cessation

XXII. Drowning

A. Pathophysiology: victim breath-holds until reflex inspiration causes aspiration or laryngospasm and hypoxemia
B. Clinical presentation
   1. Important historical elements: drowning and rescue events/timing, precipitating factors (seizure, arrhythmia, drug use)
C. Testing
   1. Chest radiographs performed unless brief, insignificant submersion
   2. Cervical spine plain films if diving, related symptoms
   3. Test end-organ function: chemistry panel, CBC, liver studies
   4. ABG: to assess respiratory status and acidosis
   5. Cranial imaging (CT, magnetic resonance imaging [MRI]): to assess cerebral edema and anoxic injury
   6. If precipitating event, consider ECG, toxicology screen
D. Management: ABCs, intubation if needed, warm patient, supportive care

XXIII. Hypothermia

A. Causes
   1. Primary hypothermia: prolonged exposure to cold (infants at increased risk)
   2. Secondary causes: sepsis, burns, hypothalamic lesions
B. Clinical features
   1. History: duration, type of exposure, precipitating factors (drug use, trauma)
   2. Physical exam: cyanosis, shivering, pupillary response, deep tendon reflexes
C. Testing
   1. ABG, chemistry panel (check for ↓ potassium), clotting factors (risk of disseminated intravascular coagulation [DIC]), CBC

QUICK HIT

Intestinal absorption is increased in malnourished children, especially with iron and calcium deficiencies.

QUICK HIT

No evidence definitively links ALTEs to subsequent sudden infant death syndrome (SIDS), and apnea is not a precursor to SIDS.

QUICK HIT

The goal of the ALTE evaluation is to distinguish those patients with a serious, potentially life-threatening cause from the majority of patients who have either a benign etiology or no identifiable cause for their ALTE.

QUICK HIT

Most patients who have had an ALTE will look well at presentation in the emergency department (ED). A detailed history from the patient's caretaker is therefore the most important means by which benign and serious causes of ALTE can be distinguished.

QUICK HIT

The diagnostic evaluation of patients with ALTE should be driven by a patient's signs and symptoms; many patients will require only minimal workup and observation.

QUICK HIT

According to the American Academy of Pediatrics (AAP), home apnea monitoring does not prevent SIDS in healthy term infants with or without a history of ALTE.

QUICK HIT

The incidence of SIDS markedly decreased after 1992, when the AAP "Back to Sleep" campaign recommended placing infants to sleep in the supine position.

QUICK HIT

There is a 2%–6% risk of a second SIDS death in a family with a previous SIDS death.

QUICK HIT

Evidence suggests that pacifier use is associated with a decreased risk of SIDS.

QUICK HIT

Terms such as "near drowning," "active/passive drowning," "secondary drowning," and "dry/wet drowning" should be avoided due to their imprecision and lack of clinical significance.

QUICK HIT

Toddlers and teenage boys are at highest risk of drowning. Toddler events usually occur in an unattended bathtub or pool, whereas teens drown in natural bodies of water.

QUICK HIT

Children who arrive hypothermic and critically ill after a very cold water submersion may survive with preserved neurologic function despite a long down time.

2. ECG findings
   a. Sinus bradycardia, atrial or ventricular fibrillation, asystole
   b. Osborn or J wave: pathognomonic (but not always present)

D. Treatment: depends on severity and etiology of hypothermia
1. Stabilize ABCs, treat lab abnormalities
2. Rewarming
   a. ≥32°C with adequate perfusion: passive rewarming (remove wet clothing, blankets)
   b. <32°C with adequate perfusion or ≥32°C with inadequate perfusion: active external rewarming (heated blankets, initial risk of ↓ BP and core cooling)
   c. <32°C with inadequate perfusion or cardiac arrest: active core rewarming (bladder/gastric/peritoneal lavage, hemodialysis with warmed fluids)

XXIV. Hyperthermia

A. Clinical features
1. Heat stroke (**hyperpyrexia** = 40°–47°C)
   a. Hot, dry skin; sweating ceases before onset of heat stroke
   b. CNS dysfunction from confusion to coma
   c. Shock

B. Laboratory findings
1. Hypernatremia or hyponatremia depending on rehydration choice
2. Elevations of BUN/creatinine, LFTs, lactate
3. DIC with prolonged prothrombin and partial thromboplastin times, elevated D-dimer, thrombocytopenia

C. Treatment
1. ABCs, aggressive rehydration with IV fluids, correct lab abnormalities
2. Cooling techniques may include ice-water immersion or placing cold water on skin with electrical fans blowing over skin

XXV. Foreign Body Aspiration (FBA) and Ingestion

A. FBA
1. Epidemiology
   a. ~80% of pediatric FBA occurs in children age <3 years
   b. 60% have objects in right lung
   c. Most common: food (especially peanuts, hot dogs, candy, popcorn)
2. Historical findings: witnessed event, duration/severity of choking
   a. Symptoms that may suggest unsuspected FBA
      i. Acute respiratory distress or wheeze in toddler
      ii. Prolonged symptoms
3. Physical examination
   a. Abnormal mental status and FBA require immediate intervention
   b. Depends on site of entrapment
      i. Larynx: hoarse voice, **stridor**
      ii. Trachea/bronchus: asymmetric decreased breath sounds/**wheezing**
4. Diagnostic evaluation
   a. Plain chest/airway radiography: object seen in only 10%, normal in 2/3
   b. Chest **expiratory** films or **lateral decubitus** films (younger children)
      i. Hyperinflation or failure of deflation distal to foreign body (FB)
   c. Airway fluoroscopy: more sensitive than plain radiography
   d. Rigid bronchoscopy for diagnosis and removal
   e. Management: Figure 18-2
   f. Complete obstruction, basic life support not successful
      i. Direct laryngoscopy to remove FB
      ii. If unable to remove FB
         (a) Above vocal cords: needle cricothyrotomy, transtracheal jet ventilation
         (b) Below cords: intubate and push FB into right main stem bronchus, ventilate left lung, then bronchoscopy
   g. Suspected FBA, asymptomatic: bronchoscopy for removal

FIGURE 18-2 **Basic life support: relief of foreign body airway aspiration.**

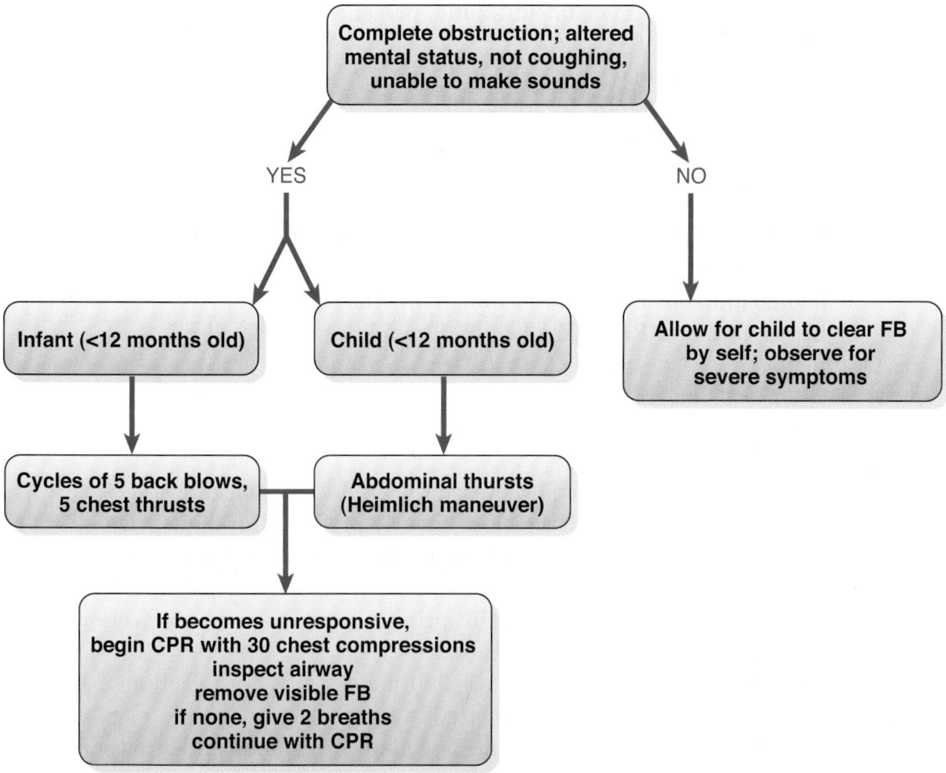

CPR, cardiopulmonary resuscitation; FB, foreign body. (Adapted from Berg MD, Schexnayder SM, Chameides L, et al. Part 13: pediatric basic life support: 2010 American Heart Association guidelines for cardiopulmonary resuscitation and emergency cardiovascular care. *Circulation*. 2010;122[18 suppl 3]:S862-S875.)

B. FB ingestion
  1. Epidemiology
    a. Usually ages 6 months–3 years
    b. Many asymptomatic
    c. Coins most commonly ingested
    d. Will pass if past the lower esophageal sphincter
  2. Pathophysiology
    a. Esophageal FBs tend to lodge in 3 areas of physiologic narrowing
      i. Thoracic inlet (cricopharyngeus muscle) (60%–80%)
      ii. Lower esophageal sphincter (10%–20%)
      iii. Level of aortic arch (5%–20%)
    b. Sharp objects may cause viscus perforation
    c. Caustic FBs (button batteries) cause injury through electrical discharge
    d. Multiple magnets (e.g., "buckyballs") may adhere across layers of bowel, causing direct mucosal injury
    e. Esophageal FBs can cause stridor/wheeze from tracheal compression
  3. Radiographic imaging
    a. ~1/3 of ingested FB are radiolucent
    b. Consider endoscopy or barium swallow if suspected and x-ray negative
  4. Management
    a. Emergent removal from esophagus or stomach
      i. Sharp or long (>5 cm) objects
      ii. Batteries or multiple magnets
      iii. Respiratory distress, unable to swallow
    b. Flexible, rigid endoscopy: common method of removal
    c. Esophageal FB lodged >24 hours should be removed
    d. Most FB of stomach and lower tract pass through in 3–8 days without complication

QUICK HIT

Cervical spine injuries are rare; immobilization should only be done if there was a concerning mechanism, such as diving into shallow water, or signs of an injury.

QUICK HIT

At lower temperatures, muscle stiffness may be so severe that it may mimic rigor mortis and make airway management extremely difficult.

QUICK HIT

Children who arrive to the ED asystolic with primary hypothermia may survive their arrest neurologically intact. The decreased metabolic rate of hypothermia may be neuroprotective.

QUICK HIT

By the time heat stroke patients reach medical attention, their temperature may be <40°C; therefore, maintain a high index of suspicion for heat stroke in all hyperthermic patients.

QUICK HIT

Risk factors for FBA include toddler age (they are mobile, curious, and prone to put things in their mouths), developmental delay and autism, and having an anatomic anomaly (e.g., esophageal stricture or congenital or surgical anomaly).

QUICK HIT

Younger children are more likely to aspirate nonfood items, whereas older children aspirate food items.

QUICK HIT

Consider a bronchial FBA in children with recurrent pneumonias, especially if pneumonia occurs in the right middle lobe.

QUICK HIT

The classic triad of wheeze, cough, and decreased breath sounds is seen in <2/3 of cases (more often if presentation is delayed) of FBA.

QUICK HIT

Do not attempt to remove an FB with a blind finger sweep, which might push it more distal.

QUICK HIT

If an FB is stuck in the mid-esophagus or if it is a food bolus, consider an anatomic anomaly (e.g., stricture or vascular ring).

QUICK HIT

Because of the rigid, incomplete, C-shaped rings of the trachea, coins and other flat objects in the trachea usually appear as circular radiolucencies on the lateral x-ray, whereas in the less rigid esophagus, they will be appear en face in the anterior-posterior x-ray.

QUICK HIT

Langer's lines are topographical lines on the human body that correspond to the orientation of collagen in the skin.

XXVI. Lacerations and Wound Care

A. Clinical features
   1. Historical findings: mechanism/timing, presence of FB, tetanus immunization
   2. Physical exam findings
      a. Laceration size, depth, location, shape
      b. Arterial injury (bright, red bleeding that is difficult to control)
      c. Presence of FB
      d. Distal motor/tendon/nerve function
      e. Laceration over joint or presence of potentially broken bone
   3. Radiology findings: radiographs rarely indicated for simple lacerations
      a. Radiopaque FBs in wound or underlying fracture
      b. Ultrasound or MRI may be helpful if radiolucent or small FB

B. Treatment
   1. Sedation and analgesia
      a. Perform before cleaning and repair
      b. Topical LET gel
      c. Deeper analgesia may require intradermal lidocaine injections
      d. Regional analgesia via nerve block may be preferred for digits, face
   2. Thorough cleaning is most important step to prevent infection, promote healing
      a. Remove devitalized tissue and FBs prior to repair to prevent infection
   3. Laceration repair (Box 18-2 and Table 18-7)
      a. Improves cosmesis and hemostasis but increases risk of infection
      b. Simple interrupted sutures preferred in simple lacerations
      c. Buried or mattress sutures for deep wounds or wounds under tension
      d. Wound edges should be apposed and everted
      e. Suture alternatives
         i. Tissue adhesive (glue): painless, fast, does not require removal; for low-tension linear wounds; not for hands, feet, joints; equivalent results to sutures

BOX 18-2

Indications to NOT Repair a Laceration

>24 hours since time of injury (this may be extended in clean facial injuries)
Human/animal bite (unless extremely large or cosmetically important)
Already infected
Small, deep punctate wound (cannot effectively irrigate)
Superficial wound that will heal without intervention (sutures will increase scarring)
Hemostasis cannot be achieved

TABLE 18-7 Laceration Repair Guidelines

Location	Closure Material	Sutures in Place for
Face	6-0 nylon or polypropylene; may use fast-absorbing gut to avoid removal in anxious children	3–5 days
Scalp	5-0 polypropylene or staples	7 days
Intraoral	5-0 fast-absorbing gut, chromic gut for deep layers	Absorbable
Upper extremities	4-0, 5-0 polypropylene	7 days
Lower extremities	4-0, 5-0 polypropylene	8–10 days
Joint	5-0 polypropylene	10–14 days

ii. Adhesive strips: painless, highest risk of dehiscence, low-tension linear wounds, must stay dry
iii. Staples: fast, frequently used on scalp wounds, poor cosmesis

f. Antibiotics: less effective than proper irrigation; may be indicated in
   i. Human or animal bites (see XXVII. Mammalian Bites)
   ii. Open fractures, joint injuries
   iii. Contaminated wound (such as barnyard injury)
   iv. >18 hours to closure
   v. Immunocompromised patient
g. Dressing: bulky/sterile, topical antibiotic ointment, splint involved joints
h. Wound care: leave initial dressing on 24–48 hours, then wash gently
i. **Tetanus booster and/or immunoglobulin**
   i. Booster if at least 3 previous tetanus vaccinations and >5 years since last immunization
   ii. For all wounds: booster necessary if <3 previous immunizations
   iii. Tetanus immunoglobulin + tetanus booster: if <3 previous tetanus immunizations *and* tetanus prone (e.g., puncture, crush, dirty, no care in >24 hours)

4. Complications
   a. Infection: especially if irrigation or wound debridement inadequate, retained FB, bite wound, avulsion injury
   b. Dehiscence: premature closure removal
   c. Poor cosmesis: keloid formation, perpendicular to **Langer's lines**
5. Duration/prognosis: full strength and final appearance in 6–8 months

XXVII. Mammalian Bites

A. Pathophysiology: dog bites cause crush injury, cat bites puncture with increased infection risk
B. Bacteriology
   1. Dog and cat bite pathogens: staph, strep, anaerobes, *Pasteurella multocida*
   2. Human bite pathogens: *Staphylococcus aureus*, *Streptococcus viridans*, anaerobes, *Eikenella* (rare, severe)
C. Acute treatment considerations
   1. Wound closure: leave open unless large or on face
   2. *Copious* irrigation for prevention of infection
   3. Antibiotic prophylaxis (amoxicillin/clavulanate) for 3–5 days: puncture wound, cat or human, hand or foot or face, delayed closure
   4. **Tetanus** therapy as per all wound management
   5. **Rabies**
      a. Rare (1–5 cases per year) but high morbidity and mortality
      b. Wild carnivores, bat bites high risk for rabies
         i. Rodents/rabbits not considered at risk for transmitting rabies
      c. Domesticated mammals considered possible rabies risk
         i. Unknown immunization status
         ii. Cannot be located for quarantine/observation
      d. In initial wound care, postexposure prophylaxis includes *both*
         i. Passive antibody (rabies immunoglobulin): 50% given into wound; 50% IM
         ii. Rabies vaccine IM
      e. 3 subsequent doses of rabies vaccine at 3, 7, and 14 days postexposure

XXVIII. Approach to Fractures

A. Common types in children
   1. **Physeal** (growth plate): 20% of all pediatric fractures, classified by Salter-Harris system (Figures 18-3 and 18-4)
      a. **Salter-Harris type I fracture**
         i. Radiographs normal: clinical diagnosis based on tenderness
         ii. Management: immobilization and orthopedic follow-up
         iii. Complications and growth disturbances are rare

> **QUICK HIT**
> Facial laceration infection rates do not increase with delayed closure in the absence of other risk factors.

> **QUICK HIT**
> If an underlying fracture is suspected, laceration repair should not occur until fracture is ruled out. An open fracture may require orthopedic consultation for possible operating room washout and antibiotics.

> **QUICK HIT**
> If an FB is identified on initial imaging, repeat images should be obtained after removal to ensure complete removal prior to repair.

> **QUICK HIT**
> With suspected joint capsule injury, inject **methylene blue** into the joint. Blue extravasation from the laceration confirms joint injury.

> **QUICK HIT**
> In some cases, families may prefer a less cosmetic result in order to minimize trauma to the patient, especially in less visible wounds or in patients with special behavioral concerns. This option should be *presented* to them, not *decided* for them.

> **QUICK HIT**
> Of mammalian bites, 85%–90% are due to dogs, 5%–10% to cats, 2%–3% to rodents and other animals, and 2%–3% to humans.

QUICK HIT

Cat bites have the highest infection rate due to the bite's deep puncture.

QUICK HIT

Mammalian bite infections often grow mixed flora.

QUICK HIT

Amoxicillin/clavulanic acid is a good choice for prophylaxis for most cat and dog bite wounds because it is effective against most pathogens.

QUICK HIT

The usual tetanus immunization schedule for children is 4 total doses between ages 2 months and 2 years (usually at 2, 4, 6, and 15 months), with boosters at ages 4–5 and 11–12 years.

QUICK HIT

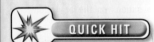

Rabies prophylaxis is not needed when the bite is by a healthy dog or cat with a known owner. Discussion with the local health department can help with decision about rabies risk.

QUICK HIT

Incomplete (e.g., greenstick, buckle, and bowing) fractures do not extend across the entire width of the bone and are more common in children than adults.

FIGURE 18-3 Salter-Harris classification system for physeal fractures.

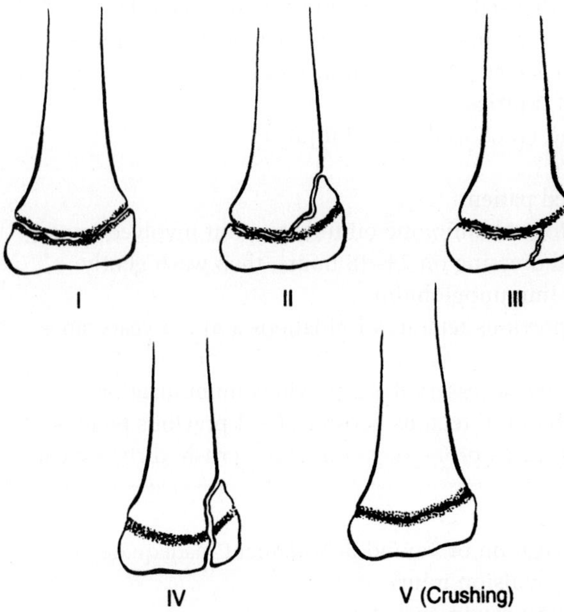

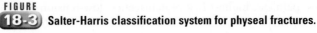

(From Harwood-Nuss A, Wolfson AB, Linden CH, et al. *The Clinical Practice of Emergency Medicine.* 3rd ed. Philadelphia: Lippincott Williams & Wilkins; 2001.)

b. Salter-Harris type II fracture
   i. Management: immobilization and orthopedic follow-up
   ii. Complications and growth disturbances are rare
c. Salter-Harris type III, IV, V fractures
   i. Management: immediate orthopedic consultation; may require surgical reduction to re-establish anatomic position and prevent growth disturbances
   ii. Increasing risk for growth disturbance

FIGURE 18-4 Anatomy of long bone.

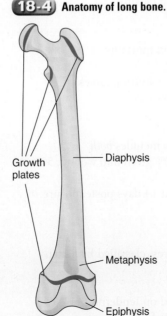

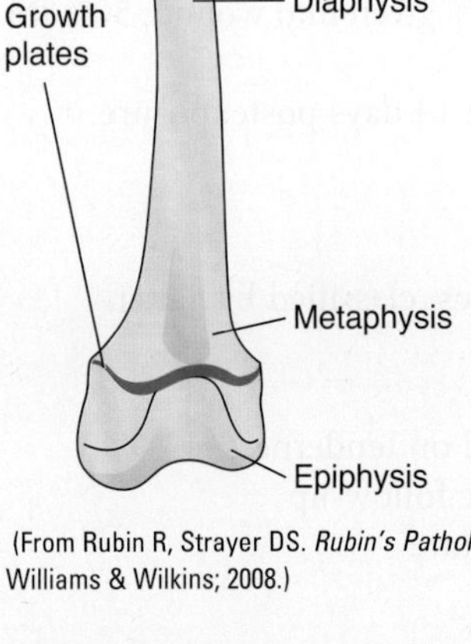

(From Rubin R, Strayer DS. *Rubin's Pathology: Clinicopathologic Foundations of Medicine.* 5th ed. Philadelphia: Lippincott Williams & Wilkins; 2008.)

2. Common pediatric fracture types
   a. **Greenstick fractures:** incomplete, not through bone (often long bone)
   b. **Buckle (torus) fractures**: compressive load buckles cortex (often distal radius from fall on outstretched hand)
   c. **Apophyseal avulsion fractures**: fragment of bone torn off by muscle contraction at tendon insertion point (often pelvis, tibial tubercle)
3. Fractures with important pediatric considerations
   a. Elbow fractures: complex because of 3 articulations, progressive ossification centers
      i. Challenging to diagnose by x-ray; look for anterior displaced fat pad: a sign of joint fluid
      ii. **Supracondylar fractures** can involve neurovascular bundle and may require emergent orthopedic involvement
   b. **Femur fractures**
      i. Assess hemodynamic status: can result in significant blood loss
      ii. Assess distal limb neurovascular status
      iii. Immediate traction and splinting to prevent blood loss
      iv. Often require operative casting and management
   c. **Toddler's fracture** (Figure 18-5)
      i. Spiral fracture through distal tibia
      ii. Occurs in young ambulatory children (usually ages 1–4 years)
      iii. Mechanism: minor fall; injury may be unwitnessed
      iv. Presentation: limp, refusal to walk, no deformity/swelling

FIGURE 18-5 **Toddler's fracture of distal tibia (*arrows*).**

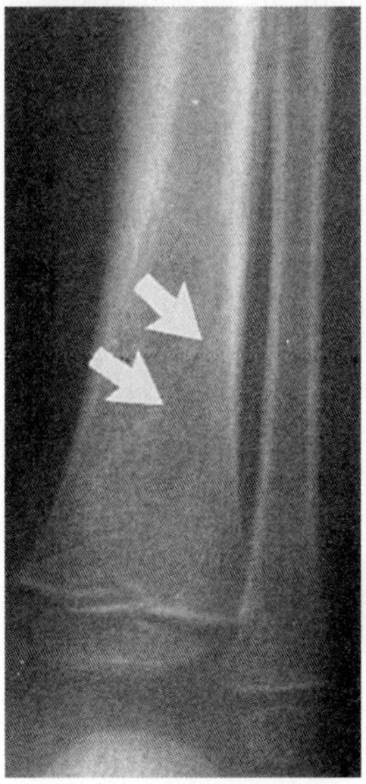

(From Fleisher GR, Ludwig S, Baskin MN. *Atlas of Pediatric Emergency Medicine.* Philadelphia: Lippincott Williams & Wilkins; 2004.)

XXIX. Child Physical Abuse and Neglect

A. Characteristics: four main types: neglect, physical abuse, sexual abuse, emotional abuse
   1. Causes are multifactorial: family stress, poor family support, societal violence, caretaker substance abuse
   2. Risk factors: colicky infants, children with disability/emotional problems, foster care
B. Clinical features
   1. Historical findings
      a. **Inconsistent or changing history**
      b. History of repeated injuries or hospitalizations
      c. Unexplained delay in seeking medical care

MNEMONIC

CRITOE: elbow ossification center appearance
Capitellum: age 1 year
Radial head: age 3 years
Internal (medial) condyle: age 5 years
Trochlea: age 7 years
Olecranon: age 9 years
External (lateral) condyle: age 11 years

QUICK HIT

Although the radiographic presence of an anterior fat pad is often normal in children, a posterior fat pad is always abnormal. A large or displaced anterior fat pad may also be abnormal.

QUICK HIT

Supracondylar fractures are the most common pediatric elbow fracture.

QUICK HIT

The common injury mechanism in a supracondylar fracture is a fall onto an outstretched hand with hyperextension of the elbow.

QUICK HIT

When femur fracture is seen in a nonambulatory child, consider nonaccidental trauma as a possible cause.

QUICK HIT

Child abuse is any recent act or failure to act that results in imminent risk of serious physical or emotional harm or death of a child (person age <18 years) by the parent or caregiver responsible for the child's welfare (Child Abuse Prevention and Treatment Act – Pub L No. 108-36).

QUICK HIT

Accidental bruising is more common in ambulatory children and usually located on bony prominences of the extremities and the forehead.

d. History of injury inconsistent with child's development
e. History does not explain physical exam findings or injuries

2. Physical exam findings
   a. Bruise characteristics associated with child abuse
      i. Any location in nonambulatory children
      ii. Concerning locations: flexor surfaces, ear pinna, torso/abdomen, neck, genitals
      iii. Patterned bruising (e.g., linear, hand marks, belt marks)
      iv. Extensive bruising, especially old + new injuries present
   b. Concerning burns
      i. Immersion burns: usually occur in hot bathwater to toddlers
         (a) Stocking or glove pattern on arms or feet
         (b) Symmetric, in genitourinary (GU) area, spares creases
      ii. Cigarette burns: deep, well-circumscribed, 8-mm diameter
      iii. Patterned burns from iron, curling iron, stove coil
   c. Human bite marks: circular lesions 1–2 inches in diameter
   d. Torn lingual frenulum: in nonambulatory children (from forced bottle)

C. Diagnosis
1. Differential diagnosis (Table 18-8)
2. Laboratory findings
   a. Rule out other causes of bruising or fracture: check CBC, coagulation studies, vitamin D levels, calcium/phosphorus/alkaline phosphatase, parathyroid hormone, screen of osteogenesis imperfecta
3. Radiology findings
   a. Skeletal injuries
      i. Complete skeletal survey in children age <2 years: to evaluate for occult fractures (unexplained or multiple/different stages of healing are all concerning)
   b. Intracranial injury
      i. All children age <12 months and suspicious injuries
         (a) MRI: asymptomatic children
         (b) CT scan: symptomatic children after stabilization
      ii. Multiple findings may be seen: subdural hematomas, skull fractures, diffuse axonal injury
   c. Abdominal imaging: indications include abdominal bruising, vomiting, severe abdominal pain, elevated liver transaminases
4. Shaken baby syndrome (more accurately called **abusive head trauma**)
   a. Cause/pathophysiology: violent shaking of infant (with or without subsequent impact) resulting in diffuse or focal brain injury/bleed

QUICK HIT

Shaken baby syndrome is a triad of subdural hemorrhage, diffuse multilayered retinal hemorrhages, and diffuse brain injury.

TABLE 18-8 Differential Diagnosis of Child Abuse

Physical Exam Finding or Injury	Differential Diagnosis
Bruising	Unintentional trauma Acquired and inherited coagulation disorders Pseudobruise from clothing dye Cultural practices: coining, cupping Birth marks, Mongolian spots
Intracranial hemorrhage	Unintentional trauma Acquired and inherited coagulation disorders Glutaric aciduria type I
Burn	Unintentional spill Contact dermatitis Bullous impetigo
Fracture	Unintentional trauma Metabolic: rickets, osteopenia Congenital: osteogenesis imperfecta, Blount disease

b. Clinical presentation: increasing head circumference, ALTE, irritability/vomiting, seizure, change in mental status

D. Treatment
1. Injuries should be treated as medically indicated
2. Medical professionals are mandated reporters of child abuse to Child Protective Services (CPS)
3. Documentation: use quotation marks, describe findings in detail, take pictures if possible
4. Prevention: pediatricians play important role by providing
   a. Education on range of normal behaviors, parenting advice
   b. Community resources
   c. Screening for adult: partner violence, maternal depression, and parental substance abuse

XXX. Sexual Abuse

A. Clinical features
1. Presentation to medical care: patients may seek care for variety of reasons
   a. Disclosure of inappropriate sexual contact
   b. Physical complaints or anogenital injury
   c. Sexually transmitted infection (STI)
   d. Pregnancy
   e. Encopresis, dysuria, abdominal pain
   f. Inappropriate sexual behaviors
   g. Other behavioral complaints: acting out, sleep disturbances and nightmares, school trouble, unwillingness to go certain places
2. Physical exam findings
   a. Usually physical exam is normal
   b. May have findings suggestive of physical abuse and neglect
   c. GU examination
      i. For patients presenting within 72 hours of sexual abuse, evidence collection may be indicated
      ii. Goal of exam is to look for evidence of trauma or infection
      iii. Examine girls in frog-leg posture or prone in knee–chest position
      iv. Frog-leg or prone knee–chest exam; internal vaginal examination only if concern for internal injury
      v. GU exam findings
         (a) Document hymen appearance and presence of normal variants (notches, clefts) or evidence of injury (tears, bruising)
         (b) Posterior fourchette scarring indicates chronic abuse with penetration
         (c) Signs of possible infection: ulcerations, genital warts, vesicles, or vaginal discharge
         (d) Vulvovaginitis
         (e) Rectal tears, discharge, injuries, asymmetric folds

B. Diagnosis
1. Differential diagnosis: varied depending on exam findings
2. Laboratory evaluation
   a. Within 72 hours of alleged sexual abuse, forensic evidence collection may be indicated
   b. Testing for STIs and pregnancy as needed

C. Treatment
1. Therapy
   a. Prophylaxis in postpubertal children presenting within 72 hours of assault
      i. Antibiotics for risk of STIs (gonorrhea, *Chlamydia*, trichomoniasis)
      ii. Hepatitis B prophylaxis: vaccinate if not fully immunized
      iii. Consider HIV prophylaxis
   b. Pregnancy prevention: levonorgestrel up to 5 days after event
2. Reporting to police and CPS depends on local laws
3. All victims of sexual abuse require psychosocial referral and follow-up

> **QUICK HIT**
> According to the Child Abuse Prevention and Treatment Act, **sexual abuse** is "a type of maltreatment that refers to the involvement of the child in sexual activity to provide sexual gratification or financial benefit to the perpetrator, including contacts for sexual purposes, molestation, statutory rape, prostitution, pornography, exposure, incest, or other sexually exploitative activities."

> **QUICK HIT**
> An STI in a child age <12 years is considered sexual abuse until proven otherwise.

> **QUICK HIT**
> Internal examination of prepubescent girls often requires anesthesia or procedural sedation.

> **QUICK HIT**
> The normal prepubescent hymen has a smooth opening, often of crescentic shape.

> **QUICK HIT**
> Accidental vaginal injury is more likely to occur anteriorly, whereas injury due to sexual abuse is more likely to be posteriorly located.

19 Disorders of the Ear, Nose, and Throat

SYMPTOM SPECIFIC

I. Approach to Stridor

A. Background information
  1. Monophonic, harsh, variable-pitched sound caused by passage of air through narrowed airway
  2. Sign of **upper airway obstruction**; not a diagnosis
  3. Can be **inspiratory**, **expiratory**, or **biphasic**
    a. Location in respiratory cycle can help determine site of obstruction (Table 19-1)
    b. Airway obstruction exaggerates normal changes in airway caliber

B. Differential diagnosis
  1. Etiologies often categorized as either *acute* or *chronic*
  2. **Acute onset**
    a. Croup (most common cause)
    b. Peritonsillar abscess (PTA) or retropharyngeal abscess (RPA)
    c. Epiglottitis (rare after universal vaccination against *Haemophilus influenzae* type b)
    d. Airway foreign body
    e. Anaphylaxis
    f. Hypocalcemic tetany
    g. Caustic ingestion or thermal burn
  3. **Chronic causes**: often result from anatomic aberrations
    a. Laryngomalacia/tracheomalacia (most common chronic cause)
    b. Vocal cord dysfunction
    c. Subglottic stenosis
    d. Mediastinal mass (e.g., tumor, tuberculosis [TB])
    e. Hemangiomas

QUICK HIT

Stertor is a low-pitched, inspiratory noise caused by nasal or nasopharyngeal obstruction, whereas **stridor** is a variable-pitched sound due to upper airway obstruction.

QUICK HIT

Tracheomalacia is the most frequent cause of expiratory stridor.

TABLE 19-1 **Pathophysiology of Stridor Based on Location of Obstruction**

Obstruction in the extrathoracic airways ↓	Supraglottic • Epiglottis • Aryepiglottic folds • False vocal cords	Inspiratory stridor caused by loose supporting structures that collapse during inspiration as a result of higher atmospheric pressure than intraluminal pressure
Thoracic inlet ↓	Glottic/subglottic • True vocal cords • Extrathoracic trachea to thoracic inlet	Rigid and noncollapsible tube that, when obstructed, causes fixed, biphasic stridor
Intrathoracic trachea	Intrathoracic trachea	During inspiration, the negative intrathoracic pressure maintains integrity; during expiration, the positive intrathoracic pressure causes airway collapse that worsens obstruction

TABLE 19-2 **Pertinent Historical Questions for Evaluating Stridor**

Questions	Significance
What is the age of the patient?	Laryngomalacia, tracheomalacia, and subglottic stenosis usually present in the 1st few weeks of life Foreign body aspiration is generally seen in an infant older than 6 months when the child is able to grab objects Croup generally occurs in children between the ages of 6 months and 3 years Retropharyngeal abscess occurs in preschool-aged children Peritonsillar abscess more commonly occurs in children and adolescents
Were there any complications after birth? Was the patient in the neonatal intensive care unit?	History of prolonged intubation may suggest **subglottic stenosis**; history of patent ductus arteriosus ligation may suggest vocal cord dysfunction from damage to recurrent laryngeal nerve
When did the symptoms begin? Have they been getting worse?	Acute onset in a toddler with no other upper respiratory infection (URI) symptoms or a choking event that was unwitnessed should suggest **foreign body aspiration** Acute onset with preceding URI symptoms now with barking cough and stridor—think croup Acute onset in a patient with known exposed allergen would suggest an allergic reaction or caustic ingestion Symptoms since birth may suggest a structural problem Symptoms worsening around 6–9 months of age may suggest a growing laryngotracheal hemangioma
Are there any associated symptoms?	Fever suggests an infectious etiology. A choking event may suggest a foreign body aspiration. Aphonia suggests bilateral vocal cord paralysis. Urticaria or emesis is seen with an allergic reaction.
Does anything seem to make the stridor worse? Better?	Stridor that is worse when crying or placed supine and improved with prone placement is typically seen with laryngomalacia

C. Historical findings: birth history
  1. Birth complications
  2. Need for intubation, age of onset, relationship of stridor with feeding and body position, voice quality, and associated symptoms (Table 19-2)

D. Physical exam findings
  1. *Rapid assessment of degree of upper airway obstruction is essential*
  2. Primary focus should be on respiratory exam
    a. Look for symptoms of respiratory distress, such as alterations in mental status, increased work of breathing, and hypoxia
    b. Note stridor quality and timing
    c. Assess symmetry of respiratory exam
    d. Note factors that make stridor better or worse
  3. Look for supporting exam findings
    a. Cough, congestion, rhinorrhea (viral croup)
    b. Drooling, trismus, torticollis, inability to extend the neck, or uvular deviation (RPA or PTA)
    c. Gray pseudomembrane covering tonsils and pharynx (diphtheria)
    d. Lip swelling and hives (anaphylaxis)
    e. Hemangiomas on skin, specifically in "beard" distribution (airway hemangioma)

E. Laboratory testing and radiologic data
  1. Radiologic testing
    a. Not routinely needed, but focused evaluation based on history and physical exam can provide diagnosis or guide management (Table 19-3)
  2. Laboratory evaluation: rarely needed
    a. In toxic-appearing children, elevations in white blood cells (WBCs) or inflammatory markers may indicate bacterial tracheitis or epiglottitis
    b. Respiratory viral polymerase chain reaction (PCR) testing may help confirm etiology in croup diagnosis (not usually necessary)

II. Approach to Epistaxis

A. Background information
  1. **Epistaxis**: nasal bleeding
    a. May arise from front of nose (**anterior epistaxis**) or back of nose and possibly into oropharynx (**posterior epistaxis**)

QUICK HIT

When assessing respiratory distress and stridor, remember your **ABCs**!

QUICK HIT

Signs of increased work of breathing include tachypnea; nasal flaring; supraclavicular, intercostal, and subcostal retractions; abdominal breathing; and grunting.

QUICK HIT

Severe respiratory distress may manifest with altered mental status, hypoventilation, and cyanosis.

QUICK HIT

Of patients with a subglottic hemangioma, 50% have a cutaneous hemangioma.

QUICK HIT

Croup is most commonly caused by infection with **parainfluenza** viruses.

QUICK HIT

In some healthy and asymptomatic children, subglottic narrowing on a chest x-ray may be seen, depending on the phase of inspiration captured.

QUICK HIT

Epistaxis is very common in school-aged children, affecting ~50% of children ages 6–10 years.

QUICK HIT

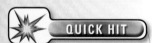

Epistaxis in children age <2 years is unusual and warrants further investigation because it may be a sign of nonaccidental trauma, a mass, or systemic illness.

QUICK HIT

Blood contains iron in its composition, which may induce nausea or vomiting if swallowed in large amounts.

TABLE 19-3 Evaluation Based on Suspected Etiology of Stridor

Diagnosis	Evaluation
Croup	Generally a clinical diagnosis, but an anteroposterior radiograph may reveal a **"steeple" sign** from subglottic narrowing
Laryngomalacia	Best diagnosed by direct observation with laryngoscopy
Tracheomalacia	Barium swallow or airway fluoroscopy will show narrowing of the trachea
Epiglottitis	Lateral neck radiograph may show a **"thumb" sign** from edema of the epiglottis
Foreign body aspiration	Lateral neck and chest radiograph may show an object if radiopaque. Air trapping may be visible on an inspiratory or forced expiratory film in an older child or on a lateral decubitus film in a younger child. Laryngoscopy or bronchoscopy may be necessary to detect objects not visible on x-ray.
Retropharyngeal abscess	Lateral neck radiograph will show widening of the prevertebral tissues. A computed tomography (CT) scan with contrast will show an abscess.
Peritonsillar abscess	Generally a clinical diagnosis; however, a CT scan with contrast can be performed to confirm the diagnosis
Vascular ring	Barium swallow may show an indentation in the esophagus. Magnetic resonance imaging or angiography of the chest is the definitive study.

b. Most cases are benign and self-limited, but bleeding can be severe and result in profound anemia and hemodynamic instability
2. Bleeding is common due to highly vascular nature of nasal mucosa
   a. It contains several venous plexuses and areas of arterial confluence
   b. Most bleeds are anterior and arise from **Kiesselbach plexus**
3. Epistaxis can develop due to a large number of causes (Box 19-1)

B. Important historical findings
1. Bleeding from nose or mouth; vomiting or spitting up blood
   a. Bleeding from nose: indicates anterior epistaxis
   b. Vomiting, spitting up blood, or bleeding from mouth: suggests posterior epistaxis, which is less common in children
2. New, recurrent, or chronic bleeding; difficulty stopping
   a. Acute, self-limited bleeds: often due to various forms of trauma (especially nose picking) or foreign body

BOX 19-1

Differential Diagnosis of Epistaxis

Local trauma (**nose picking**)
Foreign body in nose
Blunt trauma (blow to face, nasal fracture)
Inflammatory reaction
  Acute sinus or respiratory infection, chronic infection
  Allergic rhinitis or environmental
Excessively dry air
  Seasonal (winter)
  Nasal cannula oxygen (unhumidified)
Nasal polyps
Intranasal masses (nasopharyngeal tumor)
  Juvenile nasopharyngeal angiofibroma
  Pyogenic granuloma
  Rhabdomyosarcoma
  Nasopharyngeal carcinoma
Hypertension
Anatomic abnormalities (deviated septum, septal spur)
Surgery (septoplasty, endoscopic sinus surgery, turbinectomy, nasal tumor resection)
Intranasal medication/drugs (cocaine, oxymetazoline)
Systemic anticoagulation medications (aspirin, warfarin, ibuprofen)
Barotrauma (pressure differential from scuba diving, airplane descent)
Systemic diseases (anemia, vascular disorders, heart failure, connective tissue disease)
  Hereditary hemorrhagic telangiectasia
  Wegener granulomatosis
Bleeding disorders (connective tissue disease, idiopathic thrombocytopenic purpura, leukemia, von Willebrand disease)
Vitamin C or K deficiency

b. Recurrent bleeds or bleeds that are difficult to control: more likely to be associated with serious disorder or chronic medical condition
3. Prolonged bleeding with minor injuries or prior procedures (e.g., circumcision); easy bruising
   a. May indicate bleeding diathesis such as hemophilia, von Willebrand disease (VWD), or platelet aggregation problem
   b. Bruising or petechiae: often signs of thrombocytopenia
4. Associated symptoms
   a. Fever and rhinorrhea: viral respiratory infection or sinusitis
   b. Headache or progressive nasal obstruction: concerning for growing mass
5. Recent surgeries, medical conditions, or medications that may impact bleeding

C. Physical examination findings
1. Determine whether patient is hemodynamically stable and assess for signs of severe blood loss (pallor, tachycardia, orthostatic hypotension, murmur, poor perfusion)
2. Nasal and oral cavity should be examined to identify source of bleeding
   a. Look for multiple sources of bleeding, especially in patients with signs of systemic illness
   b. Flexible laryngoscopy performed by otolaryngologist: can visualize airway and identify source of bleeding, especially for posterior bleeds
3. In cases of trauma, evaluate for other signs of injury

D. Laboratory testing and radiologic imaging
1. Most cases do not require lab or radiologic evaluation
2. Laboratory investigation may be helpful in severe or chronic cases
   a. Complete blood count (CBC) to identify anemia, thrombocytopenia, or findings to suggest leukemia
   b. Type and screen if transfusion with blood products may be needed
   c. If bleeding disorder is suspected: consider prothrombin time (PT), partial thromboplastin time (PTT), international normalized ratio (INR), factor assays, bleeding time
3. Imaging: magnetic resonance angiography (MRA) or venography (MRV) or computed tomography angiography (CTA) can help determine source of bleeding if it cannot otherwise be identified

E. Treatment
1. Severe blood loss: stabilize patient with fluid resuscitation, blood transfusion, and airway protection
2. Initial treatment: pressure, ice along nasal bridge, and oxymetazoline intranasally to promote vasoconstriction
3. Silver nitrate: can be used for chemical cautery if initial treatment fails
4. If bleeding continues: use absorbable or nonabsorbable packing
5. Severe posterior bleeds: may require placement of Foley or Epistat catheter
6. Invasive interventions (e.g., **nasoendoscopy with cauterization** or **embolization**): may be needed in very severe cases
7. Long-term treatment/maintenance
   a. Continued nasal care with moisture (nasal saline, humidified air) prevents dry nasal mucosa
   b. Identify and treat any underlying contributing conditions

DISEASE SPECIFIC

III. Sinusitis

A. Characteristics
1. Definition: infection of mucosal lining of paranasal sinuses; generally, complication of allergic inflammation or viral upper respiratory infection (URI)
   a. Acute: symptoms <30 days
   b. Subacute: 4–12 weeks of symptoms
   c. Chronic: symptoms >12 weeks
2. Complicates up to 5% of URIs

> **QUICK HIT**
> **Osler-Weber-Rendu syndrome** (or hereditary hemorrhagic telangiectasia [HHT]) is a genetic disorder, resulting in abnormal blood vessel formation in the skin, mucous membranes, lungs, brain, and gastrointestinal tract. Children present with severe, frequent nosebleeds.

> **QUICK HIT**
> Suctioning with a rigid or flexible suction may remove clots to better visualize the nasal cavity but may open up clotted vessels.

> **QUICK HIT**
> Examine the skin for evidence of bruising, purpura, or petechiae, which may indicate a bleeding disorder or thrombocytopenia.

> **QUICK HIT**
> Antibiotic ointment is used to prevent toxic shock syndrome and prevent abrasion from packing.

> **QUICK HIT**
> Ethmoid and maxillary sinuses are present at birth, but the frontal and sphenoid sinuses do not develop until a child is age 4–7 years. The frontal sinus is not fully developed until adolescence.

> **QUICK HIT**
> A healthy child averages 6–8 colds/year.

> **QUICK HIT**
> Acute sinusitis and acute otitis media are caused by the same bacterial pathogens.

3. Cause: usually viral or bacterial, rarely fungal
   a. Acute infection
      i. *Streptococcus pneumoniae*
      ii. *Moraxella catarrhalis*
      iii. Nontypeable *H. influenzae*
   b. Chronic infections
      i. Acute sinusitis pathogens
      ii. Respiratory tract anaerobes
      iii. Viridans streptococci
      iv. *Staphylococcus aureus*
4. Several associated genetic disorders
   a. Cystic fibrosis (CF)
   b. Humoral immunodeficiency
      i. Bruton agammaglobulinemia
      ii. Immunoglobulin (Ig) A deficiency
      iii. Common variable immunodeficiency
   c. Immotile cilia syndrome (primary ciliary dyskinesia)
   d. Atopy
5. Risk factors for developing sinus infection
   a. URIs
   b. Allergic inflammation
   c. Mechanical obstruction of sinus ostia (trauma, foreign body)
   d. Genetic conditions listed above
   e. Smoke exposure
6. Pathophysiology
   a. Various factors may lead to retention of secretions
      i. Blockage of sinus ostia (inhibits drainage into nose) via mucosal swelling or mechanical obstruction
      ii. Impairment of mucociliary clearance
      iii. Increased secretions
   b. Nasopharyngeal bacteria enter sinuses and proliferate

> **QUICK HIT**
> Most URIs will begin to resolve by the 10th day of illness.

B. Clinical features
1. Historical findings: several presentations should raise suspicion for sinusitis
   a. Nasal discharge, congestion, and cough not improving for >10 days
   b. Purulent nasal discharge and high fever (>39°C) lasting >3–4 days
   c. URI with symptoms worsening after 5–7 days with recurrence of fever
   d. Less common complaints include malodorous breath and periorbital edema
   e. Headache and facial pain are uncommon in children
2. Physical exam findings
   a. Erythematous nasal mucosa with purulent drainage
   b. Occasional sinus tenderness in older children/adolescents

> **QUICK HIT**
> Exam findings of sinusitis are generally difficult to differentiate from those of a viral URI.

C. Diagnosis
1. Differential diagnosis
   a. Usually focused on identifying predisposing conditions
2. Radiology findings
   a. Generally not indicated unless complicated, chronic or recurrent disease, or failure to respond to therapy
   b. Computed tomography (CT) is superior to x-rays
   c. Shows opacification, mucosal thickening, or air–fluid level
3. Other laboratory data
   a. Sinus aspirate is gold standard in diagnosis but rarely needed
   b. Indicated for patients who fail to respond to antibiotics and those with chronic, recurrent, or severe disease

> **QUICK HIT**
> Always consider sinusitis in children with fever of unknown origin, insofar as presenting symptoms may be subtle.

D. Treatment
1. Therapy
   a. Antibiotics
      i. Oral medications: amoxicillin, amoxicillin-clavulanate, or 3rd-generation cephalosporins (often in combination with clindamycin)

> **QUICK HIT**
> Sinusitis is generally a clinical diagnosis.

TABLE 19-4 Complications of Sinusitis and Acute Otitis Media

Infection	Extracranial	Intracranial
Sinusitis	Periorbital cellulitis Orbital cellulitis or abscess Subperiosteal abscess Osteomyelitis Pott puffy tumor (osteomyelitis of frontal bone)	Epidural abscess Subdural empyema Cavernous or sagittal venous sinus thrombosis Brain abscess Meningitis
Acute otitis media	Perforation of the tympanic membrane Hearing impairment with speech delay Cholesteatoma* Mastoiditis Facial paralysis (rare) Intracranial spread (rare)† Facial nerve paralysis Jugular venous thrombosis†	Epidural abscess Brain abscess Meningitis Venous sinus thrombosis

*Cyst-like growth that can occur from chronic otitis.
†Usually occurs with concomitant mastoiditis.

ii. Improvement occurs within 72 hours
iii. Acute sinusitis: treat for 7 days after resolution of symptoms; usual course is 10–14 days of therapy
iv. Chronic sinusitis: requires 3–4 weeks of therapy

b. Minimal evidence for routine use of nasal saline washes, antihistamines, decongestants, or nasal steroids
c. Endoscopic sinus surgery in chronic, severe, or recurrent cases

2. Complications of sinusitis are rare but can be very severe (Table 19-4)

E. Prognosis
1. Generally can be effectively treated with oral antibiotics
2. Intracranial complications require intravenous (IV) antibiotics and surgical drainage

F. Prevention
1. Handwashing and influenza vaccine to prevent URI
2. Treatment of allergic rhinitis

> **QUICK HIT**
> FESS, or *functional endoscopic sinus surgery*, widens the sinus ostia and removes diseased mucosa and bone.

IV. Otitis Externa

A. Definition: infection or inflammation of external ear canal

B. Cause/pathophysiology
1. Associated with prolonged wetness in ear canal, dermatitis, foreign body, or trauma
2. Ear canal defenses weakened by washing away cerumen, increased desquamation, changes in normal flora (usually coagulase-negative staphylococci, micrococci, and corynebacteria), and pH changes
3. Most common causative bacteria are *Pseudomonas* species, but *Escherichia coli*, *Proteus*, *Staphylococcus aureus*, *Streptococcus*, and fungi may be involved

> **QUICK HIT**
> Otitis externa is commonly referred to as **"swimmer's ear."**

C. Clinical presentation
1. Ear pain (**otalgia**): can be severe and worsened by manipulation of outer ear, pressure on the tragus, and speculum insertion
2. Exam reveals swelling and erythema of skin of ear canal, presence of debris in canal, and normal tympanic membrane (TM); periauricular lymphadenopathy may be present
3. Complications include cellulitis progressing to mastoid area and **malignant otitis externa** (infection extending to cartilage and bone of ear canal)

> **QUICK HIT**
> Examining a child with otitis externa can be difficult due to the pain caused by moving the pinna.

D. Testing
1. Diagnosis is based on physical exam findings
2. Consider culturing ear debris, especially in atypical cases or if poor response to treatment

E. Treatment
1. Topical antibiotics: polymyxin, aminoglycosides, or fluoroquinolones
2. With extensive ear edema, wick may be inserted to allow drops to contact entire surface of ear canal
3. Removing ear debris can augment antibiotic effectiveness
4. Topical or oral analgesia for pain control
5. Infection may be prevented by drying ears well and using acetic acid preparations to acidify ear canal

V. Otitis Media

QUICK HIT

Otitis media is the most common reason antibiotics are prescribed in young children.

A. Characteristics
1. Definition: inflammation of middle ear
   a. **Acute otitis media (AOM)**: suppurative infection
   b. **Otitis media with effusion (OME)**: usually noninfectious inflammation
2. ~90% of children experience AOM before age 2 years, with peak age 6–18 months
3. Cause
   a. Usually associated with URI
   b. Common pathogens include bacteria and viruses
      i. *S. pneumoniae*
      ii. Nontypeable *H. influenzae*
      iii. *M. catarrhalis*
      iv. Viruses (often in combination with bacteria): rhinovirus, respiratory syncytial virus (RSV), parainfluenza, influenza
4. Genetics
   a. Propensity for otitis media tends to run in families
   b. Certain genetic syndromes with ear anomalies can predispose to AOM, including trisomy 21 and syndromes involving craniofacial abnormalities
5. Risk factors
   a. Daycare/exposure to other children
   b. Viral URI
   c. Winter months
   d. Young age: shorter and more horizontal eustachian tube
   e. Cleft palate and other craniofacial abnormalities
   f. Down syndrome
   g. Low socioeconomic status
   h. 2nd-hand smoke exposure

QUICK HIT

As children get older, their eustachian tubes develop a downward slant, allowing easier drainage of the middle ear; therefore, otitis media is much less common in school-aged children.

6. Pathophysiology
   a. Eustachian tube ventilates, protects, and clears middle ear
   b. Eustachian tube dysfunction (often due to edema from URI) allows buildup of fluid and reflux of nasopharyngeal secretions
   c. Effusion can be infected by nasopharyngeal bacteria

B. Clinical features
1. Historical
   a. Ear pain, manifested in young children by tugging or holding ear
   b. Fever: often >39°C
   c. Irritability
   d. Otorrhea (if TM perforation occurs)
2. Physical exam findings (Figure 19-1)
   a. Evidence of middle ear effusion
      i. Decreased or absent TM mobility with pneumatic exam
      ii. TM discoloration or opacification
      iii. TM bulging
      iv. Purulent otorrhea from perforated TM

FIGURE 19-1 **Acute otitis media: bulging tympanic membrane with increased vascular markings, distorted landmarks, marked erythema, and purulent fluid.**

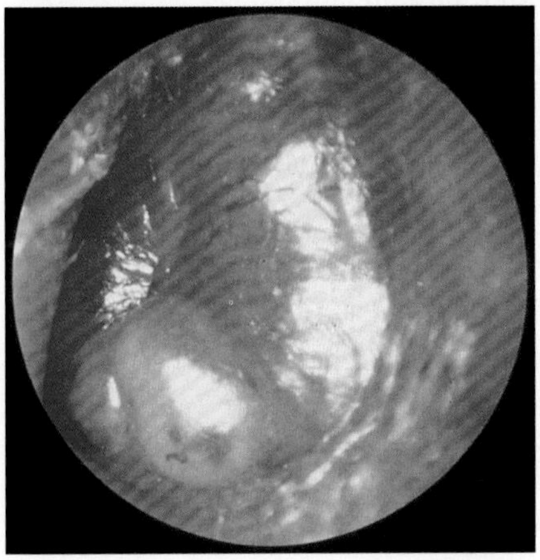

(From Moore KL, Dalley AF. *Clinically Oriented Anatomy.* 4th ed. Baltimore: Lippincott Williams & Wilkins; 1999.)

b. Evidence of inflammation
   i. Marked erythema of TM in patches or streaks
   ii. Purulent appearance to fluid
   iii. Increased vascular markings of TM
   iv. Bullous myringitis: TM with bulla

C. Diagnosis: differential diagnosis
1. OME
2. Otitis externa
3. Mastoiditis

D. Treatment
1. Therapy
   a. "Watchful waiting": in nonsevere (mild otalgia and temperature <39°C) or uncertain cases in children >6 months, appropriate to defer antibiotics for 2–3 days and monitor symptoms; many cases will spontaneously resolve (if pain and fever persist or worsen, antibiotics are initiated)
      i. Reduces antibiotic use in otitis by 40% without change in complication rate
      ii. Endorsed by American Academy of Pediatrics and American Academy of Family Physicians
      iii. Important to provide oral analgesics (acetaminophen, ibuprofen) and/or topical analgesia
   b. Antibiotic therapy
      i. Standard duration of treatment: 10 days
      ii. 1st-line therapy is high-dose amoxicillin (80–90 mg/kg/day)
      iii. Amoxicillin-clavulanate: recommended if amoxicillin fails or can be used initially in severe cases
      iv. Resistant cases: can be treated with 3 daily doses of intramuscular (IM) ceftriaxone
      v. Topical fluoroquinolone may be used if TM is perforated
      vi. Alternative regimens for children with penicillin allergy
         (a) If no history of type I reaction (urticaria, wheeze, or anaphylaxis): cefdinir, cefuroxime, or ceftriaxone
         (b) Prior type I reaction: macrolides or clindamycin
   c. Surgical management: myringotomy with tympanostomy tube insertion
      i. Considered in cases of recurrent AOM and persistent effusion
      ii. Allows topical therapy of subsequent infections and reduces duration of effusion; possibly reduces episodes of symptomatic AOM
      iii. Complications: premature tube extrusion, persistent perforation, and chronic otorrhea

QUICK HIT

The diagnosis of AOM is based on the rapid onset of symptoms and the presence of a middle ear effusion and inflammation on physical exam. Additional testing is usually unnecessary.

QUICK HIT

Most cases of AOM are caused by *S. pneumoniae*; to overcome resistance from penicillin-binding proteins, a higher dose of amoxicillin is used.

QUICK HIT

Myringotomy tube placement may improve hearing; however, long-term developmental studies have *not* shown any benefit to early tympanostomy tube placement in children with OME.

2. Treatment of AOM is aimed at limiting potential complications (see Table 19-4)
3. Duration/prognosis
   a. Most cases of AOM resolve either with or without antibiotics
   b. With antibiotics, symptoms usually improve within 72 hours
4. Prevention
   a. Breastfeeding
   b. Good handwashing and limiting contact with people with URIs
   c. Pneumococcal vaccination
   d. Avoidance of 2nd-hand smoke

QUICK HIT

TM perforation relieves the pressure of the middle ear and may actually relieve the pain.

QUICK HIT

Almost half of children still have an asymptomatic effusion 30 days after AOM diagnosis and treatment.

VI. Mastoiditis

A. Definition: suppurative infection of mastoid air cells and periosteum

B. Cause/pathophysiology
   1. AOM causes inflammation of mucoperiosteal lining of mastoid air cells, which can lead to accumulation of purulent materials and infection of periosteum
   2. Continued infection can lead to acute **mastoid osteitis** with destruction of mastoid air cells
   3. Typical bacterial pathogens are *Streptococcus pneumoniae*, group A streptococci (GAS), and *Streptococcus aureus*

QUICK HIT

Mastoiditis is almost always a complication of AOM.

C. Clinical presentation
   1. Symptoms include fever, otalgia, posterior auricular pain, redness, and swelling
   2. Physical exam findings
      a. Protrusion of auricle: pinna displaced superiorly and laterally; in infants, inferiorly and laterally (Figure 19-2)
      b. Mastoid area is swollen, red, and tender
      c. Abnormal TM
   3. Mastoiditis can lead to intra- and extracranial complications

QUICK HIT

Asymmetry of the external ears is a good way to notice subtle auricular protrusion.

D. Testing
   1. Diagnosis may be made clinically
   2. Contrast CT scan may show blurring of mastoid outline, loss of bony septa of mastoid air cells, or presence of abscess; may also demonstrate intracranial and extracranial complications

E. Therapy
   1. Antibiotics
      a. Inpatient admission to initiate IV antibiotics and monitor for complications is usually indicated; conversion to oral therapy is appropriate following clinical improvement

FIGURE 19-2 Child with mastoiditis.

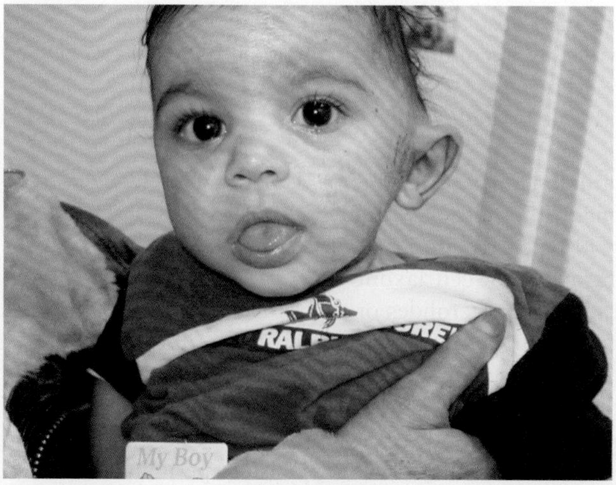

Note erythema, swelling, and protrusion of left ear. (Courtesy of Steven D. Handler, MD, MBE.)

b. Important to cover gram-positive and gram-negative organisms: 3rd-generation cephalosporins or penicillin/β-lactamase inhibitor combination with possible 2nd agent for methicillin-resistant *S. aureus* (MRSA) coverage
c. Duration of treatment: ~3 weeks
2. Surgery
a. **Myringotomy** (with or without tube placement): often performed to allow drainage of middle ear and mastoid
b. Mastoidectomy: should be performed when abscess or osteitis is present, in complicated cases, or if failure to improve with IV antibiotics

QUICK HIT

Myringotomy is therapeutic and diagnostic insofar as it allows culture of the purulent fluid in order to tailor antibiotic therapy.

VII. Pharyngitis

A. Characteristics
1. Inflammatory process of throat mucous membranes
2. Common complaint that accounts for >7 million pediatric visits each year
3. Usually due to acute infection; common pathogens listed in Table 19-5
a. Viruses: most cases
b. Group A β-hemolytic *Streptococcus* (GABHS): 20%–30% of infectious pharyngitis in children
4. Risk factors include daycare attendance and crowded living conditions
5. Pathophysiology
a. Bacterial and viral pathogens may directly invade oropharyngeal mucosa
b. Postnasal drip from viral infection can cause pharyngeal inflammation

B. Clinical features
1. History and physical vary depending on etiology (see Table 19-5)
2. Assess duration and severity of illness, associated symptoms, hydration status, and airway patency

QUICK HIT

An exanthem associated with infectious mononucleosis is seen in 5%–10% of patients. This number is increased in patients treated with amoxicillin.

TABLE 19-5 **History and Physical Exam Findings in Pharyngitis**

Organism	History	Physical
Group A β-hemolytic *Streptococcus*	Abrupt onset, fever, sore throat, headache, abdominal pain, nausea, and vomiting Lack of cough, congestion, rhinorrhea, and diarrhea	Pharyngeal erythema, tonsillar enlargement with or without exudates, palatal petechiae, and anterior cervical lymphadenopathy
Epstein-Barr virus	Malaise, fever, and sore throat	Pharyngeal erythema, tonsillar enlargement with or without exudates, prominent posterior cervical lymphadenopathy, splenomegaly
Adenovirus	Fever, rhinorrhea	+/− Exudative pharyngitis, conjunctivitis, otitis media
Coxsackie virus	Summer months, fever	Herpangina: painful, discrete, gray-white papulovesicular lesions on an erythematous base in posterior oropharynx Hand, foot, and mouth disease: painful vesicles and ulcers throughout oropharynx associated with vesicles on palms, soles, and sometimes buttocks
Herpes simplex virus	Contact with someone who has mouth sore, fever	Vesicles in anterior mouth, including lips
Influenza	Fever, myalgias	Nonexudative pharyngitis
Neisseria gonorrhoeae	Recent orogenital sexual activity	Pharyngeal erythema, cervical lymphadenopathy
Corynebacterium diphtheriae	Unimmunized child, sore throat, and low-grade fever	Gray, pseudomembrane covering the tonsils and throat, "bull neck" appearance
Rhinovirus, respiratory syncytial virus	Cough, rhinorrhea, sore throat as a secondary symptom	Congestion, may have lower respiratory tract disease

Other pathogens include group C and group G β-hemolytic streptococci, *Arcanobacterium haemolyticum, Francisella tularensis,* HIV, *Mycoplasma pneumoniae, Chlamydia pneumoniae,* and cytomegalovirus.

QUICK HIT

It is very difficult to distinguish viral pharyngitis from GAS pharyngitis clinically, so lab confirmation of GAS is encouraged to prevent overuse of antibiotics.

QUICK HIT

Rapid antigen detection testing (RADT) for GAS has a sensitivity of 70%–90% and a specificity of 95%.

QUICK HIT

If RADT is negative for GAS, a throat culture should be sent.

QUICK HIT

Patients with a history of cough, **coryza**, conjunctivitis, and diarrhea are unlikely to have GAS infection.

QUICK HIT

Of school-aged children, ~10% will be carriers of GAS. A positive streptococcal test does not distinguish a carrier of GAS from those with active infection.

QUICK HIT

A heterophile antibody may be falsely negative in the first 2 weeks of illness and in those age <4 years.

QUICK HIT

For GAS, prompt initiation of appropriate antimicrobial therapy is important to prevent **acute rheumatic fever (ARF)**.

C. Diagnosis
  1. Differentiate acute infection from other causes
    a. Noninfectious etiologies: allergic rhinitis, gastroesophageal reflux disease (GERD), malignancy, and inflammatory conditions (i.e., periodic fevers, aphthous stomatitis, pharyngitis, and adenitis [PFAPA])
    b. Consider suppurative complications such as PTA or RPA
  2. Laboratory findings
    a. GABHS
      i. Throat culture: gold standard with sensitivity of 90% and specificity of 99%
      ii. Clinical scoring systems based on findings of fever; swollen, tender anterior cervical lymph nodes; and tonsillar swelling or exudates and absence of cough: may help determine if testing is indicated
    b. Epstein-Barr virus (EBV)
      i. Heterophile antibody ("monospot") and EBV serologies are diagnostic (Table 19-6)
      ii. Supportive lab findings: atypical lymphocytosis, mild thrombocytopenia, and elevated liver enzymes
    c. Specific testing may be necessary to look for other organisms (i.e., *Neisseria gonorrhoeae* grows on Thayer-Martin medium, and *Corynebacterium diphtheriae* requires Loeffler and tellurite agars)

D. Treatment
  1. Therapy
    a. Airway management and supportive care with hydration, antipyretics, and analgesics
    b. Pharyngitis is usually self-limited process
    c. GABHS: penicillin is preferred therapy, although several alternative antimicrobial regimens are effective
    d. EBV
      i. *Avoid contact sports* until splenomegaly resolves (~4–6 weeks)
      ii. Steroids: for impending respiratory failure due to severe upper airway obstruction
    e. *N. gonorrhoeae*: IM ceftriaxone × 1; consider empiric treatment for chlamydia
  2. Complications
    a. GABHS
      i. Suppurative complications: PTA or RPA, otitis media, sinusitis, or cervical lymphadenitis
      ii. Nonsuppurative complications: acute rheumatic fever (ARF) and acute glomerulonephritis
    b. EBV
      i. Possible complications: pneumonitis, direct Coombs-positive hemolytic anemia, thrombocytopenia, icteric hepatitis, acute cerebellar ataxia, encephalitis, aseptic meningitis, myocarditis, pericarditis, and myelodysplastic syndromes
      ii. **Splenomegaly**: may lead to splenic rupture

TABLE 19-6 **Interpretation of Epstein-Barr Virus Serology**

	VCA IgM	VCA IgG	EA	EBNA
Acute infection	+	+	+	–
Recent infection	–	+/–	+/–	–
Past infection	–	+	+/–	+

EA, early antigen; EBNA, Epstein-Barr nuclear antigen; Ig, immunoglobulin; VCA, viral capsid antigen.

3. Duration/prognosis
   a. Most cases of pharyngitis resolve spontaneously within 3–4 days, but treatment of GABHS to prevent ARF requires antibiotic therapy
   b. Antibiotic treatment does not prevent glomerulonephritis
4. Prevention
   a. Patients with GABHS infection may return to school 24 hours after initiation of antibiotics

VIII. Peritonsillar Abscess

A. Definition
1. Collection of pus located between tonsillar capsule and superior pharyngeal constrictor muscle
2. Often affects preadolescents and adolescents

B. Cause/pathophysiology
1. Infectious complication of pharyngitis or tonsillitis
2. Occasionally polymicrobial
   a. GABHS
   b. *S. aureus*
   c. Oral anaerobic bacteria (*Prevotella*, *Bacteroides*, *Peptostreptococcus*)

C. Clinical presentation (Table 19-7)
1. Rapid assessment of degree of upper airway obstruction and need for emergent airway management is most critical 1st step in clinical evaluation
2. PTA is often associated with triad of trismus, uvular deviation, and "hot-potato voice" (Figure 19-3)

D. Testing
1. Diagnosis can be made clinically, without imaging
2. If warranted, CT scan with IV contrast can help distinguish cellulitis from abscess
3. Streptococcal rapid antigen detection test and/or throat culture
4. CBC may show elevated WBC count with left shift, and inflammatory markers may be increased; these findings are nonspecific and not necessary for diagnosis
5. Gram stain and culture of purulent fluid if drainage performed

E. Therapy
1. Consider hospital admission to ensure maintenance of patent airway and for surgical evaluation, IV antibiotics, and supportive care with analgesics, antipyretics, and IV hydration
2. Consultation with otolaryngology for aspiration, incision and drainage (I&D), or tonsillectomy
3. IV or oral antibiotics with clindamycin, ampicillin-sulbactam, or amoxicillin-clavulanate

QUICK HIT

N. gonorrhoeae detected in a prepubertal child is very suspicious for sexual abuse.

QUICK HIT

Poststreptococcal glomerulonephritis is not prevented by antimicrobial treatment of streptococcal pharyngitis.

QUICK HIT

Trismus is the inability to open the mouth and occurs from irritation of the internal pterygoid muscle.

TABLE 19-7 Clinical Characteristics of Peritonsillar and Retropharyngeal Abscesses

	Peritonsillar Abscess	Retropharyngeal Abscess
Age	>5 years	<5 years
Fever	Present	Present
Key historical finding	Muffled or "hot-potato" voice	Pain with neck extension
Key exam findings	Trismus, deviated uvula	Torticollis
Other noteworthy findings	Odynophagia, painful anterior cervical lymphadenopathy, drooling	Trismus, drooling, dysphagia or odynophagia, deviated uvula (occasionally), stridor (rare)

FIGURE 19-3 Physical exam findings with peritonsillar abscess.

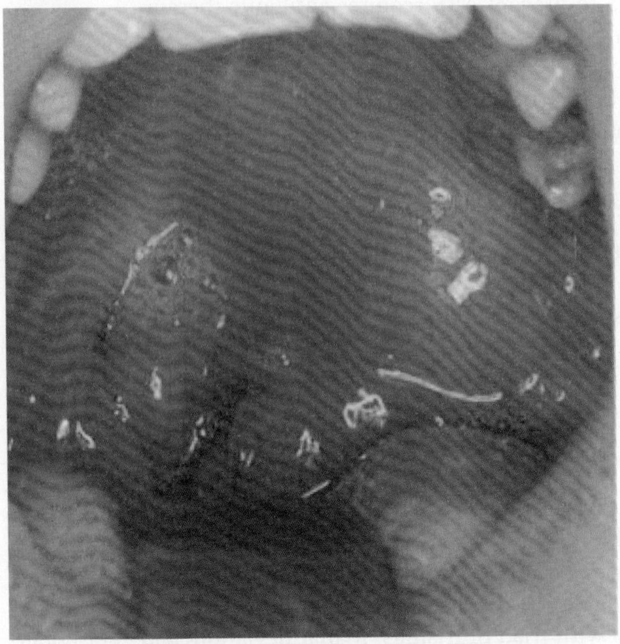

Note the erythema and swelling of the left and the uvular deviation to the right. (Courtesy of Seth Zwillenberg.)

QUICK HIT

Lymph nodes in the retropharyngeal space usually disappear by the 4th year of life; therefore, RPA in older children is uncommon.

QUICK HIT

Always assess for upper airway obstruction and the need for emergent airway management.

QUICK HIT

Although stridor is thought to be a common manifestation of RPA, a 2003 study found that it was rarely present, likely due to earlier presentation and diagnosis.

QUICK HIT

The width of the prevertebral soft tissue should be no more than the width of the vertebral body.

QUICK HIT

Many patients with RPA can be successfully treated with antibiotics alone.

IX. Retropharyngeal Abscess

A. Definition
  1. Infection of retropharyngeal lymph nodes located in space bound by posterior wall of esophagus and anterior cervical fascia
  2. Most commonly occurs in children age <5 years

B. Cause/pathophysiology
  1. Usually infectious complication of antecedent URI
  2. Less common causes: direct extension of vertebral osteomyelitis, injury from penetrating trauma to oropharynx or foreign body aspiration, or as complication of dental trauma or intubation
  3. Most infections are polymicrobial
     a. *S. aureus* and GABHS: predominant organisms
     b. Gram-negative aerobes and oral anaerobes may also be present

C. Clinical presentation (see Table 19-7)
  1. Common features include fever; ill-appearance; decreased movement of neck, particularly with extension; tender cervical lymphadenopathy; drooling
  2. Always assess for upper airway obstruction and the need for emergent airway management

D. Testing
  1. Lateral neck radiograph: may show widening of prevertebral space (Figure 19-4A,B)
  2. CT scan: most definitive imaging modality for deep neck infections
  3. Elevations in WBC count, C-reactive protein (CRP), or erythrocyte sedimentation rate (ESR) may help assess severity of illness and response to therapy
  4. Rapid antigen detection test and/or throat culture for GABHS
  5. Gram stain and cultures of purulent fluid if drainage is performed

E. Therapy
  1. Admission to hospital for airway maintenance and supportive care
  2. IV antibiotics, such as clindamycin or ampicillin-sulbactam; may transition to oral antibiotics at discharge
  3. More severe infections will require otolaryngology consultation for I&D

FIGURE 19-4 **Lateral neck x-ray in child with retropharyngeal abscess.**

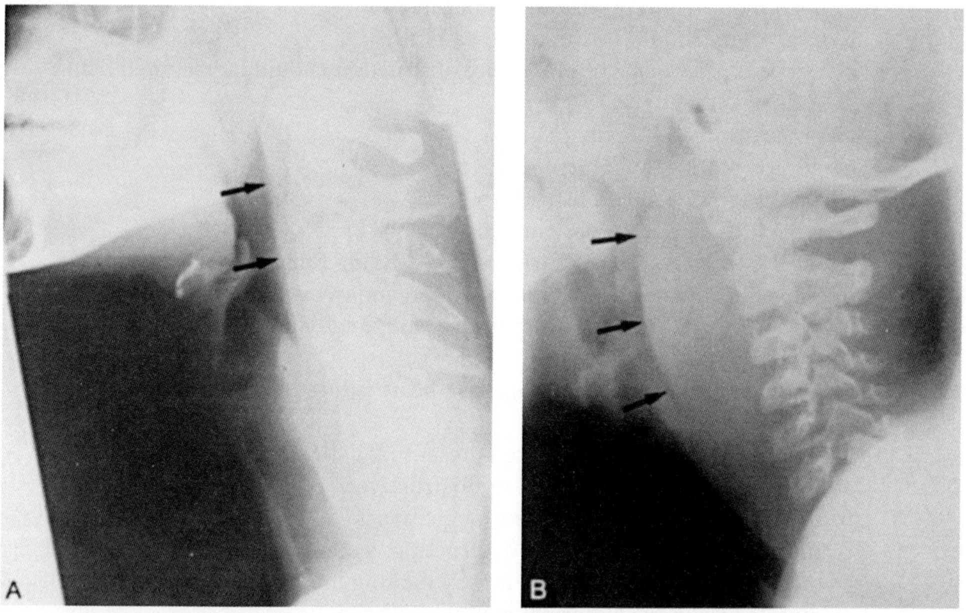

The patient in figure **(A)** has a normal lateral neck film (*arrows*), whereas the patient in figure **(B)** has a retropharyngeal abscess with marked widening of the prevertebral space. Note the lordosis and increased size of the prevertebral soft tissue compared to the adjacent vertebral bodies. (Courtesy of Dr. A. Weber, Massachusetts Eye and Ear Infirmary, Boston, MA.)

X. Tonsillar and Adenoidal Hypertrophy

A. Characteristics
  1. Tonsils and adenoids are part of the **Waldeyer ring**: ring of lymphatic tissue in nasopharynx/oropharynx
     a. Represent 1st line of immunocompetent tissue against inhaled or ingested foreign bodies
     b. Tonsils: composed primarily of B lymphocytes and involved in production of antibodies, interferon-γ, and lymphokines and in inducing secretory immunity
  2. Enlargement of lymphoid tissue occurs from swelling in response to allergens or infection (viral or bacterial)
     a. Typical viral pathogens: adenovirus, rhinovirus, influenza, coronavirus, RSV, EBV, herpes simplex virus (HSV), cytomegalovirus (CMV), and HIV
     b. Typical bacterial pathogens: GABHS, *Staphylococcus aureus, Streptococcus pneumoniae, Mycoplasma pneumoniae, Chlamydia pneumoniae*, pertussis, *Fusobacterium*, diphtheria, syphilis, and gonorrhea
  3. Tonsillar and adenoidal hypertrophy often runs in families, suggesting genetic component
  4. Pathophysiology
     a. Chronic swelling of tonsils and/or adenoids can block airway, leading to disturbances in breathing and **obstructive sleep apnea** (OSA)
     b. Children with **hypotonia**, **retrognathia**, **macroglossia**, or other underlying craniofacial abnormalities are at particular risk of OSA
     c. OSA may manifest in disturbed sleep, enuresis, daytime sleepiness, poor school performance, attention-deficit hyperactivity disorder (ADHD)
     d. Chronic oxygen deprivation may also lead to growth disturbances and failure to thrive (FTT)
     e. If untreated, may cause cardiac strain, leading to heart failure or cor pulmonale

B. Clinical features
  1. Historical findings
     a. Nighttime symptoms: sleep disturbances, snoring, gasping pauses in breath, enuresis, unusual positioning (e.g., sniff position or hyperextended neck)
     b. Daytime symptoms: persistent somnolence, poor school performance, ADHD, poor growth and FTT, hypernasal speech, dysphagia

QUICK HIT

Tonsils and adenoids grow during childhood, reaching their maximum size at ages 5–7 years, then slowly atrophying beginning in puberty.

QUICK HIT

Apnea is defined in adults as 10 seconds of pause in breathing. **Hypopneas** are episodes of shallow breathing during which airflow is decreased by at least 50%. In children, if obstruction occurs with 2 or more consecutive breaths, the event can be called an *apnea* or *hypopnea*, even if it lasts less than 10 seconds.

QUICK HIT

Children with syndromes associated with hypotonia or macroglossia, such as trisomy 21, Beckwith-Wiedemann, or congenital hypothyroidism, often develop OSA.

QUICK HIT

Obesity is an independent risk factor for developing OSA.

2. Physical examination
   a. Look for **adenoid facies**: dull facial expression, flattened nasolabial fold, open mouth, and protruding upper incisors
   b. Oral cavity should be examined carefully
   c. Size and percentage of oral cavity obstruction should be recorded using scale of 0 to 4+:
      i. 0 = tonsil in fossa
      ii. 1+ = 0%–25% obstruction
      iii. 2+ = 25%–50% obstruction
      iv. 3+ = 50%–75% obstruction
      v. 4+ = 75%–100% obstruction or "**kissing tonsils**"
   d. Signs of acute or chronic infection: red and/or swollen tonsils; white or yellow patches on tonsils; tender, stiff, and/or swollen neck; nasal congestion; or ulceration
   e. Evaluate for evidence of congestive heart failure or cor pulmonale

QUICK HIT

Tonsil size may be misinterpreted if the patient gags during the exam. A simple exam without a tongue depressor may be sufficient for most patients.

C. Diagnosis
1. Differential diagnosis for children presenting with sleep apnea
   a. Apnea may be either **central** or **obstructive**
   b. Consider seizure or other neurologic issues
   c. Alternative causes of airway obstruction: anatomic narrowing, abnormal mechanical linkage between airway dilating muscles and airway walls, muscle weakness, abnormal neural regulation
2. Laboratory findings: may reveal hypercapnia secondary to hypoventilation and chronic retention of carbon dioxide
3. Radiology findings: lateral neck x-ray will show soft tissue enlargement and determine narrowing of oropharynx and nasopharynx
4. Other findings
   a. **Flexible laryngoscopy** can assess adenoid hypertrophy and amount of airway narrowing due to tonsillar hypertrophy
      i. Sleep study: indicated when diagnosis is in doubt, when history is unclear, and for objective evaluation prior to surgery
      ii. Particularly useful for craniofacial patients, hypotonic patients, and others in which central apnea or unusual anatomy may play significant role
      iii. Determines severity of apnea using the **apnea-hypopnea index (AHI)**, which ranges from normal (<1) to severely increased (20+)
   b. Electrocardiogram (ECG), echocardiogram (echo), and chest x-ray (CXR): necessary for those with suspected heart failure or other associated cardiovascular abnormalities

QUICK HIT

A formal sleep study (**polysomnography**) is the gold standard for determining if there is true OSA versus central apnea.

D. Treatment
1. Therapy
   a. Surgical: **adenotonsillectomy (T&A)**
   b. Medical therapy: several alternative approaches may be used, especially if surgery cannot be performed (due to risk of complications or familial preference) or if symptoms of OSA persist following T&A
      i. **Intranasal steroids** and/or leukotriene receptor antagonists may modestly improve OSA symptoms; no documented benefit to systemic corticosteroids
      ii. Noninvasive mechanical ventilation with **continuous positive airway pressure (CPAP)** delivers pressure via nasal mask to help overcome upper airway obstruction during sleep; can be very effective, but success is often limited by poor adherence
2. Complications of T&A
   a. Pain
   b. Dehydration from poor oral intake related to pain
   c. Postoperative swelling is common and typically lasts 2–4 weeks; although rare, severe edema may cause obstruction of airway
   d. Changes in speech or velopharyngeal insufficiency: usually temporary and resolve in 99.5% of patients
   e. Postoperative hemorrhage: 0.5%–3%
   f. No significant immunologic consequences have ever been documented

QUICK HIT

T&A is the standard-of-care treatment for those with hypertrophic adenoids and tonsils with symptoms of OSA.

QUICK HIT

T&A is often recommended for children with multiple oropharyngeal infections; however, this remains controversial.

3. Prognosis following T&A
   a. OSA symptoms resolve in most children
   b. ~1/4 children will continue to have abnormalities on sleep study
   c. Factors associated with persistent symptoms include
      i. Obesity
      ii. Severe OSA on preoperative polysomnography
      iii. Hypotonia or underlying craniofacial abnormalities
      iv. Age >7 years
4. Prevention
   a. Maintenance of healthy weight
   b. Immunizations and good handwashing to limit infection

QUICK HIT

Due to the frequency of persistent symptoms, adenoidectomy without tonsillectomy is not recommended for patients with OSA.

XI. Nasal Polyps

A. Definitions
   1. Polyps are inflamed tissue, mobile, and nontender
   2. Large polyps can block nasal passage and lead to local infection, breathing issues, or discomfort
B. Cause/pathophysiology: many medical conditions are associated with nasal polyps
   1. Aspirin sensitivity (wheezing)
   2. Asthma
   3. CF
   4. Kartagener syndrome (primary ciliary dyskinesia)
   5. Churg-Strauss syndrome
C. Clinical presentation
   1. Symptoms: nasal obstruction, **anosmia** (loss of sense of smell), sinusitis, mouth breathing, and rhinitis
   2. Physical exam: reveals clear/grayish, boggy, grape-like mass in nasal cavity that is more pale than typical nasal mucosa
D. Testing: CT scan of sinuses will show opacification of sinuses where polypoid tissue is located and may be helpful in planning and performing FESS
E. Therapy
   1. Medications: may help relieve symptoms but rarely reduce nasal polyp size significantly
      a. Nasal steroid sprays
      b. Oral steroids can be used as short course to decrease inflammation
      c. Antibiotics helpful in cases of active infection
   2. Endoscopic sinus surgery: effective in removing nasal polyps
   3. Many patients have underlying allergic symptoms, so allergy evaluation and aggressive treatment can help decrease nasal polypoid load

QUICK HIT

Nasal polyps are abnormal growths of the mucous membranes of the nasal mucosa and/or paranasal sinuses.

QUICK HIT

CF should be considered in all children presenting with nasal polyps.

QUICK HIT

The **Samter triad** is the combination of nasal polyps, aspirin sensitivity, and asthma due to an anomaly in the arachidonic acid cascade.

QUICK HIT

Nasal polyps frequently recur, so a combination of surgical intervention and medication is typically needed for the best control of polyps.

XII. Dental Trauma

A. Definition: injury to primary or secondary tooth occurring in ~50% of children; trauma may cause
   1. Fractures: involving crown or root of tooth
   2. **Luxation injuries**: affect supporting structures (e.g., periodontal ligament)
B. Cause/pathophysiology: injury usually results from falls in younger children and sports injuries in older children and adolescents
C. Clinical presentation
   1. Symptoms vary with type of injury: tenderness, displacement, mobility, and bleeding (Table 19-8)
   2. Complications: injury to developing secondary tooth (for primary tooth trauma), abscess, and pulp necrosis
D. Testing: most injuries warrant referral to dentist and dental radiographs to assess severity of damage and potential effects on permanent teeth and to follow improvement
E. Therapy: varies for primary and secondary teeth and type of injury (see Table 19-8); extraction or root canal should be considered for all injuries resulting in **pulp necrosis**

QUICK HIT

*Avulsion of a permanent tooth is a dental emergency—*immediately reimplant the tooth! If reimplantation must be delayed, store the tooth in milk, Save-a-Tooth solution, or saliva.

QUICK HIT

Never sterilize an avulsed tooth or store in water!

QUICK HIT

Studies have shown that mouth guards are very effective in preventing dental injuries in child athletes and should be used for all contact sports.

TABLE 19-8 Common Dental Injury Types and Treatments

Injury Type	Description	Treatment
Intrusion	Displacement of tooth into alveolar bone	P: Most will spontaneously re-erupt S: Surgical or orthodontic repositioning
Subluxation	Injury to support structures causing looseness without displacement	Observation and follow-up radiographs
Luxation	Anterior, posterior, or lateral displacement of tooth	Spontaneous, surgical or orthodontic repositioning; primary teeth may be extracted if bite affected
Avulsion	Tooth is completely removed from its socket	P: **Do NOT replace tooth** S: **Reimplant immediately**
Uncomplicated fracture	Injury of crown involving enamel +/− dentin	P: Smooth edges, find fragment! S: Restoration
Complicated fracture	Crown injury with involvement of pulp	Preserve pulp with capping if possible P: Consider extraction S: Consider root canal

P, primary tooth; S, secondary tooth.

XIII. Dental Abscess

A. Definition: bacterial infection causing accumulation of pus within tooth and/or surrounding structures
B. Cause/pathophysiology
  1. Infection is usually polymicrobial
    a. Combination of aerobic and anaerobic oral flora
    b. Common organisms: *Fusobacterium*, *Bacteroides*, *Prevotella*, *Peptostreptococcus*, and *Streptococcus* species
  2. **Periapical abscess**: most common dental abscess in children
    a. Enamel defects allow bacteria to enter pulp, which leads to inflammation and necrosis, resulting in extension of infection into periapical space
    b. Usually results from **dental caries**; can also occur after trauma or dental procedures
C. Clinical presentation
  1. Pain
  2. Facial or gingival swelling
  3. Thermal sensitivity
  4. Fever
  5. Poor oral intake
  6. Tenderness to pressure or percussion
  7. Tooth mobility
  8. Gingival warmth and erythema
D. Testing
  1. Gram stain in addition to aerobic and anaerobic culture of aspirated fluid
  2. Panoramic radiography can confirm presence of abscess
  3. Severe presentations: may require CBC, blood culture, and additional imaging
    a. Lateral neck x-ray: to look for airway narrowing from abscess extension into deep neck spaces
    b. CT scan: to better delineate extent and origin of abscess
E. Treatment
  1. Secure airway, ensure adequate hydration, and optimize pain control
  2. I&D by dentist or oromaxillofacial surgeon
  3. Antibiotic therapy
    a. Indicated when I&D is not possible or the patient is immunocompromised or has evidence of systemic involvement

QUICK HIT

Potential complications of a dental abscess are sinusitis, orofacial space infections, RPA, osteomyelitis, sinus cavernous thrombosis, bacteremia, and endocarditis.

FIGURE 19-5 **Near complete congenital glottic web.**

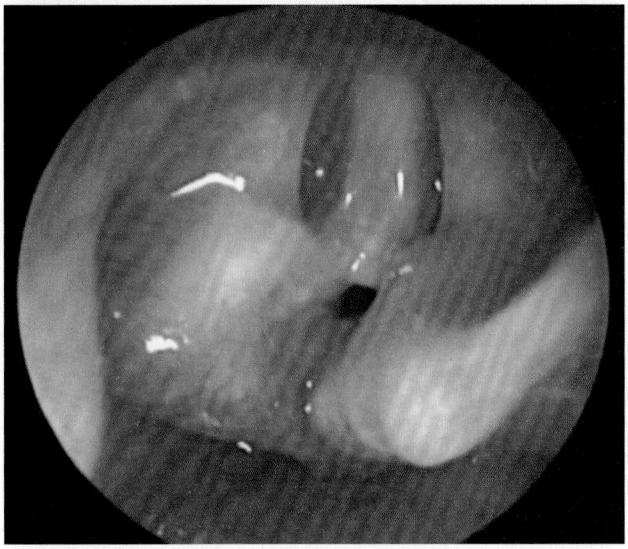

(Courtesy of Scott Rickert, MD, New York University Langone Medical Center.)

b. Preferred therapy: ampicillin-sulbactam/amoxicillin-clavulanate
c. Alternate regimens: clindamycin, cefoxitin, penicillin + metronidazole, and others

XIV. Vocal Cord Disorders

A. Characteristics
1. Voice disorders are referred to as **dysphonia** (a.k.a., hoarseness)
   a. Wide spectrum of normal voices, which may vary due to age, gender, pubertal development
   b. Different adults (parents, pediatrician, speech-language pathologist) may perceive child's voice differently and may not be in agreement with whether child is dysphonic or not
2. Prevalence of dysphonia: 6%–9% of children
3. Causes: may be congenital or acquired (Figures 19-5 and 19-6)
   a. Congenital: glottis web, vocal fold paralysis, glottic/subglottic stenosis
   b. Acquired: trauma, previous endotracheal intubation, vocal overuse

QUICK HIT

Risk factors for vocal cord pathology include prior intubation, cardiac surgery including patent ductus arteriosus repair (which could injure the recurrent laryngeal nerve), overuse (singing), and tobacco use.

FIGURE 19-6 **Bilateral vocal fold paresis seen with rigid stroboscopy.**

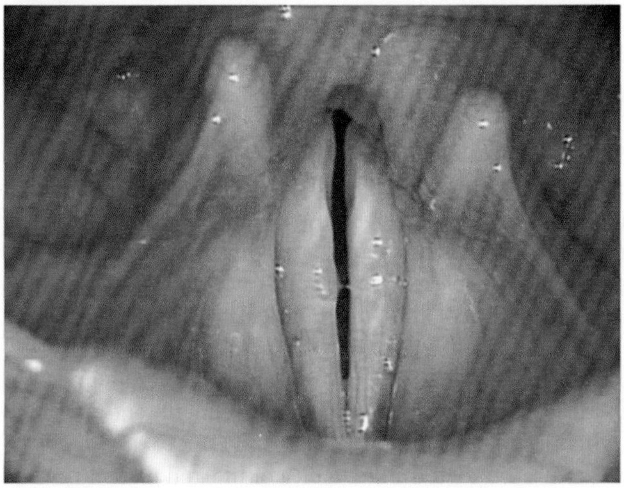

(Scott Rickert, MD, New York University Langone Medical Center.)

TABLE 19-9 **Characteristics, Pathophysiology, Evaluation, and Treatment of Common Vocal Cord Disorders**

Disorder	Key Features	Treatment
Vocal fold lesions		
Nodules	**Most common cause of childhood dysphonia** Mass of lesion causes poor contact between vocal folds and leads to dysphonia Presents with intermittent dysphonia	Voice therapy Behavioral therapy Surgery rarely indicated
Cysts	Can be mucus-filled or epidermis-filled Typically unilateral with counter-coup lesion on other vocal fold	Rarely improve with vocal therapy; often require surgical excision
Polyps	Degeneration of superficial lamina propria May occur after submucosal bleed confined to vocal fold	Rarely improve with vocal therapy; often require surgical excision
Juvenile recurrent respiratory papillomatosis (RRP)	**Most common airway neoplasm** More aggressive than adult version of RRP Associated with **HPV-6, HPV-11** Prevented with quadrivalent HPV vaccine May present with dysphonia, stridor, or respiratory distress	Removal of lesions with microlaryngoscopy Lesions frequently recur Adjuvant therapies: antiviral injections (cidofovir); systemic medications (e.g., acyclovir, interferon-α)
Laryngeal webs (see Figure 19-5)	Tethering of part of vocal folds together May be congenital or acquired Associated with genetic **deletion of 22q**	Endoscopic cold sharp dissection of web
Gastroesophageal reflux	May cause significant dysphonia Exam shows redness and swelling near posterior vocal folds, arytenoids Testing may include upper gastrointestinal series, milk scan, pH probe, impedance monitoring, or endoscopy	H_2-receptor antagonists Proton pump inhibitors Nissen fundoplication in severe cases
Vocal fold paralysis/paresis	May be due to birth trauma, cardiovascular, iatrogenic, neurogenic, infectious, or idiopathic causes Often related to **injury of recurrent laryngeal nerve** and/or superior laryngeal nerve	Mild cases may be observed Medialization to bring paralyzed vocal fold to midline position Tracheostomy may be needed for bilateral paralysis
Paradoxical vocal fold motion (vocal cord dysfunction)	**Episodic, inappropriate adduction of the vocal folds during respiration** causing obstruction of vocal folds May manifest in stress or exercise	Respiratory retraining, behavioral therapy

HPV, human papillomavirus.

4. Pathophysiology (Table 19-9): dysphonia can result from defects anywhere along vocal tract
   a. Vocal folds or glottis (main vibratory surface for voice) composed of 3 layers
      i. Vocal cover (mucosa)
      ii. Lamina propria, which is subdivided into the superficial lamina propria (SLP), a jelly-like substance that allows vocal cords to vibrate; and deep lamina propria (more collagen than SLP).
      iii. Vocal ligament (muscle layer below lamina propria)
   b. Vocal tract also includes nasal cavity (resonance), oral cavity/tongue (resonance, articulation), or pharynx (resonance), lungs/lung musculature (air support)

B. Clinical features
1. History: focuses on onset and progression of symptoms, voice variability, development, typical voice activities, psychosocial environment, and presence of other factors (e.g., allergies, medications, asthma, and GERD)
2. Several questionnaires are used to determine quality of life and disability from dysphonia

C. Diagnosis
   1. Requires evaluation by a multidisciplinary team
   2. Speech-language pathology assessment
      a. Subjective and objective assessment of voice
      b. Speech assessed on **GRBAS** (**g**rade, **r**oughness, **b**reathiness, **a**sthenia, **s**train) **scale**
      c. Aerodynamic measurements of airflow
      d. Other factors: breath support, muscle tone, alertness, social interaction
   3. Otolaryngology assessment with speech-language pathologist
      a. Thorough history and physical
      b. **Videostroboscopy**: to evaluate vocal fold pathology and motion

D. Treatment: combination of voice therapy, medical interventions, and surgery is often needed (see Table 19-9 for specific recommendations)
   1. Voice therapy: develop techniques to
      a. Augment vocal hygiene and abuse reduction
      b. Increase/decrease glottal closure
      c. Decrease muscular tension
      d. Improve coordination of respiration and phonation
      e. Raise/lower pitch
      f. Increase/decrease loudness
      g. Lower laryngeal placement
   2. Medical therapy: aimed at treatment of underlying conditions such as allergic rhinitis, asthma, GERD
   3. Surgical therapy: interventions include conservative excision of benign lesions, "cold" techniques, microlaryngeal instruments, and medialization laryngoplasty

XV. Cleft Lip/Palate (CLP)

A. Characteristics
   1. Definitions
      a. **Cleft lip with or without cleft palate (CLP)**: malformation of upper lip that may include a discontinuity of vermilion, skin, muscle, mucosa, gingiva, and bone (Figure 19-7)
         i. **Unilateral** or **bilateral**
         ii. **Complete** (entire vertical thickness of upper lip into nasal cavity) or **incomplete** (partial involvement of vertical height of lip)

FIGURE 19-7 Ventral view of the palate, gum, lip, and nose.

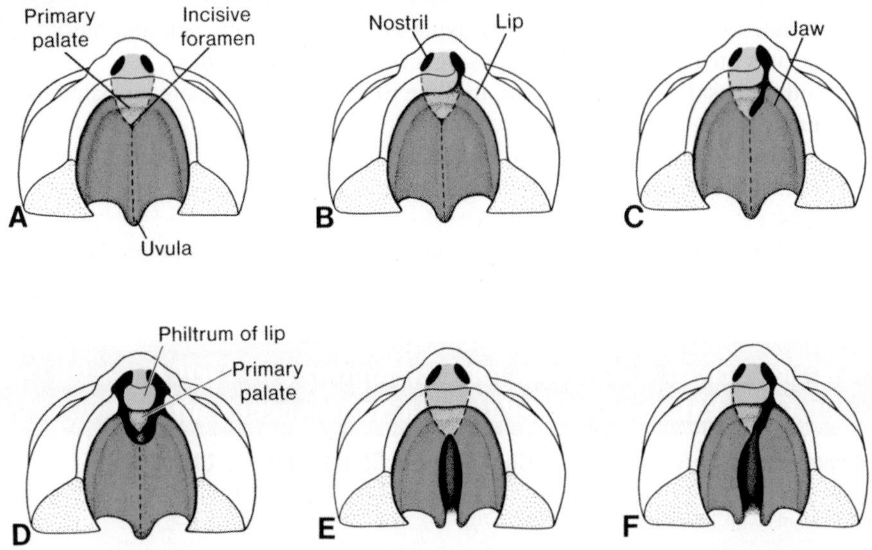

A. Normal. **B.** Unilateral cleft lip extending into the nose. **C.** Unilateral cleft involving the lip and jaw and extending to the incisive foramen. **D.** Bilateral cleft involving the lip and jaw. **E.** Isolated cleft palate. **F.** Cleft palate combined with unilateral anterior cleft lip. (From Sadler T. *Langman's Medical Embryology*. 9th ed. Baltimore: Lippincott Williams & Wilkins; 2003.)

b. **Cleft palate (CP)**: separation between 2 halves of roof of mouth, involving mucosa, muscle, and bones of hard palate (see Figure 19-7)
   i. **Unilateral** or **bilateral**
   ii. Extent can be classified as **complete** or **incomplete**
   iii. Can also be classified according to position relative to incisive foramen
      (a) Clefts of primary palate: anterior to incisive foramen
      (b) Clefts of secondary palate: posterior to incisive foramen

2. Epidemiology
   a. CLP occurs in ~1/750 Caucasian newborns
      i. Bilateral cleft lip is more often associated with CP than unilateral cleft lip
      ii. Racial predilection: Asian and Native American > Caucasian > African American
      iii. Males > females
      iv. Left side > right side
   b. Isolated CP occurs in ~1/2,500 Caucasian newborns
      i. Females > males
      ii. Does not differ among racial groups
3. Cause is multifactorial
   a. CLP has a genetic component: 1/3 of patients with CLP or CP have a positive family history (Table 19-10)
   b. Environmental: teratogens, including phenytoins, retinoids, maternal smoking, and alcohol
   c. Syndromic clefts
      i. CP is more commonly associated with syndrome than CLP
      ii. Notable associated syndromes are **microdeletions of 22q11**, Stickler, Van der Woude, and Smith-Lemli-Opitz syndromes
4. Pathophysiology
   a. Cleft lip results from failure of medial nasal and maxillary processes to fuse
   b. CP results from failure of palatine shelves to fuse

B. Clinical features
   1. Historical findings
      a. Note any possible prenatal teratogen exposure
      b. Family history: family members with CLP, isolated CP, or genetic syndrome
      c. Patient's history: feeding difficulties, weight gain, snoring, apnea, speech delays, and ear infections
   2. Physical exam findings
      a. Cleft lip: can vary from small notch in vermilion border to complete separation involving skin, muscle, mucosa, tooth, and bone
      b. Isolated CP: might involve only uvula or can extend into soft and hard palates on 1 or both sides, exposing 1 or both nasal cavities
      c. **Submucosal cleft**: bifid uvula, midline thinning of soft palate, or palpable notch at posterior of palate
      d. Associated anomalies: careful investigation for neurologic, cardiac, renal, skeletal (clubfoot), and other organ system abnormalities

C. Diagnosis
   1. Antepartum diagnosis of CLP may occur with prenatal ultrasonography, although sensitivity is poor (especially for CP)

QUICK HIT

CLP deformities are the most common congenital defects of the head.

QUICK HIT

Most clefts are *not* associated with syndromes.

QUICK HIT

The combination of micrognathia, glossoptosis, and CP is called the **Pierre-Robin sequence**.

TABLE 19-10 **Recurrent Risk Rates for Development of Cleft Lip with Cleft Palate or Cleft Palate in Subsequent Children**

Affected Family Members	Cleft Lip with Cleft Palate	Cleft Palate
2 unaffected parents with 1 affected child	3%–7%	2%–5%
1 parent affected	2%–4%	3%–7%
1 parent and sibling affected	11%–14%	15%–20%

2. Lip and palatal clefts are often initially identified on 1st physical exam
3. Exclude other anomalies that may suggest cleft is component of syndrome or chromosomal abnormality

D. Treatment
1. Therapy
   a. Goals of repair: aesthetic and functional restoration (e.g., lip closure, nasal airway, normal speech, eustachian tube function, useful dental occlusion)
   b. Multidisciplinary team: pediatrician, plastic surgeon, otolaryngologist, oral maxillofacial surgeon, geneticist, audiologist, speech-language therapist, dentist, psychologist, and social worker
   c. Airway management is crucial; severe cases may require prone positioning, nasopharyngeal airway, or tracheostomy
   d. Early feeding management: breastfeeding support, use of adaptable nipples and squeezable bottle, or supplementation with nasogastric tube feedings
   e. Surgical management
      i. Closure of cleft lip usually occurs by age 2–3 months
      ii. Closure of CP is usually done by age 1 year to help normal speech development and optimize maxillofacial growth
      iii. Alveolar bone graft is usually placed at age 7–10 years for dental eruption of canine teeth on affected side
      iv. Revision of lip and repair of nasal deformities occur in adolescence
2. Complications
   a. Airway obstruction
   b. Feeding difficulties due to inability to create negative intraoral pressure
   c. Recurrent otitis media and hearing loss
   d. Speech deficits: delayed onset, articulation disorders, velopharyngeal incompetence, or insufficiency requiring speech therapy
   e. Hypernasal speech
   f. Dental complications: malocclusion; malformed, missing, or supernumerary teeth
   g. Behavior and psychosocial problems

QUICK HIT

An adenoidectomy is contraindicated because of the adverse effect on palatal function.

20 Oncologic Diseases

SYMPTOM SPECIFIC

I. Symptoms Typical of Childhood Cancers

A. Historical findings
   1. Hematologic malignancies and certain solid tumors will often present with history of fever; therefore, differentiation from other causes of fever is important
   2. History of drenching night sweats, which are most commonly associated with Hodgkin disease or leukemia
   3. Headaches due to central nervous system (CNS)–occupying lesions typically occur in morning and may be associated with emesis
   4. History of bleeding or symptoms of anemia, which develop from cytopenias due to bone marrow infiltration/suppression
   5. Bone pain can be seen in leukemia, bone tumors, and tumors that have metastasized to bone marrow
   6. Fatigue and weight loss
   7. Family history of malignancy should be elucidated to rule out certain inherited cancer predisposition syndromes

B. Physical examination findings
   1. Fever
   2. Lymphadenopathy
      a. Lymph nodes may be enlarged secondary to infection or infiltration
      b. Lymph nodes associated with infection are usually erythematous, warm, tender, and fluctuant and should improve with appropriate antibiotics
      c. Malignant lymph nodes are firm, rubbery, nontender, and confluent
      d. Size of node or nodes in question is important; lymph nodes are considered enlarged or pathologic if they are
         i. >0.5 cm in epitrochlear region
         ii. >1 cm in cervical and axillary region
         iii. >1.5 cm in inguinal region
         iv. A left-sided supraclavicular node of any size is abnormal and should be biopsied
   3. Abdominal mass: site of lesion and age of the patient are important (Table 20-1)

QUICK HIT

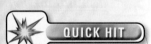

Infection is far more common in pediatrics than malignancy. A new diagnosis of pediatric cancer is not common for a practicing general pediatrician.

QUICK HIT

Growing pains can also wake a child from sleep but are usually exclusively nocturnal.

QUICK HIT

A left-sided supraclavicular lymph node (**Virchow sign**) suggests intra-abdominal malignancy.

QUICK HIT

All abdominal masses warrant evaluation, although they are usually benign in the pediatric population.

TABLE 20-1 Etiology of Abdominal Malignancies by Age

Infants	Neuroblastoma, hepatoblastoma, or teratoma
1–5 years old	Wilms tumor or neuroblastoma
>5 years old	Germ cell tumors, Hodgkin disease, or non-Hodgkin lymphoma

4. Respiratory distress can be sign of anterior mediastinal mass, which is typically associated with T-cell leukemia, Hodgkin lymphoma, or non-Hodgkin lymphoma (NHL)

C. Laboratory testing and radiologic imaging
1. Complete blood count (CBC) with differential to look for cytopenias and evaluation of peripheral blood smear for presence of blasts
2. Hypocalcemia, hyperkalemia, elevated creatinine, hyperphosphatemia, and elevated uric acid are associated with **tumor lysis syndrome (TLS)**, which is marker of rapid cell turnover in malignancies; elevated lactate dehydrogenase (LDH) is nonspecific but also suggestive of TLS
3. Tumor markers
   a. Urinary catecholamines are often elevated with neuroblastoma
   b. Serum β-human chorionic gonadotropin (β-hCG) and α-fetoprotein (AFP) should be sent in any patient with suspected germ cell tumor
   c. Serum AFP is often elevated in patients with hepatoblastoma
4. Cerebrospinal fluid (CSF) sampling for cytology (leukemia, CSF metastases)
5. Radiologic imaging
   a. Bone tumors can often be seen on plain film
   b. Magnetic resonance imaging (MRI) to evaluate brain tumors
   c. Computed tomography (CT) scan, MRI, or ultrasound of lesion is essential for solid tumors, but choice of imaging determined by type of malignancy and anatomic location
   d. Bone metastases may be seen on bone scan

QUICK HIT

If more than one hematopoietic cell line is low, it may be a sign of malignancy, bone marrow infiltration, or bone metastases.

QUICK HIT

Imaging may be indicated prior to sampling in patients with suspected brain mass, because sudden caudal depressurization of spinal fluid in patients with obstructed CSF drainage can lead to brain herniation.

Oncologic Diseases

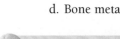

DISEASE SPECIFIC

II. Leukemia

A. Characteristics
1. Malignant transformation and proliferation of hematopoietic cells
   a. Clonal expansion of immature precursors (acute leukemias) or mature bone marrow elements (chronic leukemias)
   b. Symptoms occur from lack of normal bone marrow cell production and accumulation of malignant cells
2. Epidemiology
   a. Most common pediatric malignancy, accounting for 30% of all newly diagnosed children with cancer
   b. Slightly more common in boys than girls
3. 4 main types of leukemia occur in pediatrics
   a. **Acute lymphoblastic leukemia (ALL)**
      i. Clonal proliferation of B- and T-lymphocyte precursors
      ii. Peak age: 2–5 years
      iii. Boys > girls and more common in Caucasian children
   b. **Acute myelogenous leukemia (AML)**
      i. Clonal proliferation of myeloid precursors with many subtypes based on morphology and cytogenetic translocations
      ii. Bimodal incidence in childhood with peaks in children age <2 years and adolescents
      iii. Boys = girls
      iv. More clearly associated with toxic exposures than ALL
   c. **Chronic myelogenous leukemia (CML)**
      i. Myeloproliferative neoplasm with uncontrolled growth of myeloid cells, with relatively normal differentiation and function
      ii. Incidence increases throughout childhood and adolescence
      iii. Associated with specific fusion protein: BCR-ABL, which is constitutively active tyrosine kinase and develops from translocation between chromosomes 9 and 22
   d. **Juvenile myelomonocytic leukemia (JMML)**
      i. Very rare chronic leukemia in young children
      ii. Most cases diagnosed before age 3 years

QUICK HIT

Patients with Down syndrome have a 50-fold increase in risk for AML.

4. Cause: unknown, although it is associated with several genetic syndromes including Down syndrome, neurofibromatosis, Li-Fraumeni syndrome, and Fanconi anemia

B. Clinical features
1. Historical findings
a. AML and ALL: abrupt onset of symptoms including fatigue, lethargy, bleeding, and infection all related to cytopenias brought on by replacement of marrow precursors by leukemic cell infiltration
b. History of bone pain and refusal to bear weight secondary to marrow infiltration
c. Respiratory symptoms if mediastinal mass of leukemia cells is present (more common in T-cell ALL)
d. CML patients can be asymptomatic at diagnosis in rare cases
2. Physical exam findings
a. Fever, pallor, tachycardia, and bruising and petechiae due to cytopenias
b. Lymphadenopathy, hepatosplenomegaly, or testicular enlargement secondary to malignant cell accumulation
c. Facial swelling, wheezing, and tachypnea if mediastinal mass is present
d. Central nervous system (CNS) involvement (more common in ALL)

> **QUICK HIT**
> Leukemia should be considered in any child presenting with extremity pain out of proportion to the exam, especially when associated with fevers, fatigue, or weight loss.

C. Diagnosis
1. Laboratory findings
a. CBC with differential can show anemia, thrombocytopenia, and leukopenia, leukocytosis, or neutropenia
i. Abnormal immature lymphocytes or myelocytes ("**blasts**") are usually seen in acute leukemias
ii. CML: marked hyperleukocytosis on CBC with wide range of normal-appearing myeloid precursors, eosinophilia, and basophilia; these patients often only exhibit mild anemia and thrombocytopenia
b. Chemistry panel to evaluate for signs of TLS
c. Polymerase chain reaction testing for quantification of BCR-ABL: useful for monitoring response to therapy in patients with CML
2. Radiology findings
a. Chest radiograph: can show mediastinal mass
b. Other imaging is usually unnecessary
3. Other findings
a. Bone marrow aspiration and biopsy to confirm diagnosis are essential
i. Morphologic assessment of bone marrow can often diagnose subtype of leukemia present
ii. Flow cytometry and immunohistochemistry will identify cell surface proteins that confirm type of leukemia
iii. Cytogenetics and fluorescence in situ hybridization (FISH) studies for characteristic chromosomal abnormalities should be done to assess overall patient risk and stratify treatment
b. Lumbar puncture (LP) to evaluate CNS involvement in acute leukemias

> **QUICK HIT**
> "Blasts" are *never* a normal finding on a CBC and should always be investigated, even in an asymptomatic child.

> **QUICK HIT**
> In TLS, rapid death of cells leads to a variety of life-threatening alterations in blood chemistry, including hyperkalemia, hypocalcemia, and hyperphosphatemia.

D. Treatment
1. Therapy
a. ALL
i. Multiagent chemotherapy: given in complex administration schedule that lasts 2–3.5 years
ii. Incorporated into therapy: prophylaxis with intrathecal chemotherapy and/or radiation to sanctuary sites (CNS and testicles)
iii. Risk stratification: allows therapeutic intensity and risk of side effects to be targeted to children at more risk of treatment failure
(a) Children age >10 years and <1 year are high risk
(b) Presenting WBC count >50,000/μL considered high risk
(c) T-cell phenotype associated with higher risk
(d) Cytogenetic changes in leukemia cells
(e) Response to therapy

b. AML
  i. Multiagent intensive chemotherapy lasting 6–9 months
  ii. Hematopoietic stem cell transplant: indicated in certain subtypes of AML following initial chemotherapy
  iii. Risk factor stratification based on age at diagnosis and if patient has trisomy 21, presenting WBC count, and response to therapy
c. CML
  i. Current standard of care: single-agent therapy with tyrosine kinase inhibitors specific for BCR-ABL (e.g., imatinib)
  ii. Hematopoietic stem cell transplant is considered for poor response to tyrosine kinase inhibition
d. JMML: hematopoietic stem cell transplant is only known curative therapy

2. Prognosis
  a. ALL: excellent; overall survival ~80% (~95% in low-risk patients)
  b. AML: more guarded; overall survival ~50%; dependent on subtype
  c. CML: lifelong disorder requiring lifelong tyrosine kinase inhibitor therapy
  d. JMML: overall survival ~40% with hematopoietic stem cell transplant

III. Hodgkin Lymphoma

A. Definitions
1. B-cell neoplasm originating in germinal centers of lymph nodes
  a. Malignant cell is known as **Reed-Sternberg cell**: binucleated or multinucleated giant cell (Figure 20-1)
  b. Reed-Sternberg cell is embedded in matrix of reactive cells including lymphocytes, macrophages, eosinophils, and granulocytes
2. 3 peak time periods affected
  a. Childhood: age <10 years
  b. Adolescence/young adult: age 10–35 years
  c. Older adulthood: age >55 years

B. Cause: not known, although Epstein-Barr virus (EBV) is associated

C. Clinical presentation
1. Patients commonly present with lymphadenopathy and cough
  a. Unexplained fever, drenching night sweats, and weight loss
  b. Other symptoms: pruritus, lymph node pain with alcohol ingestion, anemia, and (rarely) nephritic syndrome
2. Lymphadenopathy: any lymph node region can be involved and/or spleen
3. Bulky mediastinal adenopathy is common, particularly with nodular sclerosing type

QUICK HIT

Patients with TLS are treated for electrolyte abnormalities and receive allopurinol, large volumes of fluid, and urine alkalinization.

QUICK HIT

The most common physical finding in Hodgkin lymphoma is painless lymphadenopathy, most commonly of the neck or supraclavicular region.

QUICK HIT

In <3% of Hodgkin lymphoma patients, involved lymph nodes are painful after alcohol consumption. Although rare, this sign is considered pathognomonic for the disease and should prompt a diagnostic evaluation.

FIGURE 20-1 **Classic Reed-Sternberg cell. Mirror-image nuclei contain large eosinophilic nucleoli.**

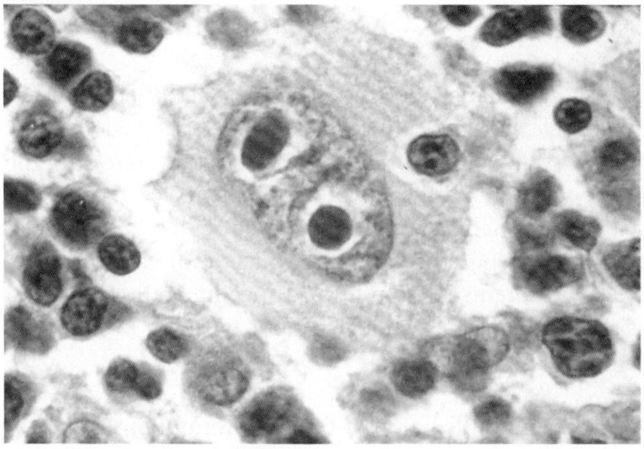

(From Rubin R, Strayer DS. *Rubin's Pathology: Clinicopathologic Foundations of Medicine.* 5th ed. Philadelphia: Lippincott Williams & Wilkins; 2008.)

D. Testing
1. Markers of inflammation commonly elevated
2. Follow erythrocyte sedimentation rate (ESR) during therapy to assess response
3. CT and positron emission tomography (PET) scans: to stage disease
4. Bone scans: performed with clinical suspicion of bone involvement (e.g., pain or high LDH) or when stage escalation would change therapy
5. Bone marrow biopsy: evaluate for marrow involvement

E. Therapy
1. Children, adolescents, and young adults should be treated using pediatric treatment regimens
2. Treatment includes combination of chemotherapy and radiation based on stage
3. Prognosis: excellent
a. 5-year, event-free survival = 85%–90%
b. Overall survival = ~95%

IV. Non-Hodgkin Lymphoma

A. Diverse collection of malignances arising from lymphoid cells and organs

B. Etiology of most childhood NHL is unknown
1. Viral infection may contribute to pathogenesis of certain NHL
a. EBV associated with endemic Burkitt lymphoma in equatorial Africa
b. HIV associated with NHL
2. NHL is associated with immunodeficiency

C. Clinical presentation
1. Rapidly progressive illness over weeks to months
2. Hepatosplenomegaly, fever, respiratory compromise from mediastinal mass, or signs of abdominal obstruction from abdominal lymphoma
3. Certain types of abdominal NHL may present with **intussusception**

D. Testing
1. Laboratory findings
a. CBC: often normal; may show cytopenias if bone marrow is involved
b. Chemistry panel can show signs of TLS
2. Radiology findings
a. Chest radiograph and abdominal ultrasound are preliminary imaging
b. CT scan of neck, chest, abdomen, and pelvis: for staging evaluation
3. Other findings
a. Biopsy of suspicious lesion is main method of diagnosis
b. Bone marrow aspiration and biopsy to evaluate for marrow involvement
c. LP performed to evaluate for CNS involvement

E. Treatment
1. Multiagent systemic chemotherapy; based on type of lymphoma
2. Prognosis is generally excellent
3. Aggressive therapy for TLS; high rate of morbidity/mortality when untreated

> **QUICK HIT**
> The most common mode of NHL presentation is painless, progressive lymphadenopathy.

> **QUICK HIT**
> NHL should be ruled out in any child age >5 years with intussusception.

> **QUICK HIT**
> TLS is fairly common in high-grade NHL, either at diagnosis or at the start of therapy.

V. Central Nervous System Tumors

A. Characteristics
1. 2nd most common pediatric malignancy; 20% of all cases of childhood cancer
2. Peak incidence in 1st decade of life; higher incidence in males; no racial predominance
3. Multiple types: classification system based on site of origin and tumor cell type
4. Specific incidence varies by type and with age; younger patients are more likely to have embryonal tumors such as **medulloblastoma**
5. Most CNS tumors in children are sporadic without risk factor or cause
6. Several genetic syndromes with predisposition toward specific brain tumors
7. Treatment and prognosis: dependent on histologic tumor type and location

B. Clinical features
1. Historical findings
a. Presentation symptoms depend on location of tumor within brain
b. Symptoms of increased intracranial pressure (ICP): morning headache, emesis, and lethargy

c. Initial signs of increased ICP can be insidious and nonlocalizing, including poor school performance, fatigue, behavioral change, weight gain or loss, increased clumsiness or walking difficulty
d. Seizures tend to be focal, medically refractory, and associated with prolonged postictal paralysis

2. Physical exam findings
   a. Infratentorial tumors
      i. More likely to present with signs of increased ICP
      ii. Cranial nerve (CN) palsies: more common with brainstem lesions
      iii. Papilledema
      iv. Ataxia due to cerebellar lesions
      v. Facial droop or weakness
      vi. Hearing loss
      vii. Diplopia
   b. Supratentorial tumors
      i. More likely to present with focal symptoms
         (a) Hemiparesis
         (b) Hemisensory loss
      ii. Hyperreflexia
      iii. Visual deficits
      iv. Seizures
      v. Hypothalamic tumors: can present with **diencephalic syndrome** including euphoria, hyperphagia, and anorexia
   c. Pineal lesions/optic chiasm tumor: defects in papillary constriction and inability to perform upward gaze (**Parinaud syndrome** or **"setting sun" sign)**

C. Diagnosis
1. Laboratory findings
   a. LP to obtain CSF for cytology is necessary for tumors that spread to CSF
   b. CSF β-hCG and AFP: can be diagnostic for CNS germ cell tumors
2. Radiologic findings
   a. MRI with gadolinium: imaging modality of choice
   b. MRI of spine: indicated for certain tumors that are known to metastasize to spine (e.g., medulloblastoma or ependymoma)
   c. CT scan: may initially identify lesion at presentation, but MRI will be needed to better characterize tumor

D. Treatment
1. Therapy and prognosis are dependent on tumor type
   a. **Medulloblastoma and primitive neuroectodermal tumor (PNET)**
      i. Medulloblastoma = PNET located in posterior fossa
         (a) ~20% of all pediatric brain tumors and 40% of all cerebellar tumors
         (b) Majority occur in 1st decade of life, peak age 5–7 years
      ii. Embryonic "small round blue cell tumors" (SRBCTs)
      iii. Treatment involves combination approach with surgical resection, radiation, and combination chemotherapy
      iv. Can metastasize throughout and outside CNS (this is quite rare)
         (a) Most likely pediatric CNS tumor to metastasize
         (b) All patients with PNET or medulloblastoma need LP for cytology and spine MRI as part of metastatic workup
      v. Prognosis: survival reported as 75%–85% for standard-risk patients and 25%–75% for high-risk patients (metastatic disease, unresectable tumors, and tumors with anaplastic features)
   b. **Ependymoma**
      i. Accounts for 10% of pediatric brain tumors; more common in 1st decade of life
      ii. Arises within ventricular system, most commonly in posterior fossa at floor of 4th ventricle
      iii. Can present with extreme emesis due to invasion of emetic chemoreceptor on dorsal medulla near 4th ventricle

QUICK HIT

Seizures as a presenting sign of a brain tumor are rare in pediatrics.

QUICK HIT

A common location for a pediatric brain tumor is in the posterior fossa, usually a medulloblastoma or primitive neuroectodermal tumor.

QUICK HIT

Infants with pineal or optic chiasm tumors can present with the **spasmus nutans triad**: unilateral or bilateral pendular nystagmus, head bobbing, and head tilt.

QUICK HIT

Avoid LP if the patient has findings of impending cerebral herniation because sudden decompression of spinal pressure can precipitate herniation and death.

QUICK HIT

A CT scan may miss smaller tumors, especially in the posterior fossa.

QUICK HIT

An SRBCT is a tumor that under the microscope has small, round, blue cells after a hematoxylin and eosin stain. These tumors include Ewing sarcoma, neuroblastoma, medulloblastoma, rhabdomyosarcoma, Wilms tumor, and retinoblastoma.

> **QUICK HIT**
> In general, pediatric brain tumors have a much higher survival rate than brain tumors in adults. However, long-term disability is common and can be very severe.

> **QUICK HIT**
> Gliomas account for ~75% of brain tumors in young children.

iv. Locally invasive with spread through spinal canal possible, but distant metastasis also reported
v. Patients need CSF sent and spine MRI for metastatic workup
vi. Surgical resection: treatment of choice and is essential for cure followed by radiation
vii. 5-year overall survival: 10%–70% depending on grade and surgical resectability

c. **Gliomas**
i. Low grade
(a) Most common of all pediatric CNS tumors
(b) Usually nonaggressive with good overall prognosis
(c) Usually do not spread, although spinal metastases are possible (5% of cases)
(d) Treatment: full surgical resection; usually full cure (~90% overall survival)
(e) Radiation and chemotherapy for unresectable or recurrent tumors

ii. High grade (anaplastic astrocytoma and glioblastoma multiforme)
(a) Represent 10% of all CNS tumors, but rare in children
(b) More commonly occur in cerebral hemispheres
(c) Regionally invasive with metastasis outside CNS
(d) Can be very difficult to surgically resect
(e) Treatment: multimodal with surgery, radiation, and chemotherapy
(f) Despite aggressive treatment, prognosis is grim
(i) Anaplastic astrocytoma: overall survival of 35%
(ii) Glioblastoma multiforme: <10% 5-year survival

iii. Diffuse pontine glioma
(a) High-grade glioma located in brainstem and therefore unresectable
(b) Accounts for 10%–20% of all pediatric brain tumors
(c) Poor prognosis: most patients die within 2 years of diagnosis
(d) Low-grade pontine lesions: better prognosis and are more likely to occur in patients with neurofibromatosis
(e) Radiation: effective in reducing tumor burden, but most patients will recur within 1 year after completing radiation therapy with progression to death
(f) Chemotherapy: not shown to improve prognosis

2. Complications: most late effects in patients with CNS tumors are related to complications from radiation therapy: growth failure, endocrinologic abnormalities, secondary brain tumors within field of radiation, vasculopathy, and long-term cognitive deficits
3. Prevention: avoidance of excessive irradiation to head (i.e., avoidance of unnecessary head CT) may reduce likelihood of future brain tumors

VI. Neuroblastoma

A. Characteristics
1. SRBCT originating from primitive neural crest cells, which normally develop into sympathetic ganglia and can present anywhere along sympathetic chain or within adrenal glands
a. Most common primary site: within adrenal gland (65% of cases)
b. Infants are more likely than older children to have cervical or thoracic primary tumor
2. Incidence
a. 90% of cases: age <5 years
b. Median age at diagnosis: 22 months
c. Accounts for 15% of all cancer-related deaths in children
3. Genetics: no specific mutation identified, although certain cytogenetic anomalies within tumor can affect prognosis
a. n-*myc* protooncogene can be amplified in neuroblastoma tumor cells
b. Amplification dramatically impairs prognosis and is used to stratify risk

> **QUICK HIT**
> Neuroblastoma is the most common malignancy in infants and the most common extracranial solid tumor of childhood.

> **QUICK HIT**
> Neuroblastoma is extremely rare in adolescence.

4. Association with Hirschsprung disease, neurofibromatosis, and Beckwith-Wiedemann syndrome
5. Metastases: liver, lymph nodes, skin, bone, and bone marrow

B. Clinical presentation
1. Historical findings
   a. Patients most commonly present with abdominal mass
   b. Constitutional symptoms possible: lethargy, weakness, irritability, weight loss, and pain due to bone metastases or local tumor invasion
   c. Bleeding or bruising secondary to bone marrow infiltration
   d. Urinary obstruction or constipation with spinal cord or pelvic involvement
2. Clinical findings
   a. Most patients have distant metastasis at diagnosis
   b. Patients will often have firm, fixed, palpable abdominal mass
   c. Hepatomegaly can be seen from liver metastasis
   d. Thoracic masses can present with **Horner syndrome** (miosis, ptosis, and anhidrosis)
   e. Paraspinal masses can present with signs of spinal cord compression including lower extremity weakness, urinary retention, and constipation
   f. Cervical masses can present with heterochromia and anisocoria
   g. Skin metastases can be seen in rare instances and appear as blue, nontender, subcutaneous nodules (more common in infants)
   h. Can metastasize to orbits, causing bilateral orbital hemorrhage commonly referred to as "**raccoon eyes**" (Figure 20-2)
   i. **Opsoclonus myoclonus syndrome**
      i. Clinical scenario characterized by jerking, rapid, involuntary eye movements, and truncal and cerebellar ataxia
      ii. Thought to be caused by autoimmune reaction to neuroblastoma cells in which antibodies react against cells of cerebellum
      iii. Highly associated with neuroblastoma; if diagnosed, patient should be evaluated for occult neuroblastoma

C. Diagnosis
1. Laboratory findings
   a. Neuroblastoma is a catecholamine-secreting tumor; >90% of patients will have elevated urinary catecholamines at diagnosis, specifically vanillylmandelic acid (VMA) and homovanillic acid (HVA)

QUICK HIT

Infants with neuroblastoma are more likely to have cervical or thoracic primary tumors than are older children.

QUICK HIT

Opsoclonus myoclonus syndrome, sometimes referred to as "dancing eyes, dancing feet syndrome," occurs in ~3% of children with neuroblastoma.

QUICK HIT

Neuroblastoma typically does not metastasize to the lungs, whereas Wilms tumor most commonly metastasizes to the lungs.

FIGURE 20-2 Periorbital neuroblastoma.

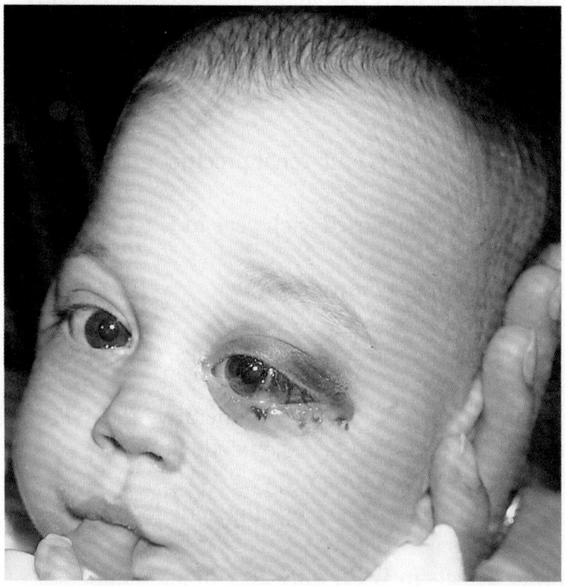

(From Fleisher GR, Ludwig W, Baskin MN. *Atlas of Pediatric Emergency Medicine*. Philadelphia: Lippincott Williams & Wilkins; 2004, with permission.)

Oncologic Diseases

b. Diagnosis: confirmed by biopsy, evaluation of histology (favorable versus unfavorable) and presence of n-*myc* amplification
c. CBC with differential: for signs of marrow infiltration
d. Ferritin: nonspecific finding that is elevated in neuroblastoma
e. Bilateral bone marrow biopsies for adequate staging
f. LP indicated with parameningeal disease

2. Radiology findings
   a. MRI/CT scan of primary tumor: to delineate extent of disease
   b. CT scan of chest, abdomen, and pelvis: necessary to stage tumor
   c. Bone scan to look for bone metastases
   d. ^{123}I metaiodobenzylguanidine (MIBG) scan
      i. Patients injected with MIBG radionucleotide
      ii. Isotope is preferentially taken up in catecholamine-producing cells
      iii. 90% of neuroblastoma cells take up isotope

QUICK HIT

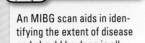

An MIBG scan aids in identifying the extent of disease and should be done in all patients newly diagnosed with neuroblastoma for adequate staging.

D. Treatment: multimodal and depends on risk status of patient
1. Risk determined by
   a. Stage (I is localized, IV is disseminated)
   b. Histology
   c. n-*myc* amplification associated with more aggressive disease
   d. DNA ploidy of tumor
   e. Other chromosomal alterations within tumor
   f. Age of patient
2. High-risk patients: treated aggressively with intensive chemotherapy, radiation, autologous stem cell transplant, surgical resection, and immunotherapy
3. Lower risk patients: observation alone after surgical resection or with less intensive chemotherapy, depending on clinical situation and overall risk status
4. Subset of patients with stage IV disease have lower risk (known as stage IV S)
   a. Age <1 year
   b. Localized primary tumor: stage I or II
   c. Metastases limited to skin, liver, and bone marrow
   d. No poor prognostic indicators
   e. Favorable prognosis with spontaneous regression of disease and event-free survival of ~90%
   f. Despite overall favorable prognosis, very large tumor burdens possible
5. Duration/prognosis
   a. Low-risk classification: good prognosis
   b. High-risk classification: guarded prognosis with event-free survival <50% despite aggressive therapy
   c. Incorporation of immunotherapy for high-risk neuroblastoma has recently been found to dramatically improve prognosis

QUICK HIT

Amplification of the proto-oncogene n-*myc* on chromosome 2 in the tumor cell dramatically worsens the overall prognosis of patients with neuroblastoma.

VII. Wilms Tumor

A. Characteristics
1. Kidney tumor arising from pluripotent embryonic renal precursor cells
2. Incidence
   a. 5%–7% of all pediatric malignancies diagnosed each year in U.S.
   b. Peak age at diagnosis: 2–3 years
3. Genetics: associated with multiple genetic syndromes
   a. **Beckwith-Wiedemann syndrome**
   b. **WAGR syndrome**: Wilms, aniridia, genitourinary anomalies, mental retardation
   c. **Denys-Drash syndrome**: pseudohermaphroditism, degenerative renal disease
   d. Associated with mutations of *WT1* and *WT2* genes; encode known transcription factors vital to kidney development
   e. Many associated genetic syndromes have deletions of genetic loci that encompass *WT1* and/or *WT2* genes
   f. Despite strong genetic link to defects in *WT1*, only 20% of all Wilms patients exhibit mutation

QUICK HIT

Wilms tumor is the most common pediatric renal malignancy.

QUICK HIT

As infants grow into school age, the incidence of Wilms tumor rises, and the incidence of neuroblastoma falls. Both are extremely rare in adolescence.

B. Clinical features
   1. Historical findings
      a. Wilms patients more likely to present with history of painless abdominal mass than any other abdominal malignancy
      b. Hematuria, weight loss, lethargy, fatigue, abdominal pain, abdominal distention, nausea, vomiting, or bleeding
   2. Physical exam findings
      a. Painless, palpable, firm, and fixed abdominal mass; tumor is extremely friable; use caution when palpating abdomen to avoid tumor rupture, which can upstage patient, require increased therapy, and affect prognosis
      b. Hypertension due to increased renin secretion
      c. Pallor secondary to anemia from bleeding into tumor or hematuria
      d. Varicoceles or inguinal hernias due to tumor compression
      e. Abdominal vein distention can occur due to tumor thrombus into inferior vena cava (IVC), obstructing blood flow
      f. Patients should be evaluated for stigmata of genetic syndromes
C. Diagnosis
   1. Laboratory findings
      a. CBC with differential: may show anemia secondary to hematuria or bleeding into tumor
      b. **Polycythemia**: secondary to increased erythropoietin secretion
      c. Urinalysis: may reveal microscopic or macroscopic hematuria
      d. Biopsy to confirm diagnosis; histology correlated to prognosis and is either classified as *favorable* or *unfavorable*
   2. Radiology findings
      a. Bilateral renal ultrasounds to diagnose
      b. CT scan of chest, abdomen, and pelvis for staging purposes; most common metastasis site is lungs, but can also metastasize to liver and lymph nodes.
D. Treatment
   1. Multimodal therapy (surgery, radiation, and chemotherapy) dependent on both stage of tumor and histology status (favorable or unfavorable)
   2. Duration/prognosis: related to stage and histology
      a. Favorable histology: excellent with conventional therapy
         i. Stage I: event-free survival >95%
         ii. Stages II/III: event-free survival between 80% and 95%
         iii. Stage IV: event-free survival ~75%
      b. Unfavorable histology: dramatically worsens overall and event-free survival
   3. Prevention: patients with known genetic syndrome that predisposes to Wilms tumor should have serial screening renal ultrasounds up to at least age 7 years

QUICK HIT

The most common presenting sign of Wilms tumor is a painless, palpable abdominal mass.

QUICK HIT

Be gentle when palpating a Wilms tumor! Rupture on exam can worsen the outcome.

QUICK HIT

Children with Beckwith-Wiedemann syndrome have hemihypertrophy and a high risk of Wilms tumor. They receive renal ultrasounds every 3 months until age 3 years and then every 6 months for early tumor detection.

QUICK HIT

Unlike with neuroblastoma, bone marrow biopsy is not indicated in Wilms tumor, which does not metastasize to the bone marrow.

QUICK HIT

Nephrectomy is performed at Wilms tumor diagnosis with full inspection of the abdomen and contralateral kidney to inspect for other disease sites.

VIII. Retinoblastoma

A. Characteristics
   1. Intraocular SRBCT that presents in infancy and is associated with genetic mutation of *Rb1* (retinoblastoma), an oncogenic tumor suppressor gene on chromosome 13q14
   2. Occurs in ~1/20,000 live births with slightly >300 cases documented in U.S. and Canada each year
   3. *Unilateral* or *bilateral*
      a. Bilateral: associated with inherited germline mutation of *Rb1*
         i. ~30% of all cases of retinoblastoma
         ii. Usually presents age <1 year
      b. Unilateral: associated with spontaneous mutation in *Rb1*
         i. ~70% of all cases
         ii. Usually presents age >2 years (ages 2–5 years)
   4. Mutation results in propensity for cellular proliferation and cell cycle dysregulation
   5. *Rb1* mutation associated with development of other tumors: osteosarcoma; soft tissue sarcomas; and adult cancers of bladder, prostate, breast, and lung

> **QUICK HIT**
> Leukocoria is sometimes identified by parents in photographs of the patient.

> **QUICK HIT**
> Early diagnosis of retinoblastoma is critical in order to salvage as much vision as possible with early treatment.

> **QUICK HIT**
> Leukocoria on physical examination of the eye is the single most common presenting sign of retinoblastoma, followed by strabismus.

> **QUICK HIT**
> The most important predictor of prognosis in patients with retinoblastoma is disease extent.

> **QUICK HIT**
> More than 90% of children with retinoblastoma survive into adulthood with conventional therapy.

6. Retinoblastoma can rarely metastasize outside eye to lungs, bones, bone marrow, or soft tissues

B. Clinical features
1. Historical findings
   a. Patients usually present with physical exam findings, although parents may report **leukocoria** in young infant
   b. Family history: rare; ~15% of cases despite inheritance pattern (most mutations that lead to disease are spontaneous)
2. Physical exam findings
   a. Leukocoria (see Chapter 17, Approach to Abnormal Red Reflex and Leukocoria): most common presenting sign
   b. Strabismus: 2nd most common presenting sign
   c. Other ocular abnormalities including decreased visual acuity, **heterochromia** (iris color does not match), rubeosis iridis (neovascularization of iris), hyphema, glaucoma, vitreous hemorrhage

C. Diagnosis
1. Laboratory findings
   a. CBC with differential: can be abnormal if there is bone marrow metastasis (although this is extremely rare)
   b. If concern for bone marrow metastasis on CBC or physical examination: bilateral bone marrow biopsies
   c. LP: if concern for spread into CNS
2. Radiologic findings
   a. Full evaluation of both eyes done under sedation by experienced ophthalmologist
   b. Ultrasound of both eyes under sedation: to document extent of disease
   c. CT and/or MRI of orbits and brain: if concerns for extraocular invasion
   d. Bone scan: only necessary if signs on history or physical examination concerning for bone metastases

D. Treatment
1. Therapy
   a. Approach prioritizes sparing as much vision as possible
   b. Multimodal combination of radiation, chemotherapy, surgery, photocoagulation, cryotherapy, thermotherapy: determined by extent of disease and degree of ocular invasion
   c. Surgical enucleation (removal of affected eye): only if 1 eye filled with tumor and no hope of restoring vision
2. Complications
   a. Inherited germline mutations: increased risk for developing other malignancies
   b. Vision loss from surgery or complications of extensive disease
   c. Secondary malignancy
      i. Radiation: causes increased risk of osteosarcoma and other soft tissue sarcomas within field of radiation
      ii. Skin cancers
3. Prognosis: metastases and increased extension into orbit toward optic nerve worsen prognosis
4. Prevention: genetic counseling may be indicated for families who have child with germline *Rb1* mutation

IX. Ewing Sarcoma

A. Definitions
1. SRBCT thought to derive from developing primitive, pluripotent, neural crest cells that are thought to normally give rise to parasympathetic ganglia
2. Can present in younger children, unlike in osteosarcoma, although still more common in adolescents
3. Much more common in Caucasian populations and extremely rare in patients of African or Asian descent

FIGURE 20-3 **Ewing sarcoma: cortical saucerization and onion skin periosteal response.**

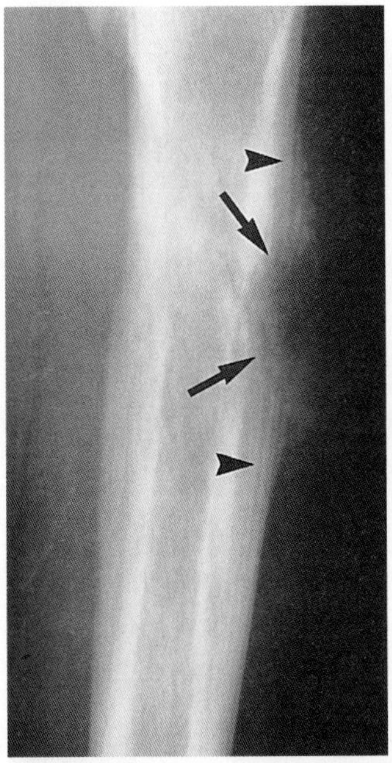

Femur: observe the permeative destruction within the medullary portion of the mid-diaphysis of the femur. Disruption in the cortex, creating a saucerization appearance, is characteristic of Ewing sarcoma (*arrows*). An additional radiographic sign of aggressive disease is the onion skin or laminated periosteal response seen adjacent to the cortical saucerization (*arrowheads*).
(From Yochum TR, Rowe LJ. *Yochum and Rowe's Essentials of Skeletal Radiology.* 3rd ed. Philadelphia: Lippincott Williams & Wilkins; 2004.)

4. Most commonly arises in any bone with extraosseous soft tissue
   a. More commonly affects flat bones of axial skeleton unlike osteosarcoma
   b. Ewing sarcoma in long bones usually arises from *diaphyses*, unlike osteosarcoma, which has predilection for *metaphyses*

B. Cause: no known cause but associated with chromosomal translocation t(11;22) found in tumor cell, which leads to chimeric protein that alters transcription, drives proliferation, and leads to aberrant cell growth
C. Clinical presentation: pathologic fracture and constitutional symptoms
D. Testing
   1. Plain film: lytic and sclerotic lesion in involved bone
      a. Soft tissue extension possible
      b. Lamellated periosteal reaction with "onion-skin" appearance
      c. Radiating spicules possible (Figure 20-3)
   2. MRI or CT scan of primary site: to guide surgical biopsy and resection
   3. Chest CT scan, bone scan, and bone marrow biopsies: to identify metastases
E. Therapy
   1. Multimodal: intensive chemotherapy, radiation, and surgical resection
   2. Prognosis
      a. Isolated: overall survival rate ~80% with conventional therapy
      b. Metastatic: overall survival rate ~20% with conventional therapy

X. Osteosarcoma

A. Definitions
   1. Pathologic diagnosis based on identification of anaplastic, spindle-shaped, stromal tumor cells with production of osteoid
   2. Associated with periods of increased linear bone growth with peak incidence in adolescence
   3. Extremely rare in children age <10 years
   4. Predilection for metaphyses of long bones

B. Cause: no known cause but associated with Li-Fraumeni syndrome, *Rb1* mutations, and prior history of radiation therapy in area of new osteosarcoma lesion

QUICK HIT
Ewing sarcoma is more likely than osteosarcoma to arise in the axial skeleton.

QUICK HIT
The most common locations for Ewing sarcoma are the pelvis, femur, humerus, ribs, and clavicle.

QUICK HIT
Patients with Ewing sarcoma most commonly present with swelling or pain in the affected area.

QUICK HIT
Osteosarcoma is the most common malignant bone tumor in children.

QUICK HIT
Osteosarcoma in the axial skeleton is extremely rare.

FIGURE 20-4 Sunburst periosteal response.

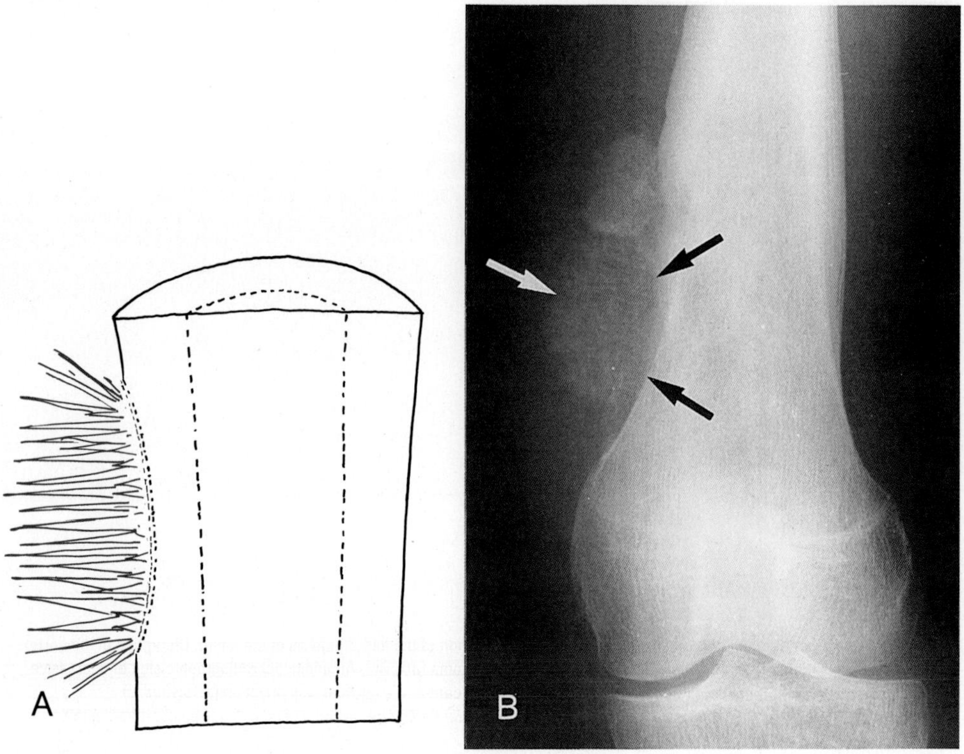

(**A and B**) Typical appearance. Note that the periosteal spicules appear to radiate away from a point source (*arrows*). The diagnosis was osteosarcoma. Note: This pattern of periosteal new bone represents an aggressively expanding lesion. (From Yochum TR, Rowe LJ. *Yochum and Rowe's Essentials of Skeletal Radiology.* 3rd ed. Philadelphia: Lippincott Williams & Wilkins; 2004.)

C. Clinical presentation: pain, swelling, and pathologic fracture at tumor site
D. Testing
   1. Plain film: classical appearance in metaphysis of long bone
      a. Soft tissue extension possible
      b. May see areas of calcification radiating from tumor known as **"sunburst sign"** (Figure 20-4)
   2. MRI of affected area: to help guide surgical biopsy
   3. Biopsy and eventual resection: biopsy must be done en bloc to avoid spillage of tumor cells, which can lead to metastatic disease
   4. Bone and chest CT scans: for staging; osteosarcoma most commonly metastasizes to other bones or lungs
E. Therapy
   1. Treatment: combination of intensive chemotherapy and surgical resection
   2. Radiation: not typically indicated; osteosarcoma not radiosensitive tumor
   3. Prognosis
      a. Nonmetastatic: overall survival ~60%–70% with conventional therapy
      b. Metastatic: overall survival ~20%

> **QUICK HIT**
> The classic presentation of osteosarcoma is pain or swelling at the affected site in an adolescent.

> **QUICK HIT**
> Osteosarcoma has a predilection for the metaphyses of long bones, whereas Ewing sarcoma more commonly presents in the diaphyses of long bones and is more likely to arise in the axial skeleton.

> **QUICK HIT**
> Without chemotherapy, osteosarcoma will recur in up to 90% of patients.

XI. Rhabdomyosarcoma

A. Definitions
   1. Most common soft tissue sarcoma of childhood; thought to arise from primitive precursor stem cells of skeletal muscle
   2. 2 major histologic variants
      a. **Embryonal rhabdomyosarcoma**: SRBCT; has improved prognosis compared to alveolar subtype
      b. **Alveolar rhabdomyosarcoma**: resembles alveoli of lung tissue; has worse prognosis than embryonal subtype

c. Other histologic subtypes (less common)
   i. **Botryoid**: classical presentation in infancy with predilection for bladder and vagina; can present with grape-like protrusion from vagina
   ii. **Undifferentiated** and **spindle cell** variants: extremely rare

B. Cause: no specific cause identified, but associations with Li-Fraumeni syndrome and neurofibromatosis have been reported

C. Clinical presentation: anywhere in body with skeletal muscle; rarely where no known skeletal muscle

D. Testing
   1. Imaging of primary lesion and diagnosis confirmed by surgical biopsy
   2. Chest CT, bone scan, and bilateral bone marrow aspirates and biopsies: staging evaluation at diagnosis; tumor can metastasize to bones, bone marrow, lymph nodes, lungs, liver, and (rarely) brain
   3. Parameningeal disease sites need a brain MRI

E. Therapy
   1. Multimodal treatment of chemotherapy, radiation, and surgery, dictated by staging system
   2. Prognosis: depends on site of origin, presence of metastases, and histologic subtype; overall 5-year survival ~70%

QUICK HIT

A rhabdomyosarcoma will most commonly present as swelling, pain, and/or mass effect in affected area.

XII. Teratomas

A. Definitions
   1. Germ cell tumors that arise from all 3 primordial germ layers
   2. Often contain tissue anatomically unrelated to site of origin; some also have immature elements
   3. Categorized as *mature* or *immature* depending on differentiation status of tumor cells
   4. Arise in midline owing to germ cell origin and predominate in 4 major areas: sacrococcygeal, mediastinum, ovary, CNS

B. Clinical presentation
   1. Sacrococcygeal teratomas: arise outside body; often diagnosed on prenatal ultrasounds or at birth (Figure 20-5)

QUICK HIT

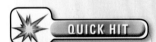

A teratoma can contain fat, teeth, hair, or other organized tissue from anywhere in the body.

FIGURE 20-5 **A large sacrococcygeal teratoma.**

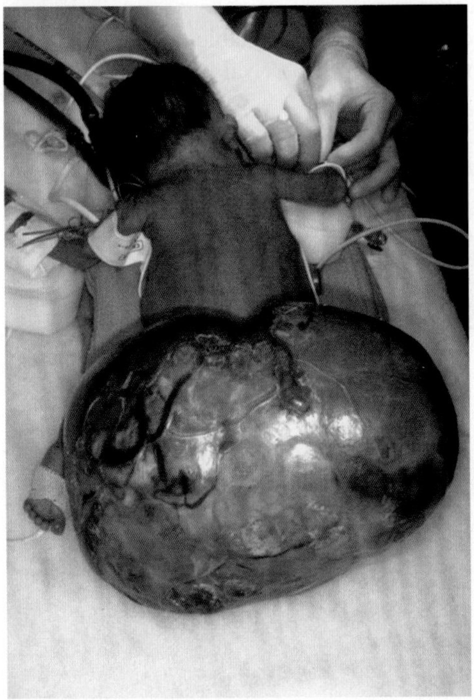

(Reprinted with permission from www.virtualpediatrichospital.org.)

2. Mediastinal teratomas: can be asymptomatic or can present with respiratory symptoms or chest pain
3. Ovarian teratomas: usually present with abdominal pain
4. CNS teratomas: symptoms similar to other CNS tumors dependent on site of origin within brain

C. Testing
1. Close pathologic evaluation of tumor is essential
2. Teratomas can have malignant or immature components, which will worsen prognosis and may require chemotherapy
3. AFP and β-hCG: sometimes elevated with certain types of malignant component

D. Therapy
1. Mature teratoma
a. Treatment usually consists of only full resection
b. Excellent overall prognosis
2. Immature teratoma and/or malignant components
a. Chemotherapy after resection may be indicated
b. More guarded prognosis, although still have 80%–90% overall survival rates with standard chemotherapy regimens

XIII. Liver Tumors

A. Definitions
1. Rare in childhood, accounting for only 1%–2% of all pediatric malignancies
2. Most are either hepatoblastoma or hepatocellular carcinoma (Table 20-2)

B. Clinical presentation
1. Most commonly present with painless, palpable mass
2. Associated abdominal distention, weight loss, fatigue, irritability, and emesis
3. Jaundice: rare presenting sign usually signifying advanced disease

C. Testing
1. Abdominal imaging, followed by biopsy to confirm diagnosis
2. Chest, abdomen, and pelvis CT scan: hepatoblastoma can metastasize to lungs and lymph nodes
3. Hepatoblastoma: elevated serum AFP in 90% of cases; levels can also be used to follow treatment efficacy and evaluate for recurrence

D. Therapy
1. Treatment
a. Surgery: most important mode of therapy
b. Liver transplant: may be indicated if tumor is unresectable
c. Chemotherapy after resection: improves overall survival in most cases of hepatoblastoma
d. Chemotherapy or radiation prior to resection: to improve odds of achieving full resection with negative margins

Oncologic Diseases

QUICK HIT

Pediatric liver tumors rarely present with jaundice; most present with a palpable abdominal mass.

TABLE 20-2 Differences between Hepatoblastoma and Hepatocellular Carcinoma

	Hepatoblastoma	Hepatocellular Carcinoma
Usual age of diagnosis	<3 years old	>10 years old
Association	Prematurity Beckwith-Wiedemann syndrome Familial adenomatous polyposis Li-Fraumeni syndrome Hemihypertrophy Trisomy 18 Meckel diverticulum	Hepatitis B Hepatitis C Inborn errors of metabolism Cirrhosis of the liver
Precursor cell	Primitive hepatocyte	Adult hepatocyte
Blood test if suspicious	α-Fetoprotein (AFP)	Carcinoembryonic antigen (CEA)

2. Prognosis
   a. Patients who achieve full resection have very good long-term outcomes
   b. Metastatic or unresectable tumors: guarded prognosis

XIV. Testicular Tumors

A. Definitions
   1. 75% of testicular tumors in children are germ cell tumors; remainder develop from supporting cells of testis
   2. Germ cell tumors derive from primordial germ cells of developing embryo, which normally develop into sperm and ova
   3. Can metastasize to lymphatic system into retroperitoneum and mediastinum
B. Cause/pathophysiology
   1. Most commonly identified risk factor: undescended testicle; if still undescended at age 6–12 months, surgically corrected
   2. Most have no identifiable associated risk factor
C. Clinical presentation: most present with isolated, irregular, nontender mass in involved testicle
D. Testing
   1. Ultrasound of affected testicle
   2. CT scan of chest, abdomen, and pelvis and bone scan: to look for metastases
   3. Certain histologic subtypes will have elevated AFP and hCG: can be followed for treatment effect and recurrence
E. Therapy
   1. Primarily surgical: radical inguinal orchiectomy
   2. Most cured with surgery alone, although some subtypes are more aggressive and require treatment with radiation and chemotherapy

QUICK HIT

Children with undescended testes are at increased risk for the development of a testicular germ cell tumor.

QUICK HIT

Early detection radically improves prognosis. Adolescent boys should be taught to perform regular self-exams of the testes through their mid-30s and to report any unusual lumps to their primary care physician.

XV. Ovarian Tumors

A. Definitions
   1. Extremely rare in pediatric population, although incidence rises in adolescence
   2. Most are germ cell tumors that develop from primordial germ cells of developing embryo, which normally develop into sperm and ova
   3. Prognosis and treatment: depend on histologic subtype
   4. Malignant ovarian tumors can metastasize to lymphatic system, lungs, liver, or bone
B. Clinical presentation
   1. Most commonly present with persistent, dull abdominal pain
   2. Subset will present with an acute abdomen due to tumor-induced ovarian torsion
D. Testing
   1. Ultrasound or abdominal/pelvic CT: sufficient to diagnose mass lesion
   2. Surgical biopsy and resection: ideally to determine diagnosis
   3. Chest CT and bone scan: to stage and determine extent of metastases
   4. AFP and β-hCG: may be elevated in certain subtypes
E. Therapy
   1. Treatment is based on histologic diagnosis and disease extent
      a. Surgical resection alone is sufficient in certain cases
      b. Malignant subtypes and/or presence of metastases will be treated with chemotherapy
   2. Prognosis: very good; 80%–90% event-free survival

XVI. Langerhans Cell Histiocytosis (LCH)

A. Characteristics
   1. Nonmalignant proliferation of immature histiocytes
   2. Incidence: 5–8 cases per million children with slight male predominance
   3. Classified as either *single system* or *multifocal* based on sites involved
   4. Pathophysiology
      a. **Histiocytes**: dendritic cells derived from bone marrow stem cells, which normally function as antigen-presenting cells
      b. In LCH, immune dysfunction likely leads to proliferation and accumulation of histiocytes in skin, bone, or other organs

QUICK HIT

Older names for LCH include Hand-Schüller-Christian disease (pituitary and skull disease), Letterer-Siwe disease (disseminated disease), and eosinophilic granulomata (bone disease).

B. Clinical features
  1. Historical findings
    a. Unifocal or multifocal bone lesions: history of pain in affected area
    b. History of persistent draining otitis
    c. History of unexplained tooth loss
    d. LCH can present with symptoms of diabetes insipidus because it has predilection for pituitary stalk (history of polyuria and polydipsia)
    e. Respiratory symptoms if lungs are involved
    f. History of fatigue, fever, or symptoms of bleeding or bruising may be present if bone marrow involvement
  2. Physical exam findings
    a. Swelling over affected bone if unifocal or multifocal bone involvement
    b. Erythematous scaly rash
      i. Particularly behind ears and around genitalia
      ii. LCH rash can appear similar to eczema
      iii. Seborrheic dermatitis often present
    c. Hepatosplenomegaly and lymphadenopathy
    d. Respiratory involvement including wheezing and spontaneous pneumothorax

QUICK HIT

Patients with new-onset diabetes insipidus should be evaluated for LCH.

C. Diagnosis
  1. Laboratory findings
    a. CBC: may reveal cytopenias with bone marrow involvement
    b. Liver function tests: can reveal elevated transaminases, elevated bilirubin, or decreased albumin
  2. Radiology findings
    a. Plain films of involved bone: will reveal lytic lesion, which may have soft tissue component
    b. Skeletal survey to determine if other bones are involved
    c. Whole-body PET scan to detect other metabolically active lesions
    d. Chest imaging: to look for pulmonary involvement
    e. If any bones in base of skull are involved, brain MRI should be done to evaluate pituitary
  3. Other findings
    a. Biopsy of suspicious lesion is key to diagnosis
      i. Pathology will show histiocytes in inflammatory milieu
      ii. Histiocytes will stain positive for CD1a and CD207
      iii. **Birbeck granules**: cell membrane derived in Langerhans cells and refer to tennis racket–shaped granules seen on electron microscopy of affected lesions
    b. Bone marrow aspiration and biopsy indicated for cytopenias or with multisystem involvement
D. Treatment
  1. Therapy
    a. Isolated bone lesions
      i. Surgical biopsy or resection with no further therapy
      ii. Intralesional injection of steroids may also be used in some cases
    b. Multisystem disease
      i. Systemic chemotherapy; depends on organs involved
      ii. Certain organs are classified as "risk organs": known to have higher risk of recurrence and require increased therapy
    c. Additional chemotherapy or hematopoietic stem cell transplant may be used for recurrent or refractory disease
  2. Complications
    a. Diabetes insipidus may present before other lesions of LCH present or years later after treatment
    b. Panhypopituitarism due to pituitary involvement
  3. Prognosis: highly variable depending on clinical presentation and response to therapy
    a. Some infants with skin-only disease will experience resolution with no therapy
    b. Single bone lesions may require only local treatment

QUICK HIT

Children with multifocal LCH disease involving "risk organs" can progress rapidly to death without treatment.

APPENDIX: Epidemiology and Biostatistics Basics

- **Basic biostatistics**
  - **Null hypothesis**: no significant difference between treatment groups
  - **Type I (α) error**: inappropriate rejection of null hypothesis when null hypothesis is true (i.e., concluding that difference exists between comparison groups when there is no difference)
  - **Type II (β) error**: incorrectly accepting null hypothesis when null hypothesis is false (i.e., concluding that no difference exists between comparison groups when difference exists)
  - **Probability (*P*) value**: chance of type I (α) error occurring (in most cases, if $P < .05$, null hypothesis is rejected)

		TRUTH	
		No Difference	**Difference**
DECISION	H_A: difference	**Type I (α) error**	Correct
	H_0: no difference	Correct	**Type II (β) error**

- **Descriptive epidemiology**
  - **Incidence** = $\frac{\text{New Cases of Disease}}{\text{Total Population at Risk}}$
    - Number of new cases of disease in given at-risk population over prescribed time period
  - **Prevalence** = $\frac{\text{Number of Existing Cases}}{\text{Total Population}}$
    - Total number of cases in population at given time
    - Reflects both incidence of disease and disease duration
      - Chronic conditions have higher prevalence than incidence because of length of disease process
      - For conditions that resolve quickly or are rapidly fatal, incidence is approximately equal to prevalence

- **Study design**
  - **Cross-sectional study**
    - Measures disease and exposure status insofar as they exist in *defined* population in 1 *specific* point in time
    - Strengths
      - Quick and easy
      - Can study multiple outcomes and multiple exposures
      - Can measure prevalence for all factors studied
      - Good for descriptive analysis and generating hypotheses
    - Weaknesses
      - Does not measure incidence
      - Cannot determine temporal association
      - Not useful for studying rare diseases and diseases with short duration
      - Susceptible to bias
  - **Case-control study**
    - Observational study in which cases (subjects with disease) and controls (subjects without disease) are identified; information about past exposure to risk factors is assessed and compared between groups using **odds ratio (OR)**

- Strengths
  - More efficient than cohort studies in setting of rare outcomes or exposures that are difficult to assess
  - Convenient for studying multiple exposures
- Weaknesses
  - Cannot measure incidence
  - Potential for selection bias due to sampling of controls

- **Cohort study**
  - Observational study of incidence comparing group of subjects with exposure to risk factor to group of subjects without exposure to risk factor
    - **Prospective**: define exposure and then follow cohorts into future to determine if disease develops
    - **Retrospective**: define exposure and review past records to determine if cohorts had disease
  - Strengths
    - Can measure incidence and prevalence
    - Allow direct measurement of incidence in exposed and unexposed groups
    - Can examine multiple outcomes of one exposure
    - Can elucidate temporal relationship between exposure and disease
  - Weaknesses
    - Inefficient in evaluation of rare diseases
    - Validity of findings can be affected by losses to follow-up
    - Knowledge of exposure status may bias classification of outcome
    - *Prospective studies*: time consuming and costly
    - *Retrospective studies*: require availability of adequate records
- **Randomized controlled clinical trial**
  - Experimental prospective study in which subjects are assigned to treatment or control group and then followed over time to determine incidence of outcome of interest
  - Clinical/therapeutic study: using *diseased* population and supplying treatment or placebo to determine effect of treatment
  - Strengths
    - Provides strongest evidence
    - Most likely to produce valid conclusions about efficacy of therapy
    - Controls for confounding through randomization
    - Blinding minimizes bias
  - Weaknesses
    - Expensive and time consuming
    - Design and analysis can be complex
    - Generalizability may be limited
    - May not be ethical in some cases to randomly assign treatment and control
    - Not efficient for study of rare diseases or diseases with delayed outcome
- **Meta-analysis**
  - Statistical combination of data from several studies
  - Strengths: can improve statistical precision
  - Weaknesses
    - Cannot prevent bias
    - Validity is dependent on quality of methodology of included studies as well as criteria used for inclusion in meta-analysis

- **Bias (Box A-1)**
  - **Selection bias**: systematic error in choosing study participants that results in incorrect estimate of association in study group than actually exists in larger population
  - **Information bias**: systematic difference in measurement and definition of exposure and/or disease status among study participants that results in incorrect estimate of association
  - **Confounding variable**: masks or distorts apparent effect of exposure and must be
    - Associated with exposure
    - Associated with disease
    - Not be caused by exposure

BOX A-1

Bias

Trial: studying association between obesity and type 2 diabetes mellitus (T2DM) in children

- Choosing subjects from endocrinology clinic would cause **selection bias** insofar as there is higher prevalence of T2DM in endocrinology clinic than in general pediatric office
- Using parental-reported weights for some subjects and office-based weights for other subjects would lead to **information bias**
- Genetics of child must be considered **confounding variable** in relationship between obesity and T2DM (i.e., genetics are associated with obesity, genetics are associated with T2DM, and obesity does not cause genetics)

- **Measures of association (Box A-2)**

	Disease +	Disease −
Exposure + (Experiment)	A	B
Exposure − (Control)	C	D

- OR: used to estimate risk in case-control studies
  - $\text{OR} = \dfrac{\text{Odds of Diseases in Exposed Group}}{\text{Odds of Diseases in Control Group}} = \dfrac{A/B}{C/D} = \dfrac{AD}{BC}$
  - Interpretation: Individuals with disease have X times the odds of having the exposure compared with individuals without the disease

QUICK HIT

In a very common disease, the OR will be much higher than the RR. Do not confuse the two.

BOX A-2

Measures of Association

Trial: examining role of antibiotic prophylaxis on recurrent urinary tract infection (UTI) in children (Craig JC, Simpson JM, Williams GJ, et al. Antibiotic prophylaxis and recurrent urinary tract infection in children. *N Engl J Med.* 2009;361[18]:1748–1759.)

- Randomized control trial in which children with ≥1 prior UTI were randomized to receive either daily antibiotic prophylaxis (trimethoprim-sulfamethoxazole) or placebo for 12 months and followed for 1 year, with primary outcome being recurrent UTI
- Results

	UTI	No UTI	Total
Antibiotic prophylaxis	36	252	288
Placebo	55	233	288

- CER = disease in control group/total number in control group = 55/288 = 19%
  - 19% of patients who received placebo developed UTI
- EER = disease in treatment group/total number in treatment group = 36/288 = 13%
  - 13% of patients who received daily antibiotic prophylaxis developed UTI
- RR = EER/CER = 0.13/0.19 = 0.68
  - Patients receiving antibiotic prophylaxis had 0.68 times the risk of developing UTI as those receiving placebo
  - Note that because RR is <1, patients in experimental group are at *less* risk of outcome
- ARR = CER − EER = 19% − 13% = 6%
  - 6% risk reduction in development of UTI with daily antibiotic prophylaxis
- NNT = 1/0.06 = 16
  - 16 patients would need to receive daily antibiotic prophylaxis over 1 year to prevent 1 UTI

- **Control event rate (CER)**: incidence of disease in controls
  - CER = C/(C + D)
- **Experimental event rate (EER)**: incidence of disease in exposed individuals
  - EER = A/(A + B)
- **Relative risk (RR)**: also called *risk ratio*
  - $RR = \frac{\text{Incidence of Disease in Exposed}}{\text{Incidence of Disease in Controls}} \frac{(EER)}{(CER)} = \frac{A/(A + B)}{C/(C + D)}$
  - Interpretation: exposed individuals have X times the risk of disease compared with nonexposed individuals
- **Absolute risk reduction (ARR)**: difference in risk between control and experimental groups
  - ARR = incidence of disease in controls minus incidence of disease in exposed

    $= [C/(C + D)] - [A/(A + B)] = CER - EER$
- **Relative risk reduction (RRR)**: percentage change relative to baseline risk
  - $RRR = \frac{[C/(C + D)] - [A/(A + B)]}{C/(C + D)} = \frac{CER - EER}{CER} = \frac{ARR}{CER} = 1 - \frac{EER}{CER} = 1 - RR$
- **Number need to treat (NNT)**: number of patients who need to receive treatment in order to prevent 1 additional case of disease
  - NNT = 1/ARR

- **Screening and test performance**

	Disease +	Disease –	
Test +	True positive (TP)	False positive (FP)	PPV = TP/(TP + FP)
Test –	False negative (FN)	True negative (TN)	NPV = TN/(TN + FN)
	Sensitivity = TP/(TP + FN)	Specificity = TN/(TN + FP)	

- **Sensitivity** = TP/(TP + FN)
  - Probability that person having disease will have positive test result
  - "Positivity in disease"
  - Sensitive test is good for ruling *out* disease; good *screening* test
- **Specificity** = TN/(TN + FP)
  - Probability that person without disease will have negative test result
  - "Negativity in health"
  - Specific test is good for ruling *in* disease; good *confirmatory* test
- **Positive predictive value (PPV)** = TP/(TP + FP)
  - Probability that individual who tests positive has disease
  - Tests for diseases with high prevalence will have high PPV (fewer FPs)
- **Negative predictive value (NPV)** = TN/(TN + FN)
  - Probability that individual who tests negative does not have disease
  - Tests for diseases with low prevalence will have high NPV (fewer FNs)
- **Reliability**: reproducibility of results
- **Validity**: appropriateness of test's measurements (i.e., test measures what it is supposed to)

- **Prevention**
  - **Primary prevention**: preventing disease from occurring in 1st place (e.g., immunizations)
  - **Secondary prevention**: detecting disease early and preventing severe consequences (e.g., newborn screening for metabolic diseases)
  - **Tertiary prevention**: preventing or reducing morbidity, impairment, or disability (e.g., rehabilitation following injury)

Index

Note: Page numbers followed by *b* indicate boxes; *f* indicates figures, and *t* indicates tables.

B

C

Index

D

G

I

N

O

P

T

U

V

W

X

Y

Z

CCS1013